Pharmacology
SECOND EDITION

Pharmacology

SECOND EDITION

George M. Brenner, Ph.D.

Professor Emeritus of Pharmacology
Oklahoma State University
Center for Health Sciences
Tulsa, Oklahoma

Craig W. Stevens, Ph.D.

Professor of Pharmacology
Oklahoma State University
Center for Health Sciences
Tulsa, Oklahoma

SAUNDERS

ELSEVIER

SAUNDERS
ELSEVIER

1600 John F. Kennedy Blvd.
Ste 1800
Philadelphia, PA 19103-2899

PHARMACOLOGY, Second Edition   ISBN 13:   978-1-4160-2984-7
Copyright © 2006, Elsevier Inc.   ISBN 10:   1-4160-2984-2

Notice

Knowledge and best practice in this field are constantly changing. As new research and experience broaden our knowledge, changes in practice, treatment and drug therapy may become necessary or appropriate. Readers are advised to check the most current information provided (i) on procedures featured or (ii) by the manufacturer of each product to be administered, to verify the recommended dose or formula, the method and duration of administration, and contraindications. It is the responsibility of the practitioner, relying on their own experience and knowledge of the patient, to make diagnoses, to determine dosages and the best treatment for each individual patient, and to take all appropriate safety precautions. To the fullest extent of the law, neither the Publisher nor the Authors assumes any liability for any injury and/or damage to persons or property arising out or related to any use of the material contained in this book.

Previous editions copyrighted: 2000

Library of Congress Cataloging-in-Publication Data
Brenner, George M.
    Pharmacology / George M. Brenner, Craig W. Stevens.—2nd ed.
      p. ; cm.
    Includes bibliographical references and index.
    ISBN 1-4160-2984-2
    1. Pharmacology.   I. Stevens, Craig W.   II. Title.
    [DNLM: 1. Pharmacology.   2. Drug Therapy.   3. Pharmaceutical Preparations. QV4 B838p 2006]
  RM300.B74 2006
  615'.1—dc22

                                             2005050031

Publishing Director: Linda Belfus
Acquisitions Editor: Alex Stibbe
Publishing Services Manager: Joan Sinclair
Developmental Editor: Katie Miller
Project Manager: Mary Stermel
Design Direction: Ellen Zanolle
Marketing Manager: John Gore
Cover Designer: Louis Forgione

Printed in the United States of America

Last digit is the print number: 9   8   7   6   5   4   3   2   1

CONTENTS

PREFACE

Medical pharmacology is primarily concerned with the mechanisms by which drugs relieve symptoms and counteract the pathophysiological manifestations of disease. It is also concerned with the factors that determine the time course of drug action, including drug absorption, distribution, biotransformation, and excretion. Students are often overwhelmed by the vast amount of pharmacologic information available today. This textbook provides the essential concepts and information that students need to be successful in their courses without an overwhelming amount of detail.

This text is primarily intended for students who are taking their first course in pharmacology, but it will also be useful for those who are preparing to take medical board examinations. Because of the large number of drugs available today, this text emphasizes the general properties of drug categories and prototypical drugs. Chapters begin with a drug classification box to familiarize students with drug categories, subcategories, and specific drugs to be discussed in the chapter.

Throughout the book, the pharmacologic information is organized in the same format, with sections on mechanisms of action, physiologic effects, pharmacokinetic properties, adverse effects and interactions, and clinical uses for each drug category. Numerous illustrations are used to depict drug mechanisms and effects, while well-organized tables compare the specific properties of drugs within a therapeutic category. At the end of each chapter, a summary of important points is provided to reinforce concepts and clinical applications that are crucial for students to remember.

Several changes have been incorporated into the second edition of this text, including the addition of a co-author, Dr. Craig W. Stevens, who brings noteworthy expertise in the field of neuropharmacology. We have revised each chapter to incorporate new drugs and drug categories, as well as to update concepts of drug mechanisms and therapeutic use. For example, recent changes in hormone replacement therapy and in the treatment of hypertension and dyslipidemia have been included in the text. In addition, review questions have been added to the end of each chapter so that students can assess their knowledge of key drugs and concepts.

This book would not have been possible without the advice and encouragement of mentors, colleagues, and editorial personnel. We would particularly like to thank Alexandra Stibbe and Katie Miller at Elsevier, Inc. for their helpful assistance and support throughout the production of this book.

George M. Brenner
Craig W. Stevens

PRINCIPLES OF PHARMACOLOGY

CHAPTER 1

Introduction to Pharmacology

PHARMACOLOGY AND RELATED SCIENCES

History and Role of Pharmacology

Although people have attempted to treat diseases with substances derived from plants, animals, and minerals for more than 4000 years, the science of pharmacology is less than 150 years old. Historically, the selection and use of drugs were based on superstition or on experience (empiricism). Knowledge of the physiologic mechanisms by which drugs produce their therapeutic effects has largely been acquired during the past century, ushering in the era of rational pharmacotherapeutics.

In the first or earliest phase of drug usage, noxious plant and animal preparations were administered to the diseased patient to rid the body of the evil spirits believed to cause illness. The Greek word *pharmakon*, from which the term *pharmacology* is derived, originally meant a magic charm for treating disease. Later, *pharmakon* came to mean a remedy or drug.

In the second phase of drug usage, experience enabled people to understand which substances were actually beneficial in relieving particular disease symptoms. The first effective drugs were probably simple external preparations, such as cool mud or a soothing leaf, and the earliest known prescriptions from 2100 BCE included salves containing thyme. Over many centuries, people learned the therapeutic value of natural products through trial and error. By 1500 BCE, Egyptian prescriptions called for castor oil, opium, and other drugs that are still used today. Dioscorides, a Greek army surgeon of the first century CE, described more than 600 medicinal plants that he collected and studied as he traveled with the Roman armies. During the Middle Ages, Islamic physicians (e.g., Avicenna) and Christian monks cultivated and studied the use of herbal medicines.

The third phase of drug usage, the rational or scientific phase, gradually evolved with important advances in chemistry and physiology that gave rise to the new science of pharmacology. At the same time, a more rational understanding of disease mechanisms provided a scientific basis for using drugs whose physiologic actions and effects were under-

stood. Some of the critical events leading to the development of pharmacology and pharmacotherapeutics are listed in Table 1–1.

The advent of pharmacology was particularly dependent on the isolation of pure drug compounds from natural sources and on the development of experimental physiology methods to study these compounds. The isolation of morphine from opium in 1804 was rapidly followed by the extraction of many other drugs from plant sources, providing a diverse array of pure drugs for pharmacologic experimentation. Advances in physiology allowed pioneers, such as François Magendie and Claude Bernard, to conduct some of the earliest pharmacologic investigations, including studies that localized the site of action of curare to the neuromuscular junction. The first medical school pharmacology laboratory was started by Rudolf Büchheim in Estonia. Büchheim and one of his students, Oswald Schmiedeberg, trained many other pharmacologists, including John Jacob Abel, who began the first pharmacology departments in the United States of America (USA).

The goal of pharmacology is to understand the mechanisms by which drugs interact with biologic systems to enable the rational use of effective agents in the diagnosis and treatment of disease. The success of pharmacology in this task has led to an explosion of new drug development, particularly in the past 50 years. Twentieth-century developments include the isolation and use of insulin for diabetes, the discovery of antimicrobial and antineoplastic drugs, and the advent of modern psychopharmacology. Recent advances in molecular biology, genetics, and drug design suggest that new drug development and pharmacologic innovations will provide even greater advances in the treatment of medical disorders in the future.

Pharmacology and Its Subdivisions

Pharmacology is the biomedical science concerned with the interaction of chemical substances with living cells, tissues, and organisms. It is particularly concerned with the mechanisms by which drugs counteract the manifestations of disease and by which drugs affect fertility. Pharmacology is not primarily concerned with the synthesis or isolation of

TABLE 1–1. **Important Persons and Events in the History of Pharmacology**

Person and Life Span	Event
Paracelsus (1493–1541)	Refuted the tenets of humoralism. Advocated the use of a specific chemical to treat a particular disease (such as the use of mercury to treat syphilis).
John Wepfer (1620–1695)	Published studies on the toxicity of drugs and poisons in animals.
Felice Fontana (1730–1805)	Studied the toxicity of crude drug preparations.
Frederick Sertürner (1783–1841)	Isolated morphine from opium in 1804, becoming the first scientist to isolate the active ingredient of a natural drug.
François Magendie (1783–1855)	Proposed that the sites of action of drugs could be localized to specific organs in the body.
Claude Bernard (1813–1878)	Localized the site of action of curare to the neuromuscular junction in 1856.
Rudolf Büchheim (1820–1879)	Established the first medical school laboratory to be used exclusively for pharmacologic studies. Proposed that drugs exert their effects via their physiochemical interaction with cell constituents.
Oswald Schmiedeberg (1838–1921)	Was a student of Büchheim and later trained many pharmacologists, including John Jacob Abel. Defined pharmacology as the science concerned with effects of chemicals on living organisms.
Paul Ehrlich (1854–1915)	Demonstrated that drugs can destroy microbes. Developed antimicrobial chemotherapy.
John Jacob Abel (1857–1938)	Was the first pharmacology professor in the USA. Started pharmacology society and journals.

drugs or with the preparation of pharmaceutical products. The sciences that deal with these subjects are described below.

Pharmacology has been divided into two subdivisions, **pharmacokinetics** and **pharmacodynamics.** The relationship between these subdivisions is shown in Fig. 1–1. Pharmacokinetics is concerned with the processes that determine the concentration of drugs in body fluids and tissues over time, including **drug absorption, distribution, biotransformation,** and **excretion.** Pharmacodynamics is the study of the actions of drugs on target organs. It is particularly concerned with the **biochemical mechanisms** by which drugs produce their physiologic effects and with the **dose-response relationship,** defined as the relationship between the concentration of a drug in a tissue and the magnitude of the tissue's response to that drug. Most drugs produce their effects by binding to macromolecular **receptors** in target tissues, a process that activates a cascade of events known as **signal transduction.** Pharmacokinetics and pharmacodynamics are discussed in greater detail in Chapters 2 and 3.

Toxicology

Toxicology is the science of poisons and toxicity. It focuses both on the harmful effects of drugs and other chemicals and on the mechanisms by which toxic agents produce pathologic changes, disease, and death. As with pharmacology, toxicology is concerned with the relationship between the dose of an agent and the resulting tissue concentration and biologic effects that the agent produces. For this reason, some authorities consider toxicology to be a subdivision of pharmacology.

Pharmacotherapeutics

Pharmacotherapeutics is the medical science concerned with the use of drugs in the treatment of disease. Pharmacology provides a rational basis for pharmacotherapeutics by explaining the mechanisms and effects of drugs on the body and the relationship between dose and drug response. Human studies known as **clinical trials** are then used to determine the efficacy and safety of drug therapy in human subjects. The purpose, design, and evaluation of human drug studies are discussed in Chapter 4.

Pharmacy and Related Sciences

Pharmacy is the science and profession concerned with the preparation, storage, dispensing, and proper use of drug products. Related sciences include pharmacognosy, medi-

Figure 1–1. Relationship between pharmacokinetics and pharmacodynamics.

cinal chemistry, and pharmaceutical chemistry. **Pharmacognosy** is concerned with the isolation and characterization of drugs from natural sources, including plants, microbes, animal tissues, and minerals. **Medicinal chemistry** is a branch of organic chemistry that specializes in the design and chemical synthesis of drugs. **Pharmaceutical chemistry,** or **pharmaceutics,** is concerned with the formulation and chemical properties of pharmaceutical products, such as tablets, liquid solutions and suspensions, and aerosols.

DRUG SOURCES AND PREPARATIONS

A **drug** can be defined as a natural product, chemical substance, or pharmaceutical preparation intended for administration to a human or animal to diagnose or treat a disease. The word *drug* is derived from the French *drogue,* which traditionally meant dried herbs and which was originally used in the context of the sale and marketing of herbs, rather than the medicinal use of these substances. **Medication** and **medicament** are terms often used synonymously with the word *drug.*

Natural Sources of Drugs

Drugs have been obtained from **plants, microbes, animal tissues,** and **minerals.** Among the various types of drugs derived from plants are **alkaloids,** which are nitrogenous substances that give an alkaline reaction in aqueous solution. Examples of alkaloids include morphine, cocaine, atropine, and quinine. **Antibiotics** have been isolated from numerous microorganisms, including *Penicillium* and *Streptomyces* species. **Hormones** are the most common type of drug obtained from animals, whereas minerals have yielded a few useful therapeutic agents, including the lithium compounds used in psychotherapy.

Synthetic Drugs

The rise of modern chemistry in the 19th century enabled scientists to synthesize new compounds and to modify naturally occurring drugs. Aspirin, barbiturates, and local anesthetics (e.g., procaine) were among the first drugs to be synthesized in the laboratory. Semisynthetic derivatives of naturally occurring compounds (e.g., morphine) have led to the development of drugs with improved pharmacokinetic and pharmacodynamic properties.

In some cases, scientists have discovered new drug compounds either by accident or by actively screening various agents for their potential pharmacologic activity. With some classes of drugs, however, scientists have been able to discern a **structure-activity relationship** (i.e., a relationship between the chemical structure and the pharmacologic activity), and this information has guided the synthesis of new compounds. Recently, chemists have developed new drugs with the aid of computer programs that model the receptor of a particular drug and facilitate the design of drug structures that best fit the three-dimensional conformation of the receptor. This approach has been used, for example, to design agents that inhibit angiotensin synthesis and agents

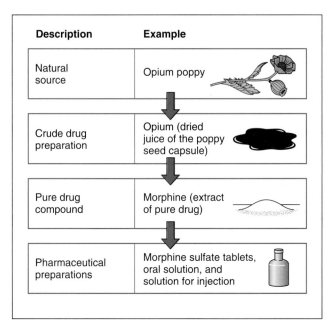

Figure 1–2. Types of drug preparations. A crude drug preparation retains most or all of the active and inactive compounds contained in the natural source from which it was derived. After a pure drug compound (e.g., morphine) is extracted from a crude drug preparation (in this case, opium), it is possible to manufacture pharmaceutical preparations that are suitable for administration of a particular dose to the patient.

that inhibit the maturation of the human immunodeficiency virus.

Drug Preparations

Drug preparations include crude drug preparations obtained from natural sources, pure drug compounds isolated from natural sources or synthesized in the laboratory, and pharmaceutical preparations of drugs intended for administration to patients. The relationship between these types of drug preparations is illustrated in Fig. 1–2.

Crude Drug Preparations

Some crude drug preparations are made by drying or pulverizing a plant or animal tissue. Others are made by extracting substances from a natural product with the aid of hot water or a solvent such as alcohol. Three familiar examples of crude drug preparations are coffee, tea, and opium (the dried juice of the poppy seed capsule). Many herbal medicines are available today in the form of crude drug preparations containing the same active and inactive ingredients found in the original source.

Pure Drug Compounds

It is difficult to identify and quantify the pharmacologic effects of crude drug preparations because these products contain multiple ingredients, the amounts of which vary from batch to batch. Hence, the development of methods to isolate pure drug compounds from natural sources was an important step in the growth of pharmacology and rational therapeutics. Frederick Sertürner, a German apothecary, isolated the first pure drug from a natural source when he extracted and purified morphine from opium in 1804 and named it after Morpheus, the Greek god of dreams. The subsequent isolation of many other drugs from natural sources provided pharmacologists with a number of pure compounds for study and characterization. One of the greatest medical achievements of the early 20th century was the isolation of insulin from the pancreas. This achievement by Frederick Banting and Charles Best led to the development of insulin preparations for treating diabetes mellitus.

Pharmaceutical Preparations

Pharmaceutical preparations or dosage forms are drug products suitable for administration of a specific dose of a drug to a patient by a particular route of administration. Most of these preparations are made from pure drug compounds, but a few are made from crude drug preparations and are often called herbal remedies.

TABLETS AND CAPSULES. Tablets and capsules are the most common preparations for oral administration because they are suitable for mass production, are stable and convenient to use, and can be formulated to release the drug immediately after ingestion or to release it over a period of hours.

In the manufacture of tablets, a machine with a punch and die mechanism compresses a mixture of powdered drug and inert ingredients into a relatively hard disk. The **inert ingredients** include specific components that provide bulk, prevent sticking to the punch and die and disintegration in the bottle, and facilitate disintegration of the tablet when it reaches gastrointestinal fluids. These ingredients are called **fillers, lubricants, adhesives,** and **disintegrants,** respectively.

A tablet must disintegrate after it is ingested, and then the drug must dissolve in gastrointestinal fluids before it can be absorbed into the circulation. Variations in the rate and extent of tablet disintegration and drug dissolution can give rise to differences in the oral bioavailability of drugs from different tablet formulations (see Chapter 4).

Tablets may have various types of coatings. **Enteric coatings** consist of polymers that will not disintegrate in gastric acid but will break down in the more alkaline intestines. Enteric coatings are used to protect drugs that would otherwise be destroyed by gastric acid. Enteric coatings are also used to slow the release and absorption of a drug when a large dose is given at one time (e.g., the product called PROZAC WEEKLY).

Sustained-release products, or **extended-release products,** release the drug from the preparation over many hours. The two methods used to extend the release of the drug are **controlled diffusion** and **controlled dissolution.** Diffusion of the drug from the drug product can be regulated by a rate-controlling membrane. Dissolution is controlled by inert polymers that gradually break down in body fluids. These polymers may be part of the tablet matrix, or they may be used as coatings over small pellets of drug enclosed in a capsule. In either case, the drug is gradually released into the gastrointestinal tract as the polymers dissolve.

Some products use **osmotic pressure** to provide a sustained release of a drug. These products contain an osmotic agent that attracts gastrointestinal fluid at a constant rate. The attracted fluid then forces the drug out of the tablet through a small laser-drilled orifice (Fig. 1–3A).

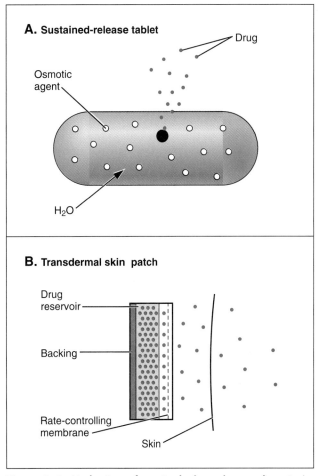

Figure 1–3. Mechanisms of sustained-release drug products. In the sustained-release tablet (A), water is attracted by an osmotic agent in the tablet, and this forces the drug out through a small orifice. In the transdermal skin patch (B), the drug diffuses through a rate-controlling membrane and is absorbed through the skin into the circulation.

Capsules are hard or soft gelatin shells enclosing a powdered or liquid medication. **Hard capsules** are used to enclose powdered drugs, whereas **soft capsules** enclose a drug in solution. The gelatin shell quickly dissolves in gastrointestinal fluids to release the drug for absorption into the circulation.

SOLUTIONS AND SUSPENSIONS. Drug solutions and particle suspensions, the most common liquid pharmaceutical preparations, can be formulated for oral, parenteral, or other routes of administration. Solutions and suspensions provide a convenient method for administering drugs to pediatric and other patients who cannot easily swallow solid dosage forms. They are less convenient than solid dosage forms, however, because the liquid must be measured each time a dose is given.

Solutions and suspensions for oral administration are often sweetened and flavored to increase palatability. Sweetened aqueous solutions are called **syrups,** whereas sweetened aqueous–alcoholic solutions are known as **elixirs.** Alcohol is included in elixirs as a solvent for drugs that are not sufficiently soluble in water alone.

Sterile solutions and suspensions are available for parenteral administration with a needle and syringe or with an intravenous infusion device. Many drugs are formulated as sterile powders for reconstitution with sterile liquids at the time the drug is to be injected, because the drug is not stable for long periods of time in solution. Sterile ophthalmic solutions and suspensions are suitable for administration with a dropper into the conjunctival sac.

SKIN PATCHES. Skin patches are drug preparations in which the drug is slowly released from the patch for absorption through the skin into the circulation. Most skin patches use a rate-controlling membrane to regulate the diffusion of the drug from the patch (Fig. 1–3B). Such devices are most suitable for drugs that are effective at a relatively low dosage and have sufficient lipid solubility to enable skin penetration.

AEROSOLS. Aerosols are a type of drug preparation administered by inhalation through the nose or mouth. They are particularly useful for treating respiratory disorders because they deliver the drug directly to the site of action and may thereby minimize the risk of systemic side effects. Some aerosol devices contain the drug dispersed in a pressurized gas and are designed to deliver a precise dosage each time they are activated by the patient. **Nasal sprays,** another type of aerosol preparation, can be used either to deliver drugs that have a localized effect on the nasal mucosa or to deliver drugs that are absorbed through the mucosa and exert an effect on another organ. For example, butorphanol, an opioid analgesic, is available as a nasal spray (STADOL NS) for the treatment of pain.

OINTMENTS, CREAMS, LOTIONS, AND SUPPOSITORIES. Ointments and creams are semisolid preparations intended for topical application of a drug to the skin or mucous membranes. These products contain an active drug that is incorporated into a vehicle (e.g., polyethylene glycol or petrolatum), which enables the drug to adhere to the tissue for a sufficient length of time to exert its effect. Lotions are liquid preparations often formulated as oil-in-water emulsions and are used to treat dermatologic conditions. Suppositories are products in which the drug is incorporated into a solid base that melts or dissolves at body temperature. Suppositories are usually intended for rectal, vaginal, or

urethral administration and may provide either localized or systemic drug therapy.

ROUTES OF DRUG ADMINISTRATION

Some routes of drug administration, such as the four enteral and parenteral routes compared in Table 1–2, are intended to elicit systemic effects and are commonly called systemic routes. Other routes of administration, such as the inhalational route, can elicit either localized effects or systemic effects, depending on the drug being administered.

Enteral Administration

The enteral routes of administration are those in which the drug is absorbed from the gastrointestinal tract. These include sublingual, buccal, oral, and rectal routes.

In **sublingual administration,** a drug product is placed under the tongue. In **buccal administration,** the drug is placed between the cheek and the gum. Both sublingual and buccal administration enable the rapid absorption of certain drugs and are not affected by first-pass drug metabolism in the liver. Drugs for sublingual and buccal administration must be given in a relatively low dosage and must have good solubility in water and lipid membranes. Larger doses might be irritating to the tissue and would likely be washed away by saliva before the drug would be absorbed. Two examples of drugs available for sublingual administration are nitroglycerin for treating ischemic heart disease and hyoscyamine for treating bowel cramps. Fentanyl, an opioid analgesic, is available in an oral transmucosal formulation (ACTIQ) for rapid absorption from the buccal mucosa in the treatment of breakthrough cancer pain.

In medical orders and prescriptions, **oral administration** is often designated as *per os* (PO), which refers to drug administration by mouth. The medication is swallowed, and the drug is absorbed from the stomach and small intestines. Because the oral route of administration is convenient and relatively safe and economical, it is the most commonly used

TABLE 1-2.	**Advantages and Disadvantages of Four Common Routes of Drug Administration**	
Route	**Advantages**	**Disadvantages**
Oral	Convenient, relatively safe, and economical.	Cannot be used for drugs that are inactivated by gastric acid, for drugs that have a large first-pass effect, or for drugs that irritate the gut.
Intramuscular	Suitable for suspensions and oily vehicles. Absorption is rapid from solutions and is slow and sustained from suspensions.	May be painful. Can cause bleeding if the patient is receiving an anticoagulant.
Subcutaneous	Suitable for suspensions and pellets. Absorption is similar to the intramuscular route but is usually somewhat slower.	Cannot be used for drugs that irritate cutaneous tissues or for drugs that must be given in large volumes.
Intravenous	Bypasses absorption to give an immediate effect. Allows for rapid titration of dosage. Has 100% bioavailability.	Poses more risks for toxicity and tends to be more expensive than other routes.

route. It does have some disadvantages, however. Absorption of orally administered drugs can vary widely because of the interaction of drugs with food and gastric acid and the varying rates of gastric emptying, intestinal transit, and tablet disintegration and dissolution. Moreover, some drugs are inactivated by the liver following their absorption from the gut, and oral administration is not suitable for use by patients who are sedated, comatose, or suffering from nausea and vomiting.

Rectal administration of drugs in suppository form can result in either a localized effect or a systemic effect. Suppositories are useful when patients cannot take medications by mouth, such as in the treatment of nausea and vomiting. They can also be administered for localized conditions such as hemorrhoids. Drugs absorbed from the rectum undergo relatively little first-pass metabolism in the liver.

Parenteral Administration

Parenteral administration refers to drug administration with a needle and syringe or with an intravenous infusion device. The most commonly used parenteral routes are the intravenous, intramuscular, and subcutaneous routes.

Intravenous administration bypasses the process of drug absorption and provides the greatest reliability and control over the dose of drug reaching the general circulation. It is often preferred for administration of a drug that has a short half-life and a drug whose dosage must be carefully titrated to the physiologic response, such as agents used to treat hypotension, shock, and acute heart failure. The intravenous route is widely used to administer antibiotics and antineoplastic drugs to critically ill patients, as well as to treat various types of medical emergencies. The intravenous route is potentially the most dangerous, because rapid administration of drugs by this route can cause serious toxicity.

Intramuscular and **subcutaneous administration** are suitable for treatment with drug solutions and particle suspensions. Solutions are absorbed more rapidly than particle suspensions, so suspensions are often used to extend the duration of action of a drug over many hours or days. Most drugs are absorbed more rapidly after intramuscular than after subcutaneous administration because of the greater circulation of blood to the muscle.

Intrathecal administration refers to injection of a drug through the theca of the spinal cord and into the subarachnoid space. In cases of meningitis, the intrathecal route is useful in administering antibiotics that do not cross the blood–brain barrier.

Other less commonly used parenteral routes include **intra-articular administration** of drugs used to treat arthritis.

Transdermal Administration

Transdermal administration refers to the application of drugs to the skin for absorption into the circulation. Application can be via a skin patch or, less commonly, via an ointment. Transdermal administration, which bypasses first-pass hepatic inactivation, is a reliable route of administration for drugs that are effective when given in a relatively low dosage and that are highly soluble in lipid membranes. Transdermal skin patches slowly release medication for periods of time that typically range from one to seven days. Two examples of transdermal preparations are the skin patches called fentanyl transdermal systems (DURAGESIC) that are used to treat chronic severe pain, and nitroglycerin ointment that is used to treat heart failure and angina pectoris.

Inhalational Administration

Inhalational administration can be used to produce either a localized or a systemic drug effect. A localized effect on the respiratory tract is obtained with drugs used to treat asthma or rhinitis, whereas a systemic effect is observed when a general anesthetic (e.g., halothane) is inhaled.

Topical Administration

Topical administration refers to the application of drugs to the surface of the body to produce a localized effect. It is often used to treat disorders of the skin, eyes, nose, mouth, throat, rectum, and vagina.

DRUG NAMES

A drug often has several names, including a chemical name, a nonproprietary name, and a proprietary name.

The **chemical name,** which specifies the chemical structure of the drug, uses standard chemical nomenclature. Some chemical names (e.g., acetylsalicylic acid) are relatively short. Others are relatively long because of the size and complexity of the drug molecule. For most drugs, the chemical name is of interest primarily to the chemist.

The **nonproprietary name,** or **generic name,** is the type of drug name most suitable for use by health care professionals. In the USA, the preferred nonproprietary names are the **United States Adopted Names** (USAN) designations. These designations, which are often derived from the chemical names of drugs, provide some indication of the class to which a particular drug belongs. For example, oxacillin can be easily recognized as a type of penicillin. The designations are selected by the USAN Council, which is a nomenclature committee representing the medical and pharmacy professions and the United States Pharmacopeia (see Chapter 4), with advisory input from the US Food and Drug Administration. The USAN is often the same as the **International Nonproprietary Name** (INN) and the **British Approved Name** (BAN). International names for drugs can vary with the language in which they are used.

The **proprietary name, trade name,** or **brand name** for a drug is a registered trademark belonging to a particular drug manufacturer and used to designate a drug product marketed by that manufacturer. Many drugs are marketed under two or more trade names, especially those drugs which are contained in combination drug products. Drugs can also be marketed under their USAN. For these reasons, it is often less confusing and more precise to use the USAN rather than a trade name for a drug. The proprietary name may provide some indication of the drug's pharmacologic or therapeutic effect. For example, DIURIL is a proprietary name for a diuretic, FLOMAX is a preparation used to increase urine flow, and MAXAIR is a product used to treat asthma.

SUMMARY OF IMPORTANT POINTS

■ The development of pharmacology was made possible by important advances in chemistry and physiology that enabled scientists to isolate and synthesize pure chemical compounds (drugs) and to design methods for identifying and quantifying the physiologic actions of the compounds.

■ Pharmacology has two subdivisions. Pharmacodynamics is concerned with the mechanisms of drug action and the dose-response relationship, whereas pharmacokinetics is concerned with the relationship between the drug dose and the plasma drug concentration over time.

■ The sources of drugs are natural products (including plants, microbes, animal tissues, and minerals) and chemical synthesis. Drugs can exist as crude drug preparations, pure drug compounds, or pharmaceutical preparations used to administer a specific dose to a patient.

■ The primary routes of administration are enteral (e.g., oral ingestion), parenteral (e.g., intravenous, intramuscular, and subcutaneous injection), transdermal, inhalational, and topical. Most routes produce systemic effects. Topical administration produces a localized effect at the site of administration.

■ All drugs (pure compounds) have a nonproprietary name (a generic name, such as a USAN designation) as well as a chemical name. Some drugs also have one or more proprietary names (trade names or brand names) under which they are marketed by their manufacturer.

Review Questions

1. Which route of drug administration avoids first-pass hepatic metabolism and is used with drug preparations that slowly release a drug for periods as long as seven days?
   (A) topical
   (B) sublingual
   (C) rectal
   (D) oral
   (E) transdermal

2. Which of the following correctly describes herbal remedies?
   (A) contain a specific quantity of a single pharmacologically active compound
   (B) the only type of drug preparation obtained from natural sources
   (C) vary in composition and potency
   (D) more safe and effective than other types of pharmaceutical preparations
   (E) pharmacologic effects are easily identified and quantitated

3. Which of the following correctly describes the intramuscular route of parenteral drug administration?
   (A) drug absorption is erratic and unpredictable
   (B) used to administer drug suspensions that are slowly absorbed
   (C) bypasses the process of drug absorption to give an immediate effect
   (D) cannot be used for drugs that undergo a high degree of first-pass metabolism
   (E) poses more risks than intravenous administration

Answers and Explanations

1. The answer is E: transdermal. The transdermal, sublingual, and parenteral routes of administration avoid first-pass hepatic drug metabolism. Sublingual administration is used when rapid absorption of a drug is required for an immediate effect, whereas transdermal administration provides for the sustained release of a drug over long periods of time. Orally administered drugs have the highest exposure to first-pass metabolism, whereas rectally administered drugs are partly absorbed into the general circulation and undergo less first-pass metabolism than orally administered drugs.

2. The answer is C: vary in composition and potency. Herbal remedies are crude drug preparations that usually contain the same active and inactive ingredients found in the natural product from which they are derived. Many herbal remedies contain several active ingredients whose composition and potency vary from batch to batch. Although the active ingredients may have beneficial therapeutic interactions, it is difficult to identify and quantitate the activity of the active principles in an herbal remedy.

3. The answer is B: used to administer drug suspensions that are slowly absorbed. After intramuscular injection of a suspension of drug particles, the particles slowly dissolve in interstitial fluid to provide sustained drug absorption over many hours or days. When a drug solution is injected intramuscularly, the drug is usually absorbed rapidly and completely.

SELECTED READINGS

Huxtable, R. J., and S. K. W. Schwarz. The isolation of morphine: first principles in science and ethics. Molecular Interventions 1:189–191, 2001.
Loudon, I., ed. Western Medicine: An Illustrated History. Oxford, Oxford University Press, 1997.
United States Pharmacopeial Convention. USP Dictionary of USAN and International Drug Names. Rockville, Md., United States Pharmacopeia, 2004.

CHAPTER 2

Pharmacokinetics

OVERVIEW

Pharmacokinetics is concerned with the relationship between the **dose** of a particular drug and the **concentration** of that drug in body fluids and tissues over time, as determined by the rates of **drug absorption, drug distribution,** and **drug elimination.** Drug elimination includes the **biotransformation** (metabolism) of a drug to one or more drug metabolites as well as the **excretion** of the drug from the body. The relationship between these processes is shown in Fig. 2–1.

To derive and use expressions for pharmacokinetic parameters, the first step is to establish a mathematical model that accurately relates the plasma drug concentration to the rates of drug absorption, distribution, and elimination. The **one-compartment model** is the simplest model of drug disposition, but the **two-compartment model** provides a more accurate representation of the pharmacokinetic behavior of many drugs (Fig. 2–2). In the two-compartment model, drugs are absorbed into the central compartment (the blood), distributed from the central compartment to the peripheral compartment (the tissues), and eliminated from the central compartment. Rate constants can be determined for each process and used to derive expressions for other pharmacokinetic parameters, such as the elimination half-life of a drug. In this chapter, each process of drug disposition is considered in greater detail.

DRUG ABSORPTION

Except for topically administered drugs that are absorbed directly into the target tissue, drug absorption refers to the passage of a drug from its site of administration into the circulation. Absorption requires the passage of drugs across one or more layers of cells. In the gut, lungs, and skin, drugs must first be absorbed through a layer of epithelial cells that have tight junctions (Fig. 2–3). Drugs injected into the subcutaneous tissue and muscle bypass the epithelial barrier and are more easily absorbed through spaces between capillary endothelial cells. For this reason, drugs face a greater barrier to absorption after oral administration than after parenteral administration.

Processes of Absorption

Most drugs are absorbed by **passive diffusion** across a biologic barrier and into the circulation. The rate of absorption is proportional to the drug concentration gradient across the barrier and the surface area available for absorption at that site. Drugs can be absorbed passively through cells either by lipid diffusion or by aqueous diffusion. **Lipid diffusion** is a process in which the drug dissolves in the lipid components of the cell membranes. This process is facilitated by a high degree of lipid solubility. **Aqueous diffusion** occurs by passage through the aqueous pores in cell membranes. Because aqueous diffusion is restricted to drugs with molecular weights lower than 200, most drugs are too large to be absorbed by this process.

A few drugs are absorbed by **active transport** or by **facilitated diffusion.** For example, some cephalosporin antibiotics are partly absorbed by the transporter for dipeptides, which is located in intestinal epithelial cells. Investigators have suggested that drug absorption could be enhanced by designing drugs that would utilize such transporters for absorption.

Effect of pH on Absorption of Weak Acids and Bases

Many drugs are weak acids or bases that exist in both ionized and nonionized forms in the body. Only the nonionized form of these drugs is sufficiently soluble in membrane lipids to be readily transferred across cell membranes (Box 2–1). The ratio of the two forms at a particular site influences the rate of drug absorption, distribution, or elimination.

The protonated form of a weak acid is nonionized, whereas the protonated form of a weak base is ionized. The ratio of the protonated form to the nonprotonated form of these drugs can be calculated using the **Henderson–Hasselbalch equation** (see Box 2–1). At a pH equal to the pK_a, equal amounts of the protonated and nonprotonated forms are present. If the pH is less than the pK_a, the protonated form predominates. If the pH is greater than the pK_a, the nonprotonated form predominates.

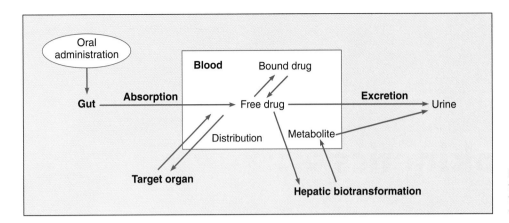

Figure 2-1. The absorption, distribution, hepatic biotransformation, and excretion of a typical drug after its oral administration.

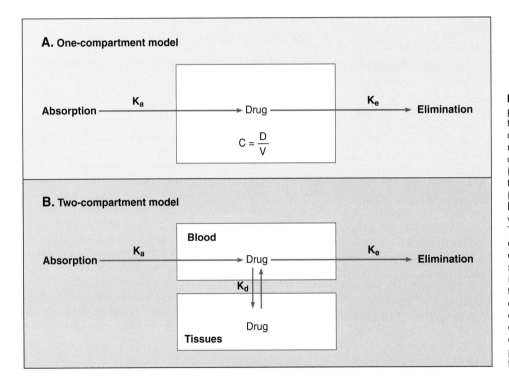

Figure 2-2. Two models of the processes of drug absorption, distribution, and elimination. K_a, K_d, and K_e are the rate constants, representing the fractional completion of each process per unit of time. (A) In the one-compartment model, the drug concentration at any time (C) is the amount of drug in the body at that time (D) divided by the volume of the compartment (V). Thus, D is a function of the dose administered and the rates of absorption and elimination represented by K_a and K_e, respectively. (B) In the two-compartment model, the drug concentration in the central compartment (the blood) is a function of the dose administered and the rates of drug absorption, distribution to the peripheral compartment (the tissues), and elimination from the central compartment.

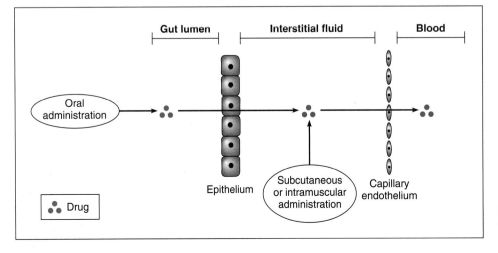

Figure 2-3. Drug absorption after oral, subcutaneous, and intramuscular administration.

BOX 2-1. EFFECT OF pH ON THE ABSORPTION OF A WEAK ACID AND A WEAK BASE

Weak acids (HA) donate a proton (H^+) to form anions (A^-), whereas **weak bases** (B) accept a proton to form cations (HB^+).

Only the **nonionized form** of a drug can readily penetrate cell membranes.

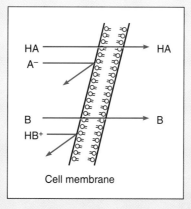

The **pK$_a$** of a weak acid or weak base is the **pH** at which there are equal amounts of the protonated form and the non-protonated form. The **Henderson–Hasselbalch equation** can be used to determine the ratio of the two forms:

$$\log \frac{[\text{Protonated form}]}{[\text{Nonprotonated form}]} = pK_a - pH$$

For **salicylic acid,** which is a weak acid with a pK$_a$ of 3, log $[HA]/[A^-]$ is 3 minus the pH. At a pH of 2, then, log $[HA]/[A^-] = 3 - 2 = 1$. Therefore, $[HA]/[A^-] = 10/1$.

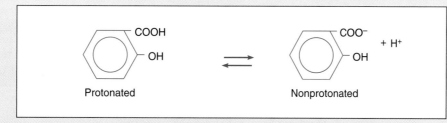

For **amphetamine,** which is a weak base with a pK$_a$ of 10, log $[HB^+]/[B]$ is 10 minus the pH. At a pH of 8, then, log $[HB^+]/[B] = 10 - 8 = 2$. Therefore, $[HB^+]/[B] = 100/1$.

Continued

BOX 2–1. EFFECT OF PH ON THE ABSORPTION OF A WEAK ACID AND A WEAK BASE—cont'd

The following are the ratios of the protonated form to the nonprotonated form at different pH levels:

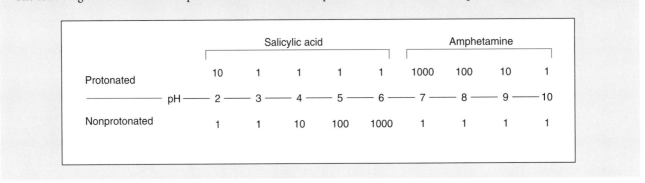

In the stomach, with a pH of 1, weak acids and bases are highly protonated. At this site, the nonionized form of weak acids (pK_a = 3–5) and the ionized form of weak bases (pK_a = 8–10) will predominate. Hence, weak acids are more readily absorbed from the stomach than are weak bases. In the intestines, with a pH of 6–7, weak bases are also mostly ionized, but much less so than in the stomach, and weak bases are absorbed more readily from the intestines than from the stomach. Weak acids can also be absorbed more readily from the intestines than from the stomach, despite their greater ionization in the intestines, because the intestines have a greater surface area than the stomach for absorption of the nonionized form of a drug, and this outweighs the influence of greater ionization in the intestines.

DRUG DISTRIBUTION

Drugs are distributed to organs and tissues via the circulation, from which they may diffuse into interstitial fluid and cells. Most drugs are not uniformly distributed throughout the total body water, and some drugs are restricted to the extracellular fluid or plasma compartment. Drugs with sufficient lipid solubility can diffuse into cells, and some drugs are concentrated in cells by the phenomenon of ion trapping, which is described below. Drugs can also be actively transported into cells. For example, some drugs are actively transported into hepatic cells, where they may undergo enzymatic biotransformation. In the intestines, drug transport by the P-glycoprotein (Pgp) and other carrier proteins in the blood-to-lumen direction leads to a secretion of various drugs into the intestinal tract, thereby serving as a detoxifying mechanism. The Pgp also removes many drugs, including anticancer drugs, from tissues throughout the body. Inhibition of Pgp by amiodarone, erythromycin, propranolol, and other drugs can increase tissue levels of these drugs and augment their pharmacologic effects.

Volume of Distribution

The volume of distribution (V_d) can be defined as the volume of fluid in which a drug would need to be dissolved to have the same concentration in that volume as it does in plasma. The V_d does not represent the volume in a particular physiologic body compartment; instead, as shown in Fig. 2–4A, it is an apparent volume that represents the relationship between the dose of a drug and the resulting plasma concentration of the drug.

Calculation

The V_d is calculated by dividing the dose of a drug (usually, the dose given intravenously) by the plasma drug concentration immediately after distribution. As shown in Fig. 2–4B, this drug concentration can be determined by extrapolating the plasma drug concentration back to time zero. The plasma drug concentration at time zero (Cp_0) represents the plasma concentration of a drug that would be obtained if it were instantaneously dissolved in its V_d. This equation can be rearranged to determine the dose of a drug that is required to establish a specified plasma drug concentration (see below).

Interpretation

Although the V_d does not correspond to a physiologic body fluid compartment, it does provide an indication of the physiologic distribution of a drug. A low V_d that approximates plasma volume or extracellular fluid volume usually indicates that the drug's distribution is restricted to a particular compartment (the plasma or extracellular fluid). When the V_d of a drug is equivalent to total body water (as occurs, for example, with ethanol ingestion), this usually indicates that the drug has reached the intracellular fluid as well. Many drugs have a V_d that is much larger than total body water. A large V_d usually indicates that the drug is concentrated intracellularly, with a resulting low concentration in the plasma.

Many weak bases, such as fluoxetine (PROZAC), have a large V_d because of the phenomenon of intracellular **ion trapping.** Weak bases are less ionized within plasma than they are within cells because intracellular fluid usually has a lower pH than extracellular fluid. After a weak base diffuses into a cell, a larger fraction is ionized in the more acidic intracellular fluid. This restricts its diffusion out of a cell and results in a large V_d.

Figure 2–4. Calculating the volume of distribution (V_d) of a drug. Unlike the physiologic distribution of a drug (A), the calculated V_d of a drug is an apparent volume that can be defined as the volume of fluid in which a drug would need to be dissolved to have the same concentration in that volume as it does in the plasma (B). The graph (C) provides an example of how the V_d is calculated. In this example, a dose of 500 mg was injected intravenously (IV) at time zero, and plasma drug concentrations were measured over time. The terminal elimination curve (β) was extrapolated back to time zero to determine that the plasma drug concentration at time zero (Cp_0) was 5 mg/L. Then the V_d was calculated by dividing the dose by the Cp_0. In this case, the result was 100 L.

A. Physiologic distribution

Plasma (4 L)

Interstitial fluid (10 L)

Intracellular fluid (28 L)

B. Apparent volume of distribution

C. Calculation of the V_d

Plasma drug concentration (mg/L)

50.00

5.00

0.50

0.05

0.00

Distribution phase (α)

Cp_0

Elimination phase (β)

Time

500 mg injected IV

$$V_d = \frac{Dose}{Cp_0} = \frac{500 \text{ mg}}{5 \text{ mg/L}} = 100 \text{ L}$$

Rate of Distribution

When drugs are administered orally, distribution occurs simultaneously with absorption, and the rate of distribution cannot be determined from the plasma drug concentration curve. After rapid intravenous drug administration, the plasma drug concentration falls rapidly at first, as the drug is distributed from the central compartment to the peripheral compartment (see Fig. 2–4C), and the rate of distribution can be determined from this portion of the curve.

Factors Affecting Distribution

Organ Blood Flow

The rate at which a drug is distributed to various organs after a drug dose is administered depends largely on the proportion of cardiac output received by the organs. Drugs are rapidly distributed to highly perfused tissues (e.g., brain, heart, liver, and kidney) and this enables a rapid onset of action of drugs affecting these tissues. Drugs are distributed more slowly to less highly perfused tissues (e.g., skeletal muscle) and even more slowly to those with the lowest blood flow (e.g., skin and adipose tissue).

Plasma Protein Binding

Almost all drugs are reversibly bound to plasma proteins, primarily albumin. The extent of binding depends on the affinity of a particular drug for protein-binding sites and ranges from less than 10% to as high as 99% of the plasma concentration. As the free (unbound) drug diffuses into interstitial fluid and cells, drug molecules dissociate from albumin to maintain the equilibrium between free drug and bound drug.

Plasma protein binding is saturable, and a drug can be displaced from binding sites by other drugs that have a higher affinity for such sites. This causes a temporary increase in the free concentration of the displaced drug and can lead to an increased tissue concentration and pharmacologic effect. This effect is usually short-lived, however, because the increased free drug concentration will accelerate drug biotransformation and excretion.

Molecular Size

Molecular size is a factor affecting the distribution of extremely large molecules, such as those in heparin. Heparin is largely confined to the plasma, although it does undergo some biotransformation in the liver.

Lipid Solubility

Lipid solubility is a major factor affecting the extent of drug distribution, particularly to the brain, where the blood–brain barrier restricts the penetration of polar and ionized molecules. The barrier is formed by tight junctions between the capillary endothelial cells and also by the glial cells that surround the capillaries and retard the penetration of polar molecules into brain neurons.

DRUG BIOTRANSFORMATION

Drug biotransformation and excretion are the two processes responsible for the decline of the plasma drug concentration over time during the terminal elimination phase (β). Drug biotransformation, often called **drug metabolism,** is the enzyme-catalyzed conversion of drugs to their metabolites. Most drug biotransformation takes place in the liver, but drug-metabolizing enzymes are found in many other tissues, including the gut, kidneys, brain, lungs, and skin.

Role of Drug Biotransformation

The primary biologic purpose of biotransformation enzymes is to inactivate and detoxify drugs and other foreign compounds (xenobiotics) that can harm the body. Drug metabolites are usually more water soluble than the parent molecule and, therefore, are more readily excreted by the kidneys. No particular relationship exists between biotransformation and pharmacologic activity. Some drug metabolites are active, whereas others are inactive. As a general rule, most conjugated drug metabolites are inactive, but a few exceptions exist.

Formation of Active Metabolites

Many pharmacologically active drugs, such as diazepam (VALIUM), are biotransformed to active metabolites. Some agents, known as **prodrugs,** are administered as inactive compounds and, subsequently, are biotransformed to active metabolites. This type of agent is usually developed because the prodrug is better absorbed than its active metabolite. For example, dipivefrin (PROPINE) is a prodrug that is converted to its active metabolite, epinephrine, by corneal enzymes after topical ocular administration. Orally administered prodrugs, such as enalapril (VASOTEC), are converted to their active metabolite by hepatic enzymes during their first pass through the liver.

First-Pass Biotransformation

Drugs that are absorbed from the gut reach the liver via the hepatic portal vein before entering the systemic circulation (Fig. 2–5). Many drugs, such as felodipine (PLENDIL), are extensively converted to inactive metabolites during their first pass through the gut wall and liver, and have low bioavailability after oral administration (see below). This phenomenon is called the first-pass effect. Drugs administered by the sublingual or rectal route undergo less first-pass metabolism and may have a higher degree of bioavailability than do drugs administered by the oral route.

Phases of Drug Biotransformation

Drug biotransformation can be divided into two phases, each composed of unique biotransformation reactions. In many cases, phase I reactions create or unmask a chemical group required for a phase II reaction. In some cases, however, drugs bypass phase I biotransformation and go directly to phase II. Although phase I metabolites often have pharmacologic activity, most phase II metabolites do not.

Phase I Biotransformation

Phase I biotransformation includes oxidative, hydrolytic, and reductive reactions (Fig. 2–6).

OXIDATIVE REACTIONS. Oxidative reactions are the most common type of phase I biotransformation. They are catalyzed by enzymes isolated in the microsomal fraction of liver homogenates (the fraction derived from the endoplasmic reticulum) and by cytoplasmic enzymes.

The **microsomal cytochrome P450 monooxygenase system** is a family of enzymes that catalyzes the biotransformation of drugs with a wide range of chemical structures. The microsomal **monooxygenase reaction** requires the following: cytochrome P450 (a hemoprotein); a flavoprotein that is reduced by nicotinamide adenine dinucleotide phosphate (NADPH), which is called NADPH—cytochrome P450 reductase; and membrane lipids in which the system is embedded. In the drug-oxidizing reaction, one atom of oxygen is used to form a hydroxylated metabolite of a drug, as shown in Fig. 2–7, whereas the other atom of oxygen forms water when combined with electrons contributed by NADPH. The hydroxylated metabolite may be the end product of the reaction or serve as an intermediate leading to the formation of another metabolite.

The most common chemical reactions catalyzed by the cytochrome P450 enzymes are aliphatic hydroxylation, aromatic hydroxylation, N-dealkylation, and O-dealkylation.

Various **cytochrome P450 isoforms** have been identified, and their role in metabolizing specific drugs is currently being elucidated. Each isoform catalyzes a different, but overlapping, spectrum of oxidative reactions. Most drug biotransformations are catalyzed by three P450 families: CYP1, CYP2, and CYP3. Each of these family members has more than 40% identical protein sequences. Each family is divided into subfamilies, the members of which have more than 55% identical protein sequences. The CYP3A subfamily catalyzes more than half of all microsomal drug oxidations.

Many drugs alter drug biotransformation by inhibiting or inducing cytochrome P450 enzymes, and **drug interactions** can occur when these drugs are administered concurrently with other drugs that are metabolized by cytochrome P450 (see Chapter 4). Two examples of **inducers of cytochrome**

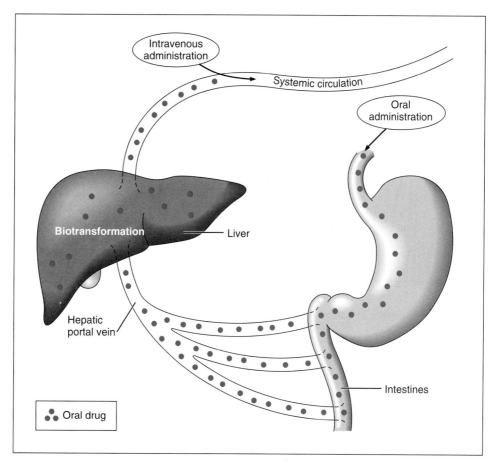

Figure 2–5. First-pass drug biotransformation. Drugs that are absorbed from the gut can be biotransformed by enzymes in the gut wall and liver before reaching the systemic circulation. This process lowers their degree of bioavailability.

P450 are phenobarbital and rifampin. The inducers stimulate the transcription of genes encoding cytochrome P450 enzymes, resulting in increased messenger RNA (mRNA) and protein synthesis. Evidence indicates that P450 enzyme inducers combine with a nuclear receptor to initiate P450 gene transcription, and other gene regulatory elements have been identified.

A few drugs are metabolized by **cytoplasmic enzymes.** For example, ethanol is oxidized by alcohol dehydrogenase, and caffeine and theophylline are biotransformed by xanthine oxidase. Other cytoplasmic oxidases include monoamine oxidase.

HYDROLYTIC REACTIONS. Esters and amides are hydrolyzed by a variety of enzymes. These include the cholinesterases and other plasma esterases that inactivate choline esters, local anesthetics, and drugs such as esmolol (BREVIBLOC), an agent that blocks cardiac β_1-adrenergic receptors.

REDUCTIVE REACTIONS. Reductive reactions are less common than are oxidative and hydrolytic reactions. Chloramphenicol and a few other drugs are partly metabolized by a hepatic nitroreductase, and this process appears to involve cytochrome P450. Nitroglycerin undergoes reductive hydrolysis catalyzed by glutathione-organic nitrate reductase.

Phase II Biotransformation

In phase II biotransformation, drug molecules undergo **conjugation reactions** with an endogenous substance such as acetate, glucuronate, sulfate, or glycine (Fig. 2–8). Conjugation enzymes, which are present in the liver and other tissues, serve to conjugate various drugs with the endogenous substance to form water-soluble metabolites that are more easily excreted. Except for microsomal glucuronosyltransferases, these enzymes are located in the cytoplasm. Most conjugated drug metabolites are pharmacologically inactive.

ACETYLATION. Acetylation is accomplished by N-acetyltransferase enzymes that utilize acetyl coenzyme A (acetyl CoA) as a source of the acetate.

GLUCURONIDE FORMATION. Glucuronide formation, the most common conjugation reaction, utilizes glucuronosyltransferases to conjugate a glucuronate molecule with a drug.

SULFATION. Sulfotransferases catalyze the conjugation of several drugs, including minoxidil and triamterene, whose sulfate metabolites are pharmacologically active.

Genetic Variations in Drug Biotransformation

Variations in Acetylation of Drugs

Individuals can exhibit slow or fast acetylation of some drugs (e.g., isoniazid and hydralazine) because of genetically determined differences in the activity of acetyltransferases located in the gut and liver. The genetic variations are attributed to different isozymes. Slow acetylation is an autosomal recessive trait, and persons with the slow phenotype are

Description	Reaction	Examples
Oxidative reactions		
Aliphatic hydroxylation		Ibuprofen, pentobarbital, and tolbutamide
Aromatic hydroxylation		Phenobarbital, phenytoin, and propranolol
N-Dealkylation	$R-NHCH_3 \longrightarrow R-NH_2 + CH_2O$	Codeine, imipramine, and theophylline
O-Dealkylation	$R-OCH_3 \longrightarrow R-OH + CH_2O$	Codeine, dextromethorphan, and indomethacin
Deamination		Amphetamine and diazepam
N-Oxidation		Chlorpheniramine
S-Oxidation		Chlorpromazine and cimetidine
Hydrolytic reactions		
Amide hydrolysis	$R_1-CNR_2 \longrightarrow R_1-COOH + R_2-NH_2$	Lidocaine and procainamide
Ester hydrolysis	$R_1-COR_2 \longrightarrow R_1-COOH + R_2-OH$	Aspirin, esmolol, and procaine
Reductive reactions		
Nitro reduction		Chloramphenicol
Reductive hydrolysis	$R-ONO_2 \longrightarrow R-OH + NO_2^-$	Nitroglycerin

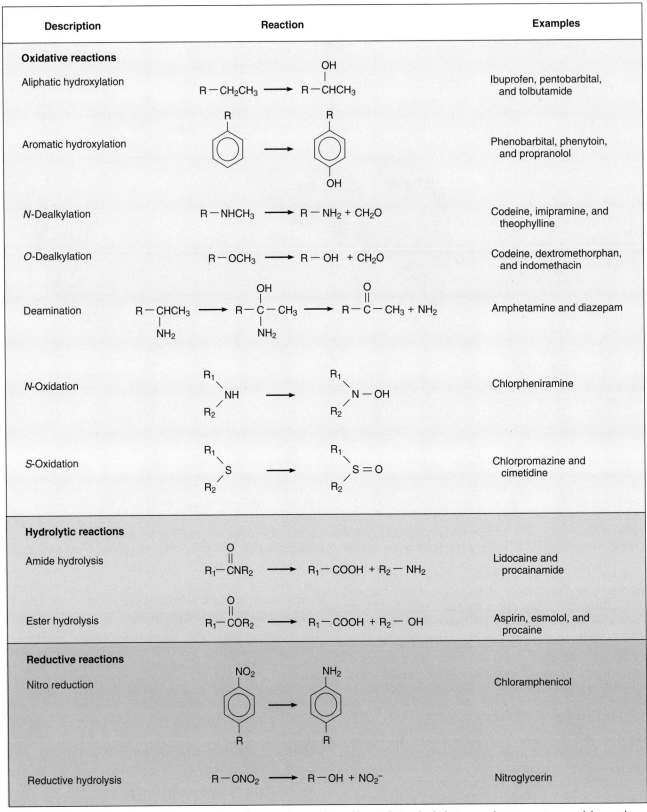

Figure 2–6. Phase I drug biotransformation. Many drugs are biotransformed by oxidative, hydrolytic, or reductive reactions and then undergo conjugation with endogenous substances. A few drugs bypass phase I reactions and directly enter phase II biotransformation.

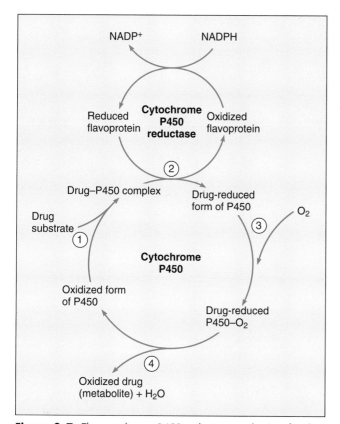

Figure 2–7. The cytochrome P450 reductase mechanism for drug oxidation. Four steps are involved in the cytochrome P450 reaction: First, the drug substrate binds to the oxidized form of P450 (i.e., Fe^{3+}). Second, the drug P450 complex is reduced by cytochrome P450 reductase, using electrons donated by the reduced form of nicotinamide adenine dinucleotide phosphate (NADPH). Third, the drug-reduced form of P450 (i.e., Fe^{2+}) interacts with oxygen. Fourth, the oxidized drug (metabolite) and water are produced.

homozygous for the slow allele (r/r). In contrast, persons with the fast phenotype are heterozygous (R/r) or homozygous dominant (R/R). The distribution of these phenotypes varies from population to population. The fast acetylation phenotype predominates in the Japanese population; the slow acetylation phenotype predominates in some Middle Eastern populations; and about half of the US population exhibits each phenotype.

Variations in Oxidation of Cytochrome P450

Variations in oxidation of some drugs have been attributed to genetic differences in certain cytochrome P450 enzymes. Genetic polymorphisms of CYP2D6 and CYP2C19 enzymes have been well characterized, and human populations of "extensive metabolizers" and "poor metabolizers" have been identified. These differences are caused by variations in the protein coding region of the P450 gene and differing rates of mRNA and protein expression that result in altered rates of catalysis. Poor metabolizers of CYP2C19 have higher plasma levels of proton pump inhibitors, such as omeprazole (PRILOSEC), whereas some extensive metabolizers of CYP2C19 require larger doses of omeprazole to cure peptic ulcer.

Most individuals are extensive metabolizers of CYP2D6, but about 7% to 10% of whites and a smaller fraction of Asians and blacks are poor metabolizers of CYP2D6. Psychiatric patients who are poor metabolizers of CYP2D6 have been found to have a higher rate of adverse drug reactions than do those who are extensive metabolizers because of higher plasma drug levels. In addition, poor metabolizers of CYP2D6 have a reduced ability to metabolize prodrug substrates to their active metabolites. For example, poor metabolizers do not convert codeine to morphine sufficiently to obtain adequate pain relief when codeine is administered for analgesia.

Other Variations in Drug Metabolism

About 1 of 3000 individuals exhibits a familial atypical cholinesterase that will not metabolize succinylcholine, a neuromuscular blocking agent, at a normal rate. Affected individuals are subject to prolonged apnea after receiving the usual dose of the drug. For this reason, patients should be screened for atypical cholinesterase before receiving succinylcholine.

Genetically determined variations in the rate of metabolism of other drugs (e.g., warfarin) have been observed, but most of these variations are relatively rare.

DRUG EXCRETION

Renal Drug Excretion

Most drugs are excreted in the urine, either as the parent compound or as a drug metabolite. Drugs, which are handled by the kidneys in the same manner as physiologic substances, undergo the processes of glomerular filtration, active tubular secretion, and passive tubular reabsorption. The amount of drug excreted is the sum of the amounts filtered and secreted minus the amount reabsorbed. The relationship between these processes, the rate of drug excretion, and renal clearance is shown in Box 2–2.

Glomerular Filtration

Glomerular filtration is the first step in renal drug excretion. In this process, the free drug enters the renal tubule as a dissolved solute in the plasma filtrate (see Box 2–2). If a drug has a large fraction bound to plasma proteins, as is the case with warfarin, it will have a low rate of glomerular filtration.

Active Tubular Secretion

Some drugs, particularly weak acids and bases, undergo active tubular secretion by transport systems located primarily in proximal tubular cells. This process is competitively inhibited by other drugs of the same chemical class. For example, the secretion of penicillins and other weak acids is inhibited by probenecid.

Active tubular secretion is not affected by plasma protein binding. This is because when the free drug is actively transported across the renal tubule, this fraction of drug is replaced by a fraction that dissociates from plasma proteins to maintain the equilibrium of free drug and bound drug.

Description	Reaction	Examples

Conjugation reactions

Acetylation — Hydralazine, isoniazid, and sulfonamides

Acetyl coenzyme A

Glucuronide formation — Acetaminophen, morphine, and oxazepam

UDP-glucuronic acid

Sulfation — Acetaminophen, minoxidil, and triamterene

3′-Phosphoadenosine-5′-phosphosulfate (PAPS)

3′-Phosphoadenosine-5′-phosphate

Figure 2–8. Phase II drug biotransformation. UDP = uridine diphosphate.

Passive Tubular Reabsorption

The extent to which a drug undergoes passive reabsorption across renal tubular cells and into the circulation depends on the **lipid solubility** of the drug. Drug biotransformation facilitates drug elimination by forming polar drug metabolites that are not as readily reabsorbed as the less-polar parent molecules.

Most nonelectrolytes, including ethanol, are passively reabsorbed across tubular cells. Ionized weak acids and bases are not reabsorbed across renal tubular cells, and they are more rapidly excreted in the urine than are nonionized drugs that undergo passive reabsorption. The proportion of ionized and nonionized drugs is affected by **renal tubular pH,** which can be manipulated to increase the excretion of a drug after a drug overdose (Box 2–3).

Biliary Excretion and Enterohepatic Cycling

Many drugs are excreted in the bile as the parent compound or a drug metabolite. Biliary excretion favors compounds with molecular weights that are higher than 300.

Numerous conjugated drug metabolites, including the glucuronate and sulfate derivatives of steroids, are excreted in the bile. After the bile empties into the intestines, a fraction of the drug may be reabsorbed into the circulation and eventually return to the liver. This phenomenon is called enterohepatic cycling (Fig. 2–9). Conjugated drugs can be hydrolyzed to the free drug by intestinal bacteria, and this facilitates the drug's reabsorption, because conjugated metabolites are more polar and less lipid-soluble than are the parent compounds.

Other Routes of Excretion

Sweat and **saliva** represent minor routes of excretion for some drugs. In pharmacokinetic studies, saliva measurements are sometimes used because the saliva concentration of a drug often reflects the intracellular concentration of the drug in target tissues.

PHARMACOKINETIC EXPRESSIONS

Most drugs exhibit **first-order kinetics,** in which the rate of drug elimination is proportional to the plasma drug concentration. A few drugs (e.g., ethanol) exhibit **zero-order kinetics,** in which the rate of drug elimination is constant and independent of plasma drug concentration. The **kinetic order** refers to the exponent of the drug concentration (0 or 1) in the expression shown in Fig. 2–10.

Pharmacokinetics concerns the relationship between the dose of a particular drug and the concentration of that drug in body fluids and tissues over time. For drugs that exhibit first-order kinetics, the plasma drug concentration can be estimated from a drug's dose and its clearance. Because the plasma drug concentration is often correlated with the magnitude of a drug's effect, it is possible to use pharmacokinetic expressions to determine and adjust drug dosages to achieve a desired therapeutic effect.

BOX 2–2. THE RENAL EXCRETION AND CLEARANCE OF A WEAK ACID, PENICILLIN G

Description and Chemical Structure

Penicillin G (benzylpenicillin) is an example of a weak acid. It has a pK_a of 2.8 and is primarily excreted via renal tubular secretion. About 60% of penicillin G is bound to plasma proteins. The pharmacokinetic calculations below are based on a urine **pH** of 5.8, a **plasma drug concentration** of 3 µg/mL, a **glomerular filtration rate** of 100 mL/min, and a **measured drug excretion rate** of 1200 µg/min. Because 40% of penicillin G is free (unbound), the **free drug plasma concentration** is 0.4×3 µg/mL = 1.2 µg/mL.

Renal Excretion

The discussion and accompanying figure illustrate the relationship between the rates of glomerular filtration, active tubular secretion, passive tubular reabsorption, and excretion.

(1) **Filtration.** The **drug filtration rate** is calculated by multiplying the glomerular filtration rate by the free drug plasma concentration: 100 mL/min × 1.2 µg/mL = 120 µg/min.

(2) **Secretion.** The **drug secretion rate** is calculated by subtracting the drug filtration rate from the drug excretion rate: 1200 µg/min − 120 µg/min = 1080 µg/min. This amount indicates that 90% of the drug's excretion occurs by the process of tubular secretion.

(3) **Reabsorption.** The ratio of the nonionized form to the ionized form of the drug in the urine is equal to the antilog of the pK_a minus the pH: antilog of 2.8 − 5.8 = antilog of −3 = 1:1000. Because most of the drug is ionized in the urine, the **drug reabsorption rate** is probably <1 µg/min.

(4) **Excretion.** The drug excretion rate was initially given as 1200 µg/min. It was determined by measuring the drug concentration in urine and multiplying it by the urine flow rate. Note that the drug excretion rate is equal to the drug filtration rate (120 µg/min) plus the drug secretion rate (1080 µg/min) minus the drug reabsorption rate (<1 µg/min).

Renal Clearance

Renal clearance is calculated by dividing the excretion rate (1200 µg/min) by the plasma drug concentration (3 µg/mL). The result is 400 mL/min, which is equal to 24 L/h.

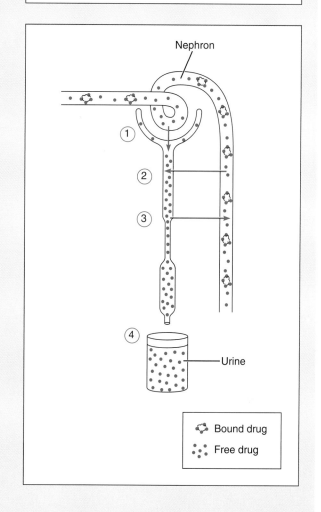

First-Order Kinetics

The following principles pertain to first-order kinetics: A drug's rate of elimination is equal to the plasma drug concentration multiplied by the drug clearance; the elimination rate declines as the plasma concentration declines (see Fig. 2–10A); and the half-life and clearance of the drug remain constant as long as renal and hepatic function do not change.

Drug Clearance

Clearance is the most fundamental expression of drug elimination. It is defined as the volume of body fluid (blood) from which a drug is removed per unit of time. Whereas a particular drug's clearance is usually constant, it is important to note that the amount of drug contained in the clearance volume will vary with the plasma drug concentration.

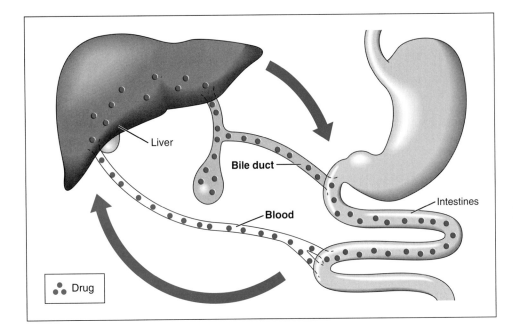

Figure 2–9. Enterohepatic cycling. Drugs and drug metabolites with molecular weights higher than 300 may be excreted via the bile, stored in the gallbladder, delivered to the intestines by the bile duct, and then reabsorbed into the circulation. This process reduces the elimination of a drug and prolongs its half-life and duration of action in the body.

B O X   2 – 3 .   URINE ACIDIFICATION AND ALKALINIZATION IN THE TREATMENT OF DRUG OVERDOSE

If a drug or other compound is a weak acid or base, its degree of ionization and rate of renal excretion will depend on its pK_a and on the pH of the renal tubular fluid. The rate of excretion of a **weak acid** can be accelerated by **alkalinizing the urine**, whereas the rate of excretion of a **weak base** can be accelerated by **acidifying the urine**. These procedures have been used to enhance the excretion of drugs and poisons, but they are not without risk to the patient, and their benefits have been established for only a few drugs.

To make manipulation of the urine pH worthwhile, a drug must be excreted to a large degree by the kidneys. The short-acting barbiturates (e.g., secobarbital) are eliminated almost entirely via biotransformation to inactive metabolites, so modification of the urine pH has little effect on their excretion. In contrast, phenobarbital is excreted to a large degree by the kidneys, so urine alkalinization is useful in treating an overdose of this drug. Urine acidification to enhance the elimination of weak bases (e.g., amphetamine), has been largely abandoned because it does not significantly increase the elimination of these drugs and poses a serious risk of metabolic acidosis.

In cases involving an overdose of aspirin or other salicylate, alkalinization of the urine produces the dual benefits of increasing drug excretion and counteracting the metabolic acidosis that occurs with serious aspirin toxicity. For patients suffering from phenobarbital overdose or from herbicide 2,4-dichlorophenoxyacetic acid (2,4-D) poisoning, alkalinization of the urine is also helpful: this is accomplished by administering sodium bicarbonate intravenously every 3 to 4 hours to increase the urinary pH to 7–8.

RENAL CLEARANCE. Renal clearance can be calculated as the renal excretion rate divided by the plasma drug concentration (see Box 2–2). Drugs that are eliminated primarily by glomerular filtration, with little tubular secretion or reabsorption, will have a renal clearance that is approximately equal to the creatinine clearance, which is normally about 100 mL/min in an adult. A renal drug clearance that is higher than the creatinine clearance indicates that the drug is a substance that undergoes tubular secretion. A renal drug clearance that is lower than the creatinine clearance suggests that the drug is highly bound to plasma proteins or that it undergoes passive reabsorption from the renal tubules.

HEPATIC CLEARANCE. Hepatic clearance is more difficult to determine than renal clearance. This is because hepatic drug elimination includes the biotransformation and biliary excretion of parent compounds. For this reason, hepatic clearance is usually determined by multiplying hepatic blood flow by the arteriovenous drug concentration difference.

Elimination Half-Life

Elimination half-life is the time required to eliminate half of the amount of a drug in the body or to reduce the plasma drug concentration by 50%. It can be calculated from the elimination rate constant, but it is usually determined from the plasma drug concentration curve (Fig. 2–11). The half-life can also be expressed in terms of the drug's clearance and volume of distribution, indicating that the drug's half-life will change when either of these factors is altered. Disease, age, and other physiologic variables can alter drug clearance or volume of distribution and thereby change the half-life (see Chapter 4).

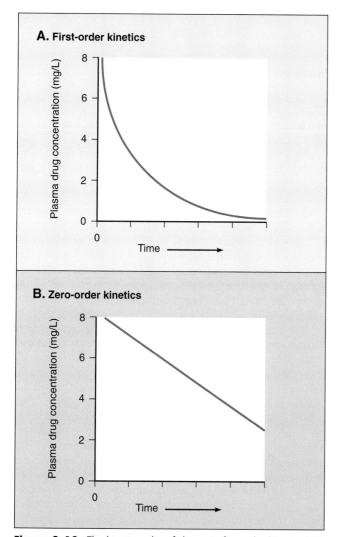

Figure 2–10. The kinetic order of drugs. In first-order kinetics **(A)**, the rate of drug elimination is proportional to the plasma drug concentration. In zero-order kinetics **(B)**, the rate of drug elimination is constant. The kinetic order of a drug is derived from the exponent, *n*, in the following expression:

$$\Delta[\text{Drug}]/\Delta t = -k[\text{Drug}]^n$$

where Δ represents change, [Drug] represents the plasma drug concentration, and *t* is time. If *n* is 1, then $\Delta[\text{Drug}]/\Delta t$ is proportional to [Drug]. If *n* is 0, then $\Delta[\text{Drug}]/\Delta t$ is constant (k), because $[\text{Drug}]^0$ equals 1.

Zero-Order Kinetics

The following principles pertain to zero-order kinetics: The rate of drug elimination is constant (see Fig. 2–10B); the drug's elimination half-life is proportional to the plasma drug concentration; the clearance is inversely proportional to the drug concentration; and a small increase in dosage can produce a disproportionate increase in the plasma drug concentration.

In many cases, the reason that the rate of drug elimination is constant is that the elimination process becomes saturated. This occurs, for example, at most plasma concen-

Figure 2–11. Drug half-life and clearance. The elimination half-life $(t_{1/2})$ is the time required to reduce the plasma drug concentration (Cp) by 50%. The formula is as follows:

$$t_{1/2} = 0.693/K_e$$

where 0.693 is the natural logarithm of 2, and K_e is the elimination rate constant. The half-life is often determined from the plasma drug concentration curve shown here. The clearance (Cl) is the volume of fluid from which a drug is eliminated per unit of time. It can be calculated as the product of the volume of distribution (V_d) and K_e. If $0.693/t_{1/2}$ is substituted for K_e, the equation is as follows:

$$Cl = 0.693\ V_d/t_{1/2}$$

Thus, a drug's clearance is directly proportional to its volume of distribution and is inversely proportional to its half-life.

trations of ethanol. In some cases, drugs exhibit zero-order elimination when high doses are administered, which occurs, for example, with aspirin and the anticonvulsant phenytoin (DILANTIN) or when a hepatic or renal disease has impaired the drug elimination processes.

SINGLE-DOSE KINETICS

Plasma Drug Concentration Curve

The plasma drug concentration curve, which plots the concentration over time, provides useful information about drug absorption, distribution, and elimination. After a single dose of drug is administered, the plasma concentration increases as the drug is absorbed, reaches a peak as absorption is completed, and then declines as the drug is eliminated (Fig. 2–12A). Except in the case of a rapid intravenous injection, the process of drug distribution occurs simultaneously with drug absorption and cannot be easily discerned from the plasma drug concentration curve.

Bioavailability

In the plasma drug concentration curve, the rate and extent of drug absorption after oral administration are indicated by the maximal plasma drug concentration (Cp_{max}), the time at which the maximal concentration occurs (t_{max}), and the area under the curve (AUC). These measures are useful for comparing the bioavailability of different pharmaceutical formulations (see Chapter 4) or of drugs given by different routes of administration.

Bioavailability is defined as the fraction of the administered dose of a drug that reaches the systemic circulation in an active form. As shown in Fig. 2–12B, the oral bioavailability of a particular drug is usually determined by dividing the AUC of an orally administered dose of the drug (AUC_{oral}) by the AUC of an intravenously administered dose of the same drug (AUC_{IV}). The assumption is that the intravenously administered drug has 100% bioavailability.

The bioavailability of orally administered drugs is of particular concern because it can be reduced by many pharmaceutical and biologic factors. Pharmaceutical factors include the rate and extent of tablet disintegration and drug dissolution. Biologic factors include the effects of food, which can sequester or inactivate a drug; the effects of gastric acid, which can inactivate a drug; and the effects of gut and liver enzymes, which can biotransform a drug during its absorption and first pass through the liver. The cytochrome P450 3A4 isozyme found in intestinal enterocytes and hepatic cells is a particularly important catalyst of first-pass drug metabolism. CYP3A4 works in conjunction with the P-glycoprotein (Pgp) described above, wherein the 3A4 isozyme located in enterocytes serves to inactivate drugs transported into the intestinal lumen by Pgp.

The bioavailability of drugs administered intramuscularly or via other routes can be determined in the same manner as the bioavailability of drugs administered orally.

CONTINUOUS- AND MULTIPLE-DOSE KINETICS

Drug Accumulation and the Steady-State Principle

When a drug that exhibits first-order pharmacokinetics is administered to a patient continuously or intermittently, the drug will accumulate until it reaches a plateau or steady-state plasma drug concentration.

The basis for this accumulation to a steady state is shown in Fig. 2–13. When the drug is first administered, the rate of administration is much greater than the rate of elimination, because the plasma concentration is so low. As the drug continues to be administered, the rate of drug elimination gradually increases, whereas the rate of administration remains constant. Eventually, as the plasma concentration rises sufficiently, the rate of drug elimination equals the rate of drug administration. At this point, the steady-state condition is achieved.

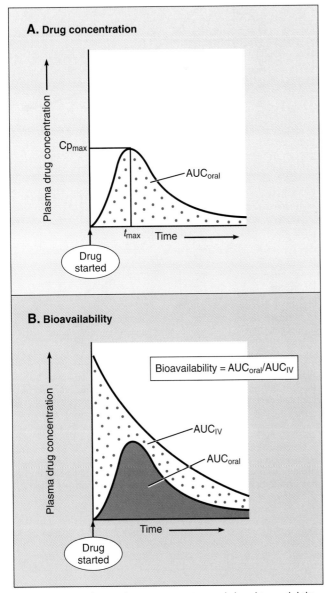

Figure 2–12. Plasma drug concentration and drug bioavailability. The plasma drug concentration curve for a single dose of a drug given orally (A) shows the maximal plasma concentration (Cp_{max}), the time at which the maximal plasma concentration occurred (t_{max}), and the area under the curve (AUC). To determine bioavailability (B), the AUC of the orally administered drug (AUC_{oral}) can be divided by the AUC of the intravenously administered drug (AUC_{IV}).

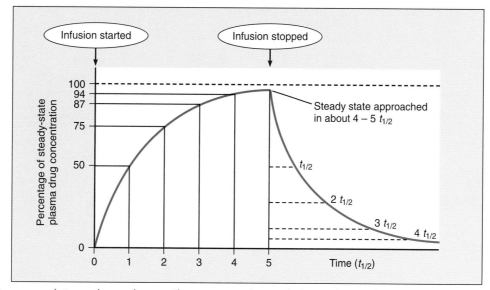

Figure 2–13. Drug accumulation to the steady state. The time required to reach the steady state depends on the half-life (t1/2); it does not depend on the dose or dose interval. The steady-state drug concentration depends on the drug dose administered per unit of time and on the drug's clearance or half-life.

Time Required to Reach the Steady-State Condition

Drug accumulation to a steady state is a first-order process and therefore obeys the rule that half of the process is completed in a defined time. Because the time to reach the steady state is dependent on the time it takes for the rate of drug elimination to equal to the rate of drug administration, the time to reach the steady state is a function of the elimination half-life of the drug. Any first-order process requires about four to five half-lives to be completed, and the time to reach the steady-state drug concentration is about four to five drug half-lives. If the half-life of a drug changes, then the time required to reach the steady-state also changes. Note that the time required to reach the steady state is independent both of the drug dose and the rate or frequency of drug administration.

Steady-State Drug Concentration

The steady-state drug concentration depends on the drug dose administered per unit of time and on the half-life of the drug. If the dose is doubled, the steady-state concentration is also doubled. Likewise, if the half-life is doubled, the steady-state concentration is doubled.

Figure 2–14 illustrates typical plasma concentration curves after drugs are administered continuously or intermittently. A drug administered intermittently will accumulate to a steady state at the same rate as a drug given by continuous infusion, but the plasma drug concentration will fluctuate as each dose is absorbed and eliminated. The average steady-state plasma drug concentration with intermittent intravenous administration will be the same as if the equivalent dose were administered by continuous infusion.

With intermittent oral administration, the fractional bioavailability will also influence the steady-state plasma concentration.

Dosage Calculations

Loading Dose

A loading dose, or **priming dose,** is given to rapidly establish a therapeutic plasma drug concentration. The loading dose can be calculated by multiplying the volume of distribution by the desired plasma drug concentration (Box 2–4). The loading dose, which is usually larger than the maintenance dose, is generally administered as a single dose, but it can be divided into fractions that are given over several hours. A divided loading dose is sometimes used for drugs that are more toxic (e.g., digitalis glycosides).

Maintenance Dose

A maintenance dose is given to establish or maintain a desired steady-state plasma drug concentration. For drugs given intermittently, the maintenance dose is one of a series of doses administered at regular intervals. The amount of drug to be given is based on the principle that at the steady state, the rate of drug administration equals the rate of drug elimination. To determine the rate of drug elimination, the drug clearance is multiplied by the average steady-state plasma drug concentration. The maintenance dose is then calculated as the rate of drug elimination multiplied by the dosage intervals. If the drug is administered orally, its fractional bioavailability must be included in the equation.

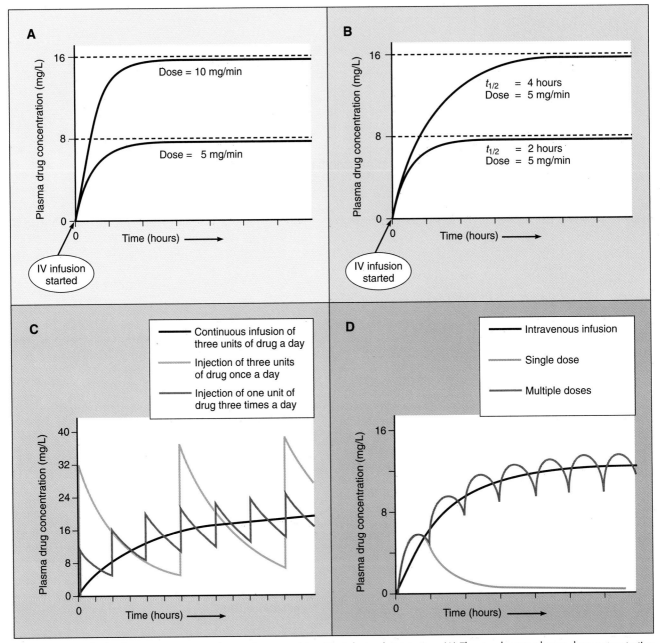

Figure 2–14. Plasma drug concentrations after continuous or intermittent drug administration. (A) The steady-state plasma drug concentration is proportional to the dose administered per unit of time. (B) The steady-state plasma drug concentration is directly proportional to the half-life (and is inversely related to clearance). (C) The average steady-state concentration is the same for intermittent infusion as it is for continuous infusion. With intermittent drug administration, however, the plasma concentrations fluctuate between doses, and the size of fluctuations increases as the dosage interval increases. (D) Plasma drug concentrations after intermittent oral administration are affected by the rates of drug absorption, distribution, and elimination. If only one dose is given, the peak in plasma drug concentration is followed by a continuous decline in the curve.

BOX 2–4. DRUG DOSAGE CALCULATIONS

Loading Dose

The loading dose, or priming dose, of a drug is determined by multiplying the **volume of distribution** (V_d) of the drug by the **desired plasma drug concentration** (desired Cp). (This information can be found in the medical literature.) For theophylline, for example, the estimated V_d for an adult weighing 70 kg is 35 L, and the desired Cp is 15 mg/L. The calculation is as follows:

$$\begin{aligned} \text{Loading dose} &= V_d \times Cp \\ &= 35 \text{ L} \times 15 \text{ mg/L} \\ &= 525 \text{ mg} \end{aligned}$$

As is discussed in Chapter 3, the patient's body weight and other characteristics affect the V_d and, therefore, should be considered in determining the appropriate loading dose for a particular patient.

Maintenance Dose

Calculations of the maintenance dose must take into consideration the **intended frequency of drug administration.** With intermittent administration, the fluctuations in Cp increase as the dosage interval increases. A twofold fluctuation in Cp will occur when the dosage interval is equal to the drug's half-life. This is because the Cp will fall 50% between doses. For many drugs, the half-life is a convenient and acceptable dosage interval.

The maintenance dose is designed to establish or maintain a **desired steady-state Cp.** The amount of drug to be given is based on the principle that at the steady state, the rate of drug administration equals the rate of drug elimination. The rate of elimination is equal to the clearance multiplied by the steady-state drug concentration. For example, if the steady-state gentamicin concentration is 2 mg/L and the clearance for gentamicin is 100 mL/min (0.1 L/min), then the elimination rate is 0.1 L/min × 2 mg/L = 0.2 mg/min. If the drug is to be administered every 8 hours, then the dosage would be calculated as follows:

$$\begin{aligned} \text{Maintenance dose} &= \text{Hourly rate} \\ &\quad \times \text{dosage interval in hours} \\ &= 0.2 \text{ mg/min} \\ &\quad \times 60 \text{ minutes in an hour} \\ &\quad \times 8 \text{ hours} \\ &= 96 \text{ mg every 8 hours} \end{aligned}$$

If a drug is to be administered orally, the calculated dose must be divided by the fractional bioavailability to determine the administered dose.

Dosage Adjustment Using Pharmacokinetic Values

First, choose the target Cp and administer the initial dose on the basis of the standard published values (general population values) for clearance or V_d. Second, measure the patient's plasma drug levels and calculate the patient's V_d and clearance. Third, revise the dosage based on the patient's V_d and clearance.

SUMMARY OF IMPORTANT POINTS

■ Most drugs are absorbed by passive diffusion across or between cells. The rate of passive diffusion of a drug across cell membranes is proportional to the drug's lipid solubility and the surface area available for absorption. Only the nonionized form of weak acids and bases is lipid soluble.

■ The ratio of the ionized form to the nonionized form of a weak acid or base can be determined from the pK_a of the drug and the pH of the body fluid in which the drug is dissolved.

■ The distribution of a drug is influenced by organ blood flow and by the plasma protein binding, molecular size, and lipid solubility of the drug. Only drugs with high lipid solubility can penetrate the blood–brain barrier.

■ The volume of distribution is the volume of fluid in which a drug would need to be dissolved to have the same concentration in that volume as it does in plasma. It is calculated by dividing the drug dose by the plasma drug concentration at time zero.

■ Many drugs are biotransformed before excretion. Drug metabolites can be pharmacologically active or inactive. Phase I reactions include oxidative, reductive, and hydrolytic reactions, whereas phase II reactions conjugate a drug with an endogenous substance. The cytochrome P450 enzymes located in the endoplasmic reticulum of liver cells are the most important oxidative biotransformation enzymes.

■ Most drugs are excreted in the urine, either as the parent compound or as drug metabolites, and undergo the processes of glomerular filtration, active tubular secretion, and passive tubular reabsorption. The renal clearance of a drug can be calculated by dividing the renal excretion rate by the plasma drug concentration.

■ Most drugs exhibit first-order kinetics, in which the rate of drug elimination is proportional to the plasma drug concentration at any given time. If drug elimination mechanisms (biotransformation and excretion) become saturated, a drug can exhibit zero-order kinetics, in which the rate of drug elimination is constant.

■ In first-order kinetics, a drug's half-life and clearance are constant as long as physiologic elimination processes are constant. The half-life is the time required for the plasma drug concentration to decrease by 50%. The clearance is the volume of plasma from which a drug is eliminated per unit of time.

■ The oral bioavailability of a drug is the fraction of the administered dose that reaches the circulation in an active form. It is determined by dividing the area under the plasma drug concentration curve (AUC) after oral administration by the AUC after intravenous administration. Factors that reduce bioavailability include incomplete tablet disintegration and first-pass and gastric inactivation of a drug.

■ With continuous or intermittent drug administration, the plasma drug concentration increases until it reaches a steady-state condition, in which the rate of drug elimination is equal to the rate of drug administration. It takes about four to five drug half-lives to achieve the steady-state condition.

■ The steady-state drug concentration can be calculated as the dose per unit of time divided by the clearance, and this equation can be rearranged to determine the dose per unit of time required to establish a specified steady-state drug concentration.

■ A loading dose is a single or divided dose given to rapidly establish a therapeutic plasma drug concentration. The dose can be calculated by multiplying the volume of distribution by the desired plasma drug concentration.

Review Questions

1. If food decreases the rate but not the extent of the absorption of a particular drug from the gastrointestinal tract, then taking the drug with food will result in a smaller
   (A) area under the plasma drug concentration-time curve
   (B) maximal plasma drug concentration
   (C) time at which the maximal plasma drug concentration occurs
   (D) fractional bioavailability
   (E) total clearance

2. If a drug exhibits first-order elimination, then
   (A) the elimination half-life is proportional to the plasma drug concentration
   (B) the drug is eliminated at a constant rate
   (C) hepatic drug metabolizing enzymes are saturated
   (D) drug clearance will increase if the plasma drug concentration increases
   (E) the rate of drug elimination (mg/minute) is proportional to the plasma drug concentration

3. After a person ingests an overdose of an opioid analgesic, the plasma drug concentration is found to be 32 mg/L. How long will it take to reach a safe plasma concentration of 2 mg/L if the drug's half-life is 6 hours?
   (A) 12 hours
   (B) 24 hours
   (C) 48 hours
   (D) 72 hours
   (E) 1 week

4. What dose of a drug should be injected intravenously every 8 hours to obtain an average steady-state plasma drug concentration of 5 mg/L if the drug's volume of distribution is 30 L and its clearance is 8 L/h?
   (A) 40 mg
   (B) 80 mg
   (C) 160 mg
   (D) 320 mg
   (E) 400 mg

Answers and Explanations

1. The answer is B: the maximal plasma drug concentration. If the rate of drug absorption is reduced, then the maximal plasma drug concentration will be less because more time will be available for drug distribution and elimination while the drug is being absorbed. Moreover, the time at which the maximal plasma drug concentration occurs will increase. If the extent of drug absorption (fraction absorbed) does not change, then the area under the curve and fractional bioavailability will not change.

2. The answer is E: the rate of drug elimination (mg/min) is proportional to the plasma drug concentration. In first-order elimination, drug half-life and clearance do not vary with the plasma drug concentration, but the rate of drug elimination (quantity per time) is proportional to plasma drug concentration at any time.

3. The answer is B: 24 hours. The half-life is the time required to reduce the plasma drug concentration 50%. In this case, it will take four drug half-lives or 24 hours to reduce the plasma level from 32 to 2 mg/L.

4. The answer is D: 320 mg. The dose required to establish a target plasma drug concentration is calculated by multiplying the clearance by the target concentration and dosage interval. In this case, it is 5 mg/L × 8 L/h × 8 hours = 320 mg.

SELECTED READINGS

Birkett, D.J. Pharmacokinetics Made Easy, 2nd ed. Roseville, Australia, McGraw-Hill Australia, 2002.
Guengerich, F.P. Cytochromes P450, drugs, and diseases. Mol Interv 3:194–204, 2003.
Levine, R. R. Pharmacology: Drug Actions and Reactions, 6th ed. New York, Parthenon, 2000.
Rowland, M., and T. N. Tozer. Clinical Pharmacokinetics: Concepts and Applications, 3rd ed. Philadelphia, Lea and Febiger, 1995.

CHAPTER 3

Pharmacodynamics

OVERVIEW

Pharmacodynamics is concerned with the detailed mechanisms of action by which drugs produce their biochemical and physiologic effects. It is also concerned with the dose-response relationship, which is the relationship between drug concentration (dose) and the magnitude of drug effect. Pharmacodynamics provides a scientific basis for the selection and use of drugs to counteract specific pathophysiologic mechanisms in particular diseases.

NATURE OF DRUG RECEPTORS

Drugs produce their effects by interacting with specific cell molecules called receptors. By far, most ligands (drugs or neurotransmitters) bind to protein receptors, although some agents act directly on DNA or membrane lipids (Table 3–1).

Types of Drug Receptors

The largest family of receptors for pharmaceutical agents is **G-protein coupled receptors, called GPCR**. These membrane-spanning proteins consist of specific extracellular, transmembrane, and intracellular domains (Fig. 3–1). Extracellular domains and, to some extent, transmembrane regions determine ligand binding and selectivity. Intracellular loops, especially the third one, mediate the receptor interaction with its **effector molecule**, a **guanine nucleotide binding protein (G protein)**.

A number of ligands inhibit the function of specific **enzymes** by competitive or noncompetitive inhibition. A ligand that binds to the same active, catalytic site as the endogenous substrate is a **competitive inhibitor.** Ligands that bind at a different site on the enzyme and alter the shape of the molecule, thereby reducing its catalytic activity, are called **noncompetitive inhibitors.**

Drugs also target **membrane transport proteins** including ligand- and voltage-gated ion channels and neurotransmitter transporters. At ligand-gated ion channels, drugs bind at the same site as the endogenous ligand and directly compete for the receptor site. Drugs can also bind at a different site (**allosteric site**) that alters the ion channel and increases or decreases the flow of ions. Neurotransmitter transporters are large, 12-transmembrane domain proteins that transfer neurotransmitter molecules out of the synapse and back to the neuron. A large group of agents, known generally as re-uptake inhibitors, target these transport proteins.

Other macromolecules that serve as receptors include the various lipids and phospholipids that make up the membrane. Some of the effects of general anesthetics and alcohol are due to interaction with membrane lipids. Steroid hormone receptors are intracellular proteins that translocate to the nucleus on ligand (steroid) binding. In the nucleus, the steroid receptor complex alters the transcription rate of specific genes. DNA is also a receptor site for ligands that bind directly to nucleic acids, most notably the antineoplastic agents.

Receptor Classification

Drug receptors are classified according to drug specificity, tissue location, and, more recently, by their molecular structure. For example, adrenergic receptors were initially divided into two types (α and β), based on their affinity for norepinephrine, epinephrine, and other agents in different tissues. Subsequently, the distinction between the types was confirmed by the development of selective antagonists that blocked either α-adrenergic or β-adrenergic receptors. Later, the two types of receptors were divided into subtypes, based on more subtle differences in agonist potency, tissue distribution, and varying effects.

At present, most receptors for drug targets and endogenous ligands are cloned and their amino acid sequences determined. Also present are numerous other receptor-like proteins predicted from gene sequencing for which an endogenous ligand is not identified, called **orphan receptors.** Families of receptors types are grouped by their sequence similarity using bioinformatics and this classification supports that from earlier *in vivo* and *in vitro* functional studies. In many cases, each type of receptor corresponds to a single, unique gene with subtypes arising from different transcripts of the same gene (alternative splicing).

TABLE 3–1. **Drug Receptors**

Types of Drug Receptors	Examples of Drugs that Bind Receptor
Hormone and Neurotransmitter Receptors	
Adrenergic receptors	Epinephrine and propranolol
Histamine receptors	Cimetidine and diphenhydramine
5-Hydroxytryptamine (serotonin) receptors	Tegaserod, ondansetron, and sumatriptan
Insulin receptors	Insulin
Muscarinic receptors	Atropine and bethanechol
Nicotinic receptors	Tubocurarine
Opioid receptors	Morphine and codeine
Steroid receptors	Cortisol, estradiol, and tamoxifen
Enzymes	
Carbonic anhydrase	Acetazolamide
Cholinesterase	Donepezil and physostigmine
Cyclooxygenase	Aspirin and celecoxib
DNA polymerase	Acyclovir and zidovudine
DNA topoisomerase	Ciprofloxacin
Human immunodeficiency virus (HIV) protease	Indinavir
Monoamine oxidase	Phenelzine
Na^+,K^+-adenosine triphosphatase	Digoxin
Xanthine oxidase	Allopurinol
Membrane transport proteins	
Ion channels	Lidocaine, quinidine, and verapamil
Ion transporters	Furosemide and hydrochlorothiazide
Neurotransmitter transporters	Amitriptyline, cocaine, and fluoxetine
Other macromolecules	
Membrane lipids	Alcohol and amphotericin B
Nucleic acids	Cyclophosphamide and doxorubicin

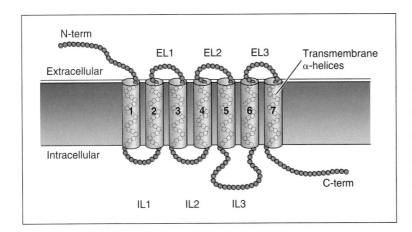

Figure 3–1. Structure of a typical GPCR. All GPCR consist of a long polypeptide chain of amino acids threaded through the cell membrane with seven transmembrane (TM) domains. These TM domains are arranged in α-helices composed of hydrophobic residues. The *N*-terminal of the receptor protein is outside the cell and the *C*-terminal on the inside. Three extracellular loops (EL) and three intracellular loops (IL) are formed by this configuration. The protein in the cell membrane forms a circle with TM1 and TM7 in close proximity but is shown here in a two-dimensional view for clarity.

DRUG-RECEPTOR INTERACTIONS

Receptor Binding and Affinity

To initiate a cellular response, a drug must first bind to a receptor. In most cases, drugs bind to their receptor by forming hydrogen, ionic, or hydrophobic (Van der Waals) bonds with a receptor site (Fig. 3–2). These weak bonds are reversible and enable the drug to dissociate from the receptor as the tissue concentration of the drug declines. The binding of drugs to receptors often exhibits stereospecificity, so that only one of the stereoisomers will form a three-point attachment with the receptor. In a few cases, drugs form relatively permanent covalent bonds with a specific receptor.

This occurs, for example, with antineoplastic drugs that bind to DNA and with drugs that irreversibly inhibit the enzyme cholinesterase.

The tendency of a drug to combine with its receptor is called affinity, which is a measure of the strength of the drug-receptor bonding. According to the law of mass action, the number of receptors [R] occupied by a drug depends on the drug concentration [D] and the drug-receptor association and dissociation rate constants (k_1 and k_2):

$$[D] + [R] \underset{k_2}{\overset{k_1}{\rightleftarrows}} [D\text{-}R] \longrightarrow \text{Effect}$$

Figure 3–2. Drug binding to receptors. (A) L-Isoproterenol, a β-adrenergic receptor agonist, forms hydrogen, ionic, and hydrophobic (Van der Waals) bonds with three sites on the β-adrenergic receptor. (B) D-Isoproterenol binds to two sites on the β-adrenergic receptor but is unable to bind with the third site. (C) L-Propranolol, a β-adrenergic receptor antagonist, binds to two sites on the receptor in the same way that L-isoproterenol does. The naphthyloxy group (N) forms weak bonds with the third receptor site, but these are not sufficiently strong for the drug to have intrinsic (agonist) activity. iC₃H₇ = isopropyl.

The ratio of k_2 to k_1 is known as the K_D and represents the drug concentration required to saturate 50% of the receptors. The lower the K_D, the greater is the drug's affinity for the receptor. Most drugs have a K_D in the micromolar to nanomolar (10^{-6} to 10^{-9} M) range of drug concentrations. As discussed below, receptor affinity is the primary determinant of drug potency.

Signal Transduction

Signal transduction describes the pathway from ligand binding to conformational changes in the receptor, receptor interaction with an effector molecule (if present), and other downstream molecules called second messengers. This cascade of receptor-mediated biochemical events ultimately leads to a physiologic effect (Table 3–2).

Membrane receptors are often coupled with a G protein, an ion channel, or an enzyme. The signal transduction pathway for GPCR is well understood. These receptors constitute a superfamily of receptors for many physiologic ligands and drugs, including receptors for acetylcholine, epinephrine, histamine, opioids, and serotonin. Fig. 3–3 illustrates signal transduction for a receptor that is coupled with G proteins.

The G proteins have three subunits known as Gα, Gβ, and Gγ. The Gα subunit serves as the site of guanosine triphosphate (GTP) hydrolysis, a process catalyzed by GTPase. Several types of Gα subunits exist, each of which determines a specific cellular response. For example, the Gα$_s$ (stimulating) subunit increases adenylyl cyclase activity and thereby stimulates the production of cyclic adenosine monophosphate (**cyclic AMP,** or cAMP). The Gα$_i$ (inhibitory) subunit decreases adenylyl cyclase activity and inhibits the production of cAMP. Another G protein (Gα$_q$) activates phospholipase C and leads to the formation of inositol triphosphate (**IP₃**) and diacylglycerol (**DAG**) from membrane phospholipids. IP₃ and DAG further cause an elevation of Ca^{+2} ions inside the cell. Several other types of Gα subunits are also present in cells and activated by receptors.

Cyclic AMP, IP₃, DAG, and other second messengers activate or inhibit unique cellular enzymes in each target cell. Cyclic AMP activates a number of tissue-specific protein kinases. When phosphorylated, these kinases regulate muscle contraction, ion channel activity, and the activity of enzymes such as glycogen phosphorylase. IP₃ and DAG evoke the release of calcium from intracellular storage sites and thereby augment calcium-induced processes such as muscle contraction and glandular secretion.

Efficacy

The ability of a drug to initiate a cellular effect is called intrinsic activity or efficacy. Efficacy is the ability of a ligand to stimulate the receptor and start the signal transduction pathway. Drugs that have both receptor affinity and efficacy are called **agonists,** whereas drugs that have receptor affinity but lack efficacy are called **antagonists.** With a few classes of drugs (e.g., the β-adrenergic receptor agonists and antagonists), the specific molecular structures responsible for affinity and efficacy have been identified. Both agonists and antagonists have common components sufficient for

TABLE 3–2.   **Examples of Receptors and Signal Transduction Pathways**

Family and Type of Receptor	Mechanism of Signal Transduction	Example of Effect in Tissue or Cell
G protein-coupled receptors		
α_1-Adrenergic receptor	Activation of phospholipase C	Vasoconstriction
α_2-Adrenergic receptor	Inhibition of adenylyl cyclase	Release of norepinephrine decreased
β-Adrenergic receptor	Stimulation of adenylyl cyclase	Heart rate increased
Muscarinic receptor	Activation of phospholipase C	Glandular secretion increased
Ligand-gated ion channels		
$GABA_A$ receptors	Chloride ion flux	Hyperpolarization of neuron
Nicotinic receptors	Sodium ion flux	Skeletal muscle contraction
Membrane-bound enzymes		
Atrial natriuretic factor receptors	Stimulation of guanylyl cyclase	Sodium excretion increased
Insulin receptors	Activation of tyrosine kinase	Glucose uptake stimulated
Nuclear receptors		
Steroid receptors	Activation of gene transcription	Reduced cytokine production
Thyroid hormone receptors	Activation of gene transcription	Oxygen consumption increased

GABA = γ-aminobutyric acid.

receptor affinity, but only agonists have the structure required for efficacy (see Fig. 3–1).

There are three types of agonists. **Full agonists** can produce the maximal response obtainable in a tissue. **Partial agonists** can only produce a submaximal response. In the presence of a full agonist, a partial agonist will act like an antagonist because it will prevent the full agonist from binding the receptor and exerting a maximal response.

Inverse agonists, which are also called **negative antagonists,** are involved in a special type of drug-receptor interaction. The effect of inverse agonists is based on the finding that signal transduction proceeds at a basal rate in the absence of any ligand binding to the receptor. A full agonist increases the rate of signal transduction when it binds to the receptor, whereas an inverse agonist decreases the rate of signal transduction. Only a few inverse agonists have been identified,

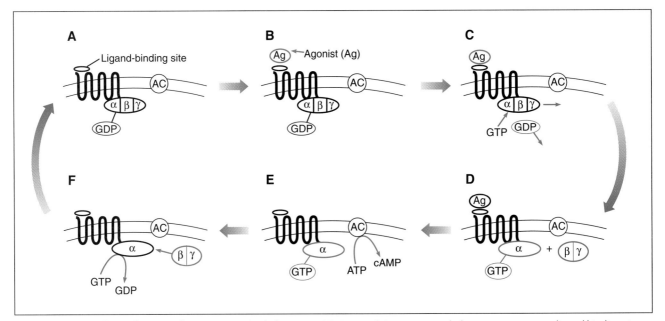

Figure 3–3. Signal transduction with a G protein-coupled receptor. (A) A typical G protein-coupled receptor contains a ligand-binding site on the external surface of the plasma membrane and a G protein-binding site on the internal surface. In the inactive state, guanosine diphosphate (GDP) is bound to the Gα subunit of the G protein. (B) and (C) When the agonist (Ag) binds to the receptor, guanosine triphosphate (GTP) binds to the G protein and causes the dissociation of GDP. (D) Activation of the Gα subunit by GTP causes the dissociation of the Gβ and Gγ subunits. (E) The Gα subunit is then able to activate adenylyl cyclase (AC) and thereby stimulate the conversion of adenosine triphosphate (ATP) to cyclic adenosine monophosphate (cAMP). (F) GTP hydrolysis, catalyzed by Gα subunit GTPase, leads to reassociation of the Gα and the Gβ and Gγ subunits.

and drugs that bind to the benzodiazepine receptor located in the central nervous system are examples. Antagonists can prevent the action of agonists and inverse agonists by occupying receptor-binding sites. **Competitive antagonists** bind to the same site as the agonist but are reversibly bound. **Noncompetitive antagonists** block the agonist site irreversibly, usually by forming a covalent bond.

Receptor Regulation and Drug Tolerance

Receptors can undergo dynamic changes with respect to their density (number per cell) and their affinity for drugs and other ligands. The continuous or repeated exposure to agonists can desensitize receptors, usually by phosphorylating serine or threonine residues in the C-terminal domain of GPCR. Phosphorylation of the receptor reduces the G-protein coupling efficiency. This acute effect of agonist exposure is called **desensitization** or **tachyphylaxis.** Phosphorylation also signals the cell to internalize the membrane receptor. By this **internalization** mechanism and by regulation of the receptor gene, the number of receptors on the cell membrane decreases. This longer-term adaptation is called **down-regulation.** In contrast, continuous or repeated exposure to antagonists initially can increase the response of the receptor, called **supersensitivity.** With chronic exposure to antagonist, the number of receptors on the membrane surface increases via **up-regulation.**

Drug tolerance is seen when the same dose of drug given repeatedly loses its effect or when greater doses are needed to achieve a previously obtained effect. Receptor downregulation is often responsible for **pharmacodynamic tolerance,** which describes adaptations to chronic drug exposure at the tissue and receptor level. Pharmacodynamic tolerance is distinct from **pharmacokinetic tolerance** in that the latter is caused by accelerated drug elimination, usually an upregulation of the enzymes that metabolize the drug.

Disease states can alter the number and function of receptors and thereby affect the response to drugs. For example, myasthenia gravis is an autoimmune disorder in which antibodies destroy the nicotinic receptors in skeletal muscle, leading to impaired neurotransmission and muscle weakness. This condition is treated by administration of nicotinic receptor agonists (see Chapter 6).

DOSE-RESPONSE RELATIONSHIPS

In pharmacodynamic studies, different doses of a drug can be tested in a group of subjects or in isolated organs, tissues, or cells. The relationship between the concentration of a drug at the receptor site and the magnitude of the response is called the dose-response relationship. Depending on the purpose of the studies, this relationship can be described in terms of a **graded** (continuous) response or a **quantal** (all-or-none) response.

Graded Dose-Response Relationships

In graded dose-response relationships, the response elicited with each dose of a drug is described in terms of a percent-

Figure 3–4. Graded dose-response relationships. (A) The dose-response curves of three agonists (R, S, and T) are compared. Drugs R and S are full agonists. Both have maximal efficacy, but R is more potent than S. Drug T is a partial agonist and, therefore, is incapable of producing the same magnitude of effect as a full agonist. T is also less potent than R and S. ED_{50} = median effective dose. (B) The effects that antagonists have on an agonist's dose-response curve are compared. X = agonist alone; Y = agonist in the presence of a competitive antagonist; and Z = agonist in the presence of a noncompetitive antagonist.

age of the **maximal response** and is plotted against the **log dose** of the drug (Fig. 3–4). Graded-dose response curves illustrate the relationship between drug dose, receptor occupancy, and the magnitude of the resulting physiologic effect. For a given drug, the maximal response is produced when all of the receptors are occupied, and the half-maximal response is produced when 50% of the receptors are occupied. In some cases, fewer than 50% of total receptors will be occupied but still give the half-maximal response. This is because only a fraction of the total receptors are needed to produce the maximal response. The remaining unbound receptors are considered to be "spare" receptors.

Potency is a characteristic of drug action useful for comparing different pharmacologic agents. It is usually expressed in terms of the **median effective dose** (ED_{50}), which is the dose that produces 50% of the maximal response. The potency of a drug varies inversely with a drug's ED_{50}, so that a drug whose ED_{50} is 4 mg is 10 times more potent than a drug whose ED_{50} is 40 mg. Potency is largely determined by the affinity of a drug for its receptor, because drugs with greater affinity require a lower dose to occupy 50% of the functional receptors.

The maximal response produced by a drug is known as its **efficacy**. A **full agonist** has maximal efficacy, whereas a **partial agonist** has less than maximal efficacy and is incapable of producing the same magnitude of effect as a full agonist, even at the very highest doses (see Fig. 3–4A). As discussed, when a partial agonist is administered with an agonist, the partial agonist may act as an antagonist by preventing the agonist from binding to the receptor and thereby reducing its effect. An antagonist, by definition, has no efficacy in this sense but can be an effective medication as in the use of an adrenergic receptor antagonist (β-blocker) to treat hypertension.

The effect that an **antagonist** has on the dose-response curve of an agonist depends on whether the antagonist is competitive or noncompetitive (see Fig. 3–4B). A **competitive antagonist** binds reversibly to a receptor, and its effects are surmountable if the dose of the agonist is increased sufficiently. A competitive antagonist shifts the agonist's dose-response curve to the right, but it does not reduce the maximal response. Although a **noncompetitive antagonist** also shifts the agonist's dose-response curve to the right, it binds to the receptor in a way that reduces the ability of the agonist to elicit a response. The amount of reduction is in proportion to the dose of the antagonist. The effects of a noncompetitive antagonist cannot be overcome or surmounted with greater doses of an agonist.

Quantal Dose-Response Relationship

In quantal dose-response relationships, the response elicited with each dose of a drug is described in terms of the cumulative percentage of subjects exhibiting a defined **all-or-none effect** and is plotted against the **log dose** of the drug (Fig. 3–5). An example of an all-or-none effect is sleep when a sedative-hypnotic agent is given. With quantal dose-response curves, the median effective dose (ED_{50}) is the dose that produces the observed effect in 50% of the subjects.

Quantal relationships can be defined for both toxic and therapeutic drug effects to allow calculation of the **therapeutic index** (TI) and the **certain safety factor** (CSF) of a drug. The TI and CSF are based on the difference between the toxic dose and the therapeutic dose in a population of subjects. The TI is defined as the ratio between the median lethal dose (LD_{50}) and the median effective dose (ED_{50}). It provides a general indication of the margin of safety of a drug, but the CSF is a more realistic estimate of drug safety. The CSF is defined as the ratio between the dose that is lethal in 1% of subjects (LD_1) and the dose that produces a therapeutic effect in 99% of subjects (ED_{99}). When phenobarbital was tested in animals, for example, it was found to have a TI of 10 and a CSF of 2. Because the dose that will kill 1% of animals is twice the dose that is required to produce the therapeutic effect in 99% of animals, the drug has a good margin of safety.

SUMMARY OF IMPORTANT POINTS

■ Most drugs form reversible, stereospecific bonds with macromolecular receptors located in target cells.

■ The tendency of a drug to bind to a receptor, called affinity, is directly related to potency. The affinity of a drug is often expressed as the K_D, which is the drug concentration required to saturate 50% of the functional receptors.

■ The ability of a drug to initiate a response is called intrinsic activity or efficacy. Agonists have both affinity and efficacy, whereas antagonists only have receptor affinity.

■ Graded dose-response curves show the relationship between the dose and the magnitude of the drug effect in a group of subjects or in a particular tissue, organ, or type of cell. The median effective dose (ED_{50}) produces 50% of the maximal response.

■ A competitive antagonist and a noncompetitive antagonist will both cause a rightward shift in the dose-response curve of an agonist, but only a noncompetitive antagonist will reduce the maximal response of the agonist.

■ Quantal dose-response curves show the relationship between the dose and the cumulative percentage of subjects exhibiting an all-or-none effect. The ratio of the median lethal dose (toxic dose) to the median effective dose (therapeutic dose) is called the therapeutic index, which is an indication of the margin of safety of a drug.

Review Questions

1. The description of molecular events initiated with the ligand binding and ending with a physiologic effect is called:
   (A) receptor down-regulation
   (B) signal transduction pathway
   (C) ligand-receptor binding
   (D) law of mass action
   (E) intrinsic activity or efficacy

Figure 3–5. Quantal dose-response relationships. The dose-response curves for a therapeutic effect (sleep) and a toxic effect (death) of a drug are compared. The ratio of the LD_{50} to the ED_{50} is the therapeutic index. The ratio of the LD_1 to the ED_{99} is the certain safety factor. ED = effective dose; and LD = lethal dose.

2. G protein-coupled receptors that activate an inhibitory Gα subunit alter the activity of adenylyl cyclase to:
   (A) increase the coupling of receptor to G protein
   (B) block the ligand from binding
   (C) initiate the conversion of GTP to GDP
   (D) generate intracellular inositol triphosphate
   (E) decrease the production of cAMP

3. The law of mass-action explains the relationship between:
   (A) dose of drug and physiologic response
   (B) concentration of drug and association/dissociation of drug-receptor
   (C) receptors and the rate of signal transduction
   (D) an enzyme and ligands that inhibit the enzyme
   (E) graded and quantal dose-response curves

4. In a log dose-response plot, drug efficacy is determined by the maximal height of the measured response on the effect axis, whereas drug potency is determined by:
   (A) number of animals exhibiting an all-or-none response
   (B) signal transduction pathway
   (C) formula, including the affinity of the drug and the number of drug receptors
   (D) position of the curve along the log-dose axis
   (E) steepness of the dose-response curve

5. A partial agonist is best described as an agent that:
   (A) has low potency but high efficacy
   (B) acts as both an agonist and antagonist
   (C) interacts with more than one receptor type
   (D) cannot produce the full effect even at high doses
   (E) blocks the effect of the antagonist

Answers and Explanations

1. The correct answer is B: the signal transduction pathway. Pharmacodynamics is the study of the detailed molecular pathway starting from the drug (ligand) binding to its receptor, the activation of effector molecules (e.g., G proteins) and the generation of second messengers, which ultimately produce an effect that can be measured at the cell, tissue, or whole animal level. This process is called the signal transduction pathway.

2. The correct answer is E: decrease the production of cAMP. Adenylyl cyclase is an enzyme that converts ATP to cyclic AMP (cAMP). GPCR that activate inhibitory Gα subunits are known to inhibit adenylyl cyclase and, therefore, reduce the generation of cAMP. cAMP is the second messenger in this system, even though in this case its levels are decreased. Activated Gα subunits also have direct effects on ion channels.

3. The correct answer is B: the relationship of the concentration of drug and the association or dissociation of drug-receptor complex. The law of mass action is used to derive the affinity of a drug for its receptor and is noted as the K_D. The K_D, which is the equilibrium dissociated constant, comes from the kinetic rate (k_2) of drug-receptor dissociation divided by the rate (k_1) of drug-receptor association.

4. The correct answer is D: the position of the curve along the log-dose axis. Potency and efficacy can be determined from a graph of the log dose-response curve be visual inspection. The height of the curve along the effect or y-axis is a measure of efficacy. The placement of the curve along the log dose axis or x-axis determines potency such that curves to the right represent more potent drugs than curves to the left. This is because curves to the right give rise to smaller doses of a drug needed to reach 50% effect or ED_{50}. The ED_{50} is a measure of the drug's potency but says nothing of efficacy. Whereas some agents are potent and efficacious, these two characteristics of drug action are not necessarily correlated. It is possible to have an agent that is highly potent but does not have great efficacy.

5. The correct answer is D: cannot produce the full effect even at high doses. An agonist acts at its receptor to activate the signal transduction pathway and produce an effect. An antagonist binds to its receptor, produces no effect at the receptor but rather blocks the receptor so that agonists cannot bind and produce an effect. A partial agonist binds to the receptor and activates the signal transduction pathway, but not to the maximal degree. Because the degree that a ligand activates its receptor is called its efficacy, it is clear that partial agonists do not have full efficacy.

SELECTED READINGS

Bissantz C. Conformational changes of G protein-coupled receptors during their activation by agonist binding. J Recept Signal Transduct Res 23:123–153, 2003.

Gainetdinov R.R., et al. Desensitization of G protein-coupled receptors and neuronal functions. Annu Rev Neurosci 27:107–144, 2004.

Fredriksson R., et al. The G-protein-coupled receptors in the human genome form five main families: phylogenetic analysis, paralogon groups, and fingerprints. Mol Pharmacol 63:1256–1272, 2003.

Kenakin T. Principles: receptor theory in pharmacology. Trends Pharmacol Sci 25:186–192, 2004.

CHAPTER 4

Drug Development and Safety

Drugs have the potential to produce harmful and beneficial effects when they are administered to humans or animals. As the Renaissance physician Paracelsus argued, "All substances are poisons: there is none which is not a poison. The right dose differentiates a poison from a remedy" (quoted in Klaassen 1996, p. 4). Indeed, investigators have not yet discovered a drug that does not have the potential to cause toxicity. This chapter begins with a description of drug development and the processes for evaluating drug safety and efficacy and then provides information on the various types of adverse effects and interactions that are caused by drugs.

DRUG DEVELOPMENT

Drug development in most countries has many features in common, beginning with the discovery and characterization of a new drug and proceeding through the clinical investigations that ultimately lead to regulatory approval for marketing the drug. Steps in the process of drug development in the USA are depicted in Fig. 4–1.

Discovery and Characterization

New drug compounds are either synthesized or isolated from a natural product in a chemical laboratory. Synthetic drugs may be patterned after other drugs with known pharmacologic activity, or their structure may be designed to bind a particular receptor and be based on computer modeling of the drug and receptor. Because the likely activity of some new compounds is relatively uncertain, they must be submitted to a battery of screening tests to determine their effects. There are cases in which a particular pharmacologic activity of a drug was discovered accidentally after the drug was administered to patients for other purposes. For example, the antihypertensive effect of clonidine was discovered when a physician administered a small dose to an office worker to treat nasal congestion (the anticipated clinical use of the drug) and found that the person experienced a profound hypotensive episode. This led to the drug's subsequent development and use in treating hypertension.

Experimental Studies

Before a new drug is administered to humans, its pharmacologic effects are thoroughly investigated in studies involving animals. The studies are designed to ascertain whether the new drug has any harmful or beneficial effects on vital organ function, including cardiovascular, renal, and respiratory function; to elucidate the drug's mechanisms and therapeutic effects on target organs; and to determine the drug's pharmacokinetic properties, thereby providing some indication of how the drug would be handled by the human body.

Federal regulations require that extensive toxicity studies in animals be conducted to predict the risks that will be associated with administering the drug to healthy human subjects and patients. The value of the experimental studies is based on the proven correlation between a drug's toxicity in animals and its toxicity in humans. As outlined in Table 4–1, the studies involve short-term and long-term administration of the drug and are designed to determine the risk of **acute, subacute, and chronic toxicity,** as well as the risk of **teratogenesis, mutagenesis,** and **carcinogenesis.** After animals are treated with the new drug, their behavior is assessed; their blood samples are analyzed for indications of tissue damage, metabolic abnormalities, and immunologic effects; their tissues are removed and examined for gross and microscopic pathologic changes; and their offspring are also studied for adverse effects.

Studies in animals do not usually reveal all of the adverse effects that will be found in human subjects, either because of the low incidence of particular effects or because of differences in susceptibility among species. This means that some toxic reactions will not be detected until the drug is administered to humans. Because the studies of long-term effects in animals may require years for completion, it is usually possible to begin human studies while animal studies are being completed if the acute and subacute toxicity studies have not revealed any abnormalities in animals.

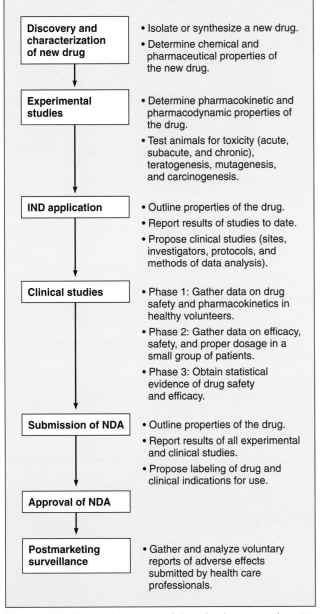

Discovery and characterization of new drug	• Isolate or synthesize a new drug. • Determine chemical and pharmaceutical properties of the new drug.
Experimental studies	• Determine pharmacokinetic and pharmacodynamic properties of the drug. • Test animals for toxicity (acute, subacute, and chronic), teratogenesis, mutagenesis, and carcinogenesis.
IND application	• Outline properties of the drug. • Report results of studies to date. • Propose clinical studies (sites, investigators, protocols, and methods of data analysis).
Clinical studies	• Phase 1: Gather data on drug safety and pharmacokinetics in healthy volunteers. • Phase 2: Gather data on efficacy, safety, and proper dosage in a small group of patients. • Phase 3: Obtain statistical evidence of drug safety and efficacy.
Submission of NDA	• Outline properties of the drug. • Report results of all experimental and clinical studies. • Propose labeling of drug and clinical indications for use.
Approval of NDA	
Postmarketing surveillance	• Gather and analyze voluntary reports of adverse effects submitted by health care professionals.

Figure 4–1. Steps in the process of drug development in the USA. IND = investigational new drug; NDA = new drug application.

THE INVESTIGATIONAL NEW DRUG (IND) APPLICATION

The **Food and Drug Administration** (FDA) must approve an application for an investigational new drug (IND) before the drug can be distributed for the purpose of conducting studies in human subjects. The IND application includes a complete description of the drug, the results of all experimental studies completed to date, and a description of the design and methods of the proposed clinical studies and the qualifications of the investigators.

Clinical Studies

Phase 1 studies seek to determine the pharmacokinetic properties and safety of an IND in healthy human subjects. In the past, most of the subjects were men. Today, women are being included in phase 1 studies to determine if gender has any influence on the properties of the IND. The subjects typically undergo physical examination, imaging studies, and chemical and pharmacokinetic analyses of samples of blood and other body fluids. The pharmacokinetic analyses provide a basis for estimating doses to be employed in the next phase of studies, and the other examinations seek to determine if the drug is safe for use in humans.

Phase 2 studies are the first studies to be performed in human subjects who have the particular disease for which the IND is to be used. These studies use a small number of patients to obtain a preliminary assessment of the drug's efficacy and safety in diseased individuals and to establish a dosage range for further clinical studies.

Phase 3 studies are conducted to compare the safety and efficacy of the IND with that of another substance or treatment approach. Phase 3 studies employ a larger group of subjects, often consisting of hundreds or even thousands of patients involving multiple clinical sites and investigators. Phase 3 studies are rigorously designed to prevent investigator bias and are often double-blind and placebo-controlled. A **double-blind study** is one in which neither the investigator nor the patient knows if the patient is receiving the IND or another substance. With some diseases, it is unethical to administer a placebo because of the proven benefits of standard drug therapy. In such cases, the IND is compared with the standard drug. Phase 3 trials often involve **crossover studies,** in which the patients receive one medication or placebo for a period of time and then are switched, after a washout period, to the other medication or placebo.

In many cases, the data are analyzed statistically at various points to determine whether the IND is sufficiently effective or toxic to justify terminating a clinical study. For example, if a statistically significant therapeutic effect can be demonstrated after 6 months in the group of patients who are receiving the IND, it is unethical to continue giving a placebo to the other group, the members of which could also benefit from receiving the IND. A clinical study is also stopped if an IND has been found to cause a significant increase in rate of mortality or serious toxicity.

The New Drug Application (NDA) and Its Approval

After phase 3 studies are completed and analyzed, the drug developer may submit a new drug application (NDA) to the FDA to request approval to market the drug. This application includes the results of all experimental and clinical studies, as well as the proposed labeling and clinical indications for the drug. The NDA typically constitutes an enormous amount of written material.

The FDA often requires a number of months to review the NDA before deciding whether to permit the drug to be marketed. Approved drugs are labeled for specific indications based on the data submitted to the FDA. Some drugs are found to have other clinical uses after the drug has been

TABLE 4–1.	**Drug Toxicity Studies in Animals**	
Type of Study	Method	Observations
Acute toxicity	Administer a single dose of the drug in two species via two routes.	Behavioral changes, LD_{50},* and mortality.
Subacute toxicity	Administer the drug for 90 days in two species via a route intended for humans.	Behavioral and physiologic changes, blood chemistry levels, and pathologic findings in tissue samples.
Chronic toxicity	Administer the drug for 6–24 months, depending on the type of drug.	Behavioral and physiologic changes, blood chemistry levels, and pathologic findings in tissue samples.
Teratogenesis	Administer the drug to pregnant rats and rabbits during organogenesis.	Anatomic defects and behavioral changes in offspring.
Mutagenesis	Perform the Ames test in bacteria. Examine cultured mammalian cells for chromosomal defects.	Evidence of chromosome breaks, gene mutations, chromatid exchange, trisomy, or other defects.
Carcinogenesis	Administer the drug to rats and mice for their entire lifetime.	Higher than normal rate of malignant neoplasms.

*The LD_{50} (the medial lethal dose) is the dose that kills half of the animals in a 14-day period after the dose is administered.

marketed. These indications are known as unlabeled or "off label" uses. For example, gabapentin (NEURONTIN) is approved for treating partial seizures but has had unlabeled use for preventing migraine headache and treating chronic pain. In some cases, manufacturers have promoted the use of a drug for an unlabeled use without adequate clinical evidence for the drug's efficacy. Gabapentin was highly promoted for treating bipolar disorder for a period of time but was later found to be ineffective for this indication.

Postmarketing Surveillance

If a drug is approved for marketing, its safety in the general patient population is monitored by a procedure known as postmarketing surveillance. The FDA seeks voluntary reporting of adverse drug reactions from health care professionals through its MedWatch program, and standard forms for this purpose are disseminated widely. Postmarketing surveillance is particularly important for detecting drug reactions that are uncommon and are therefore unlikely to be found during clinical trials.

FEDERAL DRUG LAWS AND REGULATIONS IN THE USA

There are two major types of legislation pertaining specifically to drugs. One type concerns **drug safety and efficacy** and regulates the processes by which drugs are evaluated, labeled, and marketed. The other type focuses on the **prevention of drug abuse.** In both cases, the laws and regulations reflect society's concern with minimizing the harm that may result from drug use while permitting the therapeutic use of safe and beneficial agents.

Drug Safety and Efficacy

Pure Food and Drug Act

The Pure Food and Drug Act of 1906 was the first federal legislation concerning drug product safety and efficacy in the USA. The act was passed in response to the sale of patent medicines that often contained toxic or habit-forming ingre-

dients. The legislation required accurate labeling of the ingredients in drug products and sought to prevent the adulteration of products through the substitution of inactive or toxic ingredients for the labeled ingredients. Because the courts refused to allow the use of this act to prevent fraudulent advertising, the legislation was only partially successful in eliminating unsafe drug products.

Food, Drug, and Cosmetic Act

The Food, Drug, and Cosmetic (FD&C) Act of 1938 came in response to a tragic incident in which over 100 people died after ingesting an elixir that contained sulfanilamide and ethylene glycol. The legislation, which is still in force today, made major strides by requiring evidence of drug safety before a drug product could be marketed, by establishing the FDA to enforce this requirement, and by giving legal authority to the drug product standards contained in the **United States Pharmacopeia** (USP).

First compiled in 1820, the USP has been updated and published at regular intervals by a private organization that is called the **United States Pharmacopeial Convention** and is composed of representatives of medical and pharmacy colleges and societies from each state. The USP contains information on the chemical analysis of drugs and indicates how much variance in drug content is allowable for each drug product. For example, the USP states that aspirin tablets must contain not less than 90% and not more than 110% of the labeled amount of $C_9H_8O_4$ (aspirin). In addition, the USP outlines standards for tablet disintegration and many other aspects of drug product composition and analysis.

PROVISIONS OF THE FOOD, DRUG, AND COSMETIC ACT. The FD&C Act prohibits the distribution of drug products that are adulterated, misbranded (mislabeled), or that do not have an approved New Drug Application. The act requires that drug product labels contain the name, dosage, and quantity of ingredients, and warnings against unsafe use in children or in persons with medical conditions where use of the drug might be dangerous. A drug product is said to be adulterated if it does not meet USP standards or if it is not manufactured according to defined "good manufacturing practices."

AMENDMENTS TO THE FOOD, DRUG, AND COSMETIC ACT. The FD&C Act has been amended many times. The **Durham-Humphrey Amendment** was passed in 1952 and created a legal distinction between nonprescription and prescription drugs. **Prescription drugs** are labeled "Rx Only." Agents that are classified as prescription drugs are those that are determined to be unsafe for use without the supervision of a designated health care professional. After a new drug has been marketed for a period of time, the FDA may reclassify the drug as a non-prescription drug if it has been found to be safe enough to be used without supervision. For example, topical cortisone products, antifungal drugs for treating candidiasis, proton pump inhibitors for treating acid reflux such as omeprazole (PRILOSEC), and antihistamines such as loratadine (CLARITIN) were originally classified as prescription drugs but are now classified as nonprescription drugs.

The **Kefauver-Harris Amendments** were passed in 1962, largely in response to reports of severe malformations in the offspring of women who took thalidomide during pregnancy. In fact, thalidomide had not been marketed in the USA, because a female scientist at the FDA, Frances Kelsey, had held up the drug's approval. Nevertheless, because the members of Congress believed that drug development should be regulated more strictly, they passed amendments that required the demonstration of both safety and efficacy in studies involving animals and humans before a drug product could be marketed. Although the processes of new drug development and testing have not changed substantially since this amendment was passed, the FDA review of new drugs has been streamlined in recent years.

The **Orphan Drug Amendments** were passed in 1983 to provide tax benefits and other incentives for drug manufacturers to test and produce drugs that are used in the treatment of rare diseases and are therefore unlikely to generate large profits. The act appears to have been successful, as several hundred orphan drugs are now available. Examples are drugs used for the treatment of urea cycle enzyme deficiencies, Gaucher's disease, homocystinuria, and other rare metabolic disorders.

The **Drug Price Competition and Patent Restoration Act** of 1984 extended the patent life of drug products (which at that time was 17 years) by the amount of time required for regulatory review of a new drug application. It also accelerated the approval of **generic drug products** by allowing investigators to submit an abbreviated new drug application (ANDA) in which the generic product is shown to be therapeutically equivalent to an approved brand name product. Therapeutic equivalence is demonstrated on the basis of a single-dose oral bioavailability study that compares the generic drug with the brand name drug. If the variance is within a specified range (usually ±20%), the generic drug may be approved for marketing. The cost of such a study is relatively small compared with the millions of dollars required for the development of a completely new drug.

In 1992, **accelerated drug approval** was authorized for **new drugs to treat life-threatening conditions** such as acquired immunodeficiency syndrome (AIDS) and cancer. Under the new regulations, patients with these conditions can be treated with an investigational drug before clinical trials have been completed.

Drug Abuse Prevention

Harrison Narcotics Act

The Harrison Narcotics Act of 1914 was the first major drug abuse legislation in the USA. It was prompted by the growing problem of heroin abuse, which followed the synthesis of this potent and rapid-acting derivative of morphine. The act sought to control narcotics through the use of tax stamps on legal drug products (a practice similar to the use of tax stamps on alcoholic beverages today). The Harrison Narcotics Act had a profound and controversial effect on the treatment of drug dependence in that it prohibited physicians from administering drugs to addicts as part of their treatment program.

Comprehensive Drug Abuse Prevention and Control Act

During the 1960s, the prevalence of drug abuse increased, especially among adolescents and young adults, who were using a wide range of drugs that included prescription sedatives and stimulants as well as illicit substances such as lysergic acid diethylamide (LSD), marijuana, and other hallucinogens. Believing that the drug abuse problem required a new approach, members of Congress passed the Comprehensive Drug Abuse Prevention and Control Act of 1970. This law is often called the **Controlled Substances Act (CSA).**

The CSA classified abused drugs into five schedules, based on their potential for abuse and their clinical usage. **Schedule I drugs** have a high abuse potential and no legitimate medical use, and their distribution and possession are prohibited. **Schedule II drugs** have a high abuse potential but a legitimate medical use, and their distribution is highly controlled through requirements for inventories and records and through restrictions on prescriptions. **Schedule III, IV, and V drugs** have lower abuse potential and fewer restrictions on distribution. The CSA requires that all distributors, practitioners, and medical institutions using controlled drugs register with the Drug Enforcement Agency, which is responsible for enforcing the act.

ADVERSE EFFECTS OF DRUGS

Adverse effects, or **side effects,** can be classified with respect to their mechanisms of action and predictability. Those due to excessive pharmacologic activity are the most predictable and are often the easiest to prevent or counteract. Organ toxicity caused by other mechanisms is often unpredictable, because its occurrence depends on the drug susceptibility of the individual patient, the drug dosage, and numerous other factors. Hypersensitivity reactions are responsible for a large number of adverse organ system effects. These reactions occur frequently with some drugs but only rarely with others.

Excessive Pharmacologic Effects

Drugs often produce adverse effects by the same mechanism that is responsible for their therapeutic effect on the target organ. For example, atropine may cause dry mouth and urinary retention by the same mechanism that reduces gastric acid secretion in the treatment of peptic ulcer- namely, by muscarinic receptor blockade. This type of adverse effect may be managed by reducing the drug dosage or by substituting a drug that is more selective for the target organ.

Hypersensitivity Reactions

Hypersensitivity reactions, or **drug allergies,** are responsible for a large number of organ toxicities that range in severity from a mild skin rash to major organ system failure. An allergic reaction occurs when the drug, acting as a hapten, combines with an endogenous protein to form an antigen that induces antibody synthesis. The antigen and antibody subsequently interact with body tissues to produce a wide variety of adverse effects.

In the **Gell and Coombs classification system,** allergic reactions are divided into four general types, each of which can be produced by drugs. **Type I reactions** are immediate hypersensitivity reactions that are mediated by immunoglobulin E (IgE) antibodies. Examples of these reactions are urticaria (hives), atopic dermatitis, and ana-phylactic shock. **Type II reactions** are cytolytic reactions that involve complement and are mediated by immunoglobulins G and M (IgG and IgM). Examples are hemolytic anemia, thrombocytopenia, and drug-induced lupus erythematosus. **Type III reactions** are mediated by immune complexes. The deposition of antigen-antibody complexes in vascular endothelium leads to inflammation, lymphadenopathy, and fever (serum sickness). An example is the severe skin rash seen in patients with a life-threatening form of drug-induced immune vasculitis that is known as Stevens-Johnson syndrome. **Type IV reactions** are delayed hypersensitivity reactions that are mediated by sensitized lymphocytes. An example is the ampicillin-induced skin rash that occurs in patients with viral mononucleosis.

Adverse Effects on Organs

In some cases, the adverse effects and therapeutic effects of a drug are caused by different mechanisms. For example, in patients taking aspirin, an adverse reaction such as tinnitus or hyperventilation that leads to respiratory alkalosis is caused by neurotoxic effects that do not appear to be mediated by the drug's primary mechanism of action, which is inhibition of prostaglandin synthesis. A variety of drugs (Table 4–2) produce toxicity of the liver, kidneys, or other vital organs, and this toxicity may not be readily apparent until significant organ damage has occurred. Patients receiving these drugs should be monitored with appropriate laboratory tests. For example, hepatotoxicity may be detected by monitoring serum transaminase levels, while hematopoietic toxicity may be detected by periodically performing blood cell counts.

Hematopoietic Toxicity

Bone marrow toxicity, one of the most frequent types of drug-induced toxicity, may present as **agranulocytosis, anemia, thrombocytopenia,** or a combination of these (**pancytopenia**). The effects are often reversible when the drug is withdrawn, but they may have serious consequences before toxicity can be detected. For example, patients who develop agranulocytosis may succumb to a fatal infection before the problem is recognized.

Many drugs, such as chloramphenicol, are believed to cause hematopoietic toxicity by triggering hypersensitivity reactions directed against the progenitor cells in the bone

TABLE 4–2. **Drug-Induced Organ Toxicities**

Organ Toxicity	Examples of Adverse Effects	Examples of Inducers
Cardiotoxicity	Cardiomyopathy	Daunorubicin, doxorubicin, and idarubicin
	Inflammatory fibrosis	Methysergide
Hematopoietic toxicity	Agranulocytosis*	Captopril, chlorpromazine, chlorpropamide, clozapine, and propylthiouracil
	Aplastic anemia*	Chloramphenicol and phenylbutazone
	Hemolytic anemia*	Captopril, levodopa, and methyldopa
	Thrombocytopenia*	Quinidine, rifampin, and sulfonamides
Hepatotoxicity	Cholestatic jaundice*	Erythromycin estolate and phenothiazines
	Hepatitis*	Amiodarone, captopril, isoniazid, phenytoin, and sulfonamides
Nephrotoxicity	Acute tubular necrosis	Aminoglycoside antibiotics, amphotericin B, and vancomycin
	Interstitial nephritis*	Nonsteroidal anti-inflammatory drugs (NSAIDs) and penicillins (especially methicillin)
Ototoxicity	Vestibular and cochlear disorders	Aminoglycoside antibiotics, furosemide, and vancomycin
Pulmonary toxicity	Inflammatory fibrosis	Methysergide
	Pulmonary fibrosis	Amiodarone, bleomycin, busulfan, and nitrofurantoin
Skin toxicity	All forms of skin rash*	Antibiotics, diuretics, phenytoin, sulfonamides, and sulfonylureas

*Immunologic mechanisms known or suspected.

marrow or their derivatives. Chloramphenicol also produces a reversible form of anemia by blocking the action of the enzyme ferrochelatase and thereby preventing the incorporation of iron into heme.

The most serious form of hematopoietic toxicity is **aplastic anemia,** which may be associated with several types of blood cell deficiencies and may lead to pancytopenia. Aplastic anemia is probably due to a hypersensitivity reaction and is often irreversible, although it has recently been treated by administration of hematopoietic growth factors (see Chapter 17).

Hepatotoxicity

A large number of drugs produce liver toxicity, either via an immunologic mechanism or via their direct effect on the hepatocytes. Liver toxicity can be classified as cholestatic or hepatocellular. **Cholestatic hepatotoxicity** is often caused by a hypersensitivity mechanism producing inflammation and stasis of the biliary system. **Hepatocellular toxicity** is sometimes caused by a toxic drug metabolite. For example, acetaminophen and isoniazid have toxic metabolites that may cause hepatitis. With many hepatotoxic drugs, elevated serum transaminase levels may provide an early indication of liver damage and levels should be monitored during the first 6 months of therapy and at longer intervals thereafter. Many authorities believe that if transaminase levels exceed two times the upper normal limit, a physician should consider alternative drug therapy or frequent monitoring of enzyme levels. If transaminase levels exceed 3 times the upper normal limit, the drug should usually be discontinued. Unfortunately, some patients have developed acute hepatic failure even when serum transaminase levels have been monitored appropriately. In recent years, several drugs such as troglitazone have been removed from the market due to excessive cases of fatal hepatic failure.

Nephrotoxicity

Renal toxicity is caused by various drugs, including several groups of antibiotics. The forms of renal toxicity can be classified according to site and mechanism and include **interstitial nephritis, renal tubular necrosis,** and **crystalluria** (the precipitation of insoluble drug in the renal tubules). Nephrotoxicity often reduces drug clearance, thereby elevating plasma drug concentrations and leading to greater toxicity. With some drugs that routinely cause renal toxicity, such as cisplatin, the kidneys can be protected by means of forced diuresis, in which the drug is administered with large quantities of intravenous fluid so as to lower the drug concentration in the renal tubules.

Bladder toxicity is less common than renal toxicity, but it may occur as an adverse effect of a few drugs. One example is cyclophosphamide, an antineoplastic drug whose metabolite causes **hemorrhagic cystitis.** This disorder can be prevented by administering mesna, a sulfhydryl-releasing agent that conjugates the toxic metabolite in the urine.

Other Organ Toxicities

Pulmonary toxicity occurs through a variety of mechanisms. Some drugs cause **respiratory depression** via their effects on the brain stem respiratory centers. Drugs such as bleomycin and amiodarone produce **pulmonary fibrosis,** so patients who are being treated with these agents should have periodic chest x-rays and blood gas measurements to detect early signs of fibrosis.

Relatively few drugs produce **cardiotoxicity.** Anthracycline anticancer drugs, such as doxorubicin (ADRIAMYCIN), produce adverse cardiac effects that resemble congestive heart failure. HMG-CoA reductase inhibitors such as lovastatin (MEVACOR) may cause **skeletal muscle damage** evidenced by muscle pain and sometimes leading to rhabdomyolysis.

Skin rashes of all varieties, including macular, papular, maculopapular, and urticarial rashes, may be produced by drug hypersensitivity reactions. A mild skin rash may disappear with continued drug administration. Nevertheless, because rashes may lead to more serious skin or organ toxicity, they should be monitored carefully.

Idiosyncratic Reactions

Idiosyncratic reactions are unexpected drug reactions caused by a genetically determined susceptibility. For example, patients who have glucose-6-phosphate dehydrogenase deficiency may develop hemolytic anemia when they are exposed to an oxidizing drug such as primaquine or to a sulfonamide.

DRUG INTERACTIONS

A drug interaction is defined as a change in the pharmacologic effect of a drug that results when it is given concurrently with another drug or with food. Drug interactions may be caused by changes in the pharmaceutical, pharmacodynamic, or pharmacokinetic properties of the affected drug (Table 4–3).

Pharmaceutical Interactions

Pharmaceutical interactions are due to a chemical reaction between drugs prior to their administration or absorption. Pharmaceutical interactions occur most frequently when drug solutions are combined before they are given intravenously. For example, if a penicillin solution and an aminoglycoside solution are mixed, they will form an insoluble precipitate, because penicillins are negatively charged and aminoglycosides are positively charged. Many other drugs are incompatible and should not be combined before they are administered.

Pharmacodynamic Interactions

Pharmacodynamic interactions occur when two drugs have additive, synergistic, or antagonistic effects on a tissue, organ system, microbe, or tumor cells. An **additive effect** is equal to the sum of the individual drug effects, whereas a **synergistic effect** is greater than the sum of the individual drug effects. Some pharmacodynamic interactions occur when two drugs act on the same receptor, and others occur when the drugs affect the same physiologic function through actions on different receptors. For example, epinephrine and histamine affect the same function but have **antagonistic**

TABLE 4-3. Types and Mechanisms of Drug Interactions

Type	Mechanism
Drug interactions with food	Altered drug absorption.
Pharmaceutical interactions (drug incompatibilities)	Chemical reaction between drugs prior to their administration or absorption.
Pharmacodynamic interactions	Additive, synergistic, or antagonistic effects on a microbe or tumor cells. Additive, synergistic, or antagonistic effects on a tissue or organ system.
Pharmacokinetic interactions	
Altered drug absorption	Altered gut motility or secretion. Binding or chelation of drugs. Competition for active transport.
Altered drug distribution	Displacement from plasma protein binding sites. Displacement from tissue binding sites.
Altered drug biotransformation	Altered hepatic blood flow. Enzyme induction. Enzyme inhibition.
Altered drug excretion	Altered biliary excretion or enterohepatic cycling. Altered urine pH. Drug-induced renal impairment. Inhibition of active tubular secretion.

effects. Epinephrine activates adrenergic receptors to cause bronchial smooth muscle relaxation, whereas histamine activates histamine receptors to produce bronchial muscle contraction.

Pharmacokinetic Interactions

In pharmacokinetic interactions, a drug alters the absorption, distribution, biotransformation, or excretion of another drug or drugs. Mechanisms and examples of pharmacokinetic interactions are provided in Tables 4–3 and 4–4.

Altered Drug Absorption

There are several mechanisms by which a drug may affect the absorption and bioavailability of another drug. One mechanism involves binding to another drug in the gut and preventing its absorption. Cholestyramine, for example, binds to digoxin and prevents its absorption. Another mechanism involves altering gastric or intestinal motility so as to affect the absorption of another drug. Drugs tend to be absorbed more rapidly from the intestines than from the stomach. Therefore, a drug that slows gastric emptying, such as atropine, often delays the absorption of another drug. A drug that increases intestinal motility, such as a laxative, may

reduce the time available for the absorption of another drug, thereby causing its incomplete absorption.

Altered Drug Distribution

Many drugs displace other drugs from plasma proteins and thereby increase the plasma concentration of the free (unbound) drug, but the magnitude and duration of this effect are usually small. As the free drug concentration increases, so does the drug's rate of elimination, and any change in the drug's effect on target tissues is usually short-lived.

The enterohepatic cycling of some drugs is dependent on intestinal bacteria that hydrolyze drug conjugates excreted by the bile and thereby enable the more lipid-soluble parent compound to be reabsorbed into the circulation (Fig. 4–2). Antibiotics administered concurrently with these drugs may kill the bacteria and reduce the enterohepatic cycling and plasma drug concentrations. When antibiotics are taken concurrently with oral contraceptives containing estrogen, for example, they may reduce the plasma concentration of estrogen and cause contraceptive failure.

Altered Drug Biotransformation

In some cases, biotransformation is affected by drugs that alter hepatic blood flood. In many cases, it is affected by drug interactions that either induce or inhibit drug-metabolizing enzymes (see Table 4–4).

Inducers of cytochrome P450 enzymes include barbiturates, carbamazepine, and rifampin, which bind to regulatory domains of cytochrome P450 genes and increase gene transcription. These agents induce the 1A2, 2C9, 2C19, and 3A4 isozymes, whereas the 2D6 and 2E1 enzymes are not readily induced by commonly used drugs. The rate of induction depends on the dose and frequency of adminstration. Enzyme induction is usually maximal after several days of continuing drug administration. Enzyme induction increases the clearance and reduces the half-life of drugs biotransformed by the enzyme. When the inducing drug is discontinued, the synthesis of P450 enzymes gradually returns to the pretreatment level.

A large number of drugs bind to and inhibit particular **cytochrome P450** isozymes. CYP3A4 is selectively inhibited by erythromycin, itraconazole, and doxycyline, whereas other drugs such as cimetidine, ketoconazole, and fluoxetine inhibit several isozymes. Significant interactions occur when these drugs reduce the clearance and increase the plasma concentration of other drugs. For example, itraconazole inhibits the biotransformation of HMG CoA reductase inhibitors, such as lovastatin and atorvastatin by CYP3A4. This inhibition increases plasma levels several fold, sometimes leading to severe muscle inflammation and lysis (rhabdomyolysis). Grapefruit juice has been found to contain bioflavonoid compounds that inhibit CYP3A4 and thereby elevate concentrations of drugs such as felodipine (PLENDIL) that are metabolized by this enzyme.

Altered Drug Excretion

Drugs can alter the renal or biliary excretion of other drugs by several mechanisms. A few drugs, such as carbonic anhydrase inhibitors, alter the renal pH. This in turn can change the ratio of another drug's ionized form to its nonionized

TABLE 4-4. **Management of Clinically Significant Pharmacokinetic Drug Interactions**

Examples of Inducers or Inhibitors	Examples of Affected Drugs	Management
Inducers of drug biotransformation		
Barbiturates, carbamazepine, and rifampin	Warfarin	Increase warfarin dosage as indicated by prothrombin time (international normalized ratio).
Carbamazepine	Theophylline	Monitor plasma theophylline concentration and adjust dosage as needed.
Rifampin	Phenytoin	Monitor plasma phenytoin concentration and adjust dosage as needed.
Inhibitors of drug absorption		
Aluminum, calcium, and iron	Tetracycline	Give tetracycline 1 hour before or 2 hours after giving the other agent.
Cholestyramine	Digoxin and warfarin	Give digoxin or warfarin 1 hour before or 2 hours after giving cholestyramine.
Inhibitors of drug biotransformation		
Cimetidine	Benzodiazepines, lidocaine, phenytoin, theophylline, and warfarin	Instead of giving cimetidine, substitute a histamine blocker that does not inhibit drug metabolism.
Disulfiram	Ethanol	Make sure the patient understands that disulfiram is used therapeutically to promote abstinence from alcohol (ethanol).
Erythromycin	Carbamazepine and theophylline	Lower the dose of the affected drug during erythromycin therapy.
Erythromycin, itraconazole, and ketoconazole	Lovastatin and atorvastatin	Avoid concurrent therapy and thereby avoid myopathy.
Monoamine oxidase inhibitors	Levodopa and sympathomimetic drugs	Avoid concurrent therapy, if possible; otherwise, give a subnormal dose of the affected drug.
Inhibitors of drug clearance		
Diltiazem, quinidine, and verapamil	Digoxin	Give a subnormal dose of digoxin and monitor the plasma drug concentration.
Probenecid	Cephalosporins and penicillin	Advise the patient that the combination of drugs is intended to increase the plasma concentration of the antibiotic.
Thiazide diuretics	Lithium	Give a subnormal dose of lithium and monitor the plasma drug concentration.

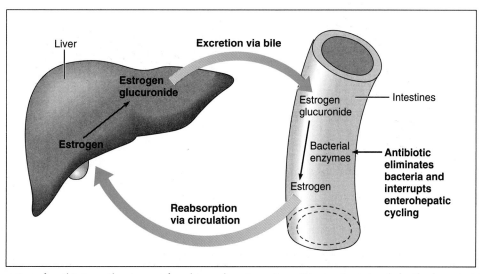

Figure 4-2. Interaction of antibiotics with estrogens found in oral contraceptives. Estrogen is conjugated with glucuronate and sulfate in the liver, and the conjugates are excreted via the bile into the intestines. Intestinal bacteria hydrolyze the conjugates, and estrogen is reabsorbed into the circulation. The enterohepatic cycling is interrupted if concurrently administered antibiotics destroy the intestinal bacteria. Contraceptive failure may result.

form and affect its renal excretion. Probenecid competes with other organic acids, such as penicillin, for the active transport system in renal tubules. Quinidine and verapamil decrease the biliary clearance of digoxin and thereby increase serum digoxin levels. Potentially nephrotoxic drugs, such as the aminoglycoside antibiotics, may impair the renal excretion of other drugs via their effect on renal function.

Clinical Significance of Drug Interactions

The clinical significance of drug interactions varies widely. In some cases, toxicity is severe and can only be prevented by avoiding the concurrent administration of drugs. In other cases, toxicity can be avoided by proper dosage adjustment and other measures (see Table 4–4). For example, when quinidine and digoxin are administered concurrently, a subnormal dose of digoxin should be used to prevent adverse effects. Fortunately, most drug interactions are of minor significance, and the interacting drugs can usually be administered concurrently without affecting their efficacy or the patient's safety. Drug interactions are more likely to occur if the affected drug has a low therapeutic index or is being used to treat a critically ill patient.

FACTORS AFFECTING DRUG SAFETY AND EFFICACY

Age, disease, pregnancy, and lactation are important biologic variables that can alter the response to drugs in particular patients.

Age

Factors affecting drug disposition in different age populations are summarized in Table 4–5.

In neonates and especially in premature infants, the capacity to metabolize and excrete drugs is often greatly reduced because of low levels of drug biotransformation enzymes. Oxidative reactions and glucuronate conjugation occur at a lower rate in neonates than in adults, whereas sulfate conjugation is well developed in neonates. Con-

sequently, some drugs that are metabolized primarily by glucuronate conjugation in adults (drugs such as acetaminophen) are metabolized chiefly by sulfate conjugation in neonates. Nevertheless, the overall rate of biotransformation of most drugs is lower in neonates and infants than it is in adults.

In comparison with children and young adults, elderly adults tend to have a reduced capacity to metabolize drugs. Biotransformation via oxidative reactions usually declines more than biotransformation via drug conjugation. Therefore, it may be safer to use drugs that are conjugated when the choice is available. For example, benzodiazepines that are metabolized by conjugation (such as lorazepam and temazepam) are believed to be safer for treatment of the elderly than are benzodiazepines that undergo oxidative biotransformation (such as diazepam).

Renal function is lower in neonates and elderly adults than it is in young adults, and this affects the renal excretion of many drugs. For example, the half-lives of aminoglycoside antibiotics are greatly prolonged in neonates. Glomerular filtration declines 35% between the ages of 20 and 90 years, with a corresponding reduction in the renal elimination of many drugs.

Because the very young and the very old tend to have increased sensitivity to drugs, the dosage per kilogram of body weight should be reduced when most drugs are used in the treatment of these populations.

Disease

Hepatic and renal disease may reduce the capacity of the liver and kidneys to biotransform and excrete drugs, thereby reducing drug clearance and necessitating a dosage reduction to avoid toxicity. Heart failure and other conditions that reduce hepatic blood flow may also reduce drug biotransformation. Oxidative drug metabolism is usually impaired in patients with hepatic disease, whereas conjugation processes may be little affected.

Guidelines for dosage adjustment in patients with hepatic or renal disease have been developed and can be found in many clinical references. Dosage adjustments are made by reducing the dose, increasing the interval between doses, or both. Adjustments for individual patients are usually based

---

TABLE 4–5. **Factors Affecting Drug Disposition in Different Age Populations**

Process of Drug Disposition	POPULATION		
	Neonates and Infants	**Children**	**Elderly Adults**
Absorption	Altered absorption of some drugs.	No major changes, but first-pass inactivation may be increased.	No major changes.
Distribution	Incomplete blood-brain barrier; higher volumes of distribution for water-soluble drugs.	No major changes.	Higher volumes of distribution for fat-soluble drugs.
Biotransformation	Lower rate of oxidative reactions and glucuronate conjugation.	Biotransformation rate for some drugs higher than in adults.	Reduced oxidative metabolism; relatively unchanged conjugation metabolism.
Excretion	Reduced capacity to excrete drugs.	No major changes.	Reduced capacity to excrete drugs.

on laboratory measurements of renal or hepatic function and on plasma drug concentration.

Pregnancy and Lactation

Drugs taken by a woman during pregnancy or lactation can cause adverse effects in the fetus or infant.

The risk of drug-induced developmental abnormalities known as **teratogenic effects** is the greatest during the period of organogenesis from the 4th to the 10th week of gestation. After the 10th week, the major risk is to the development of the brain and spinal cord. An estimated 1 to 5% of fetal malformations are attributed to drugs. Although only a few drugs have been proven to cause teratogenic effects (Table 4–6), the safety of many other drugs has not yet been determined.

The FDA has divided drugs into five categories, based on their safety in pregnant women. Drugs in categories A and B are relatively safe. Drugs in category A have been shown in clinical studies to pose no risk to the fetus, while those in category B may have shown risk in animal studies but not in human studies. For drugs in category C, adverse effects on the fetus have been demonstrated in animals but there is insufficient data in pregnant women, so risk to the fetus cannot be ruled out. Drugs in category D show positive evidence of risk to the fetus, and drugs in category X are contraindicated during pregnancy.

Drugs of choice for pregnant women are listed in clinical references and are selected on the basis of their safety to the fetus as well as their therapeutic efficacy. For example, penicillin, cephalosporin, and macrolide antibiotics (all category B drugs) are preferred for treating many infections in pregnant women, whereas tetracycline antibiotics (category D) should be avoided. Acetaminophen (category B) is usually the analgesic of choice in pregnancy, but ibuprofen and related drugs are also in category B and may be used when required. For the treatment of nausea and vomiting of pregnancy, the combination of pyridoxine (category A) in combination with doxylamine (category B) is the only medication specifically labeled for this indication by the FDA. Other drugs considered relatively safe for use in pregnancy include insulin and metformin (GLUCOPHAGE) for treating diabetes mellitus (both category B drugs), famotidine (PEPCID) and omeprazole (PRILOSEC) for reducing gastric acidity (category B drugs), diphenhydramine (BENADRYL) for treating allergic reactions (category B), and tricyclic antidepressants such as desipramine (NORPPRAMIN) for treating mood depression (category B). Most antiepileptic drugs pose some risk to the fetus and the selection of drugs for treating epilepsy in pregnant women requires careful consideration and the risks and benefits of such medication.

Some drugs can be taken by lactating women without posing a risk to their breast-fed infants. Other drugs place the infant at risk for toxicity. As a general rule, breast-feeding should be avoided if a drug taken by the mother would cause the infant's plasma drug concentration to be greater than 50 percent of the mother's plasma concentration. Clinical references provide guidelines on the use of specific drugs by lactating women.

TABLE 4–6. Examples of Teratogenic Drugs and Their Effects on the Fetus or Newborn Infant*

Drug	Adverse Effects
Alkylating agents and antimetabolites (anticancer drugs)	Cardiac defects; cleft palate; growth retardation; malformation of ears, eyes, fingers, nose, or skull; and other anomalies.
Carbamazepine	Abnormal facial features; neural tube defects, such as spina bifida; reduced head size; and other anomalies.
Coumarin anticoagulants	Fetal warfarin syndrome (characterized by chondrodysplasia punctata, malformation of ears and eyes, mental retardation, nasal hypoplasia, optic atrophy, skeletal deformities, and other anomalies).
Diethylstilbestrol (DES)	Effects in female offspring: clear cell vaginal or cervical adenocarcinoma; irregular menses; and reproductive abnormalities, including decreased rate of pregnancy and increased rate of preterm deliveries. Effects in male offspring: cryptorchidism, epididymal cysts, and hypogonadism.
Ethanol	Fetal alcohol syndrome (characterized by growth retardation, hyperactivity, mental retardation, microcephaly and facial abnormalities, poor coordination, and other anomalies).
Phenytoin	Fetal hydantoin syndrome (characterized by cardiac defects; malformation of ears, lips, palate, mouth, and nasal bridge; mental retardation; microcephaly; ptosis; strabismus; and other anomalies).
Retinoids (systemic)	Spontaneous abortions. Hydrocephaly; malformation of ears, face, heart, limbs, and liver; microcephaly; and other anomalies.
Tetracycline	Hypoplasia of tooth enamel and staining of teeth.
Thalidomide	Deafness, heart defects, limb abnormalities (amelia or phocomelia), renal abnormalities, and other anomalies.
Valproate	Cardiac defects, central nervous system defects, lumbosacral spina bifida, and microcephaly.

*Other substances known to be teratogenic: lead, lithium, methyl mercury, penicillamine, polychlorinated biphenyls, and trimethadione. Other drugs that should be avoided during the second and third trimester of pregnancy: angiotensin-converting enzyme inhibitors, chloramphenicol, indomethacin, prostaglandins, sulfonamides, and sulfonylureas. Other drugs that should be used with great caution during pregnancy: antithyroid drugs, aspirin, barbiturates, benzodiazepines, corticosteroids, heparin, opioids, and phenothiazines.

SUMMARY OF IMPORTANT POINTS

■ The process of drug development includes chemical and pharmacologic characterization, experimental studies to test for toxicity in animals, and clinical studies to determine efficacy and safety in humans.

■ Drug development is regulated by the Food and Drug Administration (FDA). An investigational new drug (IND) application must be completed before clinical studies can be started, and a new drug application (NDA) must be submitted and approved before the drug can be marketed.

■ Phase 1 studies provide data about drug safety and pharmacokinetics in healthy subjects; phase 2 studies provide data about the proper dosage and potential efficacy in a small group of patients; and phase 3 studies provide statistical evidence of efficacy and safety in a controlled clinical trial.

■ The Food, Drug, and Cosmetic Act established the FDA to regulate the development, manufacturing, distribution, and usage of drugs. Amendments have established the prescription class of drugs, stricter requirements for human drug testing, incentives for developing orphan drugs for rare diseases, and abbreviated procedures for marketing generic drug products.

■ The Comprehensive Drug Abuse Prevention and Control Act, also called the Controlled Substances Act (CSA), classifies potentially abused drugs in five categories (Schedules I through V), requires registration of legitimate drug distributors and health care professionals, and limits the prescription and distribution of controlled substances.

■ The adverse effects of drugs may be due to excessive pharmacologic effects, hypersensitivity reactions, or other mechanisms responsible for organ toxicities. The bone marrow, liver, kidney, and skin are frequent sites of drug toxicity.

■ Drug interactions occur when one drug alters the pharmacologic properties of another drug. Most interactions are due to pharmacokinetic effects, particularly inhibition or induction of drug biotransformation.

■ Age, disease, pregnancy, and lactation are factors that must be considered in drug selection and dosage. The very young and the very old tend to have an increased sensitivity to therapeutic agents, usually because of a reduced capacity to eliminate drugs. Target organs may also be more sensitive to drugs in these populations.

Review Questions

1. The 4th to the 10th week of gestation is the period of time when there is the greatest concern about drug-induced
   (A) fetal cardiac arrest
   (B) fetal hemorrhage
   (C) fetal malformations
   (D) labor
   (E) fetal jaundice

2. Which of the following drug interaction mechanisms is most likely to lead to sustained elevations of plasma drug concentrations and drug toxicity?
   (A) induction of cytochrome P450 2C19
   (B) inhibiton of cytochrome P450 3A4
   (C) displacement of a drug from plasma albumin binding sites
   (D) inhibition of the P-glycoprotein carrier protein
   (E) acceleration of gastric emptying by a "prokinetic" drug

3. Elderly persons may have altered drug disposition because of
   (A) markedly reduced absorption of many drugs
   (B) higher volumes of distribution for water-soluble drugs
   (C) accelerated renal excretion of ionized drugs
   (D) increased permeability of the blood-brain barrier
   (E) reduced capacity to oxidize drugs

Answers and Explanations

1. The answer is C: fetal malformations. The 4th to 10th week of gestation is the period when fetal organs are developed. Teratogenic drugs may cause fetal malformations if taken by a pregnant woman during this interval. These malformations include cleft palate, malformation of fingers and toes, heart defects, facial abnormalities, and skeletal deformities. Drug induced labor or jaundice is primarily of concern during the last trimester of pregnancy. Drug-induced cardiac arrest and hemorrhage are not specifically associated with the 4th to 10th week of gestation.

2. The answer is B: inhibition of cytochrome P450 3A4. Inhibition of drug metabolizing enzymes will increase the half-life and plasma concentrations of affected drugs, thereby posing a risk of toxicity. Induction of these enzymes will reduce half-life and plasma levels. Displacement of a drug from plasma proteins or inhibition of P-glycoprotein might increase plasma levels temporarily until the rate of elimination increases. Acceleration of gastric emptying might increase the rate of drug absorption but would not permanently increase plasma drug levels.

3. The answer is E: reduced capacity to oxidize drugs. Conjugative metabolism is relatively unchanged in the elderly but oxidative drug metabolism is usually reduced. The elderly tend to have a higher percentage of body fat than younger adults and therefore have increased volumes of distribution of fat soluble drugs. Drug absorption is not typically altered in the elderly and their blood-brain barrier is not noticeably impaired in most cases.

SELECTED READINGS

Bachmann, K.A., ed. Drug Interactions Handbook, 2nd ed. Hudson, OH. Lexi-Comp, 2004.

Beyth, R.J., and R.I. Shorr. Principles of drug therapy in older patients: rational drug prescribing. Clin Geriatr Med 18:577–592, 2002.

Klaassen, Curtis D. Casarett and Doull's Toxicology: The Basic Science of Poisons, 5th ed. New York, McGraw-Hill, 1996.

AUTONOMIC AND NEUROMUSCULAR PHARMACOLOGY

CHAPTER 5

Introduction to Autonomic and Neuromuscular Pharmacology

OVERVIEW OF NEUROPHARMACOLOGY

The nervous system consists of the central and peripheral nervous systems. The **central nervous system** includes the brain and spinal cord, whereas the **peripheral nervous system** includes the autonomic nervous system and the somatic nervous system.

Drugs alter nervous system function primarily by affecting **neurotransmitters** or their **receptors.** In some cases, drugs affect the synthesis, storage, release, inactivation, or neuronal reuptake of neurotransmitters. In other cases, they activate or block neurotransmitter receptors. Some drugs are relatively specific for a particular neurotransmitter or receptor, whereas other drugs affect several neurotransmitters. The spectrum of effects produced by a drug depends on the distribution of the affected neurotransmitters in the central and peripheral nervous systems. The actions of some drugs are localized to either the central or the peripheral nervous system, whereas the actions of other drugs (e.g., cocaine and amphetamine) affect both central and peripheral functions.

This chapter reviews the anatomy and physiology of the peripheral nervous system and provides an overview of the mechanisms by which drugs affect nervous system function. Drugs that act primarily on the central nervous system are discussed in the chapters of Section IV.

ANATOMY AND PHYSIOLOGY OF THE PERIPHERAL NERVOUS SYSTEM

The **autonomic nervous system** involuntarily regulates the activity of smooth muscles, exocrine glands, cardiac tissue, and certain metabolic activities, whereas the **somatic nervous system** activates skeletal muscle contraction,

thereby enabling voluntary body movements. Both the autonomic and somatic nervous systems are part of the peripheral nervous system, and both are controlled by the central nervous system. The autonomic nervous system is regulated by brain stem centers responsible for cardiovascular, respiratory, and other visceral functions. The somatic nervous system is activated by corticospinal tracts, which originate in the motor cortex, and by spinal reflexes.

Autonomic Nervous System

The autonomic nervous system consists of sympathetic and parasympathetic divisions. In the **sympathetic nervous system,** nerves arise from the thoracic and lumbar spinal cord and have a short preganglionic fiber and a long postganglionic fiber. Most of the ganglia are located in the paravertebral chain adjacent to the spinal cord, but a few prevertebral ganglia (the celiac, splanchnic, and mesenteric ganglia) are located more distally to the spinal cord. The **parasympathetic nervous system** includes portions of cranial nerves III, VII, IX, and X (the oculomotor, facial, glossopharyngeal, and vagus nerves, respectively) and some of the nerves originating from the sacral spinal cord. The parasympathetic nerves have long preganglionic fibers and short postganglionic fibers, with the ganglia often located in the innervated organs.

The origins, neurotransmitters, and receptors of the sympathetic and parasympathetic systems are shown in Fig. 5–1. The sympathetic nervous system tends to discharge as a unit, producing a diffuse activation of target organs. Preganglionic, sympathetic neurons synapse with a large number of postganglionic neurons, which contributes to widespread activation of the organs during sympathetic stimulation. In addition, the release of epinephrine and norepinephrine from the adrenal medulla into the circulation enables the activation of target tissues throughout the body, including some tissues not directly innervated by sympathetic nerves.

46

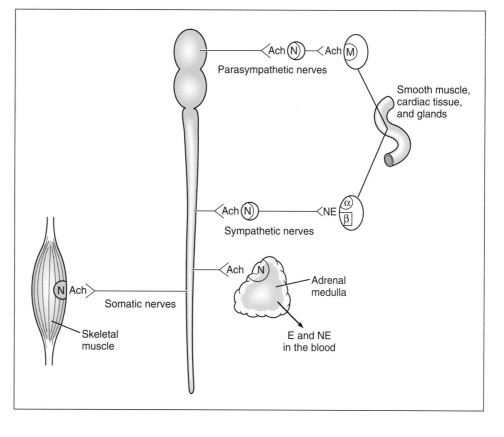

Figure 5–1. Neurotransmission in the autonomic and somatic nervous systems. The parasympathetic nervous system consists of cranial and sacral nerves with long preganglionic and short postganglionic fibers. The sympathetic nervous system consists of thoracic and lumbar nerves with short preganglionic and long postganglionic fibers. The sympathetic system includes the adrenal medulla, which releases catecholamines into the blood. The somatic nervous system consists of motor neurons to the skeletal muscle. ACh = acetylcholine; E = epinephrine; NE = norepinephrine; M = muscarinic receptors; N = nicotinic receptors; α = α-adrenergic receptors; and β = β-adrenergic receptors.

In contrast to the sympathetic system, the parasympathetic system can discretely activate specific target tissues. For example, it is possible for parasympathetic nerves to slow the heart rate without simultaneously stimulating gastrointestinal or bladder function. This is partly because a low ratio exists of postganglionic fibers to preganglionic fibers in the parasympathetic system.

As shown in Fig. 5–2, the sympathetic and parasympathetic nervous systems often have opposing effects on organ function. Activation of the sympathetic system produces the **"fight or flight" response,** which enables a person to respond to threatening situations. During this response, cardiovascular stimulation provides skeletal muscles with the oxygen and energy substrates required to support vigorous physical activity. Increases in glycogenolysis and lipolysis also help provide the required energy fuels. The parasympathetic system is sometimes called the **"rest and digest" system,** because it slows the heart rate and promotes more vegetative functions, such as digestion, defecation, and micturition. Many parasympathetic effects (including pupillary constriction, bronchoconstriction, and stimulation of gut and bladder motility) are caused by smooth muscle contraction.

Somatic Nervous System

The somatic nervous system consists of the motor neurons to the skeletal muscle. These neurons have a single nerve fiber that releases acetylcholine at the neuromuscular junction.

Enteric Nervous System

The enteric nervous system (ENS) is sometimes called the third division of the autonomic nervous system. The ENS consists of a network of autonomic nerves that are located in the gut wall and regulate gastrointestinal motility and secretion. The ENS, which includes the submucosal, myenteric, and subserosal plexuses, receives innervation from the sympathetic and parasympathetic nervous systems. The ENS has afferent fibers and efferent fibers, and it integrates input received from autonomic nerves with localized reflexes to synchronize the waves of peristalsis (the propulsive contractions of gut muscle). Parasympathetic stimulation activates the ENS, whereas sympathetic stimulation inhibits the ENS. The ENS can function independently of autonomic innervation following autonomic denervation.

NEUROTRANSMITTERS AND RECEPTORS

Neurotransmitters

The primary neurotransmitters found in the autonomic and somatic nervous systems are **acetylcholine** and **norepinephrine** (see Fig. 5–1). Acetylcholine is the transmitter at all autonomic ganglia, at parasympathetic neuroeffector junctions, and at somatic neuromuscular junctions. It is also the transmitter at a few sympathetic neuroeffector junctions, including the junctions of nerves in sweat glands and

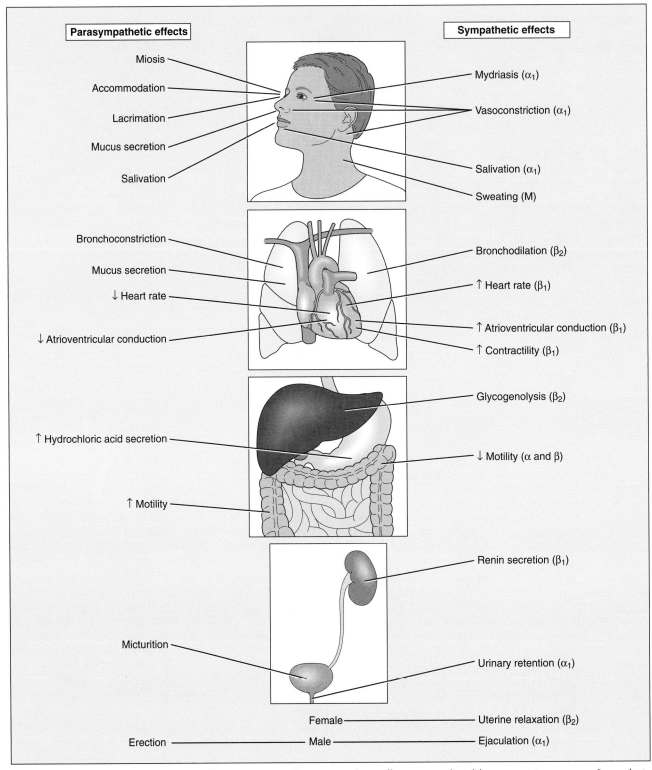

Parasympathetic effects

Miosis

Accommodation

Lacrimation

Mucus secretion

Salivation

Bronchoconstriction

Mucus secretion

↓ Heart rate

↓ Atrioventricular conduction

↑ Hydrochloric acid secretion

↑ Motility

Micturition

Erection

Sympathetic effects

Mydriasis (α_1)

Vasoconstriction (α_1)

Salivation (α_1)

Sweating (M)

Bronchodilation (β_2)

↑ Heart rate (β_1)

↑ Atrioventricular conduction (β_1)

↑ Contractility (β_1)

Glycogenolysis (β_2)

↓ Motility (α and β)

Renin secretion (β_1)

Urinary retention (α_1)

Female — Uterine relaxation (β_2)

Male — Ejaculation (α_1)

Figure 5–2. Autonomic nervous system effects on organs. All parasympathetic effects are mediated by muscarinic receptors. Sympathetic effects are mediated by α-adrenergic receptors (α), β-adrenergic receptors (β), or muscarinic receptors (M).

vasodilator fibers in skeletal muscle. The presence of acetylcholine in several types of autonomic and somatic synapses contributes to the lack of specificity of drugs acting on cholinergic neurotransmission.

Although norepinephrine is the primary neurotransmitter at most sympathetic postganglionic neuroeffector junctions, **epinephrine** is the principal catecholamine released from the adrenal medulla in response to activation of the sympathetic nervous system.

A number of other neurotransmitters have been identified in autonomic nerves called nonadrenergic-noncholinergic (NANC) neurons. These neurons are primarily found in the ENS of the gastrointestinal tract, as well as in the genitourinary tract and certain blood vessels. The transmitters released by NANC neurons include **neuropeptide Y, vasoactive intestinal polypeptide** (VIP), **enkephalin, substance P, serotonin** (5-hydroxytryptamine), **adenosine triphosphate** (ATP), and **nitric oxide** (NO). In some tissues, ATP released by so-called purinergic nerves is converted to **adenosine,** which can then activate adenosine receptors in a number of tissues (see Chapter 27). Nitric oxide is an important NANC neurotransmitter that produces vasodilatation in a many vascular beds and is also found in the ENS.

Receptors for Acetylcholine, Norepinephrine, and Epinephrine

The receptors for acetylcholine, called **cholinergic receptors**, have been divided into two types, based on their selective activation by one of two plant alkaloids. **Muscarinic (M) receptors**, which are cholinergic receptors activated by muscarine, are primarily located at parasympathetic neuroeffector junctions. **Nicotinic receptors**, which are cholinergic receptors activated by nicotine, are found in all autonomic ganglia and at somatic neuromuscular junctions. Muscarinic receptors are subdivided based on molecular and pharmacologic criteria. Activation of the M_3 muscarinic receptor produces smooth muscle contraction (except sphincters) and gland secretion. Activation of the M_2 muscarinic receptor mediates cardiac slowing. The M_1 receptor is primarily concerned with modulation of neurotransmission at central and peripheral sites. Activation of nicotinic receptors in autonomic ganglia excites neurotransmission, whereas acti-

vation of these receptors in skeletal muscle mediates muscle contraction.

The receptors for norepinephrine and epinephrine at sympathetic neuroeffector junctions are called **adrenergic receptors.** The term *adrenergic* is derived from adrenaline, another name for epinephrine. Two types of adrenergic receptors, called **α-adrenergic receptors** and **β-adrenergic receptors,** exist, which are distinguished on the basis of their selective activation and blockade by adrenergic agonists and antagonists. These receptors have been further divided into several subtypes. The α_1-adrenergic receptors mediate smooth muscle contraction, whereas β_2-adrenergic receptors mediate smooth muscle relaxation. Activation of β_1-adrenergic receptors produces cardiac stimulation. As discussed in Chapters 8 and 10, investigators have recently attributed some of the effects of α-adrenergic receptor agonists to activation of a new type of receptor called the **imidazoline receptor.**

NEUROTRANSMISSION AND SITES OF DRUG ACTION

Cholinergic and adrenergic neurotransmission have many basic similarities. In both cases, the neurotransmitter is synthesized in nerve terminals, stored in membrane-bound vesicles, and released into the synapse in response to nerve stimulation. After the neurotransmitter activates postjunctional receptors to initiate a physiologic effect, neurotransmitter action is terminated either by metabolism or neuronal reuptake. Various cholinergic and adrenergic drugs exert their effects at specific steps in the process.

Examples and sites of action for drugs that affect cholinergic and adrenergic neurotransmission are shown in Fig. 5–3, and the mechanisms of action are listed in Table 5–1.

Cholinergic Neurotransmission

Acetylcholine is synthesized from choline and acetate in the neuronal cytoplasm by choline acetyltransferase, and then it is stored in vesicles. When a cholinergic nerve is stimulated, the action potential induces calcium influx into the neuron,

TABLE 5-1. **Examples of Drugs Affecting Autonomic Neurotransmission**

Mechanism of Action	Drugs Affecting Cholinergic Neurotransmission	Drugs Affecting Adrenergic Neurotransmission
Inhibit synthesis of neurotransmitter	Hemicholinium*	Metyrosine
Prevent vesicular storage of neurotransmitter	Vesamicol*	Reserpine
Inhibit release of neurotransmitter	Botulinum toxin	Bretylium
Stimulate release of neurotransmitter	Black widow spider venom*	Amphetamine
Inhibit reuptake of neurotransmitter	—	Antidepressants and cocaine
Inhibit metabolism of neurotransmitter	Cholinesterase inhibitors	Monoamine oxidase inhibitors
Activate postsynaptic receptors	Acetylcholine, bethanechol, and pilocarpine	Albuterol, dobutamine, and epinephrine
Block postsynaptic receptors	Atropine and tubocurarine (block muscarinic and nicotinic receptors, respectively)	Phentolamine and propranolol (block α-adrenergic and β-adrenergic receptors, respectively)

*These agents have no current medical use.

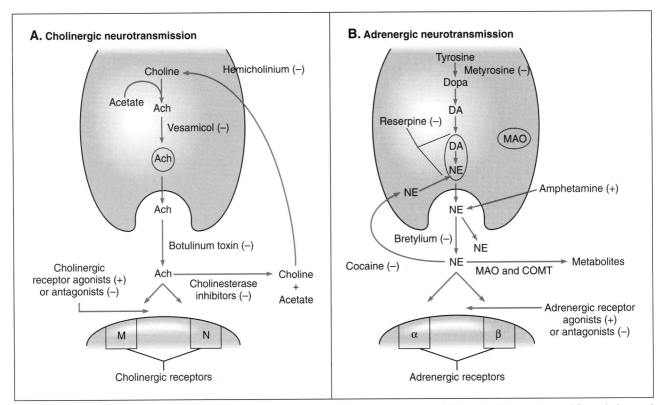

Figure 5–3. Cholinergic and adrenergic neurotransmission and sites of drug action. (A) Acetylcholine (ACh) is synthesized from choline and acetate, stored in neuronal vesicles, and released into the synapse by nerve stimulation. Hemicholinium blocks choline uptake by the neuron and inhibits ACh synthesis. Vesamicol blocks ACh storage, and botulinum toxin blocks ACh release. ACh breakdown is inhibited by cholinesterase inhibitors. Postjunctional cholinergic receptors are activated or blocked by cholinergic receptor agonists or antagonists, respectively. (B) Norepinephrine (NE) is synthesized from tyrosine in a three-step reaction: tyrosine to dopa (dihydroxyphenylalanine), dopa to dopamine (DA), and dopamine to NE. The conversion of tyrosine to dopa is inhibited by metyrosine. The vesicular storage of DA and NE is blocked by reserpine, and the release of NE in response to nerve stimulation is blocked by bretylium. After activating postsynaptic receptors, NE is sequestered by neuronal reuptake, a process blocked by cocaine. Amphetamine indirectly increases the release of NE into the synapse. Postsynaptic adrenergic receptors are activated or blocked by adrenergic receptor agonists or antagonists, respectively. M = muscarinic receptors; N = nicotinic receptors; α = α-adrenergic receptors; β = β-adrenergic receptors; MAO = monoamine oxidase; COMT = catechol-*O*-methyltransferase; (-) = inhibits; and (+) = stimulates.

and calcium mediates release of the neurotransmitter by a process called exocytosis. During exocytosis, the vesicle membrane and plasma membrane fuse, and the neurotransmitter is released into the synapse through an opening in the fused membranes. After acetylcholine activates postsynaptic cholinergic receptors, it is rapidly hydrolyzed by the enzyme cholinesterase to form choline and acetate. Choline is recycled through the process of reuptake by the presynaptic neuron. This process is mediated by a membrane protein that transports choline into the neuron. Acetylcholine can also activate presynaptic autoreceptors, which inhibits further release of the neurotransmitter by the neuron.

Drugs Affecting Cholinergic Neurotransmission

Fig. 5–3A shows the sites of various agents that affect cholinergic neurotransmission.

Hemicholinium blocks choline transport into the neuron and thereby inhibits the synthesis of acetylcholine, whereas

vesamicol prevents the vesicular storage of acetylcholine. Neither of these drugs has any current medical use.

Several toxins affect the release of acetylcholine. One example, **black widow spider venom** containing α-**latrotoxin** has been found to markedly stimulate vesicular release of acetylcholine producing excessive activation of cholinergic receptors in abdominal muscles and other tissues. Another example, **botulinum toxin A,** which is produced by *Clostridium botulinum*, has been used to treat localized spasms of various muscles including those of the eyes, face, and hands. In this application, botulinum toxin is injected directly into the muscle, where it blocks the exocytotic release of acetylcholine and inhibits neuromuscular transmission. Injections of a preparation of this toxin known as BOTOX have been shown to reduce facial wrinkles and have been widely utilized for cosmetic purposes.

After acetylcholine is released, it can activate postsynaptic muscarinic or nicotinic receptors. Many drugs, including choline esters such as **bethanechol** and plant alkaloids such as **pilocarpine,** mimic the effect of acetylcholine at these same receptors. These drugs are called **direct-acting cholinergic receptor agonists** because they directly bind and activate cholinergic receptors.

Another group of drugs, the **cholinesterase inhibitors,** prevent the breakdown of acetylcholine and thereby increase the synaptic concentration of acetylcholine. Because this action leads to an increase in the activation of cholinergic receptors by acetylcholine, these drugs are called **indirect-acting cholinergic receptor agonists** (see Chapter 6).

The most important group of drugs that inhibit cholinergic neurotransmission contains the **cholinergic receptor antagonists.** The group is divided into two subgroups. The first consists of **muscarinic receptor antagonists** and includes drugs such as atropine, whereas the second consists of **nicotinic receptor antagonists** and includes **ganglionic blocking agents** (e.g., trimethaphan) and **neuromuscular blocking drugs** (e.g., tubocurarine).

Adrenergic Neurotransmission

Norepinephrine is synthesized via the following steps: tyrosine → dopa → dopamine → norepinephrine. This pathway is illustrated in Fig. 18–3.

First, the amino acid tyrosine is converted to dopa (dihydroxyphenylalanine) by tyrosine hydroxylase, the rate-limiting enzyme in the pathway. Dopa is then converted to dopamine by L-aromatic amino acid decarboxylase (dopa decarboxylase). At this point, dopamine is accumulated by neuronal storage vesicles. Inside the vesicles, dopamine is converted to norepinephrine by dopamine-β-hydroxylase.

As with acetylcholine, norepinephrine is released into the synapse by calcium-mediated exocytosis in response to nerve stimulation. Once in the synapse, norepinephrine activates postjunctional α-adrenergic and β-adrenergic receptors. It also activates prejunctional autoreceptors that exert negative feedback and inhibit norepinephrine release.

Norepinephrine is removed from the synapse primarily by neuronal reuptake via a transport protein known as the catecholamine transporter that is localized in the presynaptic neuronal membrane. The reuptake of norepinephrine limits the duration of presynaptic and postsynaptic receptor activation and enables the neurotransmitter to be used again for neurotransmission. Once inside the neuron, norepinephrine is sequestered in storage vesicles and is recycled by adrenergic neurons in a manner similar to that used by cholinergic neurons to recycle choline. The catecholamine transporter can also sequester epinephrine and other catecholamines.

The enzymes catechol-O-methyltransferase (COMT) and monoamine oxidase (MAO) primarily serve to inactivate norepinephrine that is not sequestered by presynaptic neurons. These enzymes are found in many tissues, including the liver and gut. MAO is also located inside neuronal mitochondria and degrades cytoplasmic norepinephrine that is not accumulated by storage vesicles.

Drugs Affecting Adrenergic Neurotransmission

Fig. 5–3B shows the sites of various agents that affect adrenergic neurotransmission.

The synthesis of norepinephrine is inhibited by **metyrosine,** a drug that is a competitive inhibitor of tyrosine hydroxylase. The storage of norepinephrine in neuronal vesicles is blocked by **reserpine,** a drug that inhibits the transporter for amines located in the vesicular membrane. Bretylium blocks the release of norepinephrine in response to nerve stimulation. Drugs that block the synthesis, storage, or release of norepinephrine are called **neuronal blocking agents.**

Some endogenous substances and synthetic compounds directly activate α-adrenergic or β-adrenergic receptors and, therefore, are called **direct-acting adrenergic receptor agonists.** Examples include **albuterol, dobutamine,** and **epinephrine.** Other drugs indirectly increase the activation of adrenergic receptors by increasing the synaptic concentration of norepinephrine. These drugs are called **indirect-acting adrenergic receptor agonists,** and examples include **amphetamine** and **cocaine.** The indirect-acting agonists require the presence of a functional postganglionic neuron to exert their effects. Cocaine binds to and competitively inhibits the catecholamine transporter located in the presynaptic nerve terminal, thereby increasing the duration of action of norepinephrine at the synapse. Amphetamine and related drugs are substrates for the transporter, which transports the drugs into the presynaptic neuron where they inhibit the storage of norepinephrine by synaptic vesicles, leading to reverse transport of norepinephrine into the synapse by the catecholamine transporter. These actions serve to increase the synaptic concentration of norepinephrine and its activation of adrenergic receptors.

Another group of drugs act by inhibiting the breakdown of norepinephrine by COMT or MAO. As discussed in Chapters 21 and 22, these **catechol-O-methyltransferase inhibitors** and **monoamine oxidase inhibitors** primarily exert their effects on the central nervous system.

Drugs that inhibit sympathetic stimulation of target organs include the neuronal blocking agents (described above) and the **adrenergic receptor antagonists.** Examples of the latter are **phentolamine,** which selectively blocks α-adrenergic receptors; **propranolol,** which selectively blocks β-adrenergic receptors; and **labetalol,** which blocks both receptor types.

Drugs Modulating the Baroreceptor Reflex

In addition to exerting their primary pharmacologic actions, a number of adrenergic receptor agonists and antagonists modulate the baroreceptor reflex (Fig. 5–4).

When a drug or a physiologic action increases blood pressure, this activates stretch receptors (mechanoreceptors) located in the aortic arch and in the carotid sinus at the bifurcation of the carotid artery. Receptor activation initiates impulses that travel via afferent nerves to the brain stem vasomotor center. Stimulation of the vagal motor nucleus (via nerves from the solitary tract nucleus) leads to an increase in vagal (parasympathetic) outflow, a decrease in heart rate, and a decrease in the sympathetic nerve outflow from the vasomotor center. The effect on the heart rate is called **reflex bradycardia.**

If a drug lowers the blood pressure sufficiently, it may reduce the baroreceptor tone and thereby produce an

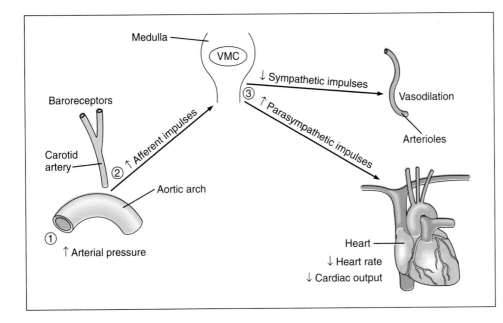

Figure 5–4. The baroreceptor reflex. (1) Increased arterial pressure activates stretch receptors in the aortic arch and carotid sinus. (2) Receptor activation initiates afferent impulses to the brain stem vasomotor center (VMC). (3) Via solitary tract fibers, the VMC activates the vagal motor nucleus, which increases vagal (parasympathetic) outflow and slows the heart. At the same time, the VMC reduces stimulation of spinal intermediolateral neurons that activate sympathetic preganglionic fibers, and this decreases sympathetic stimulation of the heart and blood vessels. By this mechanism, drugs that increase blood pressure produce reflex bradycardia. Drugs that reduce blood pressure attenuate this response and cause reflex tachycardia.

acceleration of the heart rate and activation of sympathetic vasoconstriction. In this case, the effect on the heart rate is called **reflex tachycardia.**

SUMMARY OF IMPORTANT POINTS

■ The sympathetic and parasympathetic divisions of the autonomic nervous system have opposing effects in many tissues. Drugs that activate one division often have the same effects as drugs that inhibit the other division.

■ Acetylcholine is the primary neurotransmitter at parasympathetic and somatic neuroeffector junctions, and norepinephrine is the transmitter at most sympathetic junctions. In the autonomic nervous system there are several nonadrenergic-noncholinergic neurotransmitters, including peptides, nitric oxide, and serotonin.

■ Most autonomic drugs activate or block receptors for acetylcholine or norepinephrine in smooth muscle, cardiac tissue, and glands. Activation of muscarinic and α-adrenergic receptors produces smooth muscle contraction, whereas activation of β-adrenergic receptors produces smooth muscle relaxation and mediates cardiac stimulation.

■ Some drugs have effects on neurotransmitter synthesis, storage, release, or metabolism. These are called indirect-acting drugs.

■ Indirect-acting agonists increase the concentration of a neurotransmitter at synapses, either by inhibiting transmitter inactivation (cholinesterase inhibitors), increasing transmitter release (amphetamine and tyramine), or blocking transmitter reuptake (cocaine).

■ Indirect-acting agonists require the presence of a functional postganglionic neuron to exert their effects.

Review Questions

For each numbered description of an autonomic nervous system activity or effect, select the lettered term most closely associated with it.

1. Termination of the action of synaptic norepinephrine

2. Slowing of heart rate and conduction

3. Bronchodilation

4. Synthesis of norepinephrine

5. Termination of the action of synaptic acetylcholine

   (A) acetylcholinesterase
   (B) monoamine oxidase
   (C) catecholamine transporter
   (D) tyrosine hydroxylase
   (E) muscarinic receptor activation
   (F) α-adrenergic receptor activation
   (G) β-adrenergic receptor activation

Answers and Explanations

1. The answer is C: catecholamine transporter. The synaptic actions of norepinephrine are primarily terminated by the process of neurotransmitter reuptake by the catecholamine transporter located in the presynaptic nerve terminal membrane.

2. The answer is E: muscarinic receptor activation. Activation of vagal (parasympathetic) nerve fibers innervating the heart leads to the release of acetylcholine and the activation of muscarinic M_2 receptors in the heart, thereby causing heart rate and conduction to slow.

3. The answer is G: β-adrenergic receptor activation. Activation of bronchial β_2 receptors by circulating epineph-

rine released from the adrenal medulla on sympathetic nervous system activation leads to bronchial smooth muscle relaxation and bronchodilation.

4. The answer is D: tyrosine hydroxylase. Tyrosine hydroxylase is the rate-limiting enzyme in the norepinephrine biosynthetic pathway. This enzyme, therefore, is highly regulated at both transcriptional and catalytic levels, and the enzyme contains a number of binding domains that enable enzyme activation or feedback inhibition.

5. The answer is A: acetylcholinesterase. In contrast to the sympathetic system, the action of the neurotransmitter in the parasympathetic nervous system is terminated by enzymatic inactivation rather than by neuronal reuptake.

Acetylcholinease is found throughout the peripheral and central nervous systems at synapses where acetylcholine mediates neurotransmission.

SELECTED READINGS

Brisinda, G., A. R. Bentivoglio, G. Maria, et al. Treatment with botulinum neurotoxin of gastrointestinal smooth muscles and sphincters spasms. Mov Disord 19 Suppl 8:S146–S156, 2004.

Kirstein, S. L., and P. A. Insel. Autonomic nervous system pharmacogenomics: a progress report. Pharmacol Rev 56: 31–52, 2004.

Nestler, E.J., S.E. Hyman, and R.C. Malenka. Molecular Neuropharmacology: A Foundation for Clinical Neuroscience. New York, McGraw-Hill, 2001.

CHAPTER 6

Cholinergic Receptor Agonists

CLASSIFICATION OF CHOLINERGIC RECEPTOR AGONISTS

Direct-acting Cholinergic Receptor Agonists
Choline Esters
- Acetylcholine
- Bethanechol (URECHOLINE)
- Carbachol

Plant Alkaloids
- Muscarine
- Nicotine
- Pilocarpine (SALAGEN)

Other Drugs
- Cevimeline (EVOXAC)

Indirect-acting Cholinergic Receptor Agonists
Drugs That Inhibit Cholinesterase
Reversible cholinesterase inhibitors
- Donepezil (ARICEPT)[a]
- Edrophonium (TENSILON)

- Neostigmine
- Physostigmine
- Pyridostigmine (MESTINON)

Irreversible cholinesterase inhibitors
- Echothiophate (PHOSPHOLINE)
- Isoflurophate (FLOROPRYL)
- Malathion (OVIDE)

Drugs That Augment Acetylcholine
- Sildenafil (VIAGRA)
- Tadalafil (CIALIS)
- Vardenafil (LEVITRA)

[a]also rivastigmine (EXELON) and galantamine (REMINYL)

OVERVIEW OF CHOLINERGIC PHARMACOLOGY

Cholinergic Receptors

Cholinergic receptors (cholinoceptors) are divided into two types, **muscarinic receptors** and **nicotinic receptors,** based on their selective activation by the alkaloids muscarine and nicotine.

Muscarinic Receptors

Muscarinic receptors are found in smooth muscle, cardiac tissue, and glands at parasympathetic neuroeffector junctions. They are also found in the central nervous system, on presynaptic sympathetic and parasympathetic nerves, and at autonomic ganglia. Activation of muscarinic receptors on presynaptic autonomic nerves inhibits further neurotransmitter release. The presence of muscarinic receptors on sympathetic nerve terminals provides for interaction between the parasympathetic and sympathetic nervous systems: the release of acetylcholine from parasympathetic nerves inhibits the release of norepinephrine from sympathetic nerves.

Muscarinic receptors are divided into five subtypes, M_1 through M_5, based on their selective activation or inhibition by experimental compounds and on their selective binding by radioactive compounds. The principal subtypes found in most tissues are M_1, M_2, and M_3 receptors (Table 6–1).

TABLE 6-1. **Properties of Cholinergic Receptors**

Type of Receptor	Principal Locations	Mechanism of Signal Transduction	Effects
Muscarinic			
M_1 ("neural")	Autonomic ganglia, presynaptic nerve terminals, and central nervous system	Increased inositol triphosphate (IP_3) and diacylglycerol (DAG)	Modulation of neurotransmission
M_2 ("cardiac")	Cardiac tissue (sinoatrial and atrioventricular nodes)	Increased potassium efflux or decreased cyclic adenosine monophosphate (cAMP)	Slowing of heart rate and conduction
M_3 ("glandular")	Smooth muscle and glands	Increased IP_3 and DAG	Contraction of smooth muscles and stimulation of glandular secretions
	Vascular smooth muscle	Increased cyclic guanosine monophosphate (cGMP) due to nitric oxide stimulation	Vasodilation
Nicotinic			
N_M (in muscles)	Somatic neuromuscular junctions	Increased sodium influx	Contraction of muscles
N_N (in neurons)	Autonomic ganglia	Increased sodium influx	Excitation of postganglionic neurons

The cholinergic receptor agonists that are currently available for clinical use do not selectively activate subtypes of muscarinic receptors, but an M_1 selective antagonist, pirenzepine, has been developed (see Chapter 7).

Nicotinic Receptors

Nicotinic receptors are found at all autonomic ganglia, at somatic neuromuscular junctions, and in the central nervous system. At autonomic ganglia, activation of nicotinic receptors produces neuronal excitation leading to the release of neurotransmitters at postganglionic neuroeffector junctions. At junctions of skeletal muscle and nerves, activation of nicotinic receptors depolarizes the motor end plate and leads both to the release of calcium from the sarcoplasmic reticulum and to the contraction of muscles.

Signal Transduction

Muscarinic receptor stimulation leads to the activation of guanine nucleotide-binding proteins (G proteins), which increases or decreases the formation of other second messengers (see Chapter 3). The M_1, M_3, and M_5 receptors are coupled with G_q proteins and their activation stimulates the formation of inositol triphosphate (IP_3) and diacylglycerol (DAG). The M_2 and M_4 receptors are coupled with G_i proteins and their activation increases potassium influx or decreases cyclic adenosine monophosphate (cyclic AMP, or cAMP).

Nicotinic receptors are ligand-gated sodium channels whose activation leads to sodium influx, membrane depolarization, and excitation of autonomic postganglionic neurons and skeletal muscle.

Classification of Cholinergic Receptor Agonists

The cholinergic receptor agonists can be classified as direct acting or indirect acting. The **direct-acting agonists** bind and activate cholinergic receptors, whereas the **indirect-acting agonists** increase the synaptic concentration of acetylcholine. Although most of the indirect-acting agents inhibit cholinesterase and the breakdown of acetylcholine, some of them increase the release of acetylcholine from nerve terminals.

DIRECT-ACTING CHOLINERGIC RECEPTOR AGONISTS

The direct-acting agonists include the **choline esters**, the **plant alkaloids**, and a newer synthetic drug called cevimeline. These drugs all bind and activate cholinergic receptors, but they differ with respect to their affinity for muscarinic and nicotinic receptors and their susceptibility to hydrolysis by cholinesterase (Table 6–2).

Choline Esters

The choline esters include acetylcholine and synthetic acetylcholine analogues, such as bethanechol and carbachol. Their structures are shown in Fig. 6–1A.

General Properties

The choline esters are positively charged quaternary ammonium compounds that are poorly absorbed from the gastrointestinal tract and are not distributed to the central nervous system. Acetylcholine and carbachol activate both muscarinic and nicotinic receptors, whereas bethanechol activates only muscarinic receptors. Because of their lack of specificity for muscarinic receptor subtypes, the muscarinic receptor agonists cause a wide range of effects on many organ systems.

OCULAR EFFECTS. Muscarinic receptor agonists increase lacrimal gland secretion and stimulate contraction of the iris sphincter muscle and the ciliary muscles. Contraction of the iris sphincter muscle produces pupillary constriction

TABLE 6–2. Properties and Clinical Uses of Direct-Acting Cholinergic Receptor Agonists

Drug	Receptor Specificity	Hydrolyzed by Cholinesterase	Route of Administration	Clinical Use
Choline esters				
Acetylcholine	Muscarinic and nicotinic	Yes	Intraocular Intracoronary	Miosis during ophthalmic surgery Coronary angiography
Bethanechol	Muscarinic	No	Oral or subcutaneous	Postoperative or postpartum urinary retention
Carbachol	Muscarinic and nicotinic	No	Topical ocular Intraocular	Glaucoma Miosis during ophthalmic surgery
Plant alkaloids				
Muscarine	Muscarinic	No	None	None
Nicotine	Nicotinic	No	Oral or transdermal	Smoking cessation programs
Pilocarpine	Greater affinity for muscarinic than for nicotinic	No	Topical ocular Oral	Glaucoma Xerostomia
Other drug				
Cevimeline	Muscarinic	No	Oral	Xerostomia

(miosis), whereas contraction of the ciliary muscles enables accommodation of the lens to focus on close objects (Fig. 6–2).

RESPIRATORY TRACT EFFECTS. Stimulation of muscarinic receptors increases bronchial muscle contraction and causes an increase in the secretion of mucus throughout the respiratory tract. Because muscarinic receptor agonists can cause bronchoconstriction, they should be avoided or used with extreme caution in patients with asthma and other forms of obstructive lung disease.

CARDIAC EFFECTS. Muscarinic receptor agonists decrease impulse formation in the sinoatrial node by reducing the rate of diastolic depolarization. As a result, they slow the heart rate. In addition, they slow conduction of the cardiac action potential through the atrioventricular node, and this leads to an increased PR interval on the electrocardiogram.

GASTROINTESTINAL AND URINARY TRACT EFFECTS. When muscarinic receptor agonists are taken, they stimulate salivary, gastric, and other secretions in the gastrointestinal tract. They also increase contraction of gastrointestinal smooth

Figure 6–1. Structures of selected direct-acting cholinergic receptor agonists. The choline esters include acetylcholine, bethanechol, and carbachol.

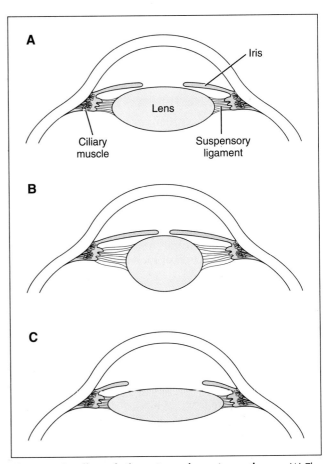

Figure 6–2. Effects of pilocarpine and atropine on the eye. (A) The relationship between the iris sphincter and ciliary muscle is shown in the normal eye. (B) When pilocarpine, a muscarinic receptor agonist, is administered, contraction of the iris sphincter produces pupillary constriction (miosis). Contraction of the ciliary muscle causes the muscle to be displaced centrally. This relaxes the suspensory ligaments connected to the lens, and the internal elasticity of the lens allows it to increase in thickness. As the lens thickens, its refractive power increases so that it focuses on close objects. (C) When atropine, a muscarinic receptor antagonist, is administered, the iris sphincter and ciliary muscles relax. This produces pupillary dilatation (mydriasis) and increases the tension on the suspensory ligaments so that the lens becomes thinner and focuses on distant objects.

muscle (except sphincters) by stimulating the enteric nervous system located in the gut wall. This, in turn, increases gastrointestinal motility. Whereas muscarinic receptor agonists stimulate the bladder detrusor muscle, they relax the internal sphincter of the bladder, and these effects promote emptying of the bladder (micturition). High or toxic doses of these agonists, therefore, can produce excessive salivation and cause diarrhea, intestinal cramps, and urinary incontinence.

Acetylcholine

CHEMISTRY AND PHARMACOKINETICS. Acetylcholine is the choline ester of acetic acid. It is rapidly hydrolyzed by cholinesterase and has an extremely short duration of action.

EFFECTS AND INDICATIONS. Because of its limited absorption, short duration of action, and lack of specificity for muscarinic or nicotinic receptors, acetylcholine has limited clinical applications.

An ophthalmic solution of acetylcholine available for intraocular use during **cataract surgery** produces miosis after extraction of the lens. The solution also can be used in other types of **ophthalmic surgery** that require rapid and complete miosis. Topical ocular administration of acetylcholine is not effective, because acetylcholine is hydrolyzed by corneal cholinesterase before it can penetrate to the iris and ciliary muscle.

In patients having **diagnostic coronary angiography,** acetylcholine can be administered by direct intracoronary injection to produce coronary vasodilatation or to provoke coronary artery spasm. The **vasodilative effect** of acetylcholine is mediated by muscarinic receptors located in vascular endothelial cells, where muscarinic stimulation causes the calcium-mediated activation of nitric oxide synthetase and the conversion of L-arginine to citrulline and nitric oxide. Nitric oxide is a gas that diffuses into vascular smooth muscle cells and activates guanylyl cyclase to increase the formation of cyclic guanosine monophosphate (cyclic GMP). Cyclic GMP then inactivates myosin light-chain kinase, leading to vascular smooth muscle relaxation and vasodilation.

The **vasospastic effect** of acetylcholine apparently is caused by stimulation of muscarinic receptors that are located on vascular smooth muscle and mediate smooth muscle contraction. In most situations, the vasodilative effect of acetylcholine is more pronounced than the vasoconstrictive effect. In patients with vasospastic angina pectoris, however, intracoronary injection of acetylcholine can provoke a localized vasoconstrictive response, and this helps establish the diagnosis of vasospastic angina.

Bethanechol and Carbachol

CHEMISTRY AND PHARMACOKINETICS. Bethanechol (URECHOLINE) and carbachol are choline esters of carbamic acid. They are resistant to hydrolysis by cholinesterase, and their duration of action is relatively short, lasting for several hours after topical ocular or systemic administration.

EFFECTS AND INDICATIONS. Bethanechol activates muscarinic but not nicotinic receptors and can be used to stimulate bladder or gastrointestinal muscle without significantly affecting heart rate or blood pressure. Although it generally has been replaced by more effective treatments, bethanechol has been given postoperatively or postpartum to increase bladder muscle tone in patients who suffer from nonobstructive, neurogenic urinary retention after receiving anesthetics or other drugs administered during childbirth or surgery. Therapeutic doses of bethanechol given orally or subcutaneously have little effect on blood pressure, but the drug should never be administered intravenously, because this can cause hypotension and bradycardia.

Carbachol is effective in the treatment of **chronic open-angle glaucoma,** but it is usually used in cases in which a patient does not respond adequately to pilocarpine (see below). Carbachol can also be used to produce miosis during **ophthalmic surgery.**

Plant Alkaloids

The plant alkaloids include muscarine, nicotine, and pilocarpine.

Muscarine and Nicotine

SOURCE AND EFFECTS. Muscarine is found in mushrooms of the genera Inocybe and Clitocybe, and the consumption of these poisonous mushrooms can cause diarrhea, sweating, salivation, and lacrimation. Muscarine is also found in trace amounts in Amanita muscaria, the original source of muscarine, but the toxicity of this mushroom is largely due to its content of ibotenic acid. Nicotine is derived from Nicotiana plants and is contained in cigarettes and other tobacco products. The effects of nicotine dependence are discussed in Chapter 24.

INDICATIONS. Muscarine has no current medical use. Nicotine is available in chewing gum, transdermal patches, and other products designed for use in smoking cessation programs.

Pilocarpine

CHEMISTRY AND PHARMACOKINETICS. Pilocarpine is a tertiary amine alkaloid that is obtained from Pilocarpus, a small shrub. The drug is well absorbed after topical ocular and oral administration.

EFFECTS AND INDICATIONS. Pilocarpine, which has greater affinity for muscarinic receptors than for nicotinic receptors, can produce all of the effects of muscarinic receptor stimulation described above.

Pilocarpine is a second-line drug for the treatment of **chronic open-angle glaucoma,** in which it lowers intraocular pressure by increasing the outflow of aqueous humor (Box 6–1). It is also used in the treatment of **acute angle-closure glaucoma,** a medical emergency in which blindness can result if the intraocular pressure is not lowered immediately. The main side effects of ocular pilocarpine administration are decreased night vision, which is caused by miosis, and difficulty in focusing on distant objects, which occurs because the lens is accommodated for close vision.

In patients with **xerostomia** (dry mouth), pilocarpine (SALAGEN) is administered orally to stimulate salivary gland secretion. Low doses can be used to produce this effect with minimal side effects in many patients because of the

In the normal eye, aqueous humor is secreted by the ciliary processes and flows through the pupillary aperture of the iris and into the anterior chamber. It then drains through the trabecular meshwork in Schlemm's canal. In patients with open-angle glaucoma, persistently elevated intraocular pressure is associated with narrowing of the anterior chamber angle, a decrease in the rate of aqueous outflow, and the gradual loss of peripheral vision. Various types of drugs can be used to reduce intraocular pressure before irreversible optic nerve damage occurs. The sites of action of these drugs are shown below.

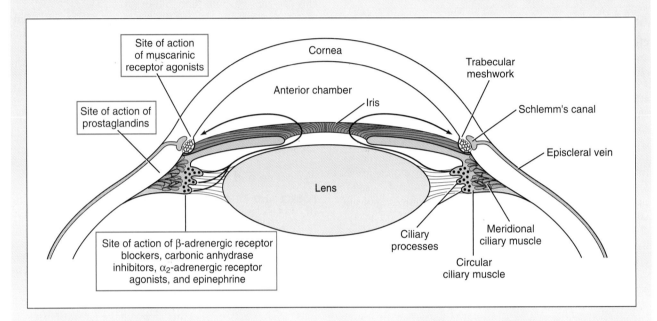

Some types of drugs act by enhancing the drainage of aqueous humor. **Muscarinic receptor agonists** (e.g., **pilocarpine**), stimulate the contraction of meridional ciliary muscle fibers that insert near the trabecular meshwork. Contraction of these fibers opens the trabecular spaces so that aqueous humor drains more easily. **Prostaglandins** (e.g., **latanoprost**) increase aqueous drainage through an alternative pathway known as the uveoscleral route. In this pathway, aqueous humor flows through the ciliary muscles into the suprachoroidal space.

Other types of drugs act by reducing the amount of aqueous humor produced by the ciliary processes. The **β-adrenergic receptor blockers** (e.g., **timolol**) and the **α₂-adrenergic receptor agonists** (e.g., **apraclonidine**) reduce the formation of cyclic adenosine monophosphate (cyclic AMP), a substance that stimulates aqueous humor production. **Carbonic anhydrase inhibitors** (e.g., **dorzolamide**) block the formation of bicarbonate by carbonic anhydrase, an enzyme that is required for aqueous humor secretion. **Epinephrine** probably acts by reducing blood flow in the ciliary processes.

high sensitivity of the salivary glands to muscarinic stimulation.

Other Drugs

Cevimeline (EVOXAC) is a new synthetic direct-acting muscarinic receptor agonist that is administered orally to treat dry mouth and is undergoing investigation for the treatment of dry eyes. The drug is used to treat these conditions in patients who have had radiation therapy for head and neck cancer and in those with Sjögren's syndrome (dry eyes, dry mouth, and arthritis). Adverse effects include increased sweating, nausea, and visual disturbances caused by drug-induced miosis. As with other cholinergic agonists, cevimeline should be used cautiously in persons with asthma or cardiac arrhythmias.

INDIRECT-ACTING CHOLINERGIC RECEPTOR AGONISTS

One group of indirect-acting agonists functions by inhibiting cholinesterase, whereas another group increases cyclic GMP levels and potentiates the vasodilative effects of acetylcholine.

DRUGS THAT INHIBIT CHOLINESTERASE

The cholinesterase inhibitors prevent the breakdown of acetylcholine at all cholinergic synapses. The shorter-acting types are referred to as **reversible cholinesterase inhibitors,** whereas the longer-acting types are called **irreversible**

TABLE 6-3.   **Properties and Clinical Uses of Reversible and Irreversible Cholinesterase Inhibitors**

Drug	Duration of Action	Route of Administration	Clinical Use
Reversible inhibitors			
Donepezil	24 hours	Oral	Alzheimer's disease
Edrophonium	10 minutes	Intravenous	Myasthenia gravis (diagnosis)
Neostigmine	2–4 hours	Oral, subcutaneous, or intramuscular	Myasthenia gravis, postoperative urinary retention, and postoperative abdominal distention
		Intravenous	Antidote for curariform drug toxicity
Physostigmine	1–5 hours	Topical ocular	Glaucoma
		Intramuscular or intravenous	Reversal of central nervous system effects of antimuscarinic drugs such as atropine
Pyridostigmine	3–6 hours	Oral, intramuscular, or intravenous	Myasthenia gravis
		Intravenous	Antidote for curariform drug toxicity
Irreversible inhibitors			
Echothiophate	1 week or more	Topical ocular	Glaucoma and accommodative esotropia
Isoflurophate	1 week or more	Topical ocular	Glaucoma and accommodative esotropia
Malathion	1 week or more	Topical	Pediculosis (lice)

cholinesterase inhibitors. The properties and clinical uses of inhibitors from each group are outlined in Table 6–3.

Reversible Cholinesterase Inhibitors

Edrophonium

CHEMISTRY AND PHARMACOKINETICS. Edrophonium (TENSILON) (Fig. 6–3A) is a positively charged quaternary alcohol that reversibly binds to a negatively charged (anionic) site on cholinesterase, but it is not a substrate for the enzyme. The reversible binding and rapid renal excretion of the drug are responsible for its short duration of action (about 10 minutes).

MECHANISMS AND EFFECTS. Edrophonium prevents the hydrolysis of acetylcholine while it is bound to cholinesterase, and it rapidly increases acetylcholine concentrations at cholinergic synapses such as the somatic neuromuscular junction.

INDICATIONS. Edrophonium is primarily used in the differential diagnosis of muscle weakness in patients suspected of having myasthenia gravis. In this autoimmune disease, antibodies are directed against nicotinic receptors in skeletal muscle. The antibodies can inactivate and destroy nicotinic receptors and thereby impair neuromuscular transmission. This causes severe fatigue and can affect any muscle, although it especially affects the muscles of the face, throat, and neck.

The muscle weakness of myasthenia gravis can result from either a deficiency or an excess of acetylcholine. In the untreated state, called a **myasthenic crisis,** muscle weakness is caused by an acetylcholine deficiency. Use of edrophonium in this situation can improve neuromuscular transmission, restore eyelid and facial tone, and improve hand grip strength. If patients with myasthenia gravis are treated with excessive doses of a cholinesterase inhibitor, however, muscle weakness can result from an acetylcholine excess that causes

prolonged depolarization of skeletal muscle. This is called a **cholinergic crisis** and should be managed by reducing the dose of cholinesterase inhibitor.

Neostigmine, Physostigmine, and Pyridostigmine

CHEMISTRY AND PHARMACOKINETICS. Neostigmine, physostigmine, and pyridostigmine (MESTINON) (see Fig. 6–3A) are esters of carbamic acid. Physostigmine, a plant alkaloid that contains a tertiary amine, is well absorbed from the gut and penetrates the blood–brain barrier. Neostigmine and pyridostigmine are synthetic quaternary amine compounds that are less well absorbed from the gut and do not cross the blood–brain barrier.

MECHANISMS AND EFFECTS. The manner in which neostigmine and related carbamates bind to cholinesterase is similar to that in which acetylcholine binds to cholinesterase (Fig. 6–4). The carbamates are slowly hydrolyzed by the enzyme and prevent the breakdown of acetylcholine for several hours.

INDICATIONS. When used in the long-term treatment of myasthenia gravis, neostigmine or pyridostigmine improves muscle tone and reduces eyelid and facial ptosis. Although either drug can also reduce diplopia (double vision) and blurred vision, diplopia is relatively resistant to treatment with tolerated doses of the cholinesterase inhibitors. If excessive doses are used, the muscle weakness can increase as a result of depolarizing neuromuscular blockade (see above). Corticosteroids and other immunosuppressant drugs reduce the formation of antibodies to the nicotinic receptor and are often used in combination with cholinesterase inhibitors to treat myasthenia gravis.

Neostigmine or pyridostigmine can be used to counteract **curariform drug toxicity,** and neostigmine is used in the treatment of **postoperative urinary retention and abdominal distention.**

Physostigmine has been used to treat **glaucoma.** In addition, it has been used to counteract seizures and other central

Figure 6–3. Structures of selected cholinesterase inhibitors. (A) The reversible cholinesterase inhibitors include edrophonium, neostigmine, and physostigmine. (B) The irreversible cholinesterase inhibitors are organophosphates and include echothiophate, isoflurophate, and malathion.

nervous system effects caused by an **atropine overdose** or an overdose of another antimuscarinic drug.

Donepezil and Related Drugs

Donepezil (ARICEPT), galantamine (REMINYL), and rivastigmine (EXELON) are centrally acting, reversible cholinesterase inhibitors that readily cross the blood–brain barrier and act to increase the concentration of acetylcholine at central cholinergic synapses. These drugs are used in the treatment of **Alzheimer's disease** and are discussed in Chapter 21.

Irreversible Cholinesterase Inhibitors

The irreversible cholinesterase inhibitors are all **organophosphates.** A few of them—including **echothiophate, isoflurophate,** and **malathion**—have been used as therapeutic agents. Most of them are used as pesticides, however, and some of them (such as soman) were developed as chemical warfare agents. Because of the widespread use of organophosphates as pesticides, they are responsible for a number of cases of accidental poisoning every year.

CHEMISTRY AND PHARMACOKINETICS. The irreversible cholinesterase inhibitors (see Fig. 6–3B) are esters of phosphoric acid. Most of these organophosphates are highly lipid-soluble and are effectively absorbed from all sites in the body, including the skin, mucous membranes, and gut. Organophosphate toxicity can occur after dermal or ocular exposure or following the oral ingestion of these compounds.

MECHANISMS AND EFFECTS. The organophosphates form a covalent bond with the catalytic site of cholinesterase. They are hydrolyzed slowly by the enzyme, and this accounts for

their long duration of action. The covalent bonding of organophosphates with cholinesterase is further stabilized through a process called "aging," in which one of the organic groups (the "leaving group") is hydrolyzed from the phosphate.

Organophosphate compounds augment cholinergic neurotransmission at both central and peripheral cholinergic synapses. Systemic exposure to these compounds can produce all of the effects of muscarinic receptor activation, including salivation, lacrimation, miosis, accommodative spasm, bronchoconstriction, bradycardia, intestinal cramps, and urinary incontinence. Excessive activation of nicotinic receptors by organophosphate compounds leads to a depolarizing neuromuscular blockade and muscle paralysis. Seizures, respiratory depression, and coma can result from cholinergic receptor activation in the central nervous system.

CLINICAL USE OF ORGANOPHOSPHATES. The clinical use of organophosphates is primarily in the treatment of ocular conditions. Echothiophate or isoflurophate has been used to treat chronic glaucoma that does not respond adequately to more conservative therapy. The long duration of action of these drugs can provide 24-hour control of intraocular pressure, a condition that can be difficult to achieve with shorter-acting agents. Echothiophate or isoflurophate has also been used to treat a form of strabismus (ocular deviation) called accommodative esotropia. In affected patients, the cholinesterase inhibitors reduce strabismus by increasing the accommodation to convergence ratio.

Although malathion is primarily used as a pesticide, it has also been used to treat head lice (**pediculosis capitis**). For this purpose it is administered as a 0.5% lotion (OVIDE) and kills ova as well as adult lice.

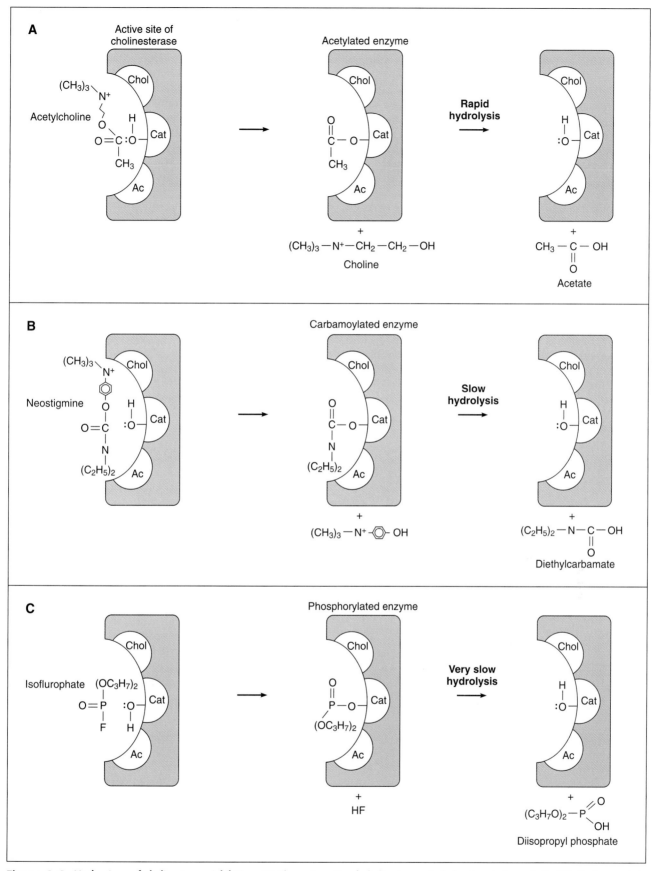

Figure 6–4. Mechanisms of cholinesterase inhibition. (A) The active site of cholinesterase includes the choline subsite (Chol), the catalytic subsite (Cat), and the acyl subsite (Ac). Acetylcholine binds to these subsites, and the acetate moiety forms a covalent bond with a serine hydroxyl group at the catalytic subsite as choline is released. The acetylated enzyme is then rapidly hydrolyzed to release acetate. (B) Carbamates (e.g., neostigmine) also bind to the active site and form a carbamoylated enzyme that is slowly hydrolyzed by cholinesterase. (C) Organophosphates (e.g., isoflurophate) form a strong covalent bond with the catalytic site of cholinesterase and are very slowly hydrolyzed by the enzyme. HF = hydrofluoric acid.

MANAGEMENT OF ORGANOPHOSPHATE POISONING. Poisoning often results from accidental exposure to organophosphate pesticides used in agricultural and gardening applications or from exposure to chemical warfare agents such as soman. Management involves the following: decontamination of the patient, support of cardiovascular and respiratory function, use of a cholinergic receptor antagonist (e.g., atropine) to block excessive acetylcholine, and use of pralidoxime to regenerate cholinesterase. Atropine can effectively counteract the muscarinic effects caused by organophosphates and other cholinesterase inhibitors. Because of the need to counteract the extremely high levels of acetylcholine at cholinergic synapses, however, the atropine doses required in the management of organophosphate poisoning are usually much higher than those used in the treatment of other medical conditions. Pralidoxime (2-PAM) is used solely to regenerate cholinesterase following organophosphate poisoning. Its high affinity for phosphorus enables it to break the phosphorus bond with cholinesterase and thereby regenerate the enzyme. It is important to administer pralidoxime as soon as possible after organophosphate exposure, because "aging" of the organophosphate reduces the ability of pralidoxime to regenerate cholinesterase.

DRUGS THAT AUGMENT EFFECTS OF ACETYLCHOLINE

Sildenafil (VIAGRA) was the first phosphodiesterase inhibitor to be developed to treat erectile dysfunction in men. Newer drugs in this class include tadalafil (CIALIS) and vardenafil (LEVITRA). These drugs potentiate the vasodilative effect of acetylcholine released from sacral parasympathetic neurons and thereby increase penile blood flow and facilitate penile erection during sexual stimulation. These drugs act by inhibiting the breakdown of cyclic GMP by **type 5 phosphodiesterase** (5-PDE). This action leads to elevated levels of cyclic GMP in the corpus cavernosum of the penis and to increased vasodilation. The effectiveness of these drugs in treating erectile dysfunction has been established in double-blind, placebo-controlled clinical trials.

PHARMACOKINETICS. Sildenafil is rapidly absorbed after oral administration and has an oral bioavailability of about 40%. The absorption of sildenafil is reduced if it is taken with a high fat meal, whereas the absorption of vardenafil and tadalafil are not affected by food. These drugs have an onset of action 30 to 60 minutes after drug administration. Sildenafil is metabolized by cytochrome P450 3A4 and its *N*-desmethyl metabolite has about half the activity of the parent compound. Whereas sildenafil and vardenafil have half-lives of about 4 hours and durations of action of 4 to 6 hours, tadalafil has a half-life of 17 hours and a duration of action of 36 hours. For this reason, men should not take more than one dose of tadalafil in a 24-hour period.

ADVERSE EFFECTS AND INTERACTIONS. The adverse effects of sildenafil and related drugs are usually mild and transient and include headache, nasal congestion, dyspepsia, myalgia, back pain, and visual disturbances.

The 5-PDE inhibitors should not be used by men who take nitroglycerin or another organic nitrate because the nitrates also increase cyclic GMP formation (see Chapter 11). Concurrent administration of 5-PDE inhibitors and nitroglycerin can cause profound hypotension, reflex tachycardia, and worsening of angina pectoris. A number of deaths occurred in men who took sildenafil and nitroglycerin. The 5-PDE inhibitors can also augment the hypotensive effects of other vasodilators including adrenergic alpha receptor antagonists (e.g., doxazosin) that are used to treat urinary retention in men with benign prostatic hyperplasia (see Chapter 9).

Sildenafil and related drugs are primarily metabolized by CYP3A4, and inhibitors of this cytochrome P450 isozyme can reduce the clearance and elevate the plasma levels of these drugs. The CYP3A4 inhibitors include cimetidine, erythromycin, ketoconazole, itraconazole, and compounds found in grapefruit juice. The initial dose of sildenafil or related drug should be reduced by 50% in men who are also taking a CYP3A4 inhibitor.

SUMMARY OF IMPORTANT POINTS

■ The direct-acting cholinergic receptor agonists include choline esters (e.g., bethanechol) and plant alkaloids (e.g., pilocarpine). Bethanechol is resistant to cholinesterase and is sufficiently selective for gut and bladder muscle to be used in treating urinary retention. Pilocarpine is primarily used to treat open-angle glaucoma.

■ The cholinesterase inhibitors indirectly activate cholinergic receptors by increasing the synaptic concentration of acetylcholine. These drugs have both parasympathomimetic and somatic nervous system effects.

■ The reversible cholinesterase inhibitors include edrophonium, which is used to diagnose myasthenia gravis, and neostigmine, which is used to treat this condition.

■ The irreversible cholinesterase inhibitors are organophosphate compounds that are widely used as pesticides and less commonly used in medical therapy. Echothiophate and isoflurophate can be used to treat ocular conditions, and malathion can be used to treat pediculosis.

■ Organophosphate toxicity is treated with atropine and a cholinesterase regenerator called pralidoxime.

■ Sildenafil and related drugs inhibit the degradation of cyclic guanosine monophosphate by type 5 phosphodiesterase and thereby potentiate the vasodilative action of acetylcholine in the penis and other tissues. These drugs are used to treat male erectile dysfunction.

Review Questions

1. Pilocarpine reduces intraocular pressure in persons with chronic open-angle glaucoma by
   (A) contracting the iris sphincter muscle
   (B) contracting the iris dilator muscle
   (C) reducing aqueous humor secretion
   (D) increasing aqueous humor outflow
   (E) relaxing the ciliary muscles

2. Sildenafil increases cyclic GMP levels in vascular smooth muscle by
   (A) inhibiting acetylcholinesterase
   (B) activating muscarinic M_3 receptors
   (C) stimulating guanylyl cyclase activity
   (D) inhibiting type 5 phosphodiesterase
   (E) increasing acetylcholine release

3. If a test dose of edrophonium causes increased muscle weakness in a woman being treated for myasthenia gravis with pyridostigmine, it indicates that
   (A) the dose of edrophonium was too large
   (B) the dose of edrophonium was too small
   (C) the patient does not have myasthenia gravis
   (D) the dose of pyridostigmine should be increased
   (E) the dose of pyridostigmine should be decreased

4. Pralidoxime improves muscle strength in persons exposed to toxic levels of an organophosphate compound by
   (A) an action that leads to increased degradation of acetylcholine
   (B) binding to and activating nicotinic receptors
   (C) increasing the elimination of organophosphate compounds
   (D) increasing acetylcholine levels at cholinergic synapses
   (E) selectively blocking muscarinic receptors

Answers and Explanations

1. The answer is D: increasing aqueous humor outflow. Cholinergic agonists such as pilocarpine and physostigmine increase aqueous humor outflow in persons with open-angle glaucoma by contracting ciliary muscles that insert near the trabecular meshwork, thereby opening the trabecular spaces to improve drainage of aqueous humor into Schlemm's canal. Cholinergic agonists also contract the iris sphincter muscle, which causes miosis and con-

tributes to problems with night vision in persons taking these drugs.

2. The answer is D: inhibiting type 5 phosphodiesterase. Sildenafil and related drugs inhibit the breakdown of cyclic GMP by type 5 phosphodiesterase, thereby increasing cyclic GMP levels in vascular smooth muscle and causing vasodilation. Acetylcholine released from sacral sympathetic nerves increases cyclic GMP formation in vascular smooth muscle.

3. The answer is E: the dose of pyridostigmine should be decreased. Edrophonium is used in the initial diagnosis of myasthenia gravis and it is also used to determine whether a patient is receiving too large or too small a dose of pyridostigmine during chronic treatment of the condition. If a test dose of edrophonium increases muscle weakness in a person being treated with pyridostigmine, it indicates that the person is receiving too large a dose of pyridostigmine.

4. The answer is A: an action that leads to increased degradation of acetylcholine. Muscle weakness in persons exposed to toxic doses of organophosphate cholinesterase inhibitors results from excessive levels of acetylcholine causing depolarizing neuromuscular blockade. Pralidoxime breaks the bond between an organophosphate compound and cholinesterase, thereby reactivating the enzyme and increasing acetylcholine degradation.

SELECTED READINGS

Burnett, A. L. The impact of sildenafil on molecular science and sexual health. Eur Urol 46:9–14, 2004.

Eyer, P. The role of oximes in the management of organophosphate pesticide poisoning. Toxicol Rev 22:165–190, 2003.

Nieuw Amerongen, A.V., and Veerman, E.C. Current therapies for xerostomia and salivary gland hypofunction associated with cancer therapies. Support Care Cancer 11:226–31, 2003.

Schecter, W. P. Cholinergic symptoms due to nerve agent attack: a strategy for management. Anesthesiol Clin North America 22:579–590, 2004.

CHAPTER 7

Cholinergic Receptor Antagonists

CLASSIFICATION OF CHOLINERGIC RECEPTOR ANTAGONISTS

Muscarinic Receptor Antagonists
Belladonna Alkaloids
- Atropine
- Hyoscyamine (LEVSIN)
- Scopolamine

Semisynthetic and Synthetic Muscarinic Receptor Antagonists
- Dicyclomine (BENTYL)
- Glycopyrrolate
- Ipratropium (ATROVENT)[a]
- Oxybutynin (DITROPAN)
- Solifenacin (VESICARE)
- Tolterodine (DETROL)
- Tropicamide (MYDRIACYL)

Nicotinic Receptor Antagonists
Ganglionic Blocking Agents
- Trimethaphan

Neuromuscular Blocking Agents
Nondepolarizing neuromuscular blocking agents
- Mivacurium[b]
- Pancuronium[c]
- Tubocurarine

Depolarizing neuromuscular blocking agents
- Succinylcholine

[a]also tiotropium (SPIRIVA)
[b]also atracurium, doxacurium
[c]also rocuronium, vecuronium

MUSCARINIC RECEPTOR ANTAGONISTS

The muscarinic receptor antagonists compete with acetylcholine for muscarinic receptors at parasympathetic neuroeffector junctions and thereby inhibit the effects of parasympathetic nerve stimulation. Because of these actions, the drugs are frequently called **muscarinic receptor blockers** or **parasympatholytic drugs.**

Some muscarinic receptor antagonists are **belladonna alkaloids** obtained from plants, whereas others are **semisynthetic or synthetic drugs.** The drugs in these two subgroups have similar effects on target organs, but they differ in their pharmacokinetic properties and clinical uses.

Belladonna Alkaloids

The belladonna alkaloids are extracted from a number of solanaceous plants found in temperate climates around the world, including *Atropa belladonna* (the deadly nightshade), *Datura stramonium* (jimson weed, or Jamestown weed), and *Hyoscyamus niger*. Belladonna, which is Italian for "fair lady," originally referred to the pupillary dilatation produced by extracts of these plants, which was considered cosmetically attractive during the Renaissance.

Atropine, scopolamine, and **hyoscyamine** are examples of belladonna alkaloids. Because they are esters of tropic acid, they are also known as the **tropane alkaloids.** The belladonna alkaloids can be highly toxic and are sometimes the cause of accidental or intentional poisonings. In fact, atropine was named after Atropos, one of the Fates in Greek

64

mythology, who was responsible for cutting the thread of life.

Atropine and Scopolamine

CHEMISTRY AND PHARMACOKINETICS. Fig. 7–1A shows the structure of atropine, which is an ester of tropic acid and a tertiary amine. Atropine and scopolamine are well absorbed from the gut and are distributed to the central nervous system. After systemic administration, they are excreted in the urine and have a fairly short half-life of about 2 hours. After topical ocular administration, they have longer-lasting effects because they bind to pigments in the iris, which slowly release the drugs over many days. People with darker irises bind more atropine and experience a more prolonged effect than do people with lighter irises. The ocular effects of

atropine gradually subside over time but are still perceptible after several days.

PHARMACOLOGIC EFFECTS. The muscarinic receptor antagonists inhibit the effects of parasympathetic nerve stimulation and thereby relax smooth muscle, increase heart rate and cardiac conduction, and inhibit exocrine gland secretion. As shown in Fig. 7–2, as the dose of atropine increases, the severity of effects increases.

(1) OCULAR EFFECTS. Atropine and other muscarinic receptor blockers relax the iris sphincter muscle, and this leads to pupillary dilatation (mydriasis). They also relax the ciliary muscle, thereby increasing the tension on the suspensory ligaments attached to the lens and causing the lens to flatten so that it is focused on distant objects. This inhibits the ability of the eye to focus on near objects, a condition that is called cycloplegia (paralysis of accommodation). Atropine also inhibits lacrimal gland secretion and can cause dry eyes.

(2) CARDIAC EFFECTS. Standard doses of atropine and related drugs increase the heart rate and atrioventricular conduction velocity by blocking the effects of the vagus nerve on the sinoatrial and atrioventricular nodes. When intravenous administration of atropine is begun, however, the low dose of the drug causes a paradoxical slowing of the heart rate. This effect probably results from stimulation of the vagal motor nucleus in the brain stem. After the full therapeutic dose has been administered, the increase in heart rate is observed.

(3) RESPIRATORY TRACT EFFECTS. In addition to producing bronchial smooth muscle relaxation and bronchodilation, atropine and other muscarinic receptor antagonists act as potent inhibitors of secretions in the upper and lower respiratory tract.

(4) GASTROINTESTINAL AND URINARY TRACT EFFECTS. Atropine reduces lower esophageal muscle tone and can cause gastroesophageal reflux. Atropine and other muscarinic receptor blockers relax gastrointestinal muscle, except sphincters, and reduce intestinal motility, thereby increasing gastric emptying time and intestinal transit time. They also inhibit gastric acid secretion. Sufficient doses of these drugs can cause constipation. Atropine relaxes the detrusor muscle of the urinary bladder and can cause urinary retention.

(5) CENTRAL NERVOUS SYSTEM EFFECTS. Atropine, scopolamine, and other tertiary amines are distributed to the central nervous system, where they can block muscarinic receptors and produce either sedation or excitement. Scopolamine, which is more sedating than is atropine, has been used as an adjunct to anesthesia. Standard doses of atropine typically cause mild stimulation, followed by a slower and longer-lasting sedative effect. With higher doses of atropine, patients can experience an acute confusional state known as delirium. Higher doses of atropine or related drugs can also cause hallucinations.

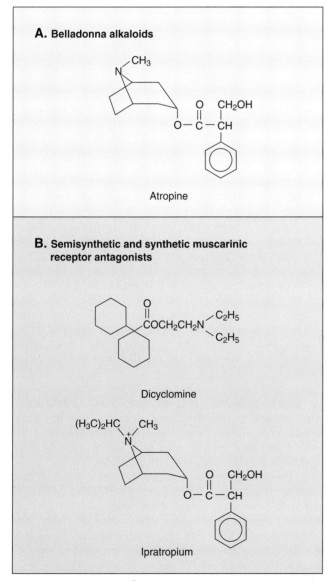

Figure 7–1. Structures of muscarinic receptor antagonists. (A) The belladonna alkaloids include atropine. (B) The semisynthetic and synthetic antagonists include dicyclomine and ipratropium. Ipratropium is the isopropyl derivative of atropine, whereas dicyclomine is a synthetic tertiary amine.

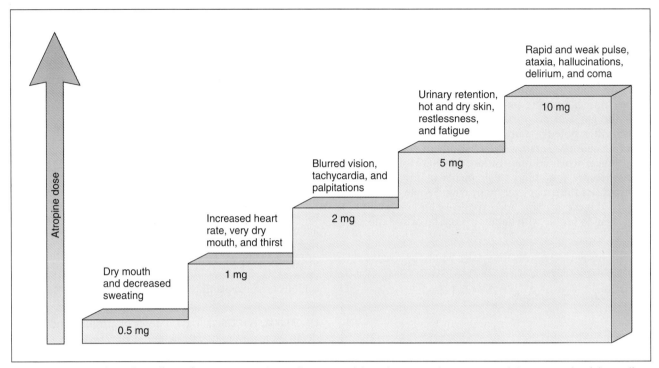

Figure 7–2. Dose-dependent effects of atropine. Low doses of atropine inhibit salivation and sweating, and the magnitude of these effects increases as the dosage increases. Higher doses produce tachycardia, urinary retention, and central nervous system effects.

(6) OTHER EFFECTS. The muscarinic receptor antagonists inhibit sweating, which can reduce heat loss and lead to hyperthermia, especially in children. The increased body temperature can cause cutaneous vasodilatation, and the skin can become hot, dry, and flushed.

INDICATIONS

(1) OCULAR INDICATIONS. To obtain a relatively localized effect on ocular tissues, atropine and other muscarinic receptor blockers are administered via topical instillation of a solution or ointment. These drugs are typically used to produce mydriasis and facilitate ophthalmoscopic examination of the peripheral retina. They can also be used to produce cycloplegia and permit the accurate determination of refractive errors, especially in younger patients with a strong accommodation. Because muscarinic receptor blockers can reduce muscle spasm and pain caused by inflammation, they are useful in the treatment of iritis and cyclitis (inflammation of the iris and ciliary muscles) associated with infection, trauma, or surgery.

(2) CARDIAC INDICATIONS. Atropine can be used to treat sinus bradycardia in cases in which the slow sinus rhythm reduces the cardiac output and blood pressure and produces symptoms of hypotension or ischemia. This type of symptomatic bradycardia sometimes occurs after a myocardial infarction. Atropine is usually administered intravenously for this purpose, but it can be injected endotracheally if a vein is not accessible. In patients with symptomatic atrioventricular block, atropine can be used to increase the atrioventricular conduction velocity.

(3) RESPIRATORY TRACT INDICATIONS. Because of its bronchodilating effects, atropine was once used to treat asthma and other obstructive lung diseases. It is no longer used for this purpose, however, because of its many adverse effects. For example, it impairs ciliary activity, thereby reducing the clearance of mucus from the lungs and causing accumulation of viscid material in the airways. As discussed below, ipratropium is now used instead of atropine to treat obstructive lung diseases. Atropine and other muscarinic receptor blockers have been used to reduce salivary and respiratory secretions and thereby prevent airway obstruction in patients who were receiving general anesthetics. Glycopyrrolate is often used for this purpose today (see below).

(4) GASTROINTESTINAL AND URINARY TRACT INDICATIONS. Atropine and related drugs are used to relieve **intestinal spasms and pain** associated with several gastrointestinal disorders, and they are also used to relieve **urinary bladder spasms in persons with overactive bladder.**

In the past, atropine was frequently used to reduce gastric acid secretion in patients with peptic ulcers. Large doses were required, however, and these doses often produced intolerable side effects, such as dry mouth, blurred vision, and urinary retention. For this reason, atropine and other nonselective muscarinic receptor blockers are seldom used to treat peptic ulcers today. As discussed later, a selective muscarinic M_1 receptor blocker, pirenzepine, is available in some countries to treat peptic ulcer disease.

(5) CENTRAL NERVOUS SYSTEM INDICATIONS. A transdermal formulation of scopolamine can be used to prevent motion sickness. The skin patch slowly releases scopolamine over a period of 3 days and is thought to work by blocking cholinergic neurotransmission from the vestibular apparatus to the vomiting center in the brain stem. As discussed in Chapter 21, muscarinic receptor blockers are also used in the treatment of Parkinson's disease.

(6) OTHER INDICATIONS. Atropine is used in two other clinical contexts. First, it is used to prevent muscarinic side effects when cholinesterase inhibitors are given to patients with myasthenia gravis. Second, as discussed in Chapter 6, it is used to reverse the muscarinic effects of cholinesterase inhibitor overdose. In this setting, supranormal doses of atropine may be required to counteract the large concentrations of acetylcholine that have accumulated at cholinergic synapses, and the atropine dosage must be titrated to the patient's response. Atropine will not counteract the effects of nicotinic receptor activation caused by cholinesterase inhibition. The muscle weakness resulting from nicotinic receptor stimulation can be attenuated by adding pralidoxime to the treatment regimen.

Hyoscyamine

Hyoscyamine, the levorotatory isomer of racemic atropine, which is the natural form of the alkaloid that occurs in plants, is primarily responsible for the pharmacologic effects of atropine. Hyoscyamine is primarily used to treat **intestinal spasms** and other gastrointestinal disorders, and it is available in preparations intended for oral or sublingual administration.

Semisynthetic and Synthetic Muscarinic Receptor Antagonists

In the search for a more selective muscarinic receptor antagonist, investigators have developed a large number of semisynthetic and synthetic blocking agents. Fig. 7–1B shows examples of their chemical structures. Although the pharmacologic effects of these agents are similar to those of atropine, their unique pharmacokinetic properties are advantageous in specific situations.

Ipratropium and Tiotropium

Ipratropium (ATROVENT) and tiotropium (SPIRIVA), quaternary amine derivatives of atropine, are administered by inhalation to patients with **obstructive lung diseases.** Because these drugs are not well absorbed from the lungs into the systemic circulation, they produce few adverse effects. For example, unlike atropine, they do not impair the ciliary clearance of secretions from the airways. This makes them particularly useful in treating patients with **emphysema** and **chronic bronchitis.** The respiratory effects and uses of these compounds are discussed more thoroughly in Chapter 27.

Dicyclomine, Oxybutynin, Solifenacin, and Tolterodine

Dicyclomine (BENTYL) is a synthetic tertiary amine used to relax intestinal smooth muscle and thereby relieve irritable bowel symptoms such as intestinal cramping. Oxybutynin (DITROPAN), tolterodine (DETROL), and solifenacin

(VESICARE) are used to reduce the four major symptoms of **hyperactive bladder:** daytime urinary frequency, nocturia, urgency, and incontinence. Tolterodine and solifenacin, which are newer drugs, are claimed to have a more selective action on the urinary bladder and to cause fewer adverse effects such as dry mouth and blurred vision. Tolterodine is available in a sustained release formulation given once daily and solifenacin is also effective with a single daily dose.

Glycopyrrolate

Glycopyrrolate blocks muscarinic receptors throughout the body. Low doses preferentially inhibit secretions and the drug is administered preoperatively to inhibit excessive salivary and respiratory tract secretions. It is also used during surgery to inhibit the secretory and vagal effects of cholinesterase inhibitors (e.g., neostigmine) that are used to reverse nondepolarizing neuromuscular blockade induced by curariform drugs.

Tropicamide

Tropicamide (MYDRIACYL) is a tertiary amine that was developed for topical ocular administration as a mydriatic. It is given just before ophthalmoscopy to facilitate **examination of the peripheral retina.** It has a short duration of action (about 1 hour) and is often preferable to atropine and scopolamine for short-term mydriasis.

Pirenzepine

Pirenzepine, a muscarinic receptor antagonist that is selective for M_1 receptors, was developed to reduce vagally stimulated gastric acid secretion in patients with **peptic ulcers.** The drug appears to act by blocking M_1 receptors on paracrine cells and thereby inhibiting the release of histamine, a potent gastric acid stimulant. Pirenzepine is currently available in Canada but not in the United States.

NICOTINIC RECEPTOR ANTAGONISTS

The nicotinic receptor antagonists include ganglionic blocking agents and neuromuscular blocking agents.

Ganglionic Blocking Agents

The ganglionic nicotinic receptor blockers (e.g., **trimethaphan**) selectively block N_N receptors at sympathetic and parasympathetic ganglia. Their effect on a particular tissue depends on whether the sympathetic or parasympathetic system is dominant in that tissue. Blockade of sympathetic ganglia causes hypotension, whereas blockade of parasympathetic ganglia produces dry mouth, blurred vision, and urinary retention.

Ganglionic blockers have been used to treat chronic hypertension, but they are no longer used for this disorder because of the advent of more effective drugs with fewer adverse effects. Trimethaphan is occasionally used in cases of **hypertensive emergency,** when extremely high blood pressures must be lowered rapidly, but other drugs have largely replaced trimethaphan for this purpose.

Neuromuscular Blocking Agents

The neuromuscular blocking agents inhibit neurotransmission at skeletal neuromuscular junctions, causing muscle weakness and paralysis. These agents can be divided into two groups, one consisting of **nondepolarizing blockers** and the other consisting of **depolarizing blockers.**

Nondepolarizing Neuromuscular Blocking Agents

General Properties

The nondepolarizing neuromuscular blocking agents, also known as **curariform drugs**, include **atracurium, doxacurium, mivacurium, pancuronium, rocuronium, tubocurarine,** and **vecuronium.** The curariform drugs were originally extracted from plants used by native South Americans as arrow poisons for hunting wild game. **Curare** is another name for the arrow poisons and their chemical derivatives.

CHEMISTRY AND PHARMACOKINETICS. Chemical structures and pharmacologic properties of curariform drugs are shown in Fig. 7–3 and Table 7–1. The curariform drugs are positively charged quaternary amines that are not well absorbed from the gut and do not cross the blood–brain barrier. Hence, they do not cause poisoning when meat containing these substances is ingested. Some of the curariform drugs (e.g., atracurium and mivacurium) are rapidly metabolized by plasma esterases and, therefore, have a shorter duration of action. Longer-acting drugs, including tubocurarine, doxacurium, and the aminosteroids (e.g., pancuronium), are eliminated by renal and biliary excretion of the unchanged compounds and hepatic metabolites.

MECHANISMS AND EFFECTS. The curariform drugs act as competitive antagonists of acetylcholine at N_M receptors in skeletal muscle, and this accounts for their muscle-relaxing effects. After a curariform drug is administered, it first paralyzes the small and rapidly moving muscles of the eyes and face and then paralyzes the larger muscles of the limbs

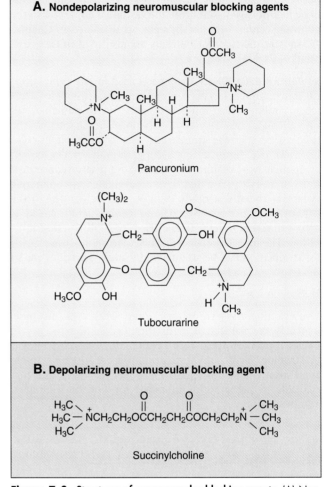

Figure 7–3. Structures of neuromuscular blocking agents. (A) Nondepolarizing neuromuscular blocking agents include pancuronium, which is an aminosteroid, and tubocurarine, which is a benzylisoquinoline. (B) Succinylcholine, the only depolarizing neuromuscular blocking agent available for clinical use today, is composed of two molecules of acetylcholine.

TABLE 7–1. Properties of Neuromuscular Blocking Agents

Drug	Depolarizing Agent	Histamine Release*	Ganglionic Blockade†	Effects Reversed by Cholinesterase Inhibitors	Duration of Action (Minutes)
Atracurium	No	Minimal	Low	Yes	30–60
Doxacurium	No	None	Low	Yes	90–120
Mivacurium	No	Minimal	Low	Yes	10–20
Pancuronium	No	None	Medium	Yes	120–180
Rocuronium	No	None	Low	Yes	30–60
Succinylcholine	Yes	Minimal	None‡	No	5–8
Tubocurarine	No	High	High	Yes	60–120
Vecuronium	No	None	Low	Yes	60–90

*May cause bronchospasm, hypotension, and excessive salivary and bronchial secretions.
†May cause hypotension and tachycardia and cardiac muscarinic receptors.
‡May cause bradycardia (by stimulating vagal ganglia) or may cause tachycardia and hypertension (by stimulating sympathetic ganglia).

and trunk. Finally, it paralyzes the intercostal muscles and diaphragm, causing respiration to cease. This sequence of paralysis is fortunate in that it enables relaxation of abdominal muscles for surgical procedures without producing apnea. Respiratory function should always be closely monitored in patients receiving a neuromuscular blocking agent, however.

Curariform drugs stimulate the release of histamine from mast cells, and they block autonomic ganglia and muscarinic receptors (see Table 7–1). These actions can cause bronchospasm, hypotension, and tachycardia. Newer drugs, such as doxacurium, mivacurium, rocuronium and vecuronium, tend to cause less histamine release and fewer autonomic side effects than do tubocurarine and pancuronium.

INTERACTIONS. The muscle-relaxing effects of curariform drugs are potentiated by various inhalational anesthetic agents (including halothane and isoflurane) and by the aminoglycoside antibiotics, tetracycline antibiotics, and calcium channel blockers. The effects are also more pronounced in patients who have neuromuscular disorders (e.g., myasthenia gravis) than they are in healthy individuals. The muscle-relaxing effects of curariform drugs can be reversed by administering a cholinesterase inhibitor (e.g., neostigmine), which acts by increasing acetylcholine levels at the neuromuscular junction and counteracting the neuromuscular blockade.

INDICATIONS. The neuromuscular blockers are primarily used to induce muscle relaxation during surgery and thereby facilitate surgical manipulations. These drugs are sometimes used as an adjunct to electroconvulsive therapy to prevent injuries that might be caused by involuntary muscle contractions. They have also been used to facilitate intubation of the respiratory tract and thereby facilitate endoscopic procedures (e.g., bronchoscopy). During the clinical use of neuromuscular blocking agents, the degree of neuromuscular blockade can be determined by monitoring the contraction of a small limb muscle in response to nerve stimulation.

Drug Selection

The selection of a nondepolarizing agent for a particular clinical application is usually based on the relative duration of action and the degree of drug-induced changes in blood pressure and heart rate. Mivacurium is used when a short-acting drug is required. Atracurium, rocuronium, and vecuronium provide an intermediate duration of action (30 to 90 minutes). All of the short- and intermediate-acting drugs have minimal effects on cardiovascular and respiratory function. Doxacurium, pancuronium, or tubocurarine might be selected when a longer duration of action is required. Tubocurarine is seldom used because its use is associated with a higher incidence of adverse effects.

Depolarizing Neuromuscular Blocking Agents

Succinylcholine, the only depolarizing agent available for clinical use today, is composed of two molecules of acetylcholine (see Fig. 7–3B). Succinylcholine binds to nicotinic receptors in skeletal muscle and causes persistent depolar-ization of the motor end plate. When the drug is first administered, it produces transient muscle contractions called fasciculations. The fasciculations are quickly followed by a sustained muscle paralysis. Succinylcholine is not hydrolyzed as rapidly by cholinesterase as acetylcholine is, and this appears to partly account for the persistent depolarization and muscle paralysis.

Table 7–1 compares the properties of succinylcholine with those of the curariform drugs. Succinylcholine has an ultra-short duration of action (5 to 10 minutes) owing to its hydrolysis by plasma cholinesterase. The sequence of muscle paralysis produced by succinylcholine is similar to that produced by the curariform drugs. The effects of succinylcholine, however, are not reversed by cholinesterase inhibitors, and no pharmacologic antidote exists to reverse an overdose of succinylcholine.

Succinylcholine is used to produce **muscle relaxation before and during surgery,** and is sometimes used to facilitate intubation of the airway. Before the drug is administered, patients should be screened for atypical cholinesterase. Individuals with this inherited disorder cannot metabolize succinylcholine at normal rates and are susceptible to prolonged neuromuscular paralysis and apnea after receiving the usual dosage of the drug.

Succinylcholine can cause hyperkalemia sufficient to cause cardiac arrest in persons with unhealed skeletal muscle injury such as follows third-degree burns, and it should not be used in these persons until the injury heals. Succinylcholine can also cause postoperative myalgia, particularly in the muscles of the neck, back, and abdomen. This effect probably results from the muscle fasciculations produced by the drug.

SUMMARY OF IMPORTANT POINTS

▪ The muscarinic receptor antagonists relax smooth muscle, increase heart rate and cardiac conduction, and inhibit exocrine gland secretion. They include belladonna alkaloids (e.g., atropine and scopolamine) and semisynthetic and synthetic drugs (e.g., ipratropium).

▪ The muscarinic receptor blockers are used to treat bradycardia, obstructive lung diseases, intestinal spasms, urinary bladder spasms, and peptic ulcers. They are also used to reduce salivary and respiratory secretions and to produce mydriasis and cycloplegia.

▪ Atropine toxicity can cause dryness of the mouth and skin, blurred vision, tachycardia, palpitations, urinary retention, delirium, and hallucinations.

▪ The nicotinic receptor antagonists include ganglionic blocking agents (e.g., trimethaphan) and neuromuscular blocking agents (e.g., the curariform drugs, which are nondepolarizing, and succinylcholine, which is depolarizing).

▪ Trimethaphan is used to produce controlled hypotension during surgery and to treat hypertensive emergencies.

■ Neuromuscular blockers are used primarily to produce muscle relaxation during surgery.

■ Curariform drugs competitively block nicotinic receptors in skeletal muscle. They do not cause muscle fasciculations, and their effects can be reversed by cholinesterase inhibitors.

■ Succinylcholine produces muscle fasciculations that are followed by muscle paralysis. The effects cannot be reversed by cholinesterase inhibitors.

Review Questions

1. Which drug produces transient muscle fasciculations followed by muscle paralysis that is not reversed by neostigmine?
   (A) rocuronium
   (B) hyoscyamine
   (C) ipratropium
   (D) succinylcholine
   (E) dicyclomine

2. Toxic doses of atropine typically cause all of the following effects EXCEPT
   (A) hallucinations
   (B) bronchospasm
   (C) hyperthermia
   (D) urinary retention
   (E) blurred vision

3. Topical ocular administration of tropicamide will cause
   (A) contraction of the ciliary muscle
   (B) vasoconstriction
   (C) miosis
   (D) relaxation of the iris sphincter muscle
   (E) lacrimation

4. The therapeutic use of tolterodine is based on its ability to
   (A) relax bronchial smooth muscle
   (B) relax urinary bladder smooth muscle
   (C) relax uterine smooth muscle
   (D) inhibit salivary secretions
   (E) relax ciliary muscle

Answers and Explanations

1. **The answer is D: succinylcholine.** Succinylcholine is a depolarizing neuromuscular blocking agent that produces persistent depolarization of the motor end plate, thereby causing transient muscle fasciculations followed by paralysis. Cholinesterase inhibitors, acting to increase acetylcholine levels, do not counteract the muscle paralysis produced by succinylcholine and can actually increase the degree of paralysis by prolonging muscle depolarization.

2. **The answer is B: bronchospasm.** Muscarinic receptor antagonists such as atropine cause relaxation of bronchial smooth muscle and bronchodilation. Atropine causes hyperthermia by inhibiting sweating, thereby leading to vasodilation and flushing. Atropine causes blurred vision by relaxing the ciliary muscle, thereby producing cycloplegia (paralysis of accommodation).

3. **The answer is D: relaxation of the iris sphincter muscle.** Tropicamide binds to muscarinic receptors and competitively blocks acetylcholine released by the parasympathetic oculomotor nerve. This action leads to relaxation of the iris sphincter muscle and dilation of the pupil (mydriasis), thereby facilitating ophthalmoscopic examination of the peripheral retina.

4. **The answer is B: relax urinary bladder smooth muscle.** Tolterodine is used to treat hyperactive bladder and relieve urgency, frequency, and incontinence. It is not used to relax uterine or bronchial smooth muscle. It can inhibit salivary secretions causing dry mouth and it can relax the ciliary muscle causing blurred vision.

SELECTED READINGS

Donati, F. Muscle relaxants: a clinical update. Can J Anaesth 50:R1–R4, 2003.

Gyermek, L. Pharmacology of Antimuscarinic Agents. Boca Raton, Fla., CRC Press, 1998.

Hashim, H., and P. Abrams. Drug treatment of overactive bladder: efficacy, cost and quality-of-life considerations. Drugs:1643–1656, 2004.

Scarpero, H. M., and R. R. Dmochowski. Muscarinic receptors: what we know. Curr Urol Reports 4:421–428, 2003.

CHAPTER 8

Adrenergic Receptor Agonists

CLASSIFICATION OF ADRENERGIC RECEPTOR AGONISTS

Direct-acting Adrenergic Receptor Agonists
Catecholamines
- Dobutamine
- Dopamine
- Epinephrine
- Isoproterenol
- Norepinephrine

Noncatecholamines
- Albuterol (PROVENTIL, VENTOLIN)[a]
- Apraclonidine[b]
- Clonidine (CATAPRES)
- Midodrine (PROAMATINE)
- Oxymetazoline

- Phenylephrine
- Ritodrine[a]
- Terbutaline (BRETHINE)[a]

Indirect-acting Adrenergic Receptor Agonists
- Amphetamine
- Cocaine

Mixed-acting Adrenergic Receptor Agonists
- Ephedrine
- Pseudoephedrine

[a]also fenoterol, formoterol, pirbuterol, salmeterol
[b]also brimonidine

OVERVIEW OF ADRENERGIC PHARMACOLOGY

The adrenergic receptor agonists are a large group of drugs whose diverse pharmacologic effects make them valuable in the treatment of a wide spectrum of clinical conditions, ranging from cardiovascular emergencies to the common cold. Although some of the agonists exert their effects on multiple organ systems, others target a specific organ. The spectrum of effects produced by a particular adrenergic receptor agonist depends on its affinity for different types of adrenergic receptors.

Adrenergic Receptors

Adrenergic receptors (adrenoceptors) have been classified as **α-adrenergic receptors** and **β-adrenergic receptors,** based on their reactions to epinephrine, norepinephrine, and other adrenergic receptor agonists in cardiac and smooth muscle. Epinephrine and norepinephrine are more potent than isoproterenol at α-adrenergic receptors located in smooth muscle, whereas isoproterenol is more potent than epinephrine and norepinephrine at β-adrenergic receptors located in cardiac muscle.

As shown in Table 8–1 and Fig. 8–1, subtypes of α- and β-adrenergic receptors have also been identified on the basis of several criteria, including differences in signal transduction and physiologic effects and differences in agonist potency and affinity at particular receptor sites. The receptor subtypes have been cloned, and their molecular structures have been determined.

α-Adrenergic Receptors

The subtypes of α-adrenergic receptors can be differentiated on the basis of their location at sympathetic neuroeffector junctions. The **α₁-adrenergic receptors** are primarily located in postjunctional smooth muscle, whereas

TABLE 8–1. Properties of Adrenergic, Dopamine, and Imidazoline Receptors

Type of Receptor	Mechanism of Signal Transduction	Effects
Adrenergic		
α_1	Increased inositol triphosphate (IP_3) and diacylglycerol (DAG)	Contraction of smooth muscles
α_2	Decreased cyclic adenosine monophosphate (cAMP)	Inhibition of norepinephrine release, decrease in secretion of aqueous humor, decrease in secretion of insulin, mediation of platelet aggregation, and mediation of central nervous system effects
β_1	Increased cAMP	Increase in secretion of renin and increase in heart rate, contractility, and conduction
β_2	Increased cAMP	Glycogenolysis, relaxation of smooth muscles, and uptake of potassium in skeletal muscles
β_3	Increased cAMP	Lipolysis
Dopamine		
D_1	Increased cAMP	Relaxation of vascular smooth muscles
D_2	Decreased cAMP, increased potassium currents, and decreased calcium influx	Modulation of neurotransmission in the sympathetic and central nervous systems
Imidazoline	Uncertain; possibly increased DAG	Natriuresis and decrease of sympathetic outflow from the central nervous system

α_2-**adrenergic receptors** are located on presynaptic neurons as well as in some postsynaptic tissues and blood platelets (see Fig. 8–1).

The α_1-receptors mediate contraction of the vascular smooth muscle, iris dilator muscle, and bladder sphincter muscle. The α_2-receptors located on sympathetic postganglionic neurons serve as **autoreceptors** whose activation leads to feedback inhibition of norepinephrine release from nerve terminals. The α_2-receptors are also found in blood platelets and in ocular, adipose, intestinal, hepatic, renal, and endocrine tissue. In blood platelets, α_2-receptors mediate platelet aggregation. In the pancreas, α_2-receptors mediate the inhibition of insulin secretion that occurs when the sympathetic nervous system is activated.

β-Adrenergic Receptors

Table 8–1 summarizes the effects of three subtypes of β-adrenergic receptors.

Activation of β_1-**adrenergic receptors** produces cardiac stimulation, leading to a positive **chronotropic effect**

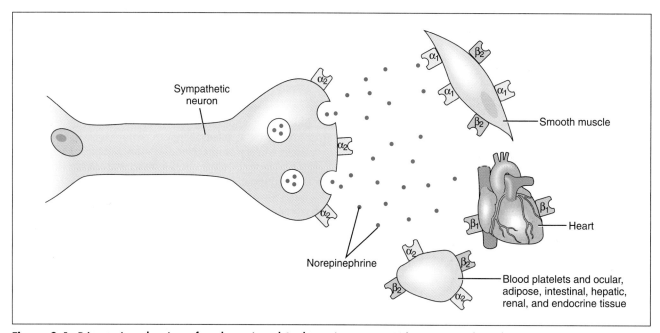

Figure 8–1. Primary tissue locations of α-adrenergic and β-adrenergic receptors. Whereas α_1- and β_2-adrenergic receptors are primarily located in smooth muscle, β_1-adrenergic receptors are predominantly found in cardiac tissue. Some α_2-adrenergic receptors are located on sympathetic neurons, where they produce feedback inhibition of neurotransmitter release. Other α_2- and β_2-adrenergic receptors are located in blood platelets and a variety of organ tissues. The α- and β-adrenergic receptors are also found in the central nervous system.

(increased heart rate), a positive **inotropic effect** (increased contractility), and a positive **dromotropic effect** (increased cardiac impulse conduction velocity). Activation of β_1 receptors also increases renin secretion from renal juxtaglomerular cells.

The **β_2-adrenergic receptors** mediate relaxation of bronchial, uterine, and vascular smooth muscle. In skeletal muscle, β_2-receptors mediate potassium uptake. In the liver, they mediate **glycogenolysis,** which increases the glucose concentration in the blood. Whereas epinephrine and norepinephrine are equally potent at β_1-receptors in cardiac tissue, epinephrine is more potent than norepinephrine at β_2-receptors in smooth muscle.

Activation of **β_3-adrenergic receptors** produces **lipolysis,** a process in which the hydrolysis of triglycerides in adipose tissue leads to the release of fatty acids into the circulation. Investigators are currently searching for selective β_3-adrenergic receptor agonists because they believe that the lipolytic effect of these agonists would be useful in the treatment of obesity.

Dopamine Receptors

Dopamine receptors are activated by dopamine but not by other adrenergic receptor agonists. Several subtypes exist, including the **D_1-receptors,** which mediate muscle relaxation in vascular smooth muscle, and the **D_2-receptors,** which modulate neurotransmitter release.

Imidazoline Receptors

Imidazoline receptors are activated by adrenergic receptor agonists and other substances that contain an imidazoline structure. One of the best-studied examples of these substances is clonidine. The imidazoline receptors are found in the central nervous system and a number of peripheral tissues. Although the antihypertensive effects of clonidine can be partly attributable to the activation of α_2-adrenergic receptors, investigators have postulated that they are also partly caused by the effects of imidazoline receptors, which act in the central nervous system to reduce sympathetic outflow to the heart and vascular smooth muscle. The pharmacologic properties of antihypertensive imidazoline drugs are discussed in greater detail in Chapter 10.

Signal Transduction

The adrenergic, dopamine, and imidazoline receptors are guanine nucleotide protein-binding (G protein-binding) receptors that are located in cell membranes of target tissues.

Activation of α_1-adrenergic receptors is coupled with activation of **phospholipase C,** which catalyzes the release of **inositol triphosphate** (IP_3) and **diacylglycerol** (DAG) from membrane phospholipids. In smooth muscle, IP_3 stimulates the release of calcium from the sarcoplasmic reticulum, and this leads to muscle contraction. This is the mechanism by which a drug can produce vasoconstriction and increase blood pressure in a patient with severe hypotension. Activation of α_2-adrenergic receptors leads to inhibition of adenylyl cyclase and a decrease in the levels of cyclic adenosine monophosphate (cAMP) in sympathetic neurons and other tissues. This is the mechanism responsible for a decrease in aqueous humor secretion and for other effects of α_2-adrenergic receptor agonists. Activation of D_2-receptors also inhibits cAMP formation.

Activation of β-adrenergic receptors and D_1-receptors leads to stimulation of adenylyl cyclase and an increase in the levels of cAMP in cardiac tissue and smooth muscle. Cyclic AMP activates **protein kinases,** which phosphorylate other proteins and enzymes. The cellular response depends on the specific type of proteins that are phosphorylated in each tissue. In cardiac tissue, calcium channels are phosphorylated, thereby augmenting calcium influx and cardiac contractility. In smooth muscle, cAMP-activated kinases produce muscle relaxation.

Classification of Adrenergic Receptor Agonists

The adrenergic receptor agonists mimic the effect of sympathetic nervous system stimulation and, therefore, are also called **sympathomimetic drugs.** These drugs can be divided into three groups on the basis of their mode of action. The **direct-acting agonists** bind to and activate adrenergic receptors. As shown in Fig. 8–2, the **indirect-acting agonists** increase the stimulation of adrenergic receptors by increasing the concentration of norepinephrine at sympathetic neuroeffector junctions in one of two ways. Cocaine binds to

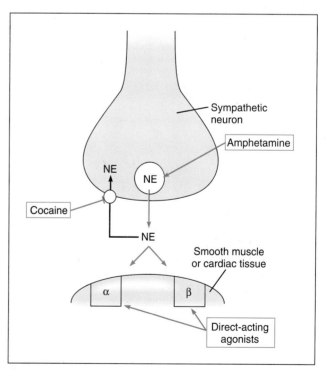

Figure 8–2. Mechanisms of indirect-acting and direct-acting adrenergic receptor agonists. Some indirect-acting agonists (e.g., cocaine) block norepinephrine reuptake, whereas other indirect-acting agonists (e.g., amphetamine) indirectly increase norepinephrine release from storage vesicles in sympathetic neurons. Direct-acting agonists bind to and activate adrenergic receptors. NE = norepinephrine; α = α-adrenergic receptor; and β = β-adrenergic receptor.

and inhibits the catecholamine transporter protein located in the plasma membrane of the presynaptic sympathetic neuron and thereby inhibits the neuronal reuptake of norepinephrine and increases its synaptic concentration. Amphetamine and related drugs, which serve as substrates for the catecholamine transporter, are transported into the sympathetic nerve terminal where they inhibit the storage of norepinephrine by neuronal vesicles, leading to reverse norepinephrine transport into the synapse by the catecholamine transporter. The **mixed-acting agonists** (e.g., ephedrine) have both direct and indirect actions.

DIRECT-ACTING ADRENERGIC RECEPTOR AGONISTS

The direct-acting agonists can be subdivided into catecholamines and noncatecholamines.

Catecholamines

The naturally occurring catecholamines include **norepinephrine,** an endogenous sympathetic neurotransmitter;

epinephrine, the principal hormone of the adrenal medulla; and **dopamine,** the precursor to norepinephrine and epinephrine. Synthetic catecholamines include **isoproterenol** and **dobutamine.**

General Properties

CHEMISTRY AND PHARMACOKINETICS. Each catecholamine consists of the catechol moiety and an ethylamine side chain (Fig. 8–3A). The catecholamines are rapidly inactivated by monoamine oxidase (MAO) and catechol-*O*-methyltransferase (COMT), enzymes found in the gut, liver, and other tissues. The drugs have low oral bioavailabilities and short plasma half-lives. For these reasons, they must be administered parenterally when a systemic action is required (e.g., in the treatment of patients who are in anaphylactic shock).

MECHANISMS AND EFFECTS. As shown in Fig. 8–3A and Table 8–2, the various catecholamines differ in their affinities and specificities for receptors. The size of the alkyl substitution on the amine nitrogen determines the relative affinity for α- and β-adrenergic receptors. Drugs with a large alkyl group (e.g., isoproterenol) have greater affinity for β-adrenergic

TABLE 8–2. **Pharmacologic Effects and Clinical Uses of Adrenergic Receptor Agonists**

Drug	Pharmacologic Effect (and Receptor)	Clinical Use
Direct-acting catecholamines		
Dobutamine	Cardiac stimulation (β_1) and vasodilation (β_2)	Cardiogenic shock, acute heart failure, and cardiac stimulation during heart surgery
Dopamine*	Renal vasodilation (D_1), cardiac stimulation (β_1), and increased blood pressure (β_1 and α_1)	Cardiogenic shock, septic shock, heart failure, and adjunct to fluid administration in hypovolemic shock
Epinephrine	Vasoconstriction and increased blood pressure (α_1), cardiac stimulation (β_1), and bronchodilation (β_2)	Anaphylactic shock, cardiac arrest, ventricular fibrillation, reduction in bleeding during surgery, and prolongation of the action of local anesthetics
Isoproterenol	Cardiac stimulation (β_1) and bronchodilation (β_2)	Asthma, refractory atrioventricular block, and refractory bradycardia
Norepinephrine	Vasoconstriction and increased blood pressure (α_1)	Hypotension and shock
Direct-acting noncatecholamines		
Albuterol	Bronchodilation (β_2)	Asthma
Apraclonidine	Decreased aqueous humor formation (α_2)	Chronic open-angle glaucoma
Clonidine	Decreased sympathetic outflow from central nervous system (α_2 and imidazoline)	Chronic hypertension
Midodrine	Vasoconstriction (α_1)	Orthostatic hypotension
Oxymetazoline	Vasoconstriction (α_1)	Nasal and ocular decongestion
Phenylephrine	Vasoconstriction, increased blood pressure, and mydriasis (α_1)	Nasal decongestion in viral and allergic rhinitis, ocular decongestion in allergic conjunctivitis, mydriasis during ophthalmologic examination, maintenance of blood pressure during surgery, and treatment of drug-induced and neurogenic shock
Ritodrine	Bronchodilation and uterine relaxation (β_2)	Asthma and premature labor
Terbutaline	Bronchodilation and uterine relaxation (β_2)	Asthma and premature labor
Indirect-acting agents		
Amphetamine	Increase in norepinephrine release	Central nervous system effects
Cocaine	Inhibition of norepinephrine uptake	Local anesthesia
Mixed-acting agents		
Ephedrine	Vasoconstriction (α_1)	Nasal decongestion in viral and allergic rhinitis
Pseudoephedrine	Vasoconstriction (α_1)	Nasal decongestion in viral and allergic rhinitis

*Dopamine is a catecholamine with mixed action.

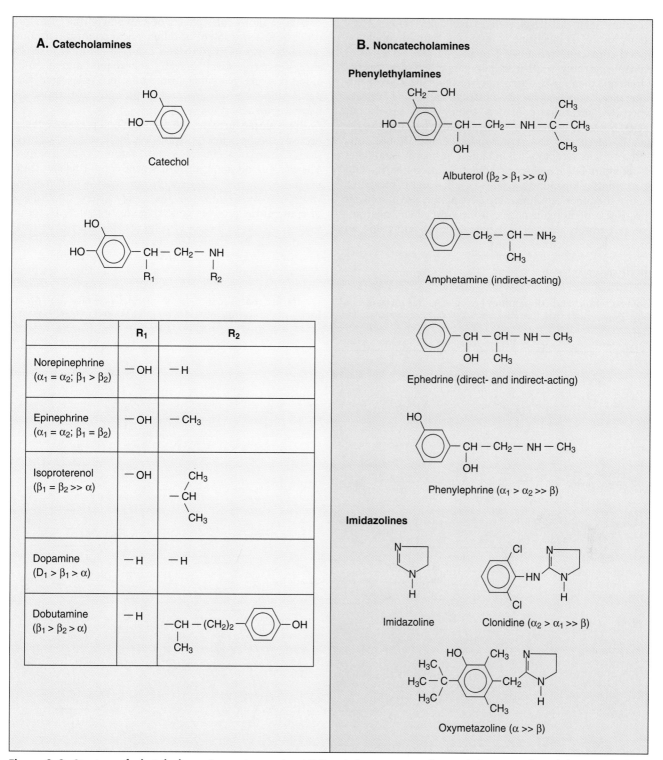

Figure 8–3. Structures of selected adrenergic receptor agonists. (A) Catecholamines contain the catechol moiety and an ethylamine side chain. The amine nitrogen substitution determines the relative affinity for α- and β-adrenergic receptors, with larger substitutions (e.g., in isoproterenol and dobutamine) decreasing the affinity for α-adrenergic receptors and increasing the affinity for β-adrenergic receptors. Note that dopamine has an even higher affinity for dopamine D_1 receptors than for adrenergic receptors. (B) One group of noncatecholamines consists of phenylethylamines, which lack one or both of the hydroxyl groups of the catechol moiety. Another group of noncatecholamines consists of imidazolines.

receptors than do drugs with a small alkyl group (e.g., epinephrine). Epinephrine is a potent agonist at all α- and β-adrenergic receptors. Norepinephrine differs from epinephrine only in that it has greater affinity for β_1-adrenergic than for β_2-adrenergic receptors. Because of this difference, norepinephrine constricts all blood vessels, whereas epinephrine constricts some blood vessels but dilates others. Isoproterenol is considered to be a selective β_1- and β_2-adrenergic receptor agonist because it has little affinity for α receptors. Dobutamine primarily stimulates β_1-receptors but has minor stimulatory effects on β_2- and α-receptors. Dopamine activates D_1-, β_1-, and α-receptors. Unlike the other catecholamines, dopamine also stimulates the release of norepinephrine from sympathetic neurons. For this reason, dopamine is both a direct-acting and an indirect-acting receptor agonist.

(1) CARDIOVASCULAR EFFECTS. Fig. 8–4 compares the cardiovascular effects when norepinephrine, epinephrine, isoproterenol, and dopamine are given by intravenous infusion.

The cardiovascular effects of norepinephrine primarily result from activation of α_1-adrenergic receptors. Activation produces vasoconstriction and increases peripheral resistance, which, in turn, increases the systolic and diastolic blood pressure. Norepinephrine can cause reflex bradycardia if blood pressure increases sufficiently to activate the baroreceptor reflex.

Epinephrine increases the systolic blood pressure but can decrease the diastolic blood pressure. Increased systolic pressure is caused by an increased heart rate and cardiac output. The effect on diastolic pressure depends on the relative stimulation of α_1- and β_2-adrenergic receptors, which mediate vasoconstriction and vasodilation, respectively. Lower doses of epinephrine produce greater stimulation of β_2-receptors than α_1-receptors, thereby causing vasodilation and decreasing diastolic blood pressure. Higher doses produce more vasoconstriction and can increase diastolic pressure.

Isoproterenol activates β_1- and β_2-adrenergic receptors and produces vasodilation and cardiac stimulation. It usually lowers the diastolic and mean arterial pressure, but it can increase the systolic pressure by increasing the heart rate and

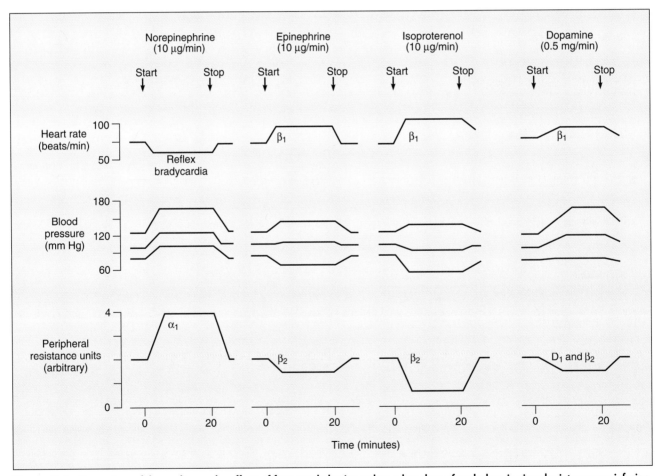

Figure 8–4. Comparison of the cardiovascular effects of four catecholamines when a low dose of each drug is given by intravenous infusion. Arrows indicate when the infusion was started and stopped. The blood pressure recordings show systolic, diastolic, and mean arterial pressure. Peripheral resistance is expressed on an arbitrary scale, ranging from 0 to 4 units. The reflex mechanism, adrenergic receptors (α_1, β_1, and β_2), or dopamine (D_1) receptors responsible for changes in the heart rate and peripheral resistance are illustrated. Norepinephrine increases peripheral resistance and blood pressure, and this leads to reflex bradycardia. Epinephrine increases heart rate while reducing peripheral resistance, and the mean arterial blood pressure increases slightly. Isoproterenol increases heart rate but significantly lowers peripheral resistance, and the mean arterial pressure declines. Dopamine increases heart rate (and increases cardiac output) while lowering vascular resistance, and the mean arterial pressure increases.

contractility. Its potent chronotropic effect can cause tachycardia and cardiac arrhythmias. For this reason, an alternative drug (e.g., dobutamine) is usually administered to increase cardiac output in cases of heart failure.

Dobutamine selectively increases myocardial contractility and stroke volume while producing a smaller increase in heart rate. These actions can increase cardiac output in persons with acute heart failure. Dobutamine also reduces vascular resistance by activating β_2-adrenergic receptors, thereby decreasing cardiac afterload. In patients with heart failure, a reduction in afterload contributes to an increased stroke volume and cardiac output.

When given in low doses, dopamine selectively activates D_1-receptors in renal and other vascular beds, thereby causing vasodilation and an increase in renal blood flow. At slightly higher doses, dopamine activates β_1-adrenergic receptors in the heart, thereby stimulating cardiac contractility and increasing cardiac output and tissue perfusion. At even higher doses, dopamine activates α_1-adrenergic receptors and causes vasoconstriction. Hence, dopamine tends to increase vascular resistance, whereas dobutamine usually decreases vascular resistance.

(2) RESPIRATORY TRACT EFFECTS. Epinephrine and isoproterenol are potent bronchodilators. Although they have been used in the treatment of asthma, more selective β_2-adrenergic receptor agonists are usually used for this purpose today.

(3) ADVERSE EFFECTS. Catecholamines can cause excessive vasoconstriction, leading to tissue ischemia and necrosis. Localized tissue ischemia can result from extravasation of an intravenous drug infusion or from the accidental injection of epinephrine into a finger when a patient is trying to stop an allergic reaction by self-injecting epinephrine into the arm or other site. The administration of excessive doses of catecholamines can reduce blood flow to vital organs, such as the kidneys, or cause excessive cardiac stimulation that leads tachycardia and other cardiac arrhythmias. The β-adrenergic receptor agonists can cause hyperglycemia secondary to glycogenolysis, and this is usually undesirable in patients with diabetes.

Specific Drugs

Catecholamines are used to treat several types of **shock.** Shock is a condition in which the circulation to vital organs is profoundly reduced as a result of inadequate blood volume (**hypovolemic shock**), inadequate cardiac function (**cardiogenic shock**), or inadequate vasomotor tone (**neurogenic shock and septic shock**). Septic shock is associated with massive vasodilation secondary to the production of toxins by pathogenic microorganisms. It is sometimes called "warm shock" to distinguish it from hypovolemic and cardiogenic shock, in which the patient's extremities are usually cold owing to inadequate blood flow. Some cases of septic shock, however, are also manifested by hypoperfusion and cold extremities. **Anaphylactic shock,** which is a manifestation of immediate hypersensitivity reactions, is usually associated with hypotension and bronchoconstriction.

Catecholamine drugs that increase blood pressure (**vasopressors**) are used in treating shock when organ function is impaired because mean arterial blood pressure is less than 60 mm Hg. **Hypovolemia** should be corrected by intra-

venous fluid administration before the use of vasopressors because vasopressors will not be effective if hypovolemia is present. In cases of cardiogenic shock, mechanical devices (e.g., the intraaortic balloon pump) are usually superior to pharmacologic agents in their ability to improve coronary artery perfusion and cardiac performance while reducing myocardial ischemia and cardiac work. Such devices are often used in conjunction with vasopressor drugs in the treatment of this condition.

Dopamine is used to treat **septic or cardiogenic shock** when patients remain hypotensive despite adequate fluid administration. Dopamine is usually started at a dose of 2 µg/kg body weight per minute and then the dose is titrated to achieve the desired blood pressure. Although low doses of dopamine can increase urine output by augmenting renal blood flow in normal subjects, ample evidence indicates that low doses of dopamine are usually not effective to prevent and treat **acute renal failure.** The most effective means of protecting the kidneys in patients with shock appears to be the maintenance of mean arterial pressure of greater than 60 mm Hg with intravenous fluids and adequate doses of a vasopressor agent.

Norepinephrine, which is a potent vasoconstrictor, is used to treat septic shock and is often given to persons with cardiogenic shock when the response to dopamine is inadequate or is accompanied by marked tachycardia. Norepinephrine is also used to treat hypotension caused by decreased peripheral resistance such as can occur in persons who have received excessive doses of a vasodilator drug. Phenylephrine is also used for this purpose, as described below.

In cases of **anaphylactic shock,** epinephrine is the treatment of choice. By producing bronchodilation and increasing blood pressure, it counteracts the effects of histamine that is released during immediate hypersensitivity reactions. Epinephrine is used as a vasoconstrictor to **reduce bleeding during surgery** and to **prolong the action of local anesthetics** by retarding their absorption into the general circulation. Epinephrine is also used as a cardiac stimulant in the treatment of **cardiac arrest** and **ventricular fibrillation.** Isoproterenol is used to treat refractory **bradycardia** and **atrioventricular block** when other measures have not been successful. Although it has been used to treat **asthma,** a selective β_2-adrenergic receptor agonist is usually preferred for this indication because it does not increase the heart rate as much as isoproterenol.

Dobutamine is a cardiac stimulant (inotropic agent) that also produces vasodilation. It is used as a **cardiac stimulant during heart surgery** and in the short-term management of **acute heart failure** and **cardiogenic shock.** Dobutamine is not routinely used in treating septic shock, however, because its vasodilator effect can further reduce vascular resistance and blood pressure. Its utility in hypotensive patients is limited to situations in which hypotension is caused by bradycardia.

Noncatecholamines

The structures of representative examples of noncatecholamines are shown in Fig. 8–3B. Because these drugs do not contain a catechol moiety, they are not substrates for

COMT. Some of the noncatecholamines are also resistant to degradation by MAO. For this reason, noncatecholamines are effective after oral administration and have a longer duration of action than do the catecholamines.

Phenylephrine

CHEMISTRY AND PHARMACOKINETICS. Phenylephrine is a phenylethylamine (see Fig. 8–3B) and a selective α_1-adrenergic receptor agonist. It is adequately absorbed after oral or topical administration and can also be administered parenterally. The drug is partly metabolized by MAO in the intestine and liver.

MECHANISMS AND EFFECTS. When phenylephrine activates α_1-adrenergic receptors, the smooth muscles contract. This produces vasoconstriction and increases vascular resistance and blood pressure. Ocular administration of phenylephrine leads to contraction of the iris dilator muscle and dilation of the pupil (mydriasis).

INDICATIONS. Phenylephrine is used as a **nasal decongestant** in patients with **viral rhinitis,** an infection that can be caused by more than a hundred serotypes of rhinovirus and is usually referred to as the common cold. It is also used by patients with **allergic rhinitis,** an inflammation of the nasal mucosa that is caused by histamine released from mast cells during allergic reactions. The drug's vasoconstrictive effect on the nasal mucosa reduces vascular congestion and mucus secretion and thereby opens the nasal passages so patients can breathe easier. Both topical and oral preparations are available for this purpose.

In patients with **allergic conjunctivitis,** an inflammation of the eyes associated with hay fever or other allergies, phenylephrine can be used as a topical **ocular decongestant.** The ocular preparation of phenylephrine is also used to induce **mydriasis** and thereby facilitate ophthalmoscopic examination. In contrast to the muscarinic receptor antagonists used for this purpose (e.g., tropicamide) phenylephrine does not affect the ciliary muscle and cause cycloplegia.

Phenylephrine can be administered intravenously to treat forms of **hypotension** and **shock** caused by decreased peripheral vascular resistance. These include hypotension caused by excessive doses of vasodilator drugs, drug-induced shock, septic shock, and neurogenic shock such as resulting from spinal cord injury. Phenylephrine is also used to **maintain blood pressure during surgery** (e.g., when hypotension is induced by anesthetic agents).

Midodrine

Midodrine (PROAMATINE) is a newer α_1-adrenergic receptor agonist used to treat postural (orthostatic) hypotension in persons who are considerably impaired by this condition (e.g., those with severe diabetic autonomic neuropathy). Midodrine has also been used to treat hypotension caused by infections in infants, hypotension induced by psychotropic agents, and hypotension in persons undergoing renal dialysis. The drug acts to increase both systolic and diastolic blood pressure in standing, sitting, and supine positions. The primary adverse effect of the drug is hypertension, particularly when persons are supine. The drug, which is rapidly absorbed after oral administration, is extensively converted to an active metabolite, desglymidodrine, in the liver and other tissues.

Albuterol, Ritodrine, Terbutaline, and Related Drugs

CHEMISTRY AND PHARMACOKINETICS. Albuterol (see Fig. 8–3B), ritodrine, and terbutaline are selective β_2-adrenergic receptor agonists that can be administered orally, parenterally, or by inhalation. Their oral bioavailability ranges from 30% to 50% because of their incomplete absorption and hepatic first-pass metabolism. They are partly metabolized to inactive compounds before undergoing renal excretion. About 50% of albuterol, for example, is converted to an inactive sulfate conjugate. To reduce their systemic absorption and adverse effects, albuterol and the related agonists are usually administered by inhalation in the treatment of asthma. The duration of action of these agonists is about 4 to 6 hours after inhalation or oral administration and is about 2 to 3 hours after intravenous administration.

MECHANISMS, EFFECTS, AND INDICATIONS. The β_2-adrenergic receptor agonists act by causing smooth muscle relaxation. As discussed in greater detail in Chapter 27, these drugs are helpful in the treatment of **asthma** and other obstructive lung diseases because they produce bronchodilation. They are also helpful in the treatment of **premature labor,** which is defined as labor that begins before the 37th week of gestation and is believed to be caused by an imbalance in hormonal regulation caused by physiologic or environmental influences. The administration of one of these agonists to a pregnant woman in premature labor will relax the uterus to bring the pregnancy as close to term as possible.

The adverse effects of albuterol and other selective β_2-adrenergic receptor agonists include tachycardia, muscle tremor, and nervousness caused by activation of β-adrenergic receptors in the heart, skeletal muscle, and central nervous system.

Several other β_2-adrenergic receptor agonists have been introduced to treat asthma, including fenoterol, formoterol, pirbuterol, and salmeterol. The distinguishing properties and clinical use of these drugs are described in Chapter 27.

Imidazolines

CHEMISTRY AND PHARMACOKINETICS. The imidazoline compounds (see Fig. 8–3B) activate α-adrenergic and imidazoline receptors. Some imidazolines are administered by topical ocular or nasal administration, whereas others are administered by systemic routes. After systemic administration, the imidazolines have a duration of action of several hours and are partly metabolized and excreted in the urine.

MECHANISMS, EFFECTS, AND INDICATIONS. Based on their clinical use, the imidazolines can be divided into three groups. The first group consists of **oxymetazoline** and similar drugs that activate α_1-adrenergic receptors to produce vasoconstriction. These drugs are used as topical **nasal and ocular decongestants.** The second group consists of **apraclonidine, brimonidine,** and other agents that activate ocular α_2-adrenergic receptors in the ciliary body and thereby reduce the level of aqueous humor secretion. These agents are used to lower intraocular pressure in patients with **chronic open-angle glaucoma,** a condition in which elevated intraocular pressure can damage the optic nerve and eventually cause blindness. The third group consists of **clonidine** and other imidazolines that activate α_2-adrenergic and imidazoline receptors in the central nervous system. The imidazoline receptors are believed to mediate a reduction in sympathetic outflow from the vasomotor center in the medulla. The drugs in this third group, which are used to treat **chronic hypertension**, are discussed in greater detail in Chapter 10.

The activation of α_2-adrenergic receptors in the central nervous system is believed to be responsible for the sedative and other central nervous system side effects of clonidine and related drugs. Oxymetazoline and similar decongestants can also cause central nervous system and cardiovascular depression if they are absorbed into the systemic circulation and distributed to the brain. For this reason, imidazolines should be used with caution in children under 6 years of age and in the elderly.

INDIRECT-ACTING ADRENERGIC RECEPTOR AGONISTS

Amphetamine and Tyramine

Amphetamine (see Fig. 8–3B) and related compounds have high lipid solubility and indirectly increase synaptic concentrations of norepinephrine in the central and peripheral nervous systems by mechanisms described above. Amphetamine produces vasoconstriction, cardiac stimulation, increased blood pressure, and central nervous system stimulation. The various **central nervous system effects** are discussed in greater detail in Chapter 24.

Tyramine is a naturally occurring amine found in a number of foods, including bananas. Under normal conditions, tyramine is rapidly degraded by MAO in the gut and liver. In patients receiving MAO inhibitors, however, tyramine can be absorbed from foods in a quantity that is high enough to exert a sympathomimetic effect and increase blood pressure. The interaction between foods containing tyramine and MAO inhibitors is discussed in greater detail in Chapter 22. Tyramine is not used as a therapeutic agent.

Cocaine

Cocaine, a naturally occurring alkaloid, acts as a local anesthetic and also stimulates the sympathetic nervous system by blocking the neuronal reuptake of norepinephrine at both peripheral and central synapses. The sympathomimetic effects of cocaine are similar to those of amphetamine. Cocaine produces both vasoconstriction and cardiac stimulation and thereby elevates blood pressure. When the drug is used as a local anesthetic, its vasoconstrictive effect serves to retard its absorption into the systemic circulation, and this prolongs its duration of action. The vasoconstrictive effect, however, can also cause ischemia and necrosis of the nasal mucosa in people who abuse cocaine. The sympathomimetic effects of cocaine also appear to be responsible for the severe hypertension and cardiac damage that occurs in susceptible people who abuse cocaine. The **central nervous system effects** and **local anesthetic effects** of cocaine are discussed further in Chapters 24 and 25, respectively.

MIXED-ACTING ADRENERGIC RECEPTOR AGONISTS

Among the drugs that activate adrenergic receptors by both direct and indirect mechanisms are dopamine (see above), ephedrine, and pseudoephedrine. These agents indirectly increase synaptic concentrations of norepinephrine in a manner similar to that of amphetamine.

Ephedrine and Pseudoephedrine

CHEMISTRY AND PHARMACOKINETICS. Ephedrine (see Fig. 8–3B) is a naturally occurring compound obtained from plants of the genus Ephedra, which is also called Ma Huang. Ephedrine is well absorbed from the gut and has sufficient lipid solubility to enter the central nervous system. Relatively resistant to metabolism by MAO and COMT, ephedrine has a duration of action of several hours. Pseudoephedrine, one of the stereoisomers of ephedrine, has been widely used as a nasal decongestant in the treatment of colds and allergies.

MECHANISM, EFFECTS, AND INDICATIONS. Ephedrine and related drugs activate both α- and β-adrenergic receptors by direct and indirect mechanisms. Via the activation of α_1-adrenergic receptors, these drugs produce vasoconstriction. This makes them useful as **nasal decongestants** in the treatment of **viral and allergic rhinitis**. Via the action of β-adrenergic receptors, the drugs produce bronchodilation. Although they have been used as a bronchodilator, a selective β_2-adrenergic receptor agonist such as albuterol is now preferred for this indication.

Side effects of ephedrine and pseudoephedrine include tachycardia caused by β_1-receptor stimulation, increased blood pressure, and urinary retention. The latter is caused by stimulation of the sphincter muscle of the bladder. These drugs also cause central nervous system stimulation and can produce insomnia. Dietary supplements containing *Ephedra* have been widely used as appetite suppressants as an aid to losing weight. The Food and Drug Administration has banned the sale of such products because fatalities caused by hypertension and excessive cardiovascular stimulation have occurred following the use of these preparations.

SUMMARY OF IMPORTANT POINTS

■ Activation of α_1-adrenergic receptors mediates smooth muscle contraction, leading to vasoconstriction, dilation of the pupils, and contraction of the bladder sphincter muscle.

■ Activation of α_2-adrenergic receptors inhibits the release of norepinephrine from sympathetic neurons, decreases the secretion of aqueous humor, and decreases the secretion of insulin.

■ Activation of β_1-adrenergic receptors produces cardiac stimulation and increases the secretion of renin, whereas activation of β_2-adrenergic receptors mediates smooth muscle relaxation.

■ The catecholamines include norepinephrine, epinephrine, isoproterenol, dopamine, and dobutamine. These drugs are rapidly metabolized, must be administered parenterally, and are primarily used to treat cardiac disorders and various types of shock.

■ In addition to activating adrenergic receptors, dopamine activates D_1-receptors and thereby increases renal blood flow.

■ Noncatecholamines (e.g., phenylephrine and albuterol) are resistant to degradation by catechol-O-methyltransferase (COMT). They are effective when given orally, have a longer duration of action than do catecholamines, and have a wide range of uses.

■ Imidazoline compounds are agents that activate both α-adrenergic and imidazoline receptors. Examples include oxymetazoline, a topical decongestant; clonidine, an antihypertensive agent; and apraclonidine, an agent used to treat glaucoma.

■ The indirect-acting adrenergic receptor agonists increase the synaptic concentration of norepinephrine. Amphetamine indirectly activates reverse norepinephrine transport by the catecholamine transporter whereas cocaine blocks the catecholamine transporter.

■ Mixed-acting agonists (e.g., pseudoephedrine) have both direct and indirect actions. They are used as a nasal decongestant.

Review Questions

Items 1–3. For each numbered patient, select the most appropriate drug treatment from the lettered choices.

1. A pregnant woman in the 28th week of gestation experiences uterine contractions every 5 to 10 minutes.

2. After being stung by a bee, a patient experiences urticaria, laryngeal edema, difficult breathing, and hypotension.

3. A 6-year-old child contracts viral rhinitis and experiences severe nasal congestion that interferes with sleep.
   (A) midodrine
   (B) apraclonidine
   (C) dobutamine
   (D) epinephrine
   (E) phenylephrine
   (F) terbutaline

Item 4. Select the single best answer from the choices provided.

4. Which effect is produced in the ciliary body after topical ocular administration of apraclonidine?
   (A) increased inositol triphosphate
   (B) increased cAMP
   (C) decreased cAMP
   (D) increased cGMP
   (E) decreased cGMP

Answers and Explanations

1. The answer is F: terbutaline. The woman is experiencing premature labor and would benefit from an adrenergic β_2 agonist such as terbutaline or ritodrine. These agents, however, must be closely monitored for fetal tachycardia. An oxytocin antagonist, atosiban, is currently under investigation to treat premature labor. It appears to reduce uterine contractions without causing fetal tachycardia.

2. The answer is D: epinephrine. The patient is experiencing an anaphylactic reaction to the bee sting that requires epinephrine administration. Anaphylactic reactions are a severe form of immediate hypersensitivity in which large quantities of histamine are released from mast cells. Epinephrine counteracts the bronchoconstriction and hypotension caused by histamine.

3. The answer is E: phenylephrine. Phenylephrine is a selective α_1 receptor agonist that produces vasoconstriction and acts as a decongestant when administered topically or systemically. It is included in a number of nonprescription products used to treat nasal congestion caused by allergies and colds.

4. The answer is C: decreased cAMP. Apraclonidine is a selective α_2-agonist that decreases aqueous humor secretion by the ciliary body and is used to treat open-angle glaucoma. The α_2-receptor is coupled with G_i, and receptor activation leads to inhibition of adenylyl cyclase and decreased levels of cAMP. Adrenergic β-receptor antagonists decrease aqueous humor secretion by blocking β_1 receptor-mediated elevation of cAMP levels in the ciliary body.

SELECTED READINGS

Lieberman, P. Use of epinephrine in the treatment of anaphylaxis. Curr Opin Aller Clin Immunol 3:13–18, 2003.

Naschitz J., D. Dreyfuss, D. Yeshurun, et al. Midodrine treatment for chronic fatigue syndrome. Postgrad Med J 80:230–232, 2004

Sharma, M., and J. R. Teerlink. A rational approach for the treatment of acute heart failure: current strategies and future options. Curr Opin Cardiol 19:254–263, 2004.

CHAPTER 9

Adrenergic Receptor Antagonists

OVERVIEW

Excessive sympathetic nervous system activity contributes to a number of diseases, including common cardiovascular disorders such as hypertension, angina pectoris, and cardiac arrhythmias. Drugs that reduce sympathetic stimulation, **sympatholytics,** are used in the management of cardiovascular diseases and other diseases such as glaucoma, migraine headache, and urinary retention. The most important group of sympatholytics consists of the adrenergic receptor antagonists. Other drugs that have a sympatholytic effect include the ganglionic-blocking agents (discussed in Chapter 7) and the sympathetic neuronal blocking agents (discussed in Chapter 5).

Adrenergic receptor antagonists can block α-adrenergic receptors, β-adrenergic receptors, or both. The **therapeutic effects** of the antagonists primarily are caused by blockade of α₁ or β₁ receptors, whereas the **adverse effects** tend to be related to blockade of α₂ or β₂ receptors. Drugs that selec-

tively block either α₁ or β₁ receptors have been developed in an effort to avoid the adverse effects caused by α₂ or β₂ receptor blockade. Blockade of α₁-receptors relaxes vascular and other smooth muscles in tissues innervated by the sympathetic nervous system, whereas blockade of β₁-receptors reduces sympathetic stimulation of the heart.

α-ADRENERGIC RECEPTOR ANTAGONISTS

The α-adrenergic receptor antagonists, or **α-blockers,** can be distinguished on the basis of their selectivity for a receptor subtypes and by their noncompetitive or competitive blockade of α receptors.

Nonselective α-Blockers

Agents that block both α₁ and α₂ receptors are called nonselective α-blockers. Phenoxybenzamine and phentolamine are examples. Phenoxybenzamine is a noncompetitive antagonist, whereas phentolamine is a competitive receptor antagonist.

Phenoxybenzamine

CHEMISTRY AND MECHANISMS. Phenoxybenzamine is a haloalkylamine whose chemical structure and mechanisms of action are similar to those of cyclophosphamide and other nitrogen mustard alkylating agents used in cancer chemotherapy. In the body, phenoxybenzamine undergoes spontaneous chemical transformation to an active electrophilic carbonium ion. The carbonium ion forms a stable covalent bond with the α-adrenergic receptor, and this results in the noncompetitive antagonism of epinephrine and other adrenergic agonists (Fig. 9–1).

PHARMACOKINETICS. When phenoxybenzamine is administered orally, it exhibits a gradual onset of action. This is because time is needed to form the active intermediate and bond covalently with α-adrenergic receptors. The drug has a duration of action of 3 to 4 days because of its stable covalent bonding with α-adrenergic receptors.

EFFECTS AND INDICATIONS. Because of its noncompetitive and relatively irreversible blockade of α-adrenergic receptors, phenoxybenzamine produces what has been called a **chemical sympathectomy.** It decreases vascular resistance; increases blood flow to the skin, mucosae, and abdominal viscera; and lowers both the supine and the standing blood pressure. It also relaxes smooth muscle in the urinary bladder neck and prostate.

As shown in Table 9–1, phenoxybenzamine is used to treat **hypertensive episodes** in patients with **pheochromocytoma.** Because this tumor of the adrenal medulla secretes huge amounts of catecholamines, patients have extremely high blood pressure and must be treated with an agent such as phenoxybenzamine to control hypertension until surgery can be performed to remove the tumor.

Phentolamine

CHEMISTRY AND PHARMACOKINETICS. Phentolamine is an imidazoline compound that is structurally related to oxymetazoline and other agents in the imidazoline class of adrenergic receptor agonists. After intravenous administration of phentolamine, the onset of action is immediate, and the duration of action is 10 to 15 minutes. After intramuscular or subcutaneous administration, the onset of action is 15 to 20 minutes, and the duration is 3 to 4 hours. The drug is chiefly metabolized in the liver before excretion in the urine.

MECHANISMS, EFFECTS, AND INDICATIONS. Phentolamine is a competitive receptor antagonist (see Fig. 9–1) that produces vasodilation, decreases peripheral vascular resistance, and decreases blood pressure. It is used in the diagnosis and treatment of **hypertensive episodes** caused by **pheochromocytoma.** In addition, it is used to treat **dermal necrosis and ischemia** caused by extravasation or accidental injection of epinephrine or other vasopressor amines. For example, if a patient who carries an epinephrine autoinjector for use in treating acute allergic reactions were to accidentally inject his or her finger and thereby cause ischemia, the patient could be treated by injecting phentolamine into the same site where epinephrine was injected. The phentolamine would competitively block the α-adrenergic receptor stimulation and vasoconstriction produced by the epinephrine.

Phentolamine and other nonselective α-blockers are not useful in treating chronic hypertension, partly because they produce too much reflex tachycardia and are associated with other adverse effects (e.g., dizziness, headache, and nasal congestion). The adverse effects are mostly caused by excessive vasodilation.

Selective α₁-Antagonists

Agents that selectively antagonize α₁-adrenergic receptors include **alfuzosin, doxazosin, prazosin, tamulosin,** and **terazosin.** Prazosin, the original drug in this class, was initially developed to treat hypertension. More recently, these drugs have also been used to treat urinary retention in men with benign prostatic hyperplasia.

General Properties

PHARMACOKINETICS. The selective α₁ receptor antagonists are administered orally and undergo varying amounts of first-pass and systemic metabolism. The drugs are highly bound to plasma proteins, including α₁-acid glycoprotein, and they are excreted in the bile, urine, and feces.

MECHANISMS, EFFECTS, AND INDICATIONS. The selective a1-blockers relax vascular and other smooth muscles, including those of the urinary bladder and prostate. Because they produce vasodilation and decrease blood pressure, they are used to treat chronic essential (primary) hypertension. The cardiovascular effects of α- and β-blockers in patients with hypertension are depicted in Fig. 9–2.

The selective α₁-blockers do not cause as much reflex tachycardia as do phentolamine and other agents that non-

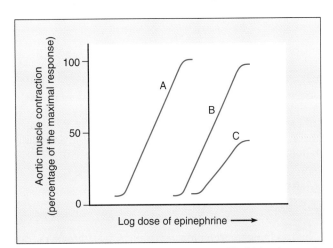

Figure 9–1. Competitive and noncompetitive blockade of epinephrine-induced aortic smooth muscle contraction by phentolamine and phenoxybenzamine. Three dose-response curves are compared. A is the curve of epinephrine alone. B is the curve of epinephrine in the presence of phentolamine. Because phentolamine is a competitive α-adrenergic receptor antagonist, epinephrine can surmount its effect. C is the curve of epinephrine in the presence of phenoxybenzamine. Because phenoxybenzamine is a noncompetitive antagonist, it reduces the maximal effect of epinephrine.

TABLE 9–1. **Mechanisms, Pharmacologic Effects, and Clinical Uses of Selected Adrenergic Receptor Antagonists***

Drug	Mechanism of Action	Pharmacologic Effect	Clinical Use
α-Blockers			
Doxazosin, Prazosin, Terazosin	Competitive α_1-blocker.	Cause vasodilation; decrease vascular resistance and blood pressure; and relax bladder neck and prostate.	Hypertension; urinary retention due to benign prostatic hyperplasia.
Alfuzosin, Tamsulosin	Competitive α_1 blocker.	Relax bladder neck and prostate.	Urinary retention due to benign prostatic hyperplasia.
Phenoxybenzamine	Noncompetitive α_1- and α_2-blocker.	Cause vasodilation; decrease vascular resistance.	Hypertensive episodes due to pheochromocytoma.
Phentolamine	Competitive α_1- and α_2-blocker.	Causes vasodilation; decreases vascular resistance and blood pressure.	Hypertensive episodes due to pheochromocytoma; necrosis and ischemia after injection of α-adrenergic receptor agonists.
β-Blockers			
Acebutolol	β_1-Blocker with ISA and MSA.	Decreases cardiac rate, output, AV node conduction, and O_2 demand; decreases blood pressure.	Hypertension; cardiac arrhythmias.
Atenolol	β_1-Blocker.	Same as acebutolol.	Hypertension; angina pectoris; acute myocardial infarction.
Esmolol	β_1-Blocker.	Same as acebutolol.	Acute supraventricular tachycardia.
Metoprolol	β_1-Blocker with MSA.	Same as acebutolol.	Hypertension; angina pectoris; acute myocardial infarction.
Nadolol	β_1- and β_2-Blocker.	Same as acebutolol.	Hypertension; angina pectoris; migraine headache.
Pindolol	β_1- and β_2-Blocker with ISA and MSA.	Same as acebutolol.	Hypertension.
Propranolol	β_1- and β_2-Blocker with MSA.	Same as acebutolol.	Hypertension; angina pectoris; cardiac arrhythmias; hypertrophic subaortic stenosis; essential tremor; migraine headache; acute thyrotoxicosis; acute myocardial infarction; pheochromocytoma.
Timolol	β_1- and β_2-Blocker.	Decreases cardiac rate, output, AV node conduction, and O_2 demand; decreases blood pressure; decreases intraocular pressure.	Hypertension; acute myocardial infarction; migraine headache; glaucoma.
α- and β-Blockers			
Carvedilol	β_1- and β_2-Blocker; α_1-blocker.	Causes vasodilation; decreases heart rate and blood pressure in patients with hypertension; increases cardiac output in patients with heart failure.	Hypertension; heart failure.
Labetalol	β_1- and β_2-Blocker with MSA; α_1-blocker.	Causes vasodilation; decreases heart rate and blood pressure.	Hypertension.

*ISA = intrinsic sympathomimetic activity (partial agonist activity); MSA = membrane-stabilizing activity (local anesthetic activity); and AV = atrioventricular.

selectively block both α_1- and α_2-receptors. This is because blockade of α_2-receptors on sympathetic neurons prevents feedback inhibition of norepinephrine release and thereby leads to increased activation of cardiac β_1-receptors and tachycardia (Fig. 9–3). The use of prazosin and other selective α_1-blockers to treat hypertension is discussed in greater detail in Chapter 10.

The ability of selective α_1-blockers to relax bladder and prostate smooth muscle has made them useful in treating **urinary retention** caused by **benign prostatic hyperplasia** and other conditions. In patients with prostatic hyperplasia, the enlarged prostate gland restricts the outflow of urine from the bladder and men with this condition complain of urinary frequency, urgency, and nocturia. By relaxing

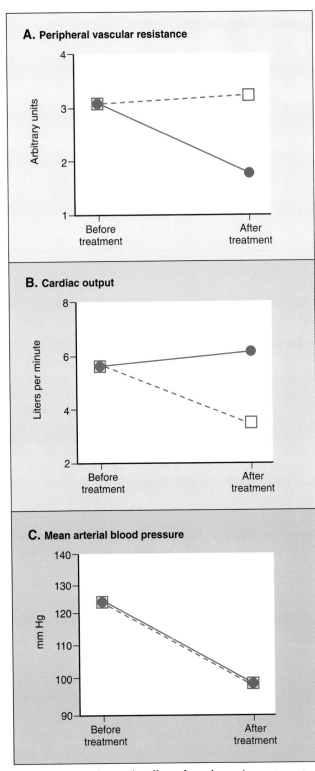

Figure 9–2. Cardiovascular effects of α₁-adrenergic receptor antagonists (solid line) and β₁-adrenergic receptor antagonists (dotted line) in patients with hypertension. (A) The α₁-blockers reduce peripheral vascular resistance. The β₁-blockers can cause a slight increase in peripheral vascular resistance, owing to reflex mechanisms. (B) The β₁-blockers reduce cardiac output. The α₁-blockers can increase cardiac output by decreasing cardiac afterload and aortic impedance to ventricular ejection of blood. (C) Both α₁-blockers and β₁-blockers reduce mean arterial blood pressure.

smooth muscle in the bladder neck and prostate, the selective α₁-blockers reduce the obstruction to urine outflow during micturition. This improves the urine flow rate, decreases the amount of urine retained, and reduces the need to urinate at night (Fig. 9–4).

The adverse effects of selective α₁-blockers are mostly caused by excessive vasodilation, which can cause hypotension, dizziness, fainting, reflex tachycardia, palpitations, and edema. The drugs often produce a greater effect on blood pressure when they are initially administered, leading to what has been called **first-dose syncope.** To prevent this phenomenon, patients should be given low doses when they begin treatment. Thereafter, doses can be increased to obtain the desired effect.

Specific Drugs

Prazosin, whose half-life is shorter than other α₁-antagonists, has a duration of action of about 6 hours. It undergoes considerable first-pass and systemic metabolism before renal and biliary excretion.

Doxazosin and terazosin are longer acting α₁-blockers that are usually administered once a day to treat hypertension or urinary symptoms of benign prostatic hyperplasia Their duration of action ranges from about 20 hours (terazosin) to about 30 hours (doxazosin).

Alfuzosin and tamulosin are newer uroselective α₁-blockers that relax bladder and prostatic smooth muscle without causing as much vasodilation and reflex tachycardia as other α₁-blockers. These drugs are only indicated for treating symptoms of urinary outflow obstruction in men with prostatic hyperplasia.

β-ADRENERGIC RECEPTOR ANTAGONISTS

The β-adrenergic receptor antagonists, or **β-blockers,** can be categorized as nonselective or selective.

Nonselective β-Blockers

The nonselective β-blockers were the first β-blockers to be developed for clinical use. In addition to blocking β₁ receptors in heart tissue, they block β₂ receptors in smooth muscle, liver, and other tissues. Examples include **nadolol, pindolol, propranolol,** and **timolol.**

General Properties

CHEMISTRY AND PHARMACOKINETICS. The β-adrenergic receptor antagonists are structural analogues of β-adrenergic receptor agonists. Fig. 9–5 shows the chemical structures and Table 9–2 outlines the pharmacologic properties of various β-blockers. All of the nonselective β-blockers can be administered orally, and propranolol can also be administered parenterally.

MECHANISMS AND EFFECTS. The nonselective β-blockers competitively block the effects of norepinephrine and other adrenergic agonists at β₁-and β₂-receptors. In addition, some of them exhibit intrinsic sympathomimetic activity (ISA)

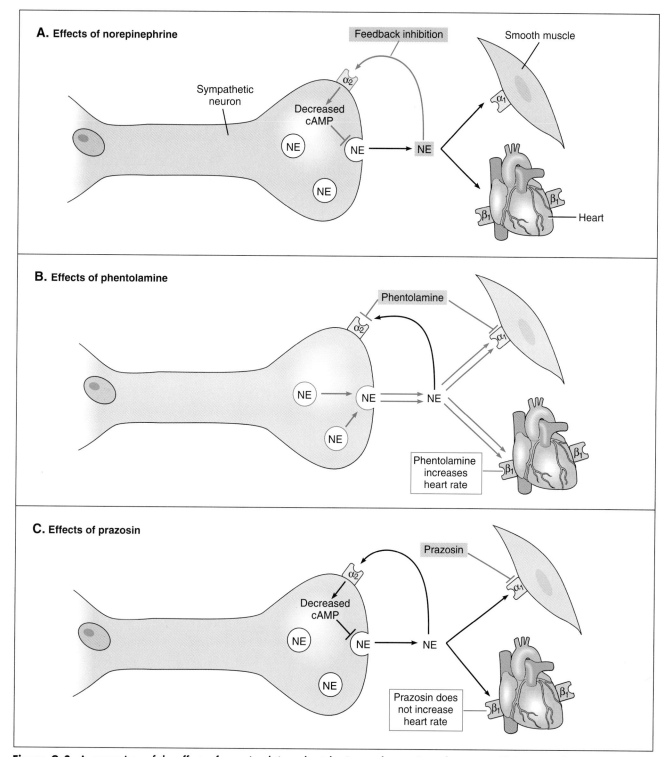

Figure 9–3. A comparison of the effects of norepinephrine, phentolamine, and prazosin on heart rate. (A) Norepinephrine (NE) activates presynaptic α_2-adrenergic receptors (α_2), and this inhibits the formation of cyclic adenosine monophosphate (cAMP) and decreases the release of NE. (B) Phentolamine blocks α_2 receptor-mediated inhibition of NE release. This increases the stimulation of cardiac β_1-adrenergic receptors (β_1) and results in tachycardia. (C) Prazosin, a selective α_1-blocker, does not block α_2 receptor-mediated inhibition of norepinephrine release. Therefore, prazosin causes less tachycardia than does phentolamine. α_1 = α_1-adrenergic receptors.

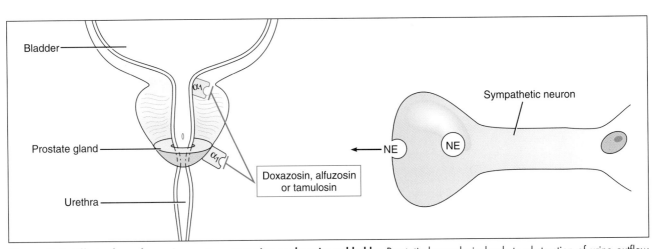

Figure 9–4. Effects of α_1-adrenergic receptor antagonists on the urinary bladder. Prostatic hyperplasia leads to obstruction of urine outflow from the bladder through the urethra. An α_1-blocker (e.g., doxazosin, alfuzosin, or tamulosin) will relax smooth muscle in the prostate and bladder neck and thereby facilitate micturition in patients with prostatic hyperplasia. $\alpha_1 = \alpha_1$-adrenergic receptors; and NE = norepinephrine.

Figure 9–5. Comparative structures of an adrenergic β-receptor agonist and β-receptor antagonists. Isoproterenol is a nonselective β_1 and β_2 receptor agonist. The β-receptor antagonists include propranolol, a nonselective β-antagonist, and atenolol, a selective β_1-antagonist. Each of these drugs contains an isopropyl group [-CH-(CH3)2] attached to the ethylamine side chain [-(CH-OH)-CH2-NH2-] that confers β-receptor selectivity. Carvedilol exerts nonselective β-blockade, α_1-receptor blockade, and antioxidant activity. The structures conferring these activities are identified in the figure.

TABLE 9–2.   **Pharmacokinetic Properties of Drugs That Cause β-Adrenergic Receptor Blockade**

Drug	Lipid Solubility	Oral Bioavailability	Elimination Half-Life	Intrinsic Sympathomimetic Activity	Membrane-Stabilizing Activity
Nonselective β-Blockers					
Nadolol	Low	35%	15–20 hours	None	None
Pindolol	Medium	75%	3–4 hours	Medium	Low
Propranolol	High	25%	4–6 hours	None	High
Timolol	Medium	50%	4–6 hours	None	None
Selective β₁-Blockers					
Acebutolol	Medium	40%	10–12 hours*	Low	Medium
Atenolol	Low	50%	6–7 hours	None	None
Esmolol	Low	—	10 minutes	None	None
Metoprolol	Medium	40%	3–4 hours	None	Low
α- and β-Blockers					
Carvedilol	Not known	30%	6–8 hours	None	None
Labetalol	Medium	20%	6–8 hours	None	Low

*Includes half-life of active metabolite.

and membrane-stabilizing (local anesthetic) activity, as outlined in Table 9–2 and defined below.

Blockade of β₁-receptors reduces sympathetic stimulation of the heart and thereby produces a negative chronotropic, inotropic, and dromotropic effect. Because the β-blockers reduce cardiac output and blood pressure (see Fig. 9–2), they can be used to treat arterial hypertension. In the kidneys, β₁-receptor blockade reduces the secretion of renin from the juxtaglomerular cells. In the eye, receptor blockade reduces aqueous humor secretion and intraocular pressure.

Blockade of β₂-receptors produces several effects that can lead to adverse reactions in some patients receiving β-blockers, such as patients with asthma or diabetes. In the lungs, antagonism of β₂-receptors can cause bronchoconstriction in patients with asthma. These patients depend on the bronchodilating effect of endogenous epinephrine to prevent bronchospasm, so agents that block β₂-receptors should be avoided or used with great caution. If a β-blocker is required to treat an asthmatic patient, a selective β₁-blocker should be used. In the liver, β₂-receptor blockade inhibits epinephrine-stimulated glycogenolysis and can thereby slow the recovery of blood glucose after a hypoglycemic episode in a patient with diabetes. The β-blockers can also mask some of the early signs of hypoglycemia (e.g., tachycardia and sweating), which would otherwise alert the diabetic patient to this problem. For these reasons, β-blockers should be used cautiously in patients with diabetes and particularly in those who have insulin-dependent diabetes and are susceptible to hypoglycemic episodes associated with excessive insulin administration.

Specific Properties

Tables 9–1 and 9–2 compare the effects, uses, and properties of four nonselective β-blockers: nadolol, pindolol, propranolol, and timolol.

Of these four drugs, only pindolol has **intrinsic sympathomimetic activity,** or **partial agonist activity,** which

enables it to exert a weak agonist effect on β-receptors. This effect is observed when the patient is resting and sympathetic tone is low, and it can result in a smaller reduction in heart rate than that caused by β-blockers without ISA. When sympathetic tone is high, pindolol acts as a competitive receptor antagonist to inhibit sympathetic stimulation of the heart in the same manner as other β-blockers.

Although pindolol and propranolol exhibit **membrane-stabilizing activity,** or **local anesthetic activity,** nadolol and timolol do not. Drugs with local anesthetic activity can block sodium channels in nerves and heart tissue and thereby slow conduction velocity.

Pindolol is used only to treat **hypertension.** In contrast, propranolol has many clinical applications. Propranolol is used, for example, to treat patients with **hypertension, angina pectoris,** or **cardiac arrhythmias** (conditions discussed in detail in the chapters of Section III); patients with **hypertrophic subaortic stenosis** (a form of hypertrophic cardiomyopathy, a condition that impedes the ejection of blood from the ventricles and reduces cardiac output); and patients with **essential tremor** (a benign condition characterized by involuntary trembling of the hands). Propranolol is also used to prevent **migraine headache** and as adjunctive therapy in the treatment of **acute thyrotoxicosis, acute myocardial infarction,** and **pheochromocytoma.** Patients with thyrotoxicosis often experience tachycardia and palpitations because thyroid hormones increase the effects of sympathetic stimulation on the heart. Propranolol is used to reduce these symptoms until the underlying thyroid disorder can be treated. Propranolol and other β-blockers are frequently administered to patients with acute myocardial infarction because clinical trials have shown that β-blockers reduce the incidence of sudden death and mortality in these patients. In patients with pheochromocytoma, propranolol is used to reduce cardiac stimulation caused by circulating catecholamines released from this adrenal medullary tumor.

Propranolol, the first β-blocker approved for clinical use, is distinguished by its high lipid solubility and central nervous system penetration, which can cause a higher incidence of central nervous system side effects in some patients. Propranolol has a greater local anesthetic effect than other β-blockers, but the clinical significance of this activity is uncertain.

Nadolol is a long-acting drug that is largely excreted unchanged in the urine. It is primarily used to treat **hypertension** and **angina pectoris** and to prevent **migraine headache.**

Timolol is administered orally to treat **hypertension,** to reduce the risk of death in patients with **acute myocardial infarction,** and to prevent **migraine headache.** Timolol was the first β-blocker to be used to treat **glaucoma** and is available as an ophthalmic solution for topical ocular administration. The drug is absorbed through the cornea and penetrates to the ciliary body. In glaucoma, which is discussed in greater detail in Chapter 6, β-blockers reduce aqueous humor secretion and intraocular pressure. Timolol was selected for ophthalmic use partly because it does not have membrane-stabilizing activity and, therefore, does not anesthetize the cornea when instilled into the eye.

Selective β₁-Blockers

General Properties

Examples of selective β₁-blockers include **acebutolol, atenolol, esmolol,** and **metoprolol.** These drugs have a greater affinity for β₁-receptors than for β₂-receptors. Because β₁-receptors are primarily located in cardiac tissue, the β₁-blockers are also known as **cardioselective β-blockers.**

In comparison with the nonselective β-blockers, the selective β₁-blockers produce less bronchoconstriction and other β₂ receptor-mediated effects. Their selectivity for β₁-receptors, however, is not absolute, and β₂-receptor blockade increases with dosage. For this reason, selective β₁-blockers should be used with caution in patients who have asthma.

Specific Properties

Tables 9–1 and 9–2 compare the effects, uses, and properties of four selective β₁-blockers.

Acebutolol is a cardioselective β-blocker with a low degree of ISA. It is converted to an active metabolite, *N*-acetyl acebutolol, which has a longer half-life than the parent compound and accounts for the drug's relatively long duration of action. Acebutolol is administered orally to treat **hypertension** and **cardiac arrhythmias** (e.g., ventricular premature beats).

Atenolol shows less variability in its oral absorption than other β-blockers and is excreted largely unchanged in the urine. It also has a lower lipid solubility and has been associated with a lower incidence of central nervous system side effects (e.g., vivid dreams, tiredness, and depression). Atenolol is administered orally or parenterally and is primarily used to treat **hypertension, angina pectoris,** and **acute myocardial infarction.**

Esmolol is administered intravenously to treat hypertension and **acute supraventricular tachycardia** in cases, for example, when this cardiac arrhythmia occurs during

surgery. Esmolol is rapidly metabolized to inactive compounds by plasma esterase enzymes and has a much shorter half-life than other β-blockers.

Metoprolol is used to treat **hypertension, angina pectoris,** and **acute myocardial infarction.** It can be administered orally or parenterally, and it is extensively metabolized by cytochrome P450 enzymes before undergoing renal excretion.

Other selective β₁-selective antagonists include bisoprolol (ZEBETA) and betaxolol (BETOPTIC, KERLONE). Both of these drugs are administered orally to treat hypertension, and betaxolol is also used to treat chronic open-angle glaucoma. Topical ocular administration of betaxolol reduces aqueous humor secretion while producing negligible blockade of systemic β-receptors.

α- AND β-ADRENERGIC RECEPTOR ANTAGONISTS

Carvedilol and **labetalol** are agents that block both α- and β-adrenergic receptors. Their effects, uses, and properties are shown in Tables 9–1 and 9–2. Carvedilol blocks β₁-, β₂-, and α₁-receptors, and possesses antioxidant activity (see Fig. 9–5). Each of these actions contributes to its cardioprotective effects in persons with myocardial infarction. The antioxidant effects of carvedilol include (1) inhibition of lipid peroxidation in myocardial membranes, (2) scavenging of free radicals, and (3) inhibition of neutrophil release of O_2. In addition, carvedilol has antiapoptotic properties that can prevent myocyte death and reduce infarct size in persons suffering from myocardial ischemia. For these reasons, carvedilol has been called a "third-generation β-blocker and neurohumoral antagonist," and its value in treating myocardial infarction has been established in clinical trials.

Carvedilol decreases blood pressure and has been used in the treatment of **hypertension.** As discussed further in Chapter 12, it also decreases cardiac afterload, increases cardiac output, and reduces mortality in patients with **heart failure.**

Labetalol is a nonselective β-blocker and a selective α₁-blocker that is primarily used in the treatment of **hypertension.** It is 5 to 10 times more potent as a β-blocker than as an α-blocker, but both actions are believed to contribute to its antihypertensive effect. Labetalol decreases heart rate and cardiac output as a result of β₁-receptor blockade, and it decreases peripheral vascular resistance as a result of α₁-receptor blockade.

SUMMARY OF IMPORTANT POINTS

■ The α-adrenergic receptor antagonists (α-blockers) relax smooth muscle and decrease vascular resistance, whereas the β-adrenergic receptor antagonists (β-blockers) reduce heart rate and cardiac output. Both α-blockers and β-blockers reduce blood pressure.

■ The nonselective α-blockers include phenoxybenzamine (a noncompetitive blocker) and phentolamine (a competitive blocker). These drugs block both α_1- and α_2-receptors and are primarily used to treat hypertensive episodes caused by pheochromocytoma.

■ The selective α_1-blockers include alfuzosin, doxazosin, prazosin, tamsulosin, and terazosin. These drugs are used to treat chronic essential (primary) hypertension or to treat urinary retention caused by benign prostatic hyperplasia and other conditions.

■ The nonselective β-blockers, which antagonize both β_1- and β_2-receptors, include nadolol, pindolol, propranolol, and timolol. In comparison with other β-blockers, pindolol has a higher degree of intrinsic sympathomimetic activity (partial agonist activity), and propranolol has a higher degree of membrane-stabilizing activity (local anesthetic activity).

■ The selective β_1-blockers include acebutolol, atenolol, esmolol, and metoprolol. These drugs cause less bronchoconstriction than do nonselective β-blockers.

■ The β-blockers have a variety of clinical applications, including the prevention of migraine headache and the treatment of hypertension, angina pectoris, cardiac arrhythmias, and glaucoma.

■ Carvedilol blocks α– and β–receptors and exerts other cardioprotective effects that make it useful in the treatment of myocardial infarction and heart failure.

Review Questions

Questions 1 to 4. For each patient described, select the most appropriate drug from the lettered choices.
(A) atenolol
(B) labetalol
(C) phenoxybenzamine
(D) phentolamine
(E) propranolol
(F) tamsulosin

1. A woman experiences pain and ischemia in her finger after accidentally injecting it with an epinephrine autoinjector that she carries for emergency treatment of allergic reactions.

2. A man complains of urinary urgency, frequency, and nocturia and is found to have benign enlargement of the prostate gland.

3. A woman with essential hypertension requires a drug that reduces both cardiac output and peripheral resistance.

4. A patient with episodic severe hypertension is found to have markedly elevated levels of epinephrine and norepinephrine metabolites in his urine, and requires a long-acting drug to lower blood pressure before surgery.

Question 5. Choose the single best answer from the lettered choices.

5. Which drug is least likely to slow recovery from hypoglycemia in a diabetic patient who has taken an excessive dose of insulin?
(A) atenolol
(B) nadolol
(C) propranolol
(D) pindolol
(E) labetalol

Answers and Explanations

1. The answer is D: phentolamine. Epinephrine and other adrenergic agonists can cause excessive vasoconstriction and ischemia when injected into fingers, toes, or other tissues because of stimulation of adrenergic α_1-receptors in vascular smooth muscle. Phentolamine is a nonselective α–receptor antagonist that can be injected directly into affected tissues to counteract the vasoconstrictive effects of adrenergic agonists.

2. The answer is F: tamsulosin. Tamsulosin is a selective α_1-receptor blocker that acts to relax smooth muscle in the bladder outflow tract and thereby relieve urinary retention caused by prostatic hyperplasia. The drug is sometimes used in combination with finasteride or other drugs that inhibit the 5α-reductase enzyme that converts testosterone to dihydrotestosterone and thereby contributes to stimulation of prostatic growth.

3. The answer is B: labetalol. Labetalol is a nonselective β-receptor antagonist and a selective α_1-receptor antagonist that is used to treat hypertension. It acts to reduce cardiac output by blocking cardiac β_1-receptors and to reduce peripheral resistance by blocking α_1-receptors in vascular smooth muscle.

4. The answer is C: phenoxybenzamine. The patient most likely has a tumor of the adrenal medulla called pheochromocytoma. This tumor secretes massive quantities of epinephrine and norepinephrine, thereby causing severe hypertension. Phenoxybenzamine is a noncompetitive, long-acting adrenergic α-receptor antagonist that is sometimes used to reduce blood pressure in patients with this condition.

5. The answer is A: atenolol. Nonselective adrenergic β–blockers (e.g., propranolol) can block epinephrine-induced glycogenolysis mediated by β_2-receptors in the liver, and thereby slow recovery from hypoglycemia. Selective β_1-blockers (e.g., atenolol) are less likely to produce this effect.

SELECTED READINGS

Chapple, C. R. Pharmacological therapy of benign prostatic hyperplasia/lower urinary tract symptoms: an overview for the practising clinician. BJU Int 94:738–44, 2004.
Dulin, B., and W. T. Abraham. Pharmacology of carvedilol. Am J Cardiol 93:3B–6B, 2004.
Lopez-Sendon, J., K. Swedberg, and J. McMurray, et al. Expert consensus document on beta-adrenergic receptor blockers. Eur Heart J 25:1341–1362, 2004.

CARDIOVASCULAR, RENAL, AND HEMATOLOGIC PHARMACOLOGY

CHAPTER 10

Antihypertensive Drugs

CLASSIFICATION OF ANTIHYPERTENSIVE DRUGS

Diuretics
Thiazide and Related Diuretics
- Hydrochlorothiazide[a]

Potassium-sparing Diuretics
- Amiloride[b]

Sympatholytics
Adrenergic Receptor Antagonists
- Atenolol (TENORMIN)[c]
- Doxazosin (CARDURA)[d]
- Labetalol (NORMODYNE, TRANDATE)
- Carvedilol (COREG)

Centrally Acting Drugs
- Clonidine[e]

Angiotensin Inhibitors
Angiotensin-converting Enzyme Inhibitors
- Enalapril (VASOTEC)[f]

Angiotensin Receptor Antagonists
- Losartan (COZAAR)[g]

Vasodilators
Calcium Channel Blockers
- Amlodipine (VORVASC)[h]

Other Vasodilators
- Hydralazine[i]

Dopamine Agonist
- Fenoldopam (CORLOPAM)

[a]also indapamide, metolazone
[b]also spironolactone, eplerenone, triamterene
[c]also betaxolol, bisoprolol, metoprolol, nadolol, pindolol, propranolol, timolol
[d]also prazosin, terazosin
[e]also guanfacine, methyldopa
[f]also benazepril, captopril, fosinopril, lisinopril, moexipril, perindopril, quinapril, ramipril, trandolapril
[g]also candesartan, eprosartan, irbesartan, telmisartan, and valsartan
[h]also diltiazem, felodipine, isradipine, nicardipine, nifedipine, nisolidpine, verapamil
[i]also minoxidil, nitroprusside

OVERVIEW

Hypertension

An estimated 50 million people in the United States of America have high blood pressure (hypertension), commonly defined as a sustained systolic blood pressure of 140 mm Hg or higher or a sustained diastolic blood pressure of 90 mm Hg or higher. Numerous studies have shown that untreated high blood pressure damages blood vessels, accelerates **atherosclerosis,** and produces **left ventricular hypertrophy.** The rate at which these changes occur is proportional to the severity of hypertension. Eventually, these abnormalities contribute to the development of **ischemic** heart disease, stroke, heart failure, and renal failure, which are the most common causes of death in patients who are hypertensive.

Over the past several decades, health professionals and public officials have increased their efforts to educate the public about the hazards of untreated hypertension, and this has led to a significant increase in the number of hypertensive individuals who are aware of their condition and treat it effectively via lifestyle modifications and pharmacologic agents. The effective treatment of high blood pressure appears to be one of the factors that has contributed to a nearly 60% reduction in the incidence of stroke and at least a 50% reduction in the mortality rate from coronary artery disease since 1970.

About 95% of the cases of hypertension are considered to be **primary hypertension** that cannot be attributed to a specific cause. The other 5% of cases are classified as **secondary hypertension**, which results from an identifiable cause such as chronic kidney disease, pheochromocytoma (a tumor of the adrenal medulla), or hyperaldosteronism. In some cases, secondary hypertension can be corrected by medication or surgery.

Although the cause of primary hypertension in any specific patient is usually unknown, numerous genetic and lifestyle factors are associated with it. These include obesity, lack of exercise, the so-called metabolic syndrome (abdominal obesity, hyperlipidemia, and insulin resistance), excessive dietary sodium intake by individuals with salt sensitivity, and excessive consumption of alcohol.

In recent years, the role of vascular **endothelial cell dysfunction** in the genesis and maintenance of hypertension has received increased attention. The endothelium is an important regulator of vascular smooth muscle tone via the synthesis and release of several relaxing factors, including **nitric oxide** (NO) and **prostacyclin** (PGI_2), as well as vasoconstricting factors such as endothelin-1 and angiotensin II. In addition to its vasoconstrictive effect, angiotensin II produces vascular injury via activation of growth factors that cause vascular smooth muscle proliferation and hypertrophy as well as fibrotic changes in the vascular wall. Oxidative stress and other pathologic stimuli appear to alter the ratio of endothelial relaxing factors and vasoconstrictive factors, thereby contributing to the development of hypertension. Several antihypertensive drugs, including carvedilol and the angiotensin inhibitors, appear to counteract endothelial cell dysfunction and thereby reduce some of the adverse consequences of hypertensive disease.

Classification of Blood Pressure

The classification of blood pressure shown in Table 10–1 was presented in the Seventh Report of the Joint National Committee on the Prevention, Detection, Evaluation, and Treatment of High Blood Pressure (JNC 7; Chobanian et al., 2003). This new classification includes the term "**prehypertension**" for those with blood pressures ranging from 120 to 139 mm Hg systolic, 80 to 89 mm Hg diastolic blood pressure, or both. This new designation was intended to identify persons in whom early adoption of **lifestyle changes** that decrease blood pressure could prevent the progression of blood pressure to hypertensive levels (see below). These persons are not candidates for drug therapy unless they have **diabetes** and a trial of lifestyle changes fails to reduce their blood pressure to the desired level of 130/80 mm Hg or less for diabetics.

The new classification includes two stages of hypertension that confer differences in follow-up recommendations and management. In addition to providing information about lifestyle modifications, stage 1 hypertension should be confirmed within 2 months and then treated appropriately. Stage 2 hypertension should be treated immediately if blood pressure is greater than 180/110 mm Hg. For lower blood pressures, stage 2 hypertension should be evaluated and treated within 1 month.

Regulation of Blood Pressure

From a systemic hemodynamic perspective, blood pressure is regulated primarily by the **sympathetic nervous system** and the **kidneys** through their influence on cardiac output and peripheral vascular resistance. There is increasing awareness that vasoactive and other substances produced within the blood vessel wall may have a substantial role in the regulation of blood pressure and in the pathophysiology of hypertension.

Cardiac output, which is the product of stroke volume and heart rate, is increased by sympathetic stimulation via activation of β_1-adrenergic receptors in the heart. Cardiac output is also influenced by the kidneys via their regulation of blood volume, which is one of the factors determining the cardiac filling pressure and stroke volume.

Peripheral vascular resistance (PVR) is chiefly determined by the resistance to blood flow through the arterioles, whose cross-sectional area depends on arteriolar smooth muscle tone in the various vascular beds. Via activation of α_1-adrenergic receptors, the sympathetic nervous system stimulates arteriolar smooth muscle contraction, and this leads to vasoconstriction. Several blood-borne substances, including vasopressin and angiotensin II, produce vasoconstriction. In addition, adenosine, serotonin, endothelin,

TABLE 10-1. **Classification of Blood Pressure for Adults and Follow-up Recommendations***

Blood Pressure Classification	SBP[1] mm Hg	DBP[2] mm Hg	Follow-up Recommendations
Normal	<120	and <80	Check again in 2 years
Prehypertension	120–139	or 80–90	Check again in 1 year
Stage 1 hypertension	140–159	or 90–99	Confirm within 2 months
Stage 2 hypertension	>160	or >100	Evaluate within 1 week to 1 month[3]

*Seventh Report of the Joint National Committee on Prevention, Detection, Evaluation, and Treatment of High Blood Pressure.
[1]Systolic blood pressure.
[2]Diastolic blood pressure.
[3]Based on blood pressure level and clinical situation.

prostaglandins, and a number of other substances produced locally in various tissues have an effect on arteriolar smooth muscle tone. These substances serve to regulate blood flow through the tissues, and they can also affect systemic arterial pressure.

The sympathetic nervous system provides **short-term regulation** of blood pressure through the **baroreceptor reflex.** This reflex modulates sympathetic stimulation of cardiac output and PVR and adjusts blood pressure in response to postural changes and altered physical activity. The kidneys are primarily responsible for the **long-term control** of blood pressure, via regulation of plasma volume and the renin-angiotensin-aldosterone axis. By these mechanisms, the sympathetic system and kidneys maintain arterial blood pressure within a fairly narrow range when a person is at rest, and they adjust blood pressure appropriately in response to postural changes and physical activity.

In normotensive individuals, an increase in blood pressure leads to a proportional increase in sodium and water excretion by the kidneys, so that blood volume is reduced and blood pressure returns to its normal "set point." In hypertensive patients, the set point at which blood pressure is controlled is higher than normal; the regulation of blood pressure is defective; and an increase in blood pressure is not followed by a proportional increase in sodium and water excretion by the kidneys. Although studies have shown that PVR is elevated in most hypertensive patients, it is not clear whether this is the cause or the result of hypertension.

Sites and Effects of Antihypertensive Drug Action

The four major categories of antihypertensive drugs are the diuretics, sympatholytics, angiotensin inhibitors, and vasodilators. Subcategories and examples are listed at the beginning of the chapter. The various antihypertensive drugs lower blood pressure through actions exerted on one or more of the following sites: kidneys, sympathetic nervous system, renin-angiotensin-aldosterone axis, or vascular smooth muscle (Fig. 10–1).

Antihypertensive drugs can be characterized in terms of their cardiovascular effects (Table 10–2) and their pharmacologic effects on serum potassium and cholesterol measurements, which are important **cardiovascular risk factors** (Table 10–3). They can also be characterized in terms of the **compensatory mechanisms** invoked by their hypotensive effect. The compensatory mechanisms tend to return blood pressure to the pretreatment level and include reflex tachycardia, fluid retention by the kidneys, and activation of the renin-angiotensin-aldosterone axis. Drugs that cause vasodilation tend to invoke compensatory mechanisms to a greater extent than do drugs that suppress cardiac output, cause diuresis, or inhibit angiotensin. For this reason, vasodilators are often combined with other types of drugs (e.g., diuretics) that prevent compensatory responses.

Whereas most antihypertensive drugs are taken orally on a long-term basis, some are administered parenterally

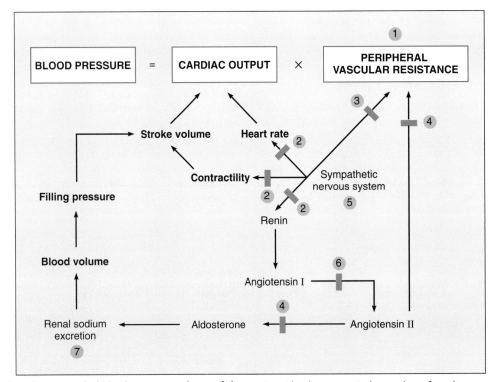

Figure 10-1. Physiologic control of blood pressure and sites of drug action. Blood pressure is the product of cardiac output and peripheral vascular resistance. These parameters are regulated on a systemic level by the sympathetic nervous system and the kidneys. Antihypertensive drugs act to suppress excessive sympathetic activity and modify renal function to counteract the mechanisms responsible for hypertension. Sites of action of the following drugs are shown: (1) vasodilators; (2) β-adrenergic receptor antagonists (β-blockers); (3) α-adrenergic receptor antagonists (α-blockers); (4) angiotensin receptor antagonists; (5) centrally acting sympatholytics; (6) angiotensin-converting enzyme (ACE) inhibitors; and (7) diuretics. The vasodilators, sympatholytics, and angiotensin inhibitors reduce peripheral vascular resistance; β-adrenergic receptor blockers reduce cardiac output; and diuretics promote sodium excretion and reduce blood volume.

TABLE 10-2. Cardiovascular Effects of Antihypertensive Drugs

Drug Classification	Peripheral Vascular Resistance	Cardiac Output	Blood Volume	Plasma Renin Activity	Left Ventricular Hypertrophy
Diuretics					
Thiazide and loop diuretics	Decrease	Decrease	Decrease	Increase	No change or decrease
Potassium-sparing diuretics	Decrease	Decrease	Decrease	Increase	No change or decrease
Sympatholytics					
α-Adrenergic receptor antagonists	Decrease	No change or increase	No change or increase	No change or decrease	Decrease
β-Adrenergic receptor antagonists	No change or decrease	Decrease	No change or decrease	Decrease	Decrease
Centrally acting drugs	Decrease	No change or decrease	Increase*	Decrease	Decrease
Angiotensin inhibitors					
Angiotensin-converting enzyme inhibitors	Decrease	No change or increase	No change	Increase	Decrease
Angiotensin receptor antagonists	Decrease	No change or increase	No change or increase	Increase	Decrease
Vasodilators					
Calcium channel blockers	Decrease	No change or increase†	No change	No change or increase	Decrease
Other vasodilators					
Hydralazine	Decrease	Increase	Increase	Increase	Increase
Minoxidil	Decrease	Increase	Increase	Increase	Increase
Nitroprusside	Decrease	Increase	Increase	Increase	No change or increase

*Two exceptions are guanabenz and guanfacine, which either cause no change in blood volume or decrease it slightly.
†An exception is verapamil, which may increase or decrease cardiac output.

TABLE 10-3. Pharmacologic Effects of Antihypertensive Drugs on Serum Potassium and Cholesterol Measurements

Drug Classification	Serum Potassium	Total Cholesterol	Low-Density Lipoproteins	High-Density Lipoproteins	Triglycerides
Diuretics					
Thiazide and loop diuretics	Decrease	Increase	Increase	No change or decrease	Increase
Potassium-sparing diuretics	Increase	Unknown	Unknown	Unknown	Unknown
Sympatholytics					
α-Adrenergic receptor antagonists	No change	Decrease	Decrease	Increase	Decrease
β-Adrenergic receptor antagonists	Slight increase	No change or increase	No change or increase	Variable	No change or increase
Centrally acting drugs	No change	No change	No change	No change	No change
Angiotensin inhibitors					
Angiotensin-converting enzyme inhibitors	Increase	No change	No change	No change	No change
Angiotensin receptor antagonists	Increase	No change	No change	No change	No change
Vasodilators					
Calcium channel blockers	No change	No change	No change	No change	No change
Other vasodilators					
Hydralazine	No change	No change	No change	No change	No change
Minoxidil	No change	No change	No change	No change	No change
Nitroprusside	No change	Not applicable*	Not applicable*	Not applicable*	Not applicable*

*Nitroprusside is used only for short-term management of hypertension.

for the management of **hypertensive emergencies**. The treatment of this condition is discussed at the end of the chapter.

DIURETICS

Chapter 13 provides detailed information about the various classes of diuretics and their uses, mechanisms of action, and pharmacologic properties. The discussion here focuses on the diuretics most commonly used to treat hypertension: the thiazide and related diuretics, and the potassium-sparing diuretics.

All diuretics cause an increase in renal sodium excretion. This so-called **natriuretic effect,** or **natriuresis,** appears to be responsible for some of their antihypertensive activity. The thiazide diuretics have a moderate natriuretic effect and are the diuretics used most frequently in the treatment of hypertension. The loop diuretics have the greatest natriuretic effect of all classes of diuretics, but are usually less effective in treating hypertension than are thiazide diuretics. Loop diuretics can be used to treat hypertension when a thiazide diuretic is not effective or is contraindicated. The potassium-sparing diuretics have a relatively low natriuretic effect and are primarily used in combination with a thiazide or loop diuretic to reduce potassium excretion and prevent hypokalemia.

Thiazide and Related Diuretics

Thiazide and related diuretics reduce blood pressure by two mechanisms, both stemming from their ability to increase sodium and water excretion. When they are first administered to a patient, the drugs decrease blood volume and thereby decrease cardiac output (Fig. 10–2 and Table 10–2). With continued administration over weeks and months, they also decrease PVR, and this appears to account for much of their long-term antihypertensive effect. The decreased PVR may result from a reduction in the sodium content of arteriolar smooth muscle cells, which decreases muscle contraction in response to vasopressor agents such as norepinephrine and angiotensin. This relationship is supported by the finding that the effect of a thiazide on PVR is reduced if patients ingest enough dietary sodium to counteract the natriuretic effect of the drug.

Use of a thiazide typically reduces the blood pressure by 10 to 15 mm Hg. **Hydrochlorothiazide** is the thiazide diuretic most often used to treat hypertension. **Indapamide, metolazone,** and other thiazide-like diuretics have equivalent efficacy in the treatment of hypertension and differ primarily in their pharmacokinetic properties. Indapamide can also cause vasodilation via calcium channel blockade.

The JNC 7 report recommends a thiazide diuretic for initial therapy of most patients with high blood pressure. Thiazide diuretics can be used alone or in combination with another type of antihypertensive agent (e.g., a sympatholytic, an angiotensin inhibitor, or a vasodilator). The two drugs usually have an additive effect on blood pressure, and the diuretic prevents the compensatory fluid retention that otherwise can be evoked by the other agent. The JNC 7

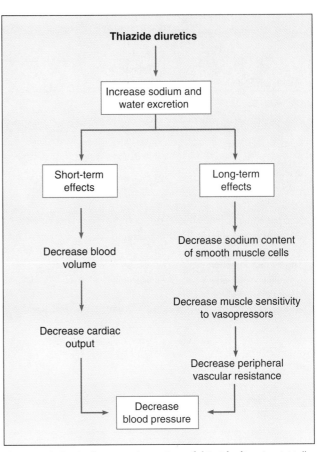

Figure 10-2. Antihypertensive actions of thiazide diuretics. Initially, thiazide diuretics decrease blood volume and thereby decrease cardiac output. Over time, the drugs decrease peripheral vascular resistance, an action that may be secondary to a reduction in the sodium content of smooth muscle cells.

report indicates that more than two thirds of patients with hypertension cannot have their condition controlled with a single drug.

The common adverse effects and interactions of thiazide diuretics and other antihypertensive agents are summarized in Table 10–4. The primary disadvantage of thiazide diuretics is their tendency to cause hypokalemia, which can lead to cardiac arrhythmias. Using a low dosage of a thiazide diuretic (e.g., 25 to 50 mg/d of hydrochlorothiazide) usually produces a maximal antihypertensive effect with minimal hypokalemia. Using a higher dosage causes more hypokalemia but does not have a greater effect on blood pressure. Thiazides elevate plasma levels of glucose, uric acid, and lipids in some patients. Less commonly, they cause hematologic toxicity and aggravate hepatic disease. They can also evoke a compensatory increase in renin secretion, and this reduces their effectiveness in some patients.

An advantage of taking thiazide diuretics is that they appear to offer protection against **osteoporosis,** a condition in which bone demineralization and loss of bone mass make patients more susceptible to fractures. Thiazides are probably beneficial in this condition because they decrease the urinary excretion of calcium.

Loop Diuretics

Despite the greater natriuretic effect of loop diuretics, they are usually less effective than thiazide diuretics in the treatment of hypertensive patients with normal renal function. For this reason, loop diuretics are usually reserved for use in hypertensive patients who have poor renal function and a serum creatinine level greater than 2.3 mg/dL.

Potassium-Sparing Diuretics

Examples of potassium-sparing diuretics are **amiloride, spironolactone,** and **triamterene.** These agents exert a mild natriuretic and antihypertensive effect. They also reduce renal potassium excretion and thereby prevent hypokalemia, a common problem caused by other diuretics.

Several drug products that contain both a thiazide diuretic and amiloride or triamterene are available. Potassium chloride tablets can also be used to prevent and treat hypokalemia.

Eplerenone is a newer aldosterone receptor antagonist that is similar to spironolactone but has fewer endocrine side effects. Eplerenone has been found to cause regression of left ventricular hypertrophy in hypertensive patients and regression of microalbuminuria in patients with type 2 diabetes. These findings open the possibility of increased use of this drug in persons with these conditions.

SYMPATHOLYTICS

The sympatholytics used in the treatment of hypertension include adrenergic receptor antagonists and the centrally acting α_2 receptor agonists. The pharmacologic effects of these drugs are summarized in Tables 10–2 and 10–3 and their common adverse effects and drug interactions are listed in Table 10–4.

Adrenergic Receptor Antagonists

The sympatholytics used most often to treat hypertension are the β-adrenergic receptor antagonists β-blockers) and α-adrenergic receptor antagonists (α-blockers). The β-blockers are among the preferred drugs for the initial treatment of hypertension (see below), whereas the α-blockers are only indicated in specific situations (e.g., in men, to treat concurrent prostatic hyperplasia).

α-Adrenergic Receptor Antagonists

The α-blockers act to inhibit sympathetic stimulation of arteriolar contraction. Selective α_1-blockers, such as **doxazosin, prazosin,** and **terazosin,** are used for the chronic treatment of primary hypertension because they produce less reflex tachycardia than do nonselective α_1- and α_2-blockers (e.g., phentolamine and phenoxybenzamine). **Phenoxybenzamine** has been used to manage patients with hypertensive episodes caused by pheochromocytoma because of its long-acting, irreversible blockade of α-receptors.

Prazosin and other α_1-blockers evoke reflex activation of the sympathetic nervous system and can increase the heart rate, contractile force, circulating norepinephrine level, and myocardial oxygen demand. These drugs do not protect the heart against ventricular arrhythmias and they are less useful in patients with ischemic heart disease. Because they also activate the renin-angiotensin-aldosterone system and can cause some fluid retention, they are frequently given in combination with a diuretic. The α_1-blockers can also cause orthostatic hypotension. For these reasons, α_1-blockers are not preferred drugs for the initial treatment of most patients with high blood pressure.

The use of a selective α_1-blocker and a diuretic causes first-dose syncope in some patients, but this can be prevented by beginning treatment with a low dose of the blocker at bedtime and withholding the diuretic for 1 day. The pharmacokinetic properties and other pharmacologic effects and uses of α-blockers are covered in Chapter 9.

β-Adrenergic Receptor Antagonists

The β-blockers are widely used in the treatment of hypertension because they are relatively safe and effective in most patients and are particularly useful in patients who suffer from angina or have a history of myocardial infarction. The drugs are cardioprotective and only rarely cause orthostatic hypotension or produce hepatic, renal, or hematopoietic toxicity. For these reasons, β-blockers provide effective therapy for many patients with mild hypertension and can be combined with other drugs to achieve greater reductions in blood pressure.

The β-blockers produce their therapeutic effects in patients with hypertension and other cardiovascular diseases by blocking β_1-adrenergic receptors in the heart and other tissues. This reduces cardiac output by decreasing the heart rate and contractility. The β-blockers inhibit renin secretion from renal juxtaglomerular cells, which, in turn, reduces the formation of angiotensin II and the subsequent release of aldosterone. The drugs also appear to reduce sympathetic outflow from the central nervous system (CNS). Hence, β-blockers have multiple actions affecting blood pressure.

Chapter 9 compares the properties of **atenolol, betaxolol, bisoprolol, esmolol, metoprolol,** and other cardioselective (β_1-selective) β-blockers with those of **nadolol, pindolol, propranolol, timolol,** and other nonselective β-blockers. Although these agents appear to be equally effective in lowering blood pressure, the selective β_1-blockers may be preferred for hypertensive patients with diabetes or chronic obstructive lung disease. The β-blockers are usually not used in asthmatic patients because they can induce bronchoconstriction by blocking the bronchodilating effect of circulating epinephrine. Atenolol is less lipophilic than propranolol and usually causes fewer CNS side effects.

Labetalol, a combined α- and β-adrenergic receptor antagonist, is used to treat both chronic hypertension and hypertensive emergencies. Because of its α-adrenergic receptor-blocking activity, it can cause orthostatic hypotension. **Esmolol** is an intravenously administered, ultrashort-acting β-blocker that is used to treat hypertension in surgical patients and in persons with hypertensive emergencies. **Carvedilol** is a unique α- and β-blocker with antioxidant properties that can protect the vascular wall from free radicals that damage blood vessels and thereby contribute to

TABLE 10–4. **Adverse Effects, Contraindications, and Drug Interactions of Antihypertensive Agents***

Drug Classification	Common Adverse Effects	Common Drug Interactions
Diuretics		
Thiazide and loop diuretics	Blood cell deficiencies, hyperlipidemia, hyperuricemia, hypokalemia, and other electrolyte changes Aggravation of diabetes	Increase serum levels of lithium. Hypotensive effect decreased by NSAIDs and augmented by ACE inhibitors
Potassium-sparing diuretics	Hyperkalemia	Hyperkalemic effect increased by ACE inhibitors and potassium supplements
Sympatholytics		
α-Adrenergic receptor antagonists	Dizziness, first-dose syncope, fluid retention, and orthostatic hypotension	Hypotensive effect increased by β-adrenergic receptor antagonists and diuretics
β-Adrenergic receptor antagonists	Bradycardia, bronchoconstriction, depression, fatigue, impaired glycogenolysis, and vivid dreams	Cardiac depression increased by diltiazem and verapamil. Hypotensive effect decreased by NSAIDs
Centrally acting drugs		
Clonidine	Dry mouth, fatigue, rebound hypertension, and sedation	Hypotensive effect decreased by tricyclic antidepressants Sedative effect increased by CNS depressants
Guanabenz	Same as clonidine	Same as clonidine
Guanfacine	Same as clonidine but milder	Same as clonidine
Methyldopa	Autoimmune hemolytic anemia, hepatitis, and lupuslike syndrome. Other adverse effects same as those of clonidine	Hypotensive effect increased by levodopa. Other interactions same as those of clonidine
Angiotensin inhibitors		
Angiotensin-converting enzyme (ACE) inhibitors	Acute renal failure, angioedema, cough, hyperkalemia, loss of taste, neutropenia, and rash	Increase serum levels of lithium. Hyperkalemic effect increased by potassium-sparing diuretics and potassium supplements. Hypotensive effect decreased by NSAIDs
Angiotensin receptor antagonists	Hyperkalemia	Serum levels of drug increased by cimetidine and decreased by phenobarbital
Vasodilators		
Calcium channel blockers		
Dihydropyridines†	Dizziness, edema, gingival hyperplasia, headache, and tachycardia	Serum levels of drug increased by azole antifungal agents, cimetidine, and grapefruit juice
Diltiazem	Atrioventricular block, bradycardia, constipation, dizziness, edema, gingival hyperplasia, headache, and heart failure	Increases serum levels of carbamazepine, digoxin, and theophylline. Decreases serum levels of lithium
Verapamil	Same as diltiazem	Same as diltiazem

TABLE 10-4. **Adverse Effects, Contraindications, and Drug Interactions of Antihypertensive Agents*—cont'd**

Drug Classification	Common Adverse Effects	Common Drug Interactions
Other vasodilators		
Hydralazine	Angina, dizziness, fluid retention, headache, lupuslike syndrome, and tachycardia	Hypotensive effect decreased by NSAIDs
Minoxidil	Angina, dizziness, fluid retention, headache, hypertrichosis, pericardial effusion, and tachycardia	Hypotensive effect decreased by NSAIDs
Nitroprusside	Dizziness, headache, increased intracranial pressure, methemoglobinemia, and thiocyanatecyanide toxicity	None

*ACE = angiotensin-converting enzyme; CNS = central nervous system; and NSAIDs = nonsteroidal anti-inflammatory drugs.
†The dihydropyridines include amlodipine, felodipine, isradipine, nicardipine, and nifedipine.

the progression of cardiovascular diseases in hypertensive patients.

Centrally Acting Drugs

The centrally acting sympatholytics include **clonidine, guanabenz, guanfacine,** and **methyldopa.** These drugs often cause more side effects than many other antihypertensive drugs and are not recommended for the initial treatment of most patients with high blood pressure. They are primarily used when other drugs are ineffective or for the treatment of hypertensive emergencies. The centrally acting drugs are α_2-adrenergic receptor agonists that reduce sympathetic outflow from the brain stem to the heart, blood vessels, and other tissues. They lower the blood pressure primarily by causing a reduction in PVR while the heart rate and cardiac output are either reduced or remain unchanged. Because tricyclic antidepressant drugs can block the effects of centrally acting sympatholytic drugs, the two classes of drugs should not be used concurrently.

Sedation, **dry mouth**, and other CNS side effects of centrally acting sympatholytics can be problematic in hypertensive patients whose work requires mental alertness, as well as in those who are elderly or have neurologic diseases. Because severe **rebound hypertension** can occur if clonidine and related drugs are discontinued abruptly, the dosage should be tapered gradually over 1 to 2 weeks if treatment is to be stopped.

In addition to activating α_2-adrenergic receptors, clonidine also activates a recently discovered class of nonadrenergic receptors in the ventrolateral medulla known as **imidazoline receptors,** which appear to be partly responsible for the drug's antihypertensive action. Selective imidazoline receptor agonists, including moxonidine and rilmenidine, reduce blood pressure and cause less sedation and dry mouth than does clonidine. Selective imidazoline receptor agonists are not currently available in the United States.

Methyldopa is similar to clonidine in its actions and effects. Unlike clonidine and other centrally acting drugs, however, methyldopa is accumulated by central noradrenergic neurons and is converted to an active metabolite, methylnorepinephrine. Methyldopa is well known for its ability to cause immunologic effects, including a Coombs-positive **hemolytic anemia** (reported in up to 2% of patients), autoimmune hepatitis, and other organ dysfunction. Methyldopa has been used to treat hypertension in pregnant women, because extensive experience has shown that it does not harm the fetus.

ANGIOTENSIN INHIBITORS

The angiotensin inhibitors include the angiotensin-converting enzyme (ACE) inhibitors and the angiotensin receptor antagonists. These drugs are effective and well tolerated and are indicated for the treatment of hypertension in persons with cardiovascular diseases and diabetes. The pharmacologic properties of these drugs are summarized in Tables 10–2 and 10–3, and their common adverse effects and drug interactions are listed in Table 10–4.

Angiotensin-Converting Enzyme Inhibitors

Drug Properties

CHEMISTRY AND PHARMACOKINETICS. Molecular techniques were used to model the active site of ACE and design drugs that inhibit ACE. The various ACE inhibitors have essentially identical mechanisms of action and pharmacologic effects, but they differ in their pharmacokinetic properties (Table 10–5). They undergo varying degrees of first-pass hepatic inactivation after oral administration, and several of the ACE inhibitors have active metabolites. Except for captopril, most of the ACE inhibitors have a duration of action of about 24

TABLE 10–5.   **Pharmacokinetic Properties of Selected Angiotensin Inhibitors**

Drug	Oral Bioavailability	Absorption Reduced by Food	Active Metabolite	Duration of Action (Hours)
Angiotensin-converting enzyme inhibitors				
Benazepril	37%	No	Benazeprilat	24
Captopril	75%	30–40%	None	6–12
Enalapril	60%	No	Enalaprilat*	24
Fosinopril	36%	No	Fosinoprilat	24
Lisinopril	25%	No	None	24
Quinapril	60%	25–30%	Quinaprilat	24
Ramipril	55%	No	Ramiprilat	24
Angiotensin receptor antagonists				
Losartan	33%	10%	Carboxylic acid metabolite	24
Valsartan	25%	40%	None	24
Candesartan	15%	No	None	24

*Enalaprilat is available as a separate drug for intravenous administration.

hours and can be administered once or twice daily to treat hypertension and other disorders.

MECHANISMS AND PHARMACOLOGIC EFFECTS. The actions of ACE inhibitors and other drugs affecting the renin-angiotensin-aldosterone axis are shown in Fig. 10–3. Three primary stimuli to renin secretion exist: (1) sympathetic nervous system activation of β_1-adrenergic receptors on renal juxtaglomerular cells, (2) a reduction in blood pressure and wall tension in renal afferent arterioles, and (3) a reduction in sodium chloride reabsorption by the renal macula densa.

When blood pressure falls and renin is released, this initiates a cascade of events that normally return blood pressure to the preexisting level. In the circulation, renin acts as a protease that converts circulating angiotensinogen to angiotensin I. ACE, a protease primarily located in the pulmonary vasculature, then converts the physiologically inactive angiotensin I to the active angiotensin II. Angiotensin II activates two types of **angiotensin receptors,** called AT_1 and AT_2. The AT_1 receptors are coupled with enzymes that

increase the formation of inositol triphosphate (IP_3) and various arachidonic acid metabolites and decrease the formation of cyclic adenosine monophosphate (cAMP). Activation of AT_1 receptors in the adrenal cortex causes the synthesis and release of aldosterone, and activation of AT_1 receptors in vascular smooth muscle causes vasoconstriction. In addition to causing these two effects via IP_3-mediated release of intracellular calcium, AT_1 receptors mediate cardiac, renal, and CNS effects. The functional significance of AT_2 receptors has not been elucidated.

In the normal chain of events, ACE converts angiotensin I to angiotensin II and also catalyzes the inactivation of **bradykinin,** an endogenous vasodilator peptide. Drugs that inhibit ACE therefore exert hypotensive effects by blocking the formation of a vasoconstrictor (angiotensin II) and the degradation of a vasodilator (bradykinin). Increased renal prostaglandin synthesis can also contribute to the hypotensive effects of these drugs. Some studies have found that angiotensin II levels can return toward pretreatment levels during long-term ACE inhibitor therapy, even though the blood pressure remains under control. This suggests

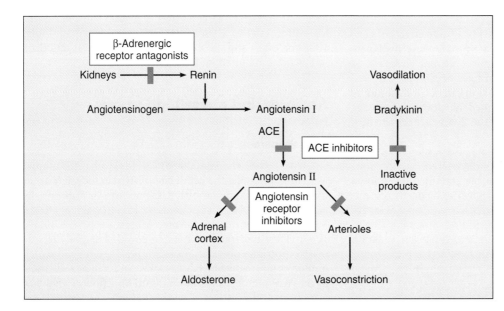

Figure 10-3. Actions of antihypertensive drugs on the renin-angiotensin-aldosterone axis. β-Adrenergic receptor antagonists inhibit sympathetic stimulation of renin secretion. Angiotensin-converting enzyme (ACE) inhibitors block the formation of angiotensin II and inhibit the breakdown of bradykinin, a vasodilator. Angiotensin receptor antagonists (e.g., losartan) block AT_1 receptors in smooth muscle and adrenal cortex.

that the effects on bradykinin and prostaglandins are an important component of the antihypertensive action of these drugs.

The antihypertensive action of ACE inhibitors is primarily caused by a reduction in PVR, with little or no change in cardiac output or blood volume (see Table 10–2). ACE inhibitors decrease both arterial pressure and venous pressure, and this in turn reduces cardiac afterload and cardiac preload, respectively. By reducing angiotensin-stimulated aldosterone secretion, ACE inhibitors prevent the compensatory increase in sodium retention and plasma volume that can occur with some other antihypertensive drugs. In patients treated with ACE inhibitors, renal sodium retention is decreased, renal potassium retention is increased, and serum potassium levels typically increase by about 0.5 mEq/L.

ADVERSE EFFECTS. ACE inhibitors can cause fetal and neonatal morbidity and mortality when administered to pregnant women, especially during the second and third trimesters. Therefore, use of these drugs should be discontinued when pregnancy is detected. ACE inhibitors can also cause renal failure in patients who have a rare condition known as bilateral renal artery stenosis, because these patients depend on angiotensin II to maintain renal blood flow and glomerular filtration, as illustrated in Fig. 10–4.

The ACE inhibitors are usually well tolerated, and epidemiologic studies have shown that they do not adversely affect the lifestyle of most hypertensive patients. The most common side effect is a **dry, nonproductive cough**, which occurs in up to 20% of patients and may be caused by increased bradykinin levels. A pruritic rash occurs in up to 10% of patients. Infrequently, ACE inhibitors cause an **abnormal taste sensation**, which appears to be related to the

Figure 10-4. Effects of angiotensin-converting enzyme (ACE) inhibitors in patients with bilateral renal artery stenosis. Renal blood flow is reduced in the presence of bilateral renal artery stenosis. In affected patients, glomerular filtration is maintained by elevating efferent arteriolar pressure via vasoconstriction produced by angiotensin II. By blocking the formation of angiotensin II, ACE inhibitors can severely impair glomerular filtration and lead to renal failure. GFR = glomerular filtration rate.

binding of zinc by the drugs. Other less common but more severe adverse effects of ACE inhibitors include **angioedema** and neutropenia. Angioedema is usually manifested as painful swelling of the lips, face, and throat.

INTERACTIONS. The antihypertensive action of ACE inhibitors is augmented by diuretics and several combination products containing an ACE inhibitor and a thiazide diuretic are available. ACE inhibitors can interact with potassium-sparing diuretics and potassium supplements to increase serum potassium levels and cause hyperkalemia. They can also increase serum lithium levels and provoke lithium toxicity in patients receiving lithium compounds for the treatment of bipolar disorder. Nonsteroidal anti-inflammatory drugs (NSAID), such as ibuprofen, can impede the effects of ACE inhibitors and other antihypertensive agents.

INDICATIONS. Because they have excellent antihypertensive action and few bothersome side effects, ACE inhibitors are used in the management of mild to severe hypertension in patients with a wide variety of traits and concomitant diseases, as outlined in Table 10–6. The drugs are of particular value in treating hypertensive patients with coexisting heart failure, myocardial infarction, chronic kidney disease, or diabetes mellitus.

Studies have shown that ACE inhibitors decrease cardiac afterload, increase cardiac output, and reduce the risk of death in patients with heart failure (see Chapter 12). These agents also increase the survival rate and reduce the incidence of overt heart failure in patients who have myocardial infarction and significant left ventricular dysfunction, as evidenced by a cardiac ejection fraction of less than 40%. (The ejection fraction is the percentage of blood that is ejected from the left ventricle during each systole.)

In diabetic patients who exhibit early signs of renal impairment (e.g., albuminuria and increased serum creatinine levels), ACE inhibitors exert a renoprotective effect. Studies indicate that the ACE inhibitor **enalapril** reduces the progression of these harbingers of renal failure and the subsequent need for renal dialysis in these patients. Moreover, if enalapril is withdrawn from treatment, the progression of nephropathy resumes quickly. Based on these findings, experts now recommend that ACE inhibitor therapy be considered for diabetic patients with albuminuria or increased serum creatinine levels, regardless of whether they have hypertension.

Specific Drugs

Three classes of ACE inhibitors have been developed. In each class, a different chemical group binds the zinc ion in ACE. The sulfhydryl (mercapto) compounds include **captopril;** the phosphoryl agents include **fosinopril;** and the carboxyl derivatives include **benazepril, enalapril, lisinopril, quinapril,** and **ramipril.** All of these drugs, except captopril and lisinopril, are enzymatically transformed to active metabolites. **Enalaprilat,** the active metabolite of enalapril, is available for intravenous administration; the other ACE inhibitors are administered orally.

The orally administered ACE inhibitors undergo considerable first-pass inactivation, and their oral bioavailability ranges from 25% to 75% (see Table 10–5). In comparison

TABLE 10-6. **Selection of Antihypertensive Drugs for Patients with Specific Traits or Concurrent Diseases***

Patient Characteristic	Most Preferred Drugs	Least Preferred Drugs
Age over 65 years	Diuretic, ACEI, CCB	Centrally acting α_2 agonist
African heritage	Diuretic, CCB	β-blocker
Pregnant	Methyldopa, labetalol	ACEI, ARB
Angina pectoris	β-blocker, CCB	Hydralazine, minoxidil
Myocardial infarction	β-blocker, ACEI, aldosterone antagonist	
Congestive heart failure	Diuretic, ACEI, ARB, β-blocker	
Recurrent stroke prevention	Diuretic, ACEI, ARB	
Chronic kidney disease	ACEI, ARB	
Diabetes	Diuretic, ACEI, ARB, β-blocker, CCB	
Asthma	CCB, ACEI	β-blocker
Benign prostatic hyperplasia	α-blocker	
Migraine headache	β-blocker, CCB	
Osteoporosis	Diuretic	

*Diuretic = thiazide diuretic; ACEI = angiotensin converting enzyme inhibitor; ARB = angiotensin receptor blocker; α-blocker = adrenergic α blocker; β-blocker = adrenergic β blocker; CCB = calcium channel blocker.

with other ACE inhibitors, which are administered one or two times a day, captopril has a shorter half-life and must be administered two or three times a day. Some studies indicate that captopril causes a higher incidence of rash, which may be related to its sulfhydryl structure.

Angiotensin Receptor Blockers

A newer approach to angiotensin inhibition has been the development of angiotensin receptor blockers (ARB). These drugs block AT_1 receptors in vascular smooth muscle and in the adrenal cortex, thereby causing vasodilation and decreasing aldosterone secretion.

Many orally effective ARB are now available, including candesartan, irbesartan, **losartan, valsartan,** and others. In the treatment of hypertension, these drugs appear to be as effective as the ACE inhibitors but only rarely cause the chronic cough that is a frequent problem with ACE inhibitors. The ARB are relatively free of other adverse effects, and most patients tolerate them well. Recent clinical trials have found that the ARB can be particularly useful in reducing the risk of cardiovascular consequences of hypertension (see Waugh and Keating, 2003). In these studies, losartan produced a greater reduction of **left ventricular hypertrophy** and the risk of stroke and new onset diabetes than did atenolol.

The ARB do not increase serum glucose, uric acid, or cholesterol levels. Occasional abnormalities in the test results of patients taking these drugs have included **hyperkalemia,** neutropenia, and elevated serum levels of hepatic aminotransferase enzymes. As with the ACE inhibitors, the angiotensin receptor blockers can cause **fetal injury and death** and should not be used during pregnancy.

VASODILATORS

The vasodilators include the calcium channel blockers and other agents such as hydralazine, minoxidil, and nitroprusside. The pharmacologic effects, adverse effects, and drug interactions of these agents are summarized in Tables 10–2, 10–3, and 10–4.

Calcium Channel Blockers

Calcium channel blockers are used to treat hypertension, angina pectoris, and cardiac arrhythmias. Chapter 11 discusses the pharmacologic properties of these drugs in detail, but this chapter focuses on their antihypertensive actions.

By blocking calcium ion channels in the plasma membranes of smooth muscle, the calcium channel blockers relax vascular smooth muscle and thereby cause vasodilation. Calcium channel blockers have a greater effect on arteriolar smooth muscle than on venous smooth muscle, and their effect on blood pressure is primarily caused by a reduction in PVR, with relatively little impact on venous capacitance, cardiac filling pressure, and cardiac output. Some studies indicate that calcium channel blockers have a natriuretic effect that may contribute to their ability to lower blood pressure.

Whereas all of the calcium channel blockers relax vascular smooth muscle, **diltiazem** and **verapamil** also have significant effects on cardiac tissue and can reduce the heart rate and cardiac output. Most of the other calcium channel blockers, including **amlodipine, felodipine, isradipine, nicardipine,** and **nifedipine,** belong to the dihydropyridine class. The dihydropyridines have relatively little effect on cardiac tissue at usual therapeutic levels; however, they can evoke reflex tachycardia.

The calcium channel blockers, which are effective in the management of all forms of hypertension, are among the most widely used antihypertensive agents. They do not alter levels of serum glucose, lipids, uric acid, or electrolytes. They are relatively free of adverse effects, and they are particularly useful in treating hypertensive patients who have asthma or are of African heritage (see Table 10–6).

Other Vasodilators

Hydralazine and Minoxidil

Hydralazine and minoxidil are orally effective vasodilators primarily used in combination with other antihypertensive drugs to treat moderate to very severe hypertension. When used alone, they often evoke reflex tachycardia and cause fluid retention, and they can precipitate angina in susceptible patients. To prevent these problems, hydralazine or minoxidil is usually given in combination with two other drugs: a diuretic plus either a β-adrenergic receptor antagonist or another sympatholytic agent. Hydralazine has been associated with a **lupus-like syndrome,** whereas minoxidil can cause hypertrichosis (excessive hair growth), particularly in women. In fact, minoxidil has been marketed as a topical formulation for the treatment of several forms of **alopecia** (baldness) in men and women.

Nitroprusside

Sodium nitroprusside is one of several drugs used in the management of hypertensive emergencies. The drug is administered by intravenous infusion and has a short half-life. Nitroprusside is rapidly metabolized to cyanide in erythrocytes and other tissues. Cyanide is then converted to thiocyanate in the presence of a sulfur donor. Both thiocyanate and cyanide gradually accumulate during nitroprusside infusion. For this reason, the duration of therapy with this drug is usually limited to a few days. During drug administration, the patient's blood pressure should be monitored frequently, and thiocyanate levels should be checked every 72 hours to detect potential toxicity.

Fenoldopam

Fenoldopam represents a new class of antihypertensive drugs. It is an agonist at dopamine D_1-like receptors, with moderate affinity for adrenergic α_2-receptors. Fenolodopam is a rapid acting, intravenously administered drug used to treat hypertensive emergencies (see below). It causes arteriolar vasodilation in systemic vascular beds, including coronary, renal, and mesenteric vessels. In the kidney, fenoldopam dilates both afferent and efferent arterioles, thereby increasing renal blood flow. The drug is rapidly converted to inactive glucuronide and other conjugates and has a short half-life of about 5 minutes. Fenoldopam can reduce serum potassium levels, which should be monitored at 6-hour intervals during drug infusion.

THE MANAGEMENT OF HYPERTENSION

Lifestyle Modifications

Patients with hypertension should be encouraged to pursue lifestyle changes that will improve their general health and can substantially lower their blood pressure. Effective strategies include exercise and weight loss, reduction of alcohol intake, and institution of a diet that is low in sodium and provides an adequate intake of potassium, calcium, and magnesium. Patients should be encouraged to consume a diet rich in fruits and vegetables and low in saturated and total fat. Unless hypertension is severe, patients should be encouraged to try lifestyle modifications for several months before instituting drug therapy.

Single- and Multiple-Drug Therapy

The JNC 7 report recommends that a **thiazide diuretic** be used for initial therapy for most patients with hypertension.

This recommendation is based on the unsurpassed ability of thiazide diuretics to prevent the cardiovascular complications of hypertension, including stroke and coronary artery disease. Numerous clinical trials have shown that thiazide diuretics are effective and relatively safe when serum potassium, glucose, uric acid, and lipid levels are monitored appropriately. In addition, thiazides are among the least expensive agents available for treating hypertension.

Other drug classes that can be considered for the initial treatment of hypertension include (1) **angiotensin converting enzyme inhibitors**, (2) **angiotensin receptor blockers**, (3) **adrenergic β-blockers**, and (4) **calcium channel blockers**. Selection of one of these drugs is recommended for initial therapy when a thiazide diuretic cannot be used or when a **compelling indication** is present that requires the use of a specific drug. Compelling indications for particular drugs include heart failure, post-myocardial infarction, diabetes, chronic kidney disease, and recurrent stroke prevention (see Table 10–6). When single drug therapy fails to control blood pressure adequately, the addition of a second drug from one of the classes listed above should be initiated.

A number of **combination drug products** are now available to treat hypertension, most of which can be taken once or twice daily. These products are usually less expensive and more convenient to use than two single drug products, and they enhance patient compliance with the treatment regimen. The JNC 7 report found that the initiation of therapy with more than one drug increases the likelihood of achieving a desired blood pressure in a timely manner. Moreover, drug combinations often achieve blood pressure reduction with lower doses of the component drugs, thereby causing fewer adverse effects. Unless intolerable side effects occur or hypertension is severe, drugs should be given a trial of several weeks before evaluating their effectiveness or changing medications.

Patients with Specific Traits or Diseases

Table 10–6 summarizes the most preferred and least preferred drugs for hypertensive patients with specific traits or concurrent diseases. These recommendations are only guidelines and individual patient characteristics should always been considered when selecting drug therapy.

In hypertensive patients over 65 years of age, the use of a thiazide diuretic, an ACE inhibitor, or a dihydropyridine calcium channel blocker may be preferred for initial therapy. In some patients over 70 years of age, β-blockers may reduce cardiac output too much. The cardioprotective effect of β-blockers, however, may still justify their use in this population if they are tolerated. In elderly black patients, β-blockers are often less effective than diuretics, so a diuretic or calcium channel blocker should be used.

Whenever possible, patients with hypertension and a coexisting disorder should be treated with drugs that are potentially beneficial to both conditions, and agents that can exacerbate the coexisting disorder should be avoided. Most patients with **ischemic heart disease,** including those with **angina pectoris** or **myocardial infarction,** should be treated with a β-blocker as well as an ACE inhibitor or angiotensin receptor blocker unless they are contraindicated. The β-blockers protect against sudden death in these patients and are among the drugs that reduce ventricular hypertrophy.

For patients with **diabetes mellitus,** the JNC 7 report recommends that blood pressure be controlled to the level of 130/80 mm Hg or lower. This is because rigorous control of blood pressure is essential for reducing the progression of **diabetic nephropathy** to end-stage renal disease. Clinical trials show that ACE inhibitors, angiotensin receptor blockers, β-blockers, and calcium antagonists have demonstrated benefits in both type 1 and type 2 diabetics. Thiazide diuretics are also beneficial in diabetics. The Antihypertensive and Lipid-Lowering Treatment to Prevent Heart Attack Trial (ALLHAT) found that thiazides reduced the incidence of fatal coronary artery disease and myocardial infarction to the same extent as an ACE inhibitor or calcium antagonist. Although diuretics can aggravate hyperglycemia, the effect is slight and easily managed in most patients.

The ACE inhibitors and angiotensin receptor blockers are important components of antihypertensive regimens for diabetic patients because of their ability to reduce the progression of diabetic nephropathy. Adrenergic β-blockers are also beneficial in diabetic patients as part of multidrug therapy, particularly in patients who also have coronary artery disease. Although β-blockers can mask symptoms of hypoglycemia and slow recovery from hypoglycemia by blocking glycogenolysis, these problems are usually managed easily and are not absolute contraindications for β-blocker use in patients with diabetes.

In patients with **asthma,** treatment with β-blockers should be avoided, because these agents can cause bronchoconstriction. Use of a calcium channel blocker or ACE inhibitor is usually preferred. Calcium channel blockers can relax bronchial smooth muscle and thereby reduce bronchoconstriction in patients with asthma.

Hypertensive Emergencies and Urgencies

Hypertensive emergencies are characterized by severe elevations in blood pressure (>180/120 mm Hg) complicated by target organ dysfunction (e.g., encephalopathy or intracranial hemorrhage). These situations require immediate reduction in blood pressure to limit target organ damage. **Hypertensive urgencies** are situations with severe elevations of blood pressure without target organ dysfunction, such as with persons who have upper levels of stage 2 hypertension associated with severe headache, shortness of breath, or severe anxiety.

The initial goal of treatment of hypertensive emergencies is to reduce blood pressure by no more than 25% within minutes to 1 hour, and then to 160/100 mm Hg within the next 2 to 6 hours. If this level of blood pressure is well tolerated, gradual reductions to normal blood pressure can be implemented in the next 24 to 48 hours. Excessive reductions in blood pressure can precipitate renal, cerebral, or coronary ischemia and should be avoided. For this reason, short-acting nifedipine is no longer an acceptable treatment for hypertensive emergencies or urgencies.

A number of drugs can be used to treat hypertensive emergencies and urgencies. Parenterally administered drugs are usually used, although oral **clonidine** can be used for less

severe hypertensive urgencies because it slowly reduces blood pressure to a safe level. The drugs most often used in treating most types of hypertensive emergencies include **fenoldopam, nicardipine, labetalol,** and **sodium nitroprusside. Hydralazine** has been used for hypertension associated with **eclampsia** of pregnancy. **Nitroglycerin** is used for hypertensive emergencies in persons with **acute coronary ischemia,** and **enalaprilat** may be of value in patients with acute **left ventricular failure** (but not acute myocardial infarction). **Esmolol** is useful in persons with **aortic dissection** and **perioperative hypertension.**

SUMMARY OF IMPORTANT POINTS

■ The four major classes of antihypertensive drugs are the diuretics, sympatholytics, angiotensin inhibitors, and vasodilators.

■ Thiazide diuretics and potassium-sparing diuretics are often used to treat hypertensive patients. The thiazides initially reduce blood volume and cardiac output, but their long-term effect on blood pressure is primarily caused by decreased peripheral vascular resistance (PVR).

■ Sympatholytics used in the treatment of hypertension include α-adrenergic receptor antagonists, β-adrenergic receptor antagonists, and centrally acting drugs. Except for the β-blockers, which reduce cardiac output, the sympatholytics reduce blood pressure primarily by decreasing PVR.

■ The two types of angiotensin inhibitors are the angiotensin-converting enzyme (ACE) inhibitors (e.g., captopril) and the angiotensin receptor antagonists (e.g., losartan). These drugs reduce PVR and aldosterone levels, with little effect on blood volume or cardiac output in patients who do not have heart failure.

■ Among the vasodilators used to treat hypertension are the calcium channel blockers, hydralazine, minoxidil, and nitroprusside. These drugs reduce PVR, and some of them provoke reflex tachycardia and fluid retention.

■ The management of high blood pressure begins with lifestyle modifications and then proceeds to the use of a diuretic, β-blocker, ACE inhibitor, angiotensin receptor blocker, or calcium channel blocker for most patients.

Review Questions

For each numbered drug description, select the corresponding drug from the lettered choices.

1. This drug reduces circulating levels of angiotensin II and increases bradykinin levels.

2. Abrupt discontinuation of this drug results in markedly elevated levels of circulating norepinephrine and rebound hypertension.

3. This drug inhibits renin secretion and decreases cardiac output.

4. This drug can cause orthostatic hypotension and reflex tachycardia.

5. This peripherally acting drug causes vasodilation and decreases cardiac output.

(A) clonidine
(B) verapamil
(C) doxazosin
(D) hydrochlorothiazide
(E) atenolol
(F) enalapril
(G) candesartan

Answers and Explanations

1. The answer is F: enalapril. ACE inhibitors such as enalapril inhibit the formation of angiotensin II and the degradation of bradykinin. β-blockers such as atenolol can reduce renin secretion and angiotensin II formation but they do not increase bradykinin levels. Candesartan blocks angiotensin II receptors but does not reduce angiotensin II levels or increase bradykinin levels.

2. The answer is A: clonidine. Clonidine and related α_2-agonists reduce sympathetic outflow from the brain stem and thereby decrease circulating norepinephrine levels. Abrupt discontinuation of these drugs results in a rebound elevation of circulating norepinephrine levels and markedly high blood pressure.

3. The answer is E: atenolol. Selective β_1-blockers such as atenolol inhibit renin secretion, thereby reducing angiotensin II formation. They also block cardiac β_1-receptors and decrease heart rate, contractility, and cardiac output. All of these actions can contribute to their antihypertensive effect.

4. The answer is C: doxazosin. Doxazosin and other α_1-blockers cause vasodilatation leading to decreased blood pressure and reflex tachycardia. Verapamil, a non-dihydropyridine calcium channel blocker, also produces vasodilation but it does not cause reflex tachycardia because of its direct cardiosuppressant effect.

5. The answer is B: verapamil. Verapamil and diltiazem are non-dihydropyridine calcium channel blockers that decrease vascular resistance and cardiac output. Dihydropyridine calcium channel blockers such as amlodipine lower blood pressure primarily by reducing vascular resistance and do not decrease cardiac output.

SELECTED READINGS

ALLHAT Officers and Coordinators for the ALLHAT Collaborative Research Group. Major outcomes in high-risk hypertensive patients randomized to angiotensin-converting enzyme inhibitor or calcium channel blocker vs diuretic: The Antihypertensive and Lipid-Lowering Treatment to Prevent Heart Attack Trial (ALLHAT) JAMA 288:2981–2997, 2002.

Brewster, L. M., G. A. van Montfrans, and J. Kleijnen. Systematic review: antihypertensive drug therapy in black patients. Ann Intern Med 141:614–627, 2004.

Chobanian, A. V., G. L. Bakris, and H. R. Black, et al. The seventh report of the Joint National Committee (JNC) on Prevention, Detection, Evaluation, and Treatment of High Blood Pressure. Hypertension 42:1206–1252, 2003.

Dandona, P., A. Chaudhuri, and A. Aljada. Endothelial dysfunction and hypertension in diabetes mellitus. Med Clin North Am 88:911–931, 2004.

Shah, S. U., S. Anjum, and W. A. Littler. Use of diuretics in cardiovascular disease: (2) hypertension. Postgrad Med J 80:271–276, 2004.

Waugh, J., and G. M. Keating. Losartan: in the reduction of stroke risk in patients with hypertension and left ventricular hypertrophy. Am J Cardiovasc Drugs 3:371–377, 2003.

Antianginal Drugs

OVERVIEW

Ischemic Heart Disease

Ischemic heart disease has two primary forms, angina pectoris and myocardial infarction (Fig. 11–1). **Angina pectoris**, which is usually a chronic condition, is characterized by episodic chest discomfort that occurs during transient coronary ischemia. In contrast, **myocardial infarction** is the result of an acute and complete occlusion of a coronary artery, which is most frequently caused by coronary thrombosis.

The symptoms of angina pectoris, often described as resembling a heavy weight or pressure on the chest, occur when the oxygen supply to the myocardium is not sufficient to provide the energy required by the tissue. The imbalance between oxygen supply and oxygen demand can result from the following: an acute disruption of coronary blood flow caused by coronary vasospasm or platelet aggregation; an increased demand for oxygen evoked by physical exertion in the face of a limited oxygen supply; or a combination of pathophysiologic mechanisms, such as vasospasm and platelet aggregation occurring in association with coronary atherosclerosis.

Typical angina occurs when the myocardial oxygen demand increases in association with exercise or stress but the coronary blood flow and oxygen supply are limited by the presence of coronary atherosclerosis that partially occludes a major coronary vessel. The condition is characterized as **stable angina** if angina attacks have similar characteristics and occur under the same circumstances each time. It is characterized as **unstable angina** if the frequency and severity of attacks increase (crescendo). Unstable angina, which is usually caused by the occlusion of coronary vessels by small thrombi and ruptured atheromatous plaque, is often the forerunner of myocardial infarction. **Variant angina (Prinzmetal's angina)** is caused by acute coronary vasospasm and often occurs at rest or during sleep. Variant angina is sometimes considered a form of unstable angina.

Table 11–1 lists four classes of drugs and compares their efficacy in treating different forms of ischemic heart disease. This chapter focuses on the first three classes: organic nitrites and nitrates, calcium channel blockers (CCB), and β-adrenergic receptor antagonists (β-blockers), which are the primary agents used to treat angina. Chapter 16 discusses antithrombotic drugs (e.g., aspirin) and fibrinolytic drugs that are useful in treating unstable angina and myocardial infarction.

Mechanisms and Effects of Antianginal Drugs

The pharmacologic treatment of angina pectoris seeks to restore the balance between myocardial oxygen supply and

TABLE 11-1. Efficacy of Drugs Used in the Treatment of Ischemic Heart Disease*

Drug or Drug Class	TYPICAL ANGINA PECTORIS		Variant Angina Pectoris	Myocardial Infarction
	Stable Angina	Unstable Angina		
Organic nitrites and nitrates	++	++	++	+
Calcium channel blockers	++	0 to ++	+++	0
β-Adrenergic receptor antagonists	++	++	0	+++
Antithrombotic drugs**	+	+++	0	+++

*Ratings range from 0 (not efficacious) to +++ (highly efficacious). **Includes antiplatelet, anticoagulant, and fibronolytic drugs.

demand, either by increasing oxygen supply or decreasing oxygen demand. The factors that determine supply and demand are illustrated in Fig. 11–2.

Myocardial oxygen supply is primarily determined by **coronary blood flow** and **regional flow distribution** but is also influenced by **oxygen extraction.** In patients with coronary artery disease, the subendocardial tissue is more likely to suffer from ischemia because it is not as well perfused as the subepicardial tissue. The use of nitrates or CCB (vasodilator drugs) can reduce ischemia by increasing both the total coronary flow and the distribution of coronary flow

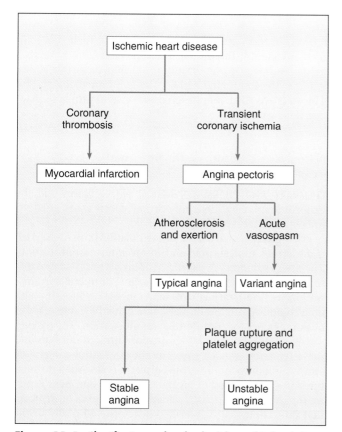

Figure 11-1. Classification and pathophysiology of ischemic heart disease. Variant angina, also called Prinzmetal's angina, is considered a form of unstable angina if the angina attacks occur with increasing severity or frequency.

to ischemic subendocardial tissue. The drugs increase the distribution of blood flow to subendocardial tissue by dilating collateral vessels and by decreasing intraventricular pressure and the resistance to perfusion of this tissue. The use of β-blockers may improve the distribution of coronary flow by reducing intraventricular pressure. Cardiac tissue extracts a higher percentage of oxygen from blood than does any other tissue, and this factor is not affected by existing drugs.

Myocardial oxygen demand is largely determined by the amount of energy required to support the work of the heart. The factors that influence cardiac work include the **heart rate, cardiac contractility,** and **myocardial wall tension.** Contractility is directly related to the amount of cytosolic calcium that is available to stimulate the shortening of myocardial fibers. As contractility increases, the velocity of fiber shortening and the peak systolic muscle tension also increase. Myocardial wall tension is equal to the product of ventricular volume (radius) and pressure, divided by wall thickness. Ventricular wall tension is primarily determined by arterial and venous blood pressure.

Antianginal drugs act by several mechanisms to reduce myocardial oxygen demand. The β-blockers and some of the CCB decrease heart rate and contractility, whereas the vasodilators reduce wall tension via their effects on ventricular volume and pressure. Dilation of veins decreases venous pressure, cardiac filling pressure, and ventricular diastolic pressure (preload). Dilation of arteries decreases arterial and aortic pressure and thereby reduces ventricular systolic pressure (afterload). The organic nitrates act primarily on venous tissue and predominantly affect preload, whereas the CCB act mostly on arteriolar muscle to reduce afterload.

In **typical angina,** which is caused by increased oxygen demand in the face of a limited oxygen supply, vasodilators and β-blockers act primarily by decreasing oxygen demand through the mechanisms described above. They can also increase the perfusion of ischemic subendocardial tissue. In **variant angina,** chest pain usually occurs at rest (when oxygen demand is relatively low), and ischemia results in a reduction in oxygen supply secondary to coronary artery spasm. Under these conditions, vasodilators increase oxygen supply by relaxing coronary smooth muscle and restoring normal coronary flow. The β-blockers are not effective in the treatment of variant angina, because they cannot counteract vasospasm and increase coronary blood flow. The β-blockers may actually reduce coronary blood flow by blocking the

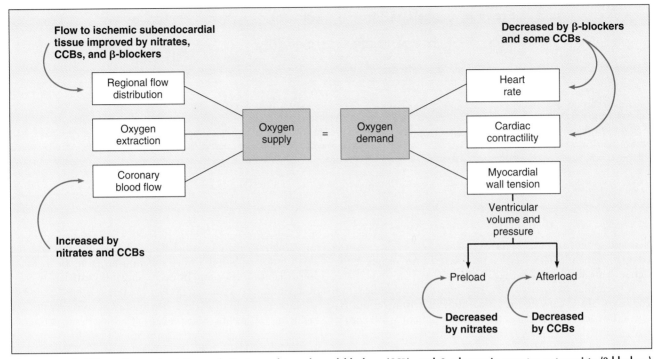

Figure 11–2. Effects of organic nitrites and nitrates, calcium channel blockers (CCB), and β-adrenergic receptor antagonists (β-blockers) on myocardial oxygen supply and demand.

vasodilative effect of epinephrine, an effect that is mediated by β₂-adrenergic receptors in coronary smooth muscle.

VASODILATORS

Two classes of vasodilators are used in the management of angina pectoris. The first consists of organic nitrites and nitrates and the second consists of calcium channel blockers.

Organic Nitrites and Nitrates

The organic nitrites and nitrates are polyol esters of nitrous acid and nitric acid, respectively (Fig. 11–3A). Amyl nitrite, the only nitrite compound used to treat angina, is administered by inhalation. Nitroglycerin (glyceryl trinitrate), isosorbide dinitrate, and isosorbide mononitrate are nitrate compounds with sufficient solubility in water and lipids to enable rapid dissolution and absorption following sublingual, oral, or transdermal administration. The onset and duration of action of these drugs varies with their physical properties, route of administration, and rate of biotransformation. Amyl nitrite has the most rapid onset and the shortest duration of action, whereas isosorbide compounds have the slowest onset and the longest duration. Nitroglycerin has an intermediate onset and duration. All of these compounds are extensively metabolized in the liver.

Amyl Nitrite

Amyl nitrite is a volatile liquid that can be inhaled and absorbed through the lungs. Its action is rapid in onset (within 30 seconds) and brief in duration (3 to 5 minutes). Amyl nitrite is effective in the **treatment of acute angina**

attacks, as well as in the **initial management of cyanide poisoning.** In patients with cyanide poisoning, amyl nitrite is used until intravenous sodium nitrite and sodium thiosulfate can be administered. The nitrites oxidize hemoglobin to methemoglobin. In comparison with hemoglobin, methemoglobin has a greater affinity for cyanide, and this allows it to trap the compound in the form of cyanmethemoglobin. Thiosulfate is then administered to convert cyanide to inactive thiocyanate.

Nitroglycerin, Isosorbide Dinitrate, and Isosorbide Mononitrate

CHEMISTRY AND PHARMACOKINETICS. Nitroglycerin and the isosorbide preparations are nitrate compounds used to **prevent and treat angina attacks.**

Nitroglycerin is available in formulations for sublingual, transdermal, topical, oral, and intravenous administration. The drug's solubility in water and lipids permits its rapid dissolution and absorption after sublingual or buccal administration for the treatment of acute angina attacks. Its high lipid solubility and low dosage have enabled the formulation of skin patches for transdermal administration. The patches slowly release the drug for absorption through the skin into the circulation and are used in the prevention of angina attacks. In ointment form, nitroglycerin is absorbed through the skin over a period of several hours. The ointment is primarily used in hospitalized patients with **angina** or **myocardial infarction.** Nitroglycerin is administered orally in the form of sustained-release capsules that are used to prevent angina attacks. The drug is well absorbed from the gut but undergoes considerable first-pass inactivation, thereby necessitating the use of larger doses when administered

Figure 11-3. Structures of selected antianginal drugs. Three groups of antianginal drugs exist. Representative structures of one group, the β-adrenergic receptor antagonists, are depicted in Fig. 9–5. Examples of the other two groups are shown here. (A) The organic nitrites and nitrates include amyl nitrite, isosorbide compounds, and nitroglycerin. The unshaded portion of isosorbide dinitrate is enzymatically removed in the formation of isosorbide mononitrate. (B) The calcium channel blockers belong to several chemical classes. Nifedipine is a dihydropyridine compound; diltiazem and verapamil are non-dihydropyridine drugs. The unshaded portion of nifedipine is the dihydropyridine moiety.

orally. Nitroglycerin is also available as an intravenous solution that is used chiefly to reduce preload but also to reduce afterload in patients who have **acute heart failure** associated with myocardial infarction and other conditions.

Isosorbide dinitrate can be administered sublingually or orally and is used for both the prevention and the treatment of angina attacks. Isosorbide dinitrate produces the same pharmacologic effects as nitroglycerin, but it has a slightly slower onset of action and a greater duration of action (Fig. 11–4). It is converted to an active compound, isosorbide mononitrate, which is now available as a separate drug preparation for the prevention of angina attacks.

MECHANISMS AND PHARMACOLOGIC EFFECTS. The organic nitrates are believed to act by releasing **nitric oxide (NO)** in vascular smooth muscle cells (Fig. 11–5), although some evidence indicates that they directly activate guanylyl cyclase. The precise mechanisms by which nitroglycerin and other organic nitrates release NO are still under investigation. Some evidence suggests the involvement of thiol (–SH) compounds in the bioactivation of organic nitrates. Recent evidence supports the involvement of **aldehyde dehydrogenase** in the release of NO as well as in the development of nitrate tolerance (see below).

Nitric oxide is a gas that activates guanylyl cyclase, forming **cyclic guanosine monophosphate** (cGMP). Cyclic GMP is believed to relax vascular smooth muscle by inacti-

vating myosin light-chain kinase or by stimulating dephosphorylation of myosin phosphate.

The organic nitrates preferentially relax venous smooth muscle and have a relatively smaller effect on arteriolar smooth muscle. This leads to venous pooling of blood, a decrease in venous blood return to the heart, and a decrease in ventricular volume, pressure, and wall tension. By these mechanisms, the nitrates reduce cardiac work and oxygen demand and thereby relieve or prevent angina pectoris. By reducing cardiac preload, the nitrates also reduce cardiac output and thereby contribute to a reduction in blood pressure. If blood pressure falls sufficiently, reflex tachycardia can be invoked. The nitrates do not have any direct effects on myocardial tissue.

TOLERANCE. Continuous administration of nitroglycerin and other organic nitrates often leads to pharmacodynamic tolerance to their vasodilative effects. It has been demonstrated to occur with intravenous, transdermal, and oral administration of the nitrates, including sustained-release preparations of them. To prevent nitrate tolerance and loss of therapeutic effect, skin patches should be removed for at least 10 hours each day, and long-acting oral medications should be administered only once or twice a day.

Several mechanisms have been proposed to explain nitrate tolerance but none has been proved conclusively.

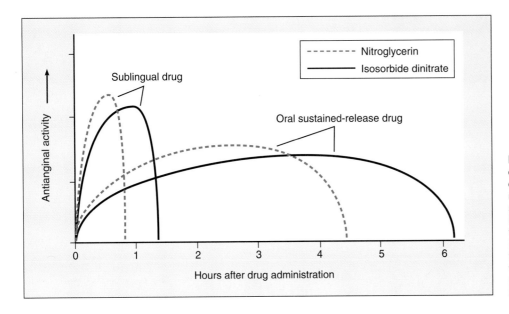

Figure 11–4. Pharmacokinetics of nitroglycerin and isosorbide dinitrate. Nitroglycerin is more rapidly absorbed and has a shorter duration of action, partly because it is quickly converted to two metabolites that are less active (glyceryl mononitrate and dinitrate). Isosorbide dinitrate is converted to a metabolite that is active and has a longer half-life (isosorbide mononitrate).

Recent studies have shown that mitochondrial **aldehyde dehydrogenase** participates in the release of NO from nitroglycerin, and that this process is accompanied by the formation of superoxide anion free radicals (O_2^-) that, in turn, inactivate aldehyde dehydrogenase and thereby lead to tolerance (Sydow et al., 2004).

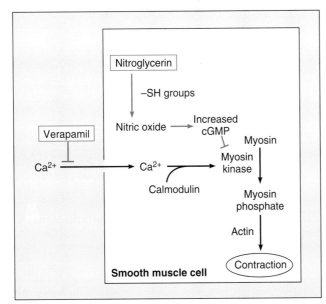

Figure 11–5. Mechanisms of action of vasodilators in smooth muscle. Actions of nitroglycerin (an organic nitrate) and verapamil (a calcium channel blocker) are shown. Organic nitrates form nitric oxide in the presence of thiol (SH) compounds. Nitric oxide activates guanylyl cyclase and thereby stimulates the formation of cyclic guanosine monophosphate (cGMP). Investigators believe that cGMP causes smooth muscle relaxation either by inactivating myosin kinase or by dephosphorylating myosin phosphate. When calcium (Ca^{2+}) enters the smooth muscle via calcium channels, it binds to calmodulin and thereby activates myosin kinase. Myosin kinase phosphorylates the light chains of myosin, enabling it to interact with actin to cause muscle contraction. Verapamil works by blocking calcium channels.

ADVERSE EFFECTS AND INTERACTIONS. The most common adverse effects of organic nitrates, which are caused by excessive vasodilation, include headache, hypotension, dizziness, and reflex tachycardia. Tachycardia increases oxygen demand and can counteract the beneficial effects of nitrates, so patients should be cautioned to avoid excessive doses of these drugs. To prevent reflex tachycardia, a β-blocker can be used together with an organic nitrate or other type of vasodilator. In combination, the drugs have a synergistic therapeutic effect.

Calcium Channel Blockers

Calcium channel blockers belong to numerous chemical classes. **Amlodipine, felodipine, isradipine, nicardipine, nifedipine,** and **nimodipine** belong to the dihydropyridine class and have similar pharmacologic properties. **Bepridil, diltiazem,** and **verapamil** each belong to a different chemical class and they are the only member of their class currently available for clinical use.

All of the CCB, except bepridil and nimodipine, are indicated for the treatment of **hypertension** (see Chapter 10). Diltiazem and verapamil are also used to treat certain types of **cardiac arrhythmias** (see Chapter 14). Nimodipine is indicated for the treatment of **subarachnoid hemorrhage,** which is one of the causes of stroke. In this setting, the drug is believed to dilate small cerebral vessels and thereby increase collateral circulation. Nimodipine can also reduce neuronal damage caused by an excessive release of calcium invoked by cerebral ischemia.

The discussion below focuses on the CCB used in the management of **angina pectoris.** These antianginal CCB include several dihydropyridines (amlodipine, felodipine, nicardipine, and nifedipine), bepridil, diltiazem, and verapamil.

Drug Properties

CHEMISTRY AND PHARMACOKINETICS. Structures of selected CCB are shown in Fig. 11–3B, and the pharmacokinetic

TABLE 11-2. Pharmacokinetic Properties of Calcium Channel Blockers Used in the Treatment of Angina Pectoris*

Drug	Oral Bioavailability	Excreted Unchanged in Urine	Elimination Half-Life (Hours)
Dihydropyridines			
Amlodipine	75%	10%	40
Felodipine	20%	1%	14
Nicardipine	35%	1%	3
Nifedipine	60%	1%	3
Other calcium channel blockers			
Bepridil	60%	5%	25
Diltiazem	55%	3%	5
Verapamil	25%	3%	5

*Values shown are the mean of values reported in the literature.

properties of the seven antianginal CCB are summarized in Table 11–2. These CCB are well absorbed after oral administration, but most of them undergo significant first-pass metabolism. Diltiazem, nicardipine, nifedipine, and verapamil, which have relatively short half-lives, are available in immediate-release preparations (which require multiple daily doses) and in sustained-release preparations (which require one or two doses a day). Amlodipine and bepridil are newer CCB that have longer half-lives and are administered once or twice a day.

MECHANISMS AND PHARMACOLOGIC EFFECTS. The **calcium ion channels** are located in the plasma membrane of smooth muscle and cardiac tissues. The influx of calcium through these channels leads to membrane depolarization and initiates or strengthens muscle contraction. CCB bind to these channels and alter their conformation in a way that prevents the entry of calcium into cells (see Fig. 11–5). By this mechanism, CCB produce smooth muscle relaxation and suppress cardiac activity.

Calcium channels are classified on the basis of their electrophysiologic properties. The two main types of voltage-activated calcium channels are the L (long) type and the T (transient) type. **L-type calcium channels** are high-voltage channels that are slowly inactivated, and their calcium influx has a relatively long duration. **T-type calcium channels** are low-voltage channels that are rapidly inactivated, and their calcium influx is more transient. Both L-type and T-type channels are found in vascular smooth muscle and in the sinoatrial (SA) and atrioventricular (AV) nodes. Only L-type channels, however, are found in the muscle cells of the heart. CCB differ in their affinity for the different types of calcium channels. All of the currently available CCB selectively bind to L-type channels. Mibefradil, a drug that selectively binds to T-type channels, was removed from the market because of excessive problems with drug interactions.

Whereas all CCB cause vascular smooth muscle to relax, they differ markedly in their effects on cardiac tissue (Table 11–3). The dihydropyridines, which are potent vasodilators, can reduce blood pressure sufficiently to evoke reflex tachycardia. At therapeutic doses, the dihydropyridines do not suppress cardiac function as much as the other CCB do. Diltiazem and verapamil decrease SA node automaticity, cardiac contractility, and AV node conduction velocity to a greater degree than the other CCB do and can significantly reduce cardiac output in patients with heart failure.

ADVERSE EFFECTS. The most common side effects of CCB in general are fatigue, headache, dizziness, flushing, **peripheral edema**, and other manifestations of vasodilation and hypotension. Several epidemiologic studies have suggested that CCB are also associated with an increased risk of adverse cardiovascular events and gastrointestinal bleeding. These drugs occasionally cause **gingival hyperplasia**.

In retrospective case-control studies, investigators found a higher incidence of myocardial infarction, congestive heart failure, and deaths from coronary heart disease in the group of patients who took immediate-release forms of nifedipine and other short-acting CCB than in the control group. In a prospective clinical trial called the Multicenter Isradipine Diuretic Atherosclerosis Study (MIDAS), investigators found a statistically significant increase in angina attacks, transient ischemic attacks, and nonfatal arrhythmias in the group of patients treated with isradipine. They also found a higher

TABLE 11-3. Cardiovascular Effects of Calcium Channel Blockers Used in the Treatment of Angina Pectoris

Drug	Coronary Blood Flow	Sinoatrial Node Automaticity*	Cardiac Contractility*	Atrioventricular Node Conduction Velocity*
Dihydropyridines				
Amlodipine	Increases	None	None	None
Nicardipine	Increases	None	None	None
Nifedipine	Increases	None	None	None
Felodipine	Increases	None	None	None
Other calcium channel blockers				
Bepridil	Increases	Decreases slightly	Decreases slightly	Dereases slightly
Diltiazem	Increases	Decreases	Decreases slightly	Decreases
Verapamil	Increases	Decreases	Decreases	Decreases

*Direct effects may be counteracted by reflex activity.

rate of myocardial infarction, stroke, congestive heart failure, angina, and sudden death in the isradipine-treated group than in the control group, but these differences were not statistically significant.

Amlodipine and Related Drugs

Amlodipine, felodipine nicardipine, and nifedipine are the dihydropyridine CCB approved for the treatment of angina. Amlodipine has a long elimination half-life and is administered once a day. It has little or no direct effect on the heart rate, AV node conduction, and cardiac contractility. Nicardipine and nifedipine have relatively short half-lives, and the immediate-release preparations must be administered several times a day in the treatment of angina. Felodipine, which has an intermediate half-life, is available in extended-release tablets administered once daily.

The dihydropyridines, which are potent vasodilators, can evoke reflex tachycardia and cause cardiac arrhythmias in some patients. Unlike diltiazem and verapamil, the dihydropyridines do not affect digoxin serum levels significantly.

Bepridil

Unlike the other CCB, which block only calcium channels, bepridil also blocks sodium channels in cardiac tissue. Bepridil slows the heart rate slightly and reduces AV node conduction while increasing the AV node refractory period. Bepridil also causes prolongation of the QT interval, which can evoke cardiac arrhythmias such as torsade de pointes (polymorphic ventricular tachycardia). For this reason, the drug is usually reserved for use in patients who have not responded to other antianginal drugs.

Diltiazem and Verapamil

Diltiazem or verapamil can be used in the treatment of typical or variant angina. Because these drugs can suppress cardiac contractility, caution should be exercised when administering either of them to patients with heart failure. In patients who have typical angina without heart failure, the drugs have the advantage of reducing the heart rate and contractility in addition to their effects on myocardial wall tension.

Verapamil and other calcium channel blockers can cause constipation, probably because of relaxation of gastrointestinal smooth muscle and reduced peristalsis. Both verapamil and diltiazem reduce the clearance of digoxin and can thereby increase serum digoxin levels and precipitate digoxin toxicity. Digoxin doses should be reduced in patients receiving these drugs.

β-ADRENERGIC RECEPTOR ANTAGONISTS

The pharmacologic properties of β-adrenergic receptor antagonists, or β-blockers, are discussed in Chapter 9, and their use in the treatment of hypertension and arrhythmias is discussed in Chapters 10 and 14, respectively.

Among the β-blockers used in the management of angina are **atenolol, metoprolol, nadolol,** and **propranolol.** These β-blockers have a significant role in the management of **typical angina pectoris** and **acute myocardial infarction,**

but they are not used in the management of variant angina or acute anginal attacks. In typical angina, they are used as prophylactic agents because of their ability to prevent exercise-induced tachycardia and increased myocardial oxygen demand. They can also prevent reflex tachycardia induced by either organic nitrates or dihydropyridine CCB.

Atenolol, metoprolol, and propranolol are often used in myocardial infarction to reduce sudden death caused by acute ventricular arrhythmias.

The β-blockers have a negative inotropic effect that can be hazardous to patients with heart failure. Because the combination of verapamil and a β-blocker is particularly likely to reduce cardiac contractility and cardiac output, it should be used with great caution. The combination of a β-blocker and diltiazem is less hazardous.

DRUGS THAT MODIFY MYOCARDIAL METABOLISM

A new group of antianginal drugs called the **partial fatty acid oxidation (pFOX) inhibitors** act by modifying myocardial metabolism. One of the new drugs, trimetazidine, is available in France and another agent, ranolazine, has completed clinical trials in the United States.

The heart uses glucose, fatty acids, and lactate as sources of energy. Although fatty acids are the major fuel for the heart, glucose is metabolized more efficiently and generates about 15% more energy. Inhibition of fatty acid oxidation by pFOX inhibitors leads to increased glucose oxidation and increased efficiency of oxygen utilization by the heart. Ranolazine appears to improve exercise capacity, decrease electrocardiographic evidence of ischemia, and reduce the frequency of angina attacks and the need for nitroglycerin use. The drug has no effect on heart rate, blood pressure, or coronary blood flow, and appears to act solely by modifying myocardial metabolism. Long-term studies to establish the clinical efficacy and safety of the pFOX inhibitors are currently underway.

MANAGEMENT OF ANGINA PECTORIS

In patients with a history of angina pectoris, the primary objectives of drug therapy are to relieve acute symptoms, to prevent ischemic attacks, improve the quality of life, and to reduce the risks of myocardial infarction and other potential cardiovascular problems, as illustrated in Box 11–1. Treatment of concurrent hypertension, hyperlipidemia, diabetes mellitus, and obesity can slow coronary artery disease progression in persons with angina, whereas antithrombotic agents (e.g., aspirin) reduce the risk of coronary thrombosis and myocardial infarction. In fact, aspirin has been shown to prolong the life of persons with chronic angina.

If a patient has only an occasional angina episode, sublingual nitroglycerin can be used as needed to relieve acute symptoms. If episodes occur predictably with exertion, sublingual nitroglycerin or isosorbide dinitrate can be taken as a prophylactic measure just before exertion. If the severity of angina requires regular use of sublingual nitroglycerin,

Case Presentation

A 57-year-old construction foreman who is a heavy smoker complains of a pressurelike discomfort in the retrosternal area. He says the problem began about a month ago and occurs two or three times a week. When questioned about the discomfort, he says that it occurs only when he is working, disappears when he rests, does not radiate to his left arm or jaw, and has never lasted for more than 15 minutes. Except for a blood pressure of 150/100 mm Hg, his results on physical examination and electrocardiogram are normal.

Case Management

After ruling out other causes of the patient's chest discomfort, the physician makes a provisional diagnosis of typical angina pectoris and prescribes sublingual nitroglycerin, 0.3 mg, as needed for acute chest discomfort. Because the patient has hypertension and angina but does not have diabetes, asthma, or heart failure, the physician also prescribes a β-adrenergic receptor antagonist, atenolol, for the treatment of hypertension and the prevention of angina. The patient is encouraged to monitor his blood pressure regularly and is scheduled to see his physician again in 3 weeks.

Case Comments

β-Adrenergic receptor antagonists are the preferred therapy for patients with hypertension and angina, because these drugs are effective in the management of both conditions and provide protection against ischemia-induced arrhythmias. Patients with chronic stable angina should be evaluated for hypercholesterolemia and treated appropriately with dietary restrictions and drug therapy to retard the progression of atherosclerosis. Control of blood pressure will also reduce atherogenesis. Patients with angina should be considered for angiographic evaluation of their coronary arteries to determine whether angioplasty or coronary artery bypass grafting is appropriate.

believed that they prevent sudden cardiac death in persons with angina. Because of this cardioprotective effect, authorities consider β-blockers the drugs of choice in treating most patients who have angina pectoris and especially those who have unstable angina. The β-blockers also have the advantage of preventing reflex tachycardia induced by organic nitrates or dihydropyridine CCB, because many patients with chronic angina require more than one antianginal medication.

Patients with unstable angina have a high risk of myocardial infarction and should also receive aspirin or other antithrombotic drugs to prevent platelet aggregation and thrombus formation. CCB are less suitable than β-blockers for patients with unstable angina or a recent myocardial infarction, because the dihydropyridine CCB have the potential to cause reflex tachycardia and because verapamil and diltiazem have the potential to suppress cardiac contractility and can increase the frequency of heart failure in persons with ventricular systolic dysfunction

The β-blockers are ineffective in treating variant angina, which is caused by coronary vasospasm. This condition is often treated with a calcium channel blocker (e.g., verapamil). Bepridil, however, is not approved for the treatment of vasospastic angina.

In patients who have angina and concomitant asthma, a CCB is usually preferred because of its potential ability to relax bronchial smooth muscle. The β-blockers should usually be avoided in persons with asthma because of their tendency to cause bronchconstriction by blocking β_2-receptors in bronchial smooth muscle. In patients with diabetes, a CCB is often used; however, if a β-blocker is chosen, it should be a cardioselective (β_1-selective) blocker (e.g., atenolol), which has less potential to interfere with β_2-mediated glycogenolysis and thereby slow the recovery from insulin-induced hypoglycemia. In many patients with heart failure, a long-acting nitrate may be preferred for angina prophylaxis. The low doses of β-blockers used initially in persons with heart failure may not adequately control angina (see Chapter 12).

however, long-term prophylactic therapy should be considered. In some cases, angiography should also be performed to determine if angioplasty or coronary artery bypass grafting is appropriate.

For patients who have stable angina and require long-term treatment, either a β-blocker, a long-acting nitrate, or a CCB can be chosen for initial therapy, with other drugs added or substituted depending on the response Most patients with chronic, stable angina benefit from receiving a β-blocker. The β-blockers are highly effective in preventing exercise-induced angina, improving exercise capacity, and preventing ischemic episodes. The β-blockers are the only antianginal drugs that have been proved to reduce the incidence of ventricular arrhythmias that cause sudden death in patients who have had a myocardial infarction, and it is

SUMMARY OF IMPORTANT POINTS

■ In patients with typical angina, the antianginal drugs act by decreasing myocardial oxygen demand. The organic nitrites and nitrates and the calcium channel blockers (CCB) decrease myocardial wall tension, whereas the β-adrenergic receptor antagonists (β-blockers) and some CCB decrease the heart rate and contractility.

■ Nitrates and dihydropyridine CCB have the potential to cause reflex tachycardia, but this effect can be prevented by concurrent administration of a β-blocker.

■ Continuous exposure to nitrates leads to tolerance. Nitrate tolerance is caused by inactivation of aldehyde dehydrogenase and decreased release of nitric oxide.

■ All CCB have similar vasodilating activity. Verapamil and diltiazem also produce significant cardiac depression, and verapamil has a greater effect than diltiazem on cardiac contractility. Verapamil and diltiazem can increase serum digoxin levels and cause digitalis toxicity.

■ In patients with a history of myocardial infarction, the β-blockers have been found to reduce the incidence of ventricular arrhythmias that cause sudden death. This cardioprotective effect adds to their value in the treatment of angina.

■ Some vasodilators are effective in the treatment of variant angina, but β-blockers are not.

Review Questions

For each numbered pharmacologic effect, select the lettered drug that is most likely associated with it.

1. Increases coronary blood flow while slowing heart rate

2. Increases venous capacity and decreases preload

3. Decreases cardiac oxygen demand but does not cause vasodilation

   (A) atenolol
   (B) felodipine
   (C) nitroglycerin
   (D) diltiazem
   (E) amlodipine

Choose the single best answer from the choices provided.

4. After beginning treatment for angina pectoris, a man complains of constipation. Which of the following is the most likely cause of this adverse reaction?

   (A) metoprolol
   (B) verapamil
   (C) nitroglycerin
   (D) propranolol
   (E) isosorbide mononitrate

5. Nitroglycerin should not be administered continuously for periods exceeding 12 to 14 hours to avoid which of the following?
   (A) headache and dizziness
   (B) induction of cytochrome P450 enzymes
   (C) hypotension and reflex tachycardia
   (D) accumulation of nitric oxide
   (E) drug tolerance

Answers and Explanations

1. The answer is D: diltiazem. Diltiazem and verapamil are non-dihydropyridine calcium channel blockers (CCB) that relax coronary smooth muscle and increase coronary blood flow while also decreasing heart rate. Dihydropyridine CCB, (e.g., amlodipine and felodipine) increase coronary blood flow but do not decrease heart rate, and sometimes cause reflex tachycardia.

2. The answer is C: nitroglycerin. Nitroglycerin preferentially relaxes venous smooth muscle, causing venodilation and reducing venous pressure and cardiac preload. Nitroglycerin has no direct effect on the heart but can cause reflex tachycardia. Calcium channel blockers relax arterial smooth muscle more than venous smooth muscle and usually reduce cardiac afterload rather than preload. Adrenergic β-blockers do not relax vascular smooth muscle.

3. The answer is A: atenolol. Adrenergic β-receptor antagonists (e.g., atenolol) decrease heart rate and contractility and thereby reduce myocardial oxygen demand. The β-blockers do not relax vascular smooth muscle or increase coronary blood flow and they do not reduce cardiac wall tension (stress).

4. The answer is B: verapamil. All calcium channel blockers can relax intestinal smooth muscle and thereby cause constipation, but verapamil is most likely to cause this effect. Adrenergic β-blockers and organic nitrates are not associated with constipation.

5. The answer is E: drug tolerance. Continuous administration of nitroglycerin for periods exceeding 12 to 14 hours can lead to drug tolerance by decreasing the release of nitric oxide that produces the vasodilative effect of this drug. Nitroglycerin skin patches and oral extended release preparations are usually removed or withheld at bedtime in order to avoid this effect. Headache, dizziness, hypotension, and reflex tachycardia are adverse effects of nitroglycerin whose occurrence may indicate a need to reduce dosage.

SELECTED READINGS

Bales, A. C. Medical management of chronic ischemic heart disease. Selecting specific drug therapies, modifying risk factors. Postgrad Med 115:39–46, 2004.

Eisenberg, M. J., A. Brox, and A. N. Bestawros. Calcium channel blockers: an update. Am J Med 116: 35–43, 2004.

Fung, H. L. Biochemical mechanism of nitroglycerin action and tolerance: is this old mystery solved? Ann Rev Pharmacol Toxicol 44:67–85, 2004.

Noronha, B., E. Duncan, and J. A. Byrne. Optimal medical management of angina. Curr Cardiol Rep 5:259–265, 2003.

Sydow, K., A. Daiber, M. Oelze, et al. Central role of mitochrondrial aldehyde-dehydrogenase and reactive oxygen species in nitroglycerin tolerance and cross-tolerance. J Clin Invest 113:482–489, 2004.

CHAPTER 12

Drugs for Heart Failure

CLASSIFICATION OF DRUGS FOR HEART FAILURE

Positively Inotropic Drugs
Digitalis Glycosides
- Digoxin

Adrenergic Receptor Agonists
- Dobutamine

Phosphodiesterase Inhibitors
- Inamrinone
- Milrinone (PRIMACOR)

Vasodilators
Angiotensin Inhibitors
- Enalapril (VASOTEC)[a]
- Valsartan (DIOVAN)[b]

Other Vasodilators
- Hydralazine

- Isosorbide dinitrate
- Nesiritide (NATRECOR)

Aldosterone Antagonists
- Spironolactone
- Eplerenone (INSPRA)

Adrenergic β-Blockers
- Carvedilol (COREG)[c]

DIURETICS

- Furosemide (LASIX)[d]

[a]also lisinopril, ramipril, and others
[b]also candesartan and others
[c]also bisoprolol, metoprolol
[d]also bumetanide, torsemide

OVERVIEW

In the United States of America, **heart failure** (HF) affects nearly 5 million individuals, is the primary cause of more than 40,000 deaths per year, and is a contributing factor in another 220,000 deaths. The overall mortality rate in patients with HF is about eight times as high as that in the normal population, and the 5-year mortality rate for patients with heart failure approaches 50%.

Pathophysiology of Heart Failure

Heart failure is the end-stage of a number of cardiovascular disorders that ultimately impair the ability of the ventricle to fill with blood or to eject blood into the circulation. **Ischemic heart disease** is the most common cause of HF. Other important causes of HF include hypertension, valvular disorders, arrhythmias, viral and congenital cardiomy-

opathy, and constrictive pericarditis. Less commonly, HF results from severe anemia, thiamine deficiency, or the use of certain anticancer drugs, such as doxorubicin (see Chapter 45). Over time, these disorders produce molecular and cellular changes in cardiac myocytes and connective tissue that lead to a series of structural and functional alternations in the ventricular wall. This process, known as **cardiac or ventricular remodeling,** is characterized by cardiac dilatation, ventricular wall thinning, interstitial fibrosis, and wall stiffness. These changes impair the ability of the heart to relax or contract.

Cardiac remodeling is believed to result primarily from the activation of neurohumoral systems in response to myocardial ischemia, excessive stretch of muscle fibers, or other pathologic stimuli. The neurohumoral systems implicated in this process include the renin-angiotensin-aldosterone axis, sympathetic nervous system, various inflammatory cytokines, and local mediators such as endothelin. These mediators activate biochemical pathways that induce myocyte hypertrophy, apoptosis, collagen production, fibrosis, and other effects that lead to cardiac remodeling and loss of ventricular function. For example, angiotensin II, which is formed locally in the myocardium in response to mechanical stretch and other stimuli, can induce collagen production and proliferation of fibroblasts. Chronic sympathetic nervous system stimulation of the injured myocardium produces myocyte hypertrophy, increased production of myocardial cytokines (e.g., tumor necrosis factor-α) and ultimately leads to myocyte death via activation of apoptotic pathways.

The hallmark of heart failure is a **reduction in stroke volume and cardiac output** at any given diastolic muscle fiber length, as determined by measuring the ventricular end-diastolic pressure (preload). The reduced stroke volume can be caused by **diastolic dysfunction** or **systolic dysfunction** and is manifested as an inability of the ventricles either to fill properly or to empty properly, respectively. Systolic dysfunction can result from decreased cardiac contractility secondary to a dilated or ischemic myocardium. Diasto-

lic dysfunction can result from decreased compliance (increased stiffness) of ventricular tissue secondary to left ventricular hypertrophy or fibrosis. Hence, both systolic and diastolic heart failure can be caused or exacerbated by the process of cardiac remodeling.

In cases of **left ventricular failure (left-sided heart failure),** the left ventricle does not adequately pump blood forward, so the pressure in the pulmonary circulation increases. When the increased pressure forces fluid into the lung interstitium, this causes **congestion** and **edema** (Fig. 12–1). **Pulmonary edema** reduces the diffusion of oxygen and carbon dioxide between alveoli and the pulmonary capillaries. This causes **hypoxemia** (deficient oxygenation of the blood) and can lead to **dyspnea** (difficulty in breathing), including **exertional dyspnea** (dyspnea provoked by exercise), **orthopnea** (intensified dyspnea when lying flat), and **paroxysmal nocturnal dyspnea** (edema-induced bronchoconstriction when sleeping).

The combination of edema-related hypoxemia and the heart's failure to pump sufficient blood to adequately perfuse the tissues can lead to generalized tissue hypoxia and organ

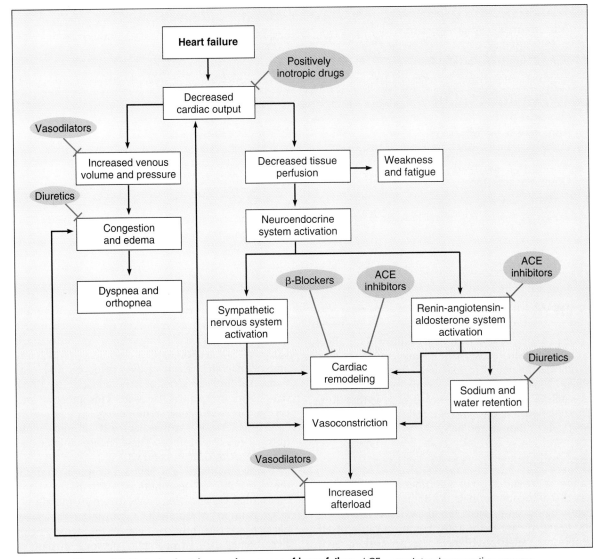

Figure 12–1. Pathophysiology and treatment of heart failure. ACE = angiotensin-converting enzyme.

dysfunction. For this reason, patients with heart failure often experience symptoms of weakness and fatigue and have reduced exercise capacity.

In cases of **right ventricular failure (right-sided heart failure),** congestion in the peripheral veins leads to **ankle edema** in the ambulatory patient and to **sacral edema** in the bedridden patient. It also leads to **hepatojugular reflux,** characterized by an increase in jugular vein distention when pressure is applied over the liver. Ultimately, right-sided failure can lead to left-sided failure as the left ventricle is forced to work harder in an attempt to maintain cardiac output.

The reduction in cardiac output that occurs in heart failure triggers a cascade of **compensatory neurohumoral responses.** Although these responses attempt to restore cardiac output via the Frank-Starling mechanism (see Fig. 12–1), they are often maladaptive and counterproductive. The reduction in tissue perfusion activates both the sympathetic nervous system and the renin-angiotensin-aldosterone system, both of which in turn stimulate vasoconstriction. Arterial vasoconstriction increases aortic impedance to left ventricular ejection and thereby decreases cardiac output, especially in patients with a weak, dilated heart. When angiotensin II stimulates the secretion of aldosterone and antidiuretic hormone, this increases the amount of sodium and water retention, the plasma volume, and the venous pressure. In addition, angiotensin II and sympathetic activation lead to cardiac remodeling and ventricular wall thinning or fibrosis, which often reduce systolic and diastolic function. Hence, the net result of the neurohumoral responses is often a further reduction in cardiac output and an increase in circulatory congestion.

Mechanisms and Effects of Drugs for Heart Failure

The primary goals of drug therapy for HF are to improve symptoms, slow or reverse deterioration in myocardial function, and prolong survival. Drugs can also be used to treat underlying conditions, control arrhythmias, prevent thrombosis, and treat anemia.

The pharmacologic agents used to treat HF include drugs that (1) increase cardiac output, (2) reduce pulmonary and systemic congestion, and (3) slow or reverse cardiac remodeling. Cardiac output can be increased by positively inotropic drugs that increase cardiac contractility and by vasodilators that reduce cardiac afterload and the impedance to left ventricular ejection. Vasodilators also reduce venous pressure, circulatory congestion, and edema. Diuretics are used to mobilize edematous fluid and reduce plasma volume, thereby decreasing circulatory congestion. Angiotensin and sympathetic inhibitors have been shown to favorably influence cardiac remodeling and increase survival in persons with HF.

Table 12–1 compares the cardiovascular effects of drugs discussed in this chapter. Each of these drugs partly counteracts the loss of myocardial function and the maladaptive responses that occur during heart failure; however, none of the current therapies, either alone or in combination, has been completely satisfactory. Because HF has such a high incidence and poor prognosis, a much effort has been ex-

pended in the search for better means to treat it. The most significant development in recent decades has been the use of angiotensin inhibitors, adrenergic β-blockers, and other agents that attenuate cardiac remodeling and reduce the mortality rate in patients with HF. Ultimately, however, the successful treatment of patients with HF may require the development of novel drugs that activate genes capable of repairing or replacing myocardial tissue.

POSITIVELY INOTROPIC DRUGS

Derived from the Greek words for fiber (*inos*) and changing (*tropikos*), the term *inotropic* refers to a change in muscle contractility. Drugs that increase cardiac contractility are said to have a **positive inotropic effect,** whereas drugs that decrease contractility have a **negative inotropic effect.** Drugs with a positive effect include members of three groups: digitalis glycosides, adrenergic β-receptor agonists, and phosphodiesterase inhibitors. The calcium sensitizing agents represent a new class of inotropic drugs that are currently under investigation for the treatment of HF. These include pimobendan and levosimendan.

All of the currently available inotropic agents increase calcium influx into cardiac muscle cells, thereby increasing cardiac contractility. The β-receptor agonists and phosphodiesterase inhibitors increase calcium influx by increasing intracellular cyclic AMP (cAMP) levels. β-agonists increase cAMP formation by activating adenylyl cyclase, whereas the phosphodiesterase inhibitors inhibit cAMP degradation. The mechanism by which digitalis glycosides increase calcium influx is described below.

Digitalis Glycosides

Despite the fact that the digitalis glycosides have been used to treat HF for more than 200 years, their effectiveness and place in therapy have been difficult to determine. Recent clinical trials indicate that digoxin provides a definite, yet limited, benefit to patients with HF caused by systolic dysfunction.

Drug Properties

Many digitalis glycosides have been isolated from plant and animal sources, including the leaves of *Digitalis* (foxglove) plants and the skin secretions of certain toads. Digoxin is the only digitalis glycoside that is extensively used today, having replaced digitoxin and crude digitalis leaf preparations in the treatment of HF and other cardiac disorders.

CHEMISTRY AND PHARMACOKINETICS. The digitalis glycosides are composed of a steroid nucleus, a lactone ring, and three sugar residues linked by glycosidic bonds (Fig. 12–2A). The stereochemical configuration of the steroid nucleus of digitalis glycosides is different than that of human steroids, and the digitalis glycosides lack most of the effects produced by gonadal or adrenal steroids.

As shown in Table 12–2, digoxin is adequately absorbed from the gut and has a long half-life of about 36 hours. It is primarily eliminated by renal excretion of the parent com-

TABLE 12–1. **Cardiovascular Effects of Drugs Used in the Treatment of Heart Failure***

Drug	Cardiac Contractility	Heart Rate	Preload Reduction	Afterload Reduction	Risk of Arrhythmia	Other Effects
Positively inotropic drugs						
Digitalis glycosides						
Digoxin	+	−	++	0 to +	++	Increases parasympathetic tone and decreases sympathetic tone.
Adrenergic receptor agonists						
Dobutamine	++	+ to ++	0 to +	+ to ++	+ to ++	
Phosphodiesterase inhibitors						
Inamrinone and Milrinone	+	0 to ++	++	++	++	
Vasodilators						
Angiotensin-converting enzyme inhibitors						
Captopril	0	0	++	++	0	
Enalapril	0	0	++	++	0	
Lisinopril	0	0	++	++	0	
Other vasodilators						
Hydralazine	0	+ (R)	0	++	+	Reduces blood pressure.
Isosorbide dinitrate	0	+ (R)	++	+	0	Reduces pulmonary congestion.
Loop-Acting Diuretics						
Bumetanide	0	0	+	0	0	Reduces edema and congestion.
Furosemide	0	0	+	0	0	Reduces edema and congestion.
Torsemide	0	0	+	0	0	Reduces edema and congestion.
Adrenergic β-blocker						
Carvedilol	0	0 to −	0	+	0	Blocks α- and β-adrenergic receptors.

*Effects are indicated as follows: decrease (−); no change or variable (0); increase ranging from small (+) to large (++); and reflex (R).

pound. Because digoxin has a low therapeutic index, serum concentrations are useful in assessing the adequacy of the dosage and evaluating potential toxicity and should be in the range of 0.5 to 2 ng/mL.

MECHANISMS AND PHARMACOLOGIC EFFECTS. The direct and indirect actions of digoxin produce a unique constellation of effects on the cardiovascular system. It has a positive inotropic effect (an increase in the force of contraction), a negative chronotropic effect (a decrease in the heart rate), and a negative dromotropic effect (a decrease in conduction velocity). Among the various types of positively inotropic drugs, digoxin is unique in its ability to strengthen cardiac contraction while decreasing heart rate. Moreover, digoxin indirectly increases parasympathetic tone while reducing sympathetic tone. This contributes to its effects on heart rate and conduction velocity and may partly account for its important role in the treatment of HF and other cardiac disorders.

(1) POSITIVE INOTROPIC EFFECT. Digoxin produces a modest positive inotropic effect that is caused by an increase in

intracellular calcium and is secondary to inhibition of the sodium pump (Na$^+$,K$^+$-ATPase) in the plasma membrane (sarcolemma). When the sodium pump is inhibited, the concentration of intracellular sodium is increased, thereby increasing the activity of the sodium-calcium exchanger and causing more calcium to enter the cardiac myocyte (Fig. 12–3). The increase in cytoplasmic calcium stimulates the release of additional calcium from the sarcoplasmic reticulum and leads to greater myofibril shortening (contraction).

The positive inotropic effect of digoxin increases the velocity of cardiac muscle contraction and the peak systolic muscle tension. These actions increase stroke volume and cardiac output at any given diastolic fiber length (preload), as shown in Fig. 12–4. The stroke volume is the amount of blood pumped by the ventricle during each systole, and the cardiac output is the amount of blood ejected from either ventricle of the heart per minute.

(2) ELECTROPHYSIOLOGIC AND ELECTROCARDIOGRAPHIC EFFECTS. Digoxin has several indirect effects on cardiac electrophysiology. It causes an increase in parasympathetic (vagal) tone, and this decreases the heart rate and atrioventricular (AV)

Figure 12–2. Structures of two examples of positively inotropic drugs for heart failure. (A) One group of positively inotropic drugs, the digitalis glycosides, includes digoxin. G denotes a glycosidic bond. (B) Two other groups of positively inotropic drugs consist of phosphodiesterase inhibitors (e.g., inamrinone, a bipyridine, shown here) and adrenergic receptor agonists (e.g., dobutamine, shown in Fig. 8–3).

node conduction velocity while increasing the AV node refractory period (Fig. 12–5). At the same time, it causes a decrease in sympathetic tone. In patients with HF, the reduction in sympathetic tone is caused partly the withdrawal of reflex sympathetic stimulation secondary to the improved cardiac output produced by digoxin. The drug also appears to directly inhibit sympathetic nerve activity. The reduction in sympathetic tone augments the effect of vagal activation on the sinoatrial and AV nodes, and it also decreases sympathetic vasoconstriction and thereby counteracts the direct vasoconstrictive effect of digoxin. The effects of digoxin on the AV node account for its ability to slow the ventricular rate in patients with atrial fibrillation (see below).

Digoxin also has direct effects on cardiac electrophysiology. Of particular importance is the drug's ability to increase abnormal impulse formation by evoking spontaneous **afterdepolarizations** (see Fig. 12–5). These abnormal depolarizations occur during or immediately after normal cardiac repolarization and lead to **extrasystoles** (premature or coupled beats) and **tachycardia** (rapid beating of the heart). The afterdepolarizations appear to be caused by excessive calcium influx into cardiac cells, and they are more likely to occur after higher doses of digoxin are given.

Digoxin has several electrocardiographic effects (see Fig. 12–5). It shortens the ventricular action potential duration by accelerating repolarization, and this decreases the QT interval. It reduces the AV node conduction velocity and thereby increases the PR interval. Finally, it causes ST segment depression, which gives rise to the so-called "hockey stick" configuration of the ST segment.

ADVERSE EFFECTS. The most common adverse effects of digoxin are gastrointestinal, cardiac, and neurologic reactions. Frequently, the earliest signs of toxicity are anorexia,

TABLE 12–2. Pharmacokinetic Properties of Positively Inotropic Drugs*

Drug	Oral Bioavailability	Onset of Action	Duration of Action	Elimination Half-Life	Excreted Unchanged in Urine	Therapeutic Serum Level
Digitalis glycosides						
Digoxin	75%	1 hour	24 hours	36 hours	60%	0.5–2 ng/ml
Adrenergic receptor agonists						
Dobutamine	NA	1 minute	<10 minutes	2 minutes	0%	NA
Phosphodiesterase inhibitors						
Inamrinone and Milrinone	NA	3 minutes	Variable	4 hours	60%	NA

*Values shown are the mean of values reported in the literature. NA = not applicable (not administered orally).

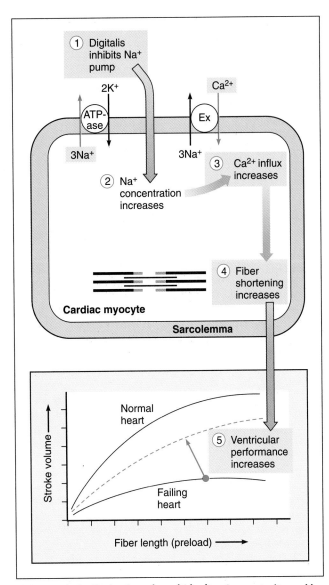

Figure 12–3. Mechanisms by which digoxin exerts its positive inotropic effect on the heart. Digoxin inhibits the sodium pump (ATPase) in the sarcolemma and increases the concentration of intracellular sodium. The high sodium concentration increases the activity of the sodium-calcium exchanger (Ex), thereby causing more calcium to enter the cardiac myocyte. Calcium activates muscle fiber shortening and increases cardiac contractility, which, in turn, increases stroke volume at any given fiber length (preload).

nausea, and vomiting. These reactions are often associated with elevated serum concentrations and may forewarn of more serious toxicity.

Arrhythmias, usually the most serious manifestation of digoxin toxicity, can include AV block and various tachyarrhythmias. Atrial tachycardia with 2:1 or 3:1 AV block is one of the most common types of digitalis-induced arrhythmia, but digoxin can also cause ventricular arrhythmias. Hypokalemia can precipitate arrhythmias in patients receiving digoxin, and the serum potassium level should be determined immediately if arrhythmias occur in these patients.

The neurologic effects of digoxin include blurred vision and yellow, green, or blue chromatopsia (a condition in which objects appear unnaturally colored). Severe digoxin toxicity can precipitate seizures.

Because digoxin has some estrogenic activity, it occasionally causes gynecomastia (excessive growth of male mammary glands).

INTERACTIONS. Several drugs can interact with digoxin and thereby affect its efficacy and toxicity (Table 12–3). Because antacids and cholestyramine can reduce the absorption of digoxin and decrease its therapeutic effects, their administration should be separated from the administration of digoxin by at least 2 hours. Diltiazem, quinidine, and verapamil reduce digoxin clearance and increase serum digoxin levels, which can cause digitalis toxicity. When digoxin is used concurrently with these drugs, only 50% of the usual dose of digoxin should be given, and serum digoxin levels should be monitored. Diuretics should be used cautiously with digoxin. Diuretic-induced hypokalemia can precipitate digitalis toxicity because the reduced serum potassium concentration increases digitalis binding to the sodium pump. Hypokalemia can also contribute directly to arrhythmias.

INDICATIONS. Digitalis glycosides have been used to treat **heart failure** for centuries, but their benefits have been uncertain, whereas their toxicity has been substantial. The improvement produced by digoxin in patients with systolic HF probably results from a combination of a modest positive inotropic effect and attenuation of the neurohumoral consequences of HF. As discussed above, digoxin augments parasympathetic tone while reducing sympathetic tone, and these actions reduce heart rate, sympathetic vasoconstriction, and cardiac afterload. Digoxin is generally not used to treat diastolic HF because contractility is not impaired in this disorder.

In patients with HF, clinical trials have shown that although digoxin treatment does not prolong survival, it reduces symptoms and the need for hospitalization, and thereby improves the quality of life of persons with HF. Moreover, patients who have been withdrawn from digoxin exhibit worsening of HF. Hence, digitalis will probably continue to have a role in treating HF in combination with angiotensin inhibitors, diuretics, adrenergic β-receptor antagonists, and other drugs.

The most certain indication for digoxin, however, appears to be the treatment of patients with **both heart failure and atrial fibrillation.** In these patients, the ventricular rate is often rapid and irregular, thereby causing palpitations and reducing cardiac output. By slowing the AV node conduction velocity and increasing the AV node refractory period, digoxin reduces the number of ectopic impulses that are transmitted from the atria to the ventricles and thereby slows the ventricular rate.

Digoxin Immune Fab

An antidote for serious digoxin toxicity is available in the form of **digoxin immune Fab.** This antibody preparation is administered intravenously and can rapidly reverse severe digoxin toxicity.

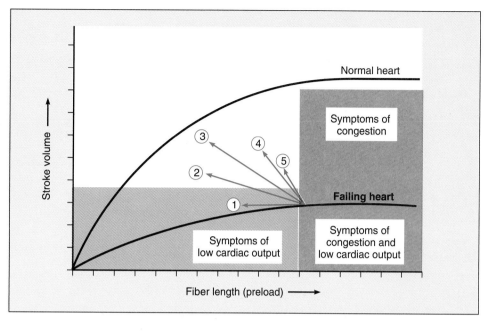

Figure 12–4. Effect of drug treatment on ventricular performance. Effects of the following drugs or drug combinations are shown: (1) a diuretic or a nitrate; (2) nitroprusside or an angiotensin-converting enzyme (ACE) inhibitor; (3) a positively inotropic drug plus a vasodilator; (4) dobutamine; and (5) digoxin. The positively inotropic drugs increase stroke volume at any given fiber length and thereby decrease venous pressure and preload. Some vasodilators (e.g., ACE inhibitors) decrease afterload and thereby increase stroke volume. Vasodilators can also decrease preload.

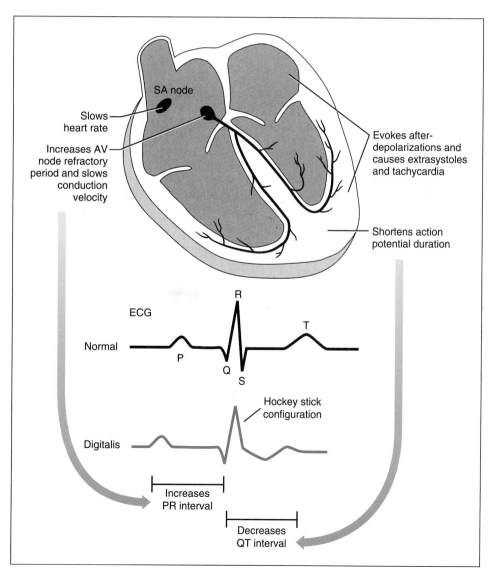

Figure 12–5. Electrophysiologic and electrocardiographic effects of digoxin. Digoxin causes an increase in parasympathetic (vagal) tone and a decrease in sympathetic tone. These actions slow the heart rate by decreasing sinoatrial (SA) node automaticity. The increased vagal tone and decreased sympathetic tone also slow the atrioventricular (AV) node conduction velocity while increasing the AV node refractory period. The reduced AV conduction velocity increases the PR interval on the electrocardiogram (ECG). In ventricular tissue, digoxin shortens the action potential duration, and this decreases the QT interval. Toxic concentrations of digoxin may evoke afterdepolarizations throughout the heart and thereby cause extra systoles and tachycardia. Digoxin also causes ST segment depression, which gives rise to the so-called hockey stick configuration on the ECG.

TABLE 12-3. **Adverse Effects, Contraindications, and Drug Interactions of Positively Inotropic Drugs**

Drug	Common Adverse Effects	Common Drug Interactions
Digitalis glycosides		
Digoxin	Anorexia, nausea, and vomiting; arrhythmias; blurred vision; chromatopsia; gynecomastia; and seizures	Digitalis absorption inhibited by antacids and cholestyramine Digitalis clearance reduced by diltiazem, quinidine, and verapamil. Diuretic-induced hypokalemia precipitates digitalis toxicity
Adrenergic receptor agonists		
Dobutamine	Excessive vasoconstriction and tachyarrhythmias	Activity affected by other agonists and antagonists
Phosphodiesterase inhibitors		
Inamrinone	Arrhythmias; hypotension; and thrombocytopenia	Incompatible with furosemide in intravenous solutions
Milrinone	Arrhythmias; hypotension; and thrombocytopenia	Unknown

Adrenergic β-receptor Agonists

Dobutamine is the adrenergic β-receptor agonist most frequently used in patients with HF. This agent must be administered by continuous intravenous infusion, and this usually restricts its use to the short-term management of **acute heart failure** and **cardiogenic shock.** Symptomatic improvement has been documented in patients with HF receiving a continuous infusion of dobutamine for 3 to 5 days, and some patients may benefit from dobutamine administration for up to 30 days. No evidence indicates that such treatments improve survival and intermittent high dose dobutamine can increase mortality. Hence, some authorities believe dobutamine and other intravenous inotropes should be limited to the short-term management of patients with severe decompensated HF.

Dobutamine selectively stimulates cardiac contractility and usually causes less tachycardia than other β-adrenergic receptor agonists, such as isoproterenol. Dobutamine also activates adrenergic β$_2$-receptors in vascular smooth muscle and thereby decreases vascular resistance and cardiac afterload.

The properties and effects of dobutamine are summarized in Tables 12–1, 12–2, and 12–3 and are described in greater detail in Chapter 8.

Phosphodiesterase Inhibitors

The phosphodiesterase inhibitors used in treating HF are **inamrinone** (see Fig. 12–2B) and **milrinone.** These bipyridine drugs inhibit **type III phosphodiesterase,** an enzyme that catalyzes the conversion of cyclic adenosine monophosphate (cAMP) to the inactive 5′-AMP. By inhibiting phosphodiesterase, the drugs increase the concentration of cAMP in cardiac tissue and smooth muscle and thereby increase cardiac contractility and relax vascular smooth muscle to cause vasodilation.

Inamrinone and milrinone are used only for the short-term management of **acute HF** or **acute exacerbations of chronic HF** in patients who are not responsive to other drugs. Intravenous administration of inamrinone and milrinone can provide both hemodynamic and symptomatic improvement in persons with advanced HF. Clinical studies have shown that the long-term use of these drugs can cause serious adverse effects, including thrombocytopenia and ventricular arrhythmias, and is associated with an increased mortality rate in patients with severe HF (Table 12–4).

VASODILATORS

The vasodilators used in treating HF include the angiotensin inhibitors and the combination of hydralazine and isosorbide dinitrate. The angiotensin inhibitors include the angiotensin converting enzyme (ACE) inhibitors and the angiotensin receptor antagonists. Vasodilators are useful in the treatment of HF because of their ability to reduce venous and arterial pressure. The reduction in venous pressure decreases edema, while the dilation of arteries reduces cardiac afterload and increases cardiac output. In addition, the angiotensin inhibitors slow or reverse **cardiac remodeling,** which is probably responsible for their beneficial effect on the survival of patients with HF.

Angiotensin-Converting Enzyme Inhibitors

The ACE inhibitors reduce the formation of angiotensin II and are used in the treatment of **diabetic nephropathy,**

TABLE 12–4. **Findings in Clinical Studies of Drugs Used in the Treatment of Heart Failure**

Drug	Study	Findings
Positively inotropic drugs		
Amrinone	Packer et al.[1]	Amrinone increased mortality rate in patients with severe heart failure.
Digoxin versus milrinone	DiBianco et al.[2]	Digoxin was superior to milrinone; milrinone caused arrhythmia in more patients.
Digoxin versus placebo	DIG[3]	Digoxin did not decrease mortality rate but decreased rate of hospitalization admissions for heart failure and other causes.
Digoxin withdrawal	PROVED[4]	Clinical worsening of heart failure occurred with digoxin withdrawal.
	RADLANCE[5]	Clinical worsening of heart failure occurred with digoxin withdrawal.
Milrinone	PROMISE[6]	Milrinone increased mortality rate in patients with severe heart failure.
Vasodilators		
Captopril	SAVE[7]	Captopril decreased risk of congestive heart failure by 37% in post–myocardial infarction patients with left ventricular dysfunction.
Enalapril	CONSENSUS[8]	Enalapril decreased mortality rate by 40% at 6 months in patients with severe heart failure.
Enalapril	SOLVD[9]	Enalapril decreased mortality rate by 18% in patients with mild to moderate heart failure; also decreased risk of congestive heart failure by 37% in patients with asymptomatic left ventricular dysfunction.
Enalapril versus combination of nitrate plus hydralazine versus placebo	V-HeFT-II[10]	Enalapril decreased risk of sudden death by 36% in patients with chronic heart failure; nitrate plus hydralazine decreased mortality rate more than placebo did but less than enalapril did.
Other drugs		
Carvedilol	AUZ-NZ[11]	Carvedilol decreased mortality rate and improved ejection fractions but did not change exercise tolerance or global assessment in patients with congestive heart failure.
Carvedilol	PRECISE[12]	Carvedilol increased exercise tolerance and improved ejection fractions in patients with congestive heart failure.
Carvedilol	US mild CHF[13]	Carvedilol decreased mortality rate, decreased rate of hospital admissions, increased exercise tolerance, and improved global assessment in patients with mild congestive heart failure.
Carvedilol versus metoprolol	COMET[14]	Carvedilol reduced mortality more than did metoprolol.
Candesartan plus ACE Inhibitor	CHARM-Added[15]	Addition of candesartan reduced mortality.
Spironolactone	RALES[16]	Spironolactone decreased mortality 30% at 24 months.

[1]Packer, M., et al. Circulation 70:1038–1047, 1984.
[2]BiBianco, R., et al. N Engl J Med 320:677–683, 1989.
[3]Digitalis Investigational Group. N Engl J Med 336:525–533, 1997.
[4]Uretsky, B. F., et al. J Am Coll Cardiol 22:955–962, 1993.
[5]Packer, M., et al. N Engl J Med 329:1–7, 1993.
[6]Packer, M., et al. N Engl J Med 325:1468–1475, 1991.
[7]Pfeffer, M. A., et al. N Engl J Med 327:669–677, 1992.
[8]CONSENSUS Trial Study Group. N Engl J Med 316:1429–1435, 1987.
[9]SOLVD Investigatiors. N Engl J Med 325:293–302, 1991.
[10]Cohn, J. N., et al. N Engl J Med 325:293–302, 1991.
[11]Australia–New Zealand Heart Failure Research Collaborative Group. Lancet 349:375–380, 1997.
[12]Packer, M., et al. Circulation 94:2793–2799, 1996.
[13]Pakcer, M., et al. N Engl J Med 334:1349–1355, 1996.
[14]Poole-Wilson, P. A., et al. Lancet 362:7–13, 2003.
[15]McMurray, J. J., et al. Lancet 362:767–771, 2003
[16]Pitt, B., et al. N Engl J Med 341:709–717, 1999.

hypertension, and **heart failure.** The general pharmacologic properties of these drugs are described in Chapter 10.

Angiotensin II has several actions that contribute to the pathogenesis of HF, including vasoconstriction and increased secretion of aldosterone and antidiuretic hormone. **Ramipril, enalapril, lisinopril,** and other ACE inhibitors act by producing venous and arterial dilation and decreasing the secretion of these two hormones. These actions in turn reduce the plasma volume, venous pressure, and level of edema, and they can increase cardiac output by reducing arterial pressure and cardiac afterload. In addition, ACE inhibitors can counteract the adverse effects of angiotensin that contribute to cardiac (ventricular) remodeling in patients with HF.

As described in Table 12–4, enalapril and other vasodilators have been shown to decrease the mortality rate in patients with HF. The Cooperative North Scandinavian Enalapril Survival Study (CONSENSUS) trial found that enalapril reduced the mortality rate by 40% in patients with **severe heart failure.** The Vasodilator Heart Failure Trial (V-HeFT-II) trial showed that treatment with enalapril reduced the mortality rate more than did treatment with the combination of a nitrate and hydralazine in patients with **chronic HF.** The Survival and Ventricular Enlargement (SAVE) and Studies of Left Ventricular Dysfunction (SOLVD) studies showed that treatment with captopril or enalapril can prevent the transition from asymptomatic to overt HF, thereby supporting the early use of an ACE inhibitor in patients with **asymptomatic heart failure.**

In patients with **acute myocardial infarction,** treatment with an ACE inhibitor has been found to improve the survival rate when it is administered within 24 hours of the onset of symptoms. Investigators believe that this benefit is partly caused by the inhibition of angiotensin II-induced cardiac remodeling, which would otherwise lead to cardiac dilatation, wall thinning, and expansion of the infarct zone in these patients.

Angiotensin Receptor Blockers

Angiotensin II receptor blockers (ARB), such as valsartan and candesartan, selectively reduce the binding of angiotensin II to AT_1 receptors and have pharmacologic and clinical effects that are similar to those of the ACE inhibitors. Unlike ACE inhibitors, ARB do not inhibit bradykinin degradation, an effect that may be responsible for some of the beneficial as well as adverse effects of ACE inhibitors (see Chapter 10). For example, ARB do not induce chronic cough, an effect that occurs in 3% to 20% of persons treated with ACE inhibitors.

Clinical trials have found that valsartan and candesartan reduce mortality and hospitalization in persons with HF. The ARB appear to be as effective or possibly slightly less effective than ACE inhibitors in treating HF, and most authorities recommend that ARB should not be used in preference to an ACE inhibitor to treat HF. The ARB are particularly indicated in patients with HF who cannot tolerate an ACE inhibitor, and valsartan is approved by the US Food and Drug Administration (FDA) for this indication. In addition, the Assessment of Reduction in Mortality and Morbidity (CHARM-added) trial showed that patients receiving an ACE inhibitor benefited from the addition of an ARB, and some authorities recommend adding an ARB to HF therapy in patients who are stable on ACE inhibitors and β-blockers.

Hydralazine and Nitrates

Isosorbide dinitrate primarily relaxes venous smooth muscle, whereas hydralazine preferentially relaxes arterial smooth muscle. The combined use of these two drugs reduces cardiac preload and afterload, leading to reduced venous pressure and edema and to increased cardiac output, respectively. Hence, the effects of isosorbide dinitrate plus hydralazine are similar to those produced by the angiotensin inhibitors. The V-HeFT trials (Table 12–4) found that this drug combination decreased mortality more than placebo but less than enalapril. For this reason, the hydralazine-isosorbide dinitrate combination is sometimes used to treat patients with HF who cannot tolerate an angiotensin inhibitor.

In the V-HeFT trials, black patients had a lesser benefit from ACE inhibitors than whites, whereas the effect of hydralazine plus isosorbide dinitrate was greater in black patients. The recently completed African-American Heart Failure Trial provided further evidence of the beneficial effects of hydralazine-isosorbide dinitrate on the survival of black patients with HF.

Nesiritide

Nesiritide (NATRACOR) is a form of **human B-type natriuretic peptide** (hBNP) obtained from *Escherichia coli* using recombinant DNA technology. It is approved for the treatment of patients with acutely decompensated HF who have shortness of breath (dyspnea) at rest or with minimal activity.

Nesiritide binds to a guanylate cyclase receptor in vascular smooth muscle and endothelial cells, leading to increased intracellular concentrations of cyclic guanosine monophosphate (cGMP). Cyclic GMP acts as a second messenger to dilate venous and arterial smooth muscle thereby leading to reductions in venous and arterial pressure in patients with HF. Clinical trials show that nesiritide reduced pulmonary capillary wedge pressure, a clinical measure of venous pressure and cardiac preload, and thereby decreased vascular congestion and dyspnea in decompensated patients with HF. The most common adverse effect of nesiritide is hypotension, although most cases were not symptomatic. Because nesiritide is a peptide drug, it must be given intravenously and it is primarily eliminated by intracellular proteolysis. The drug can be used alone or with other standard therapies for HF.

β-ADRENERGIC RECEPTOR ANTAGONISTS

Once contraindicated in HF because of their negative inotropic effect, the β-adrenergic receptor antagonists (β-blockers) have emerged as one of the newer treatments for this cardiac condition. This paradigm shift resulted from advances in the understanding of the role of the sympathetic nervous system in cardiac remodeling and the progression of heart failure.

Excessive sympathetic nervous system activity contributes to cardiac remodeling in several ways. Sympathetic activation of cardiac β-receptors produces tachycardia and increased oxygen demand, thereby increasing infarct size and the propensity for cardiac remodeling in persons with myocardial infarction. Sympathetic activation also increases activation of the renin-angiotensin-aldosterone system, whose role in cardiac remodeling is described above. In addition, chronic stimulation of cardiac β-receptors leads to both myocyte hypertrophy and apoptosis in a manner that contributes to cardiac dilatation and ventricular wall thinning. Finally, activation of the sympathetic system increases production of cardiac cytokines, including tumor necrosis factor-α and interleukins. These cytokines also induce myocyte hypertrophy and apoptosis, and produce alterations in the intracellular matrix that contribute to fibrosis and ventricular wall stiffness.

The benefits of therapy with β-blockers are caused by the ability of these drugs to reduce excessive sympathetic stimulation of the heart and circulation in patients with HF. Several clinical trials have shown that some β-blockers, particularly carvedilol, metoprolol, and bisoprolol, benefit patients with mild to moderate HF caused by left ventricular systolic dysfunction.

Much of the attention concerning β-blocker therapy in HF has been focused on carvedilol. Carvedilol is a third-generation β₁- and β₂-blocker that also produces vasodilation via α₁-receptor blockade. In addition, carvedilol and its metabolites have antioxidant properties described in Chapter 9, and it also exhibits antiinflammatory and anti-apoptotic properties that can contribute to its beneficial effects in HF. For these reasons, carvedilol has been called a **multiple-action neurohumoral antagonist.**

In several clinical trials, carvedilol has been found to increase left ventricular ejection fraction, improve symptoms, and slow disease progression. These studies show that carvedilol reduces both hospitalization and mortality in persons with HF when it is added to a standard treatment regimen. Carvedilol is currently recommended for all patients with symptomatic HF who do not have significant hypotension, pulmonary congestion, or atrioventricular block. Patients should be monitored for the adverse effects of carvedilol, which include bradycardia, worsening heart failure, and dizziness or light-headedness caused by vasodilation and decreased blood pressure.

Metoprolol and bisoprolol have also been shown to produce beneficial effects in patients with HF. Some studies, however, suggest that these drugs are not as beneficial as carvedilol in some patients with HF. In the COMET study of patients with HF, carvedilol reduced mortality more than did metoprolol. This study has been criticized with respect to whether the doses of the β-blockers used in the study produced the same degree of β-blockade. Further clinical trials may help decide whether carvedilol is superior to other beta blockers.

The initiation of β-blocker therapy in patients with HF requires careful attention to dosage titration. Because the beneficial effects of β-blockers in HF have a delayed onset of action, whereas potential adverse cardiac effects can occur immediately, patients are started on low doses of a β-blocker and the dose is then gradually titrated upward every 2 to 3 weeks until the target dose is achieved over a period of several months. Patients should be monitored regularly during the titration period and informed that β-blockers can lead to increased symptoms for 4 to 10 weeks before any improvement is noted.

ALDOSTERONE ANTAGONISTS

Spironolactone and eplerenone (INSPRA) are aldosterone antagonists that compete with aldosterone for the mineralocorticoid receptor in renal tubules and other tissues. These drugs act on the kidneys to increase sodium excretion, decrease potassium excretion, and exert a moderate diuretic effect. For this reason, spironolactone has been classified as a potassium-sparing diuretic and its pharmacologic properties and use are described in Chapter 13.

The RALES clinical trial found that spironolactone reduced mortality in persons with severe HF. This benefit has been attributed to the prevention of the adverse effects of excessive aldosterone levels on the heart and to an elevation of the serum potassium level. The survival benefits of these drugs were in addition to those provided by angiotensin inhibitors and β-blockers. Current guidelines recommend using an aldosterone antagonist only for the treatment of severe HF. Following the RALES study, many physicians began using aldosterone antagonists in patients with mild to moderate heart failure. The increased use of these drugs in elderly patients who may have renal insufficiency has been associated with about a 100% increase in the incidence of hospitalization and death caused by hyperkalemia. This illustrates one of the differences between clinical trials, in which patients are carefully selected and monitored, and typical medical care practices.

Aldosterone produces endocrine side effects resulting from its binding to androgen and progesterone receptors leading to gynecomastia and impotence in some male patients. Eplerenone produces fewer endocrine side effects than spironolactone (1% versus 10% in clinical trials). Eplerenone is much more expensive, however, and it seems reasonable to begin with spironolactone and switch to eplerenone if endocrine side effects develop.

DIURETICS

In patients with HF, diuretics are used to reduce plasma volume and edema and thereby relieve the symptoms of circulatory congestion such as shortness of breath (dyspnea).

Loop diuretics (e.g., **bumetanide, furosemide,** and **torsemide**) have more natriuretic activity than other types of diuretics and are the preferred diuretics for reducing plasma volume to control symptoms of circulatory congestion in most cases of HF. Loop diuretics must be used carefully to avoid excessive diuresis, dehydration, and electrolyte imbalances. Hypokalemia predisposes patients to digoxin toxicity and patients with HF should be closely monitored for this condition. Thiazide diuretics can be used when a lesser degree of diuresis is required in the treatment of HF.

The pharmacologic properties of diuretics are described in Chapter 13.

MANAGEMENT OF HEART FAILURE

In patients with HF, the goals are to (1) relieve the symptoms of disease, (2) prevent disease progression, and (3) prolong survival. Acute HF usually requires hospitalization and the administration of intravenous vasodilators, positively inotropic drugs, diuretics, and oxygen. Once stabilized, patients with chronic HF are usually managed with oral medications, dietary restrictions, and exercise guidelines. Although bed rest may relieve symptoms of HF during the early course of therapy, many patients benefit from an incremental exercise program after their condition is stabilized by medications.

The selection of medications for chronic HF depends on the severity of the condition and the particular signs and symptoms exhibited by the patient. The standard drug therapy for chronic HF caused by systolic dysfunction consists of the following types of medications: (1) an ACE inhibitor in combination with an adrenergic β-blocker to slow progression of HF and improve survival, (2) spironolactone or eplerenone (if spironolactone is not tolerated) to improve survival in persons with severe HF or with left ventricular dysfunction after an acute myocardial infarction, (3) a loop diuretic to reduce plasma volume and thereby control edema and shortness of breath, and (4) digoxin to improve symptoms of weakness and fatigue caused by low cardiac output, and to reduce the need for hospitalization.

Angiotensin receptor blockers can be used in persons who cannot tolerate an ACE inhibitor, and some patients taking ACE inhibitors benefit from the addition of an ARB to the drug regimen. Several other classes of drugs are currently under investigation, and the treatment of HF will continue to evolve as new drugs with unique mechanisms of action are developed.

SUMMARY OF IMPORTANT POINTS

■ Heart failure is a common manifestation of ischemic heart disease, chronic hypertension, valvular disorders, and other cardiovascular conditions.

■ Angiotensin inhibitors and adrenergic β-blockers slow cardiac remodeling and disease progression while increasing cardiac output and survival in persons with HF.

■ In patients with HF, digoxin increases cardiac contractility and cardiac output, and reduces symptoms of weakness and fatigue and the need for hospitalization.

■ Digoxin augments parasympathetic tone and thereby slows the atrioventricular (AV) node conduction velocity and increases the AV node refractory period. These actions slow the ventricular rate in patients with atrial fibrillation.

■ Digoxin is primarily eliminated by renal excretion and has a relatively long half-life.

■ The adverse gastrointestinal, cardiac, and neurologic effects of digoxin include anorexia, nausea, vomiting, arrhythmias, blurred vision, chromatopsia, and seizures.

■ Digoxin immune Fab can be used to treat life-threatening digoxin toxicity.

■ Loop-acting diuretics are used to mobilize edematous fluid in patients with HF.

■ Positively inotropic drugs (e.g., dobutamine) and vasodilators (e.g., nesiritide, a recombinant human B-type natriuretic peptide) are used in the treatment of acute decompensated HF.

Review Questions

Choose the single best answer from the choices provided.

1. Which of the following causes digoxin to slow the ventricular heart rate in some persons with atrial fibrillation?
   (A) increase in cardiac output
   (B) decrease in vagal tone
   (C) decrease in atrial depolarizations
   (D) increase in atrioventricular node refractory period
   (E) decrease in ventricular preload

2. Which of the following drugs improves survival in persons with chronic heart failure?
   (A) digoxin
   (B) enalapril
   (C) dobutamine
   (D) milrinone
   (E) furosemide

3. Which of the following options is not a characteristic of carvedilol?
   (A) produces vasodilation by blocking adrenergic α_1-receptors
   (B) increases cardiac output by blocking adrenergic β_2-receptors
   (C) reduces cardiac remodeling
   (D) improves survival in patients with heart failure
   (E) has antioxidant properties

4. What is the preferred vasodilator for treatment of heart failure in black persons?
   (A) hydralazine plus isosorbide dinitrate
   (B) an angiotensin-converting enzyme inhibitor
   (C) an angiotensin receptor blocker
   (D) a phosphodiesterase inhibitor
   (E) nesiritide

Answers and Explanations

1. The answer is D: increasing atrioventricular refractory period. Digoxin increases the atrioventricular (AV) refractory period by increasing parasympathetic (vagal) tone and reducing sympathetic tone at the AV node. By this action, it reduces the number of atrial impulses that can be transmitted to the ventricles per minute and thereby reduces the ventricular rate in persons with atrial fibrillation.

2. The answer is B: enalapril. Enalapril and other ACE inhibitors have been shown to improve survival in chronic heart failure. This effect probably results from a reduction in cardiac remodeling that would otherwise lead to further deterioration in ventricular performance. Digoxin and furosemide improve symptoms but do not increase survival in chronic heart failure, whereas milrinone and inamrinone improve symptoms in acute heart failure but decrease survival in chronic heart failure.

3. The answer is B: increases cardiac output by blocking adrenergic β_2-receptors. Carvedilol is a nonselective adrenergic β_1- and β_2-blocker and a selective α_1-blocker. It is believed to reduce cardiac remodeling and improve survival in heart failure by blocking cardiac β_1-receptors. β_2-receptor blockade is not associated with any therapeutic effect, but might cause bronchoconstriction in asthmatic patients.

4. The answer is A: hydralazine plus isosorbide dinitrate. This drug combination has been shown to increase survival in black persons with heart failure, whereas the ACE inhibitors were less beneficial in black patients than hydralazine plus isosorbide dinitrate.

SELECTED READINGS

Ertl, G., and J. Bauersachs. Endothelin receptor antagonists in heart failure: current status and future directions. Drugs 64:1029–1040, 2004.

Krum, H., and D. Liew. Eplerenone in the treatment of chronic heart failure. Expert Rev Cardiovasc Ther 2:315–320, 2004.

Lehtonen, L. A., S Antila, and P. J. Pentikainen. Pharmacokinetics and pharmacodynamics of intravenous inotropic agents. Clin Pharmacokinet 43:187–203, 2004.

Udelson, J. E. Ventricular remodeling in heart failure and the effect of β-blockade. Am J Cardiol 93(Suppl 9A):43B–48B, 2004.

CHAPTER 13

Diuretics

CLASSIFICATION OF DIURETICS

Thiazide and Related Diuretics
- Hydrochlorothiazide
- Indapamide (LOZOL)
- Metolazone

Loop Diuretics
- Bumetanide (BUMEX)
- Ethacrynic acid
- Furosemide (LASIX)
- Torsemide (DEMADEX)

Potassium-sparing Diuretics
- Amiloride
- Spironolactone (ALDACTONE)
- Triamterene (DYRENIUM)

Osmotic Diuretics
- Glycerol
- Mannitol

Carbonic Anhydrase Inhibitors
- Acetazolamide (DIAMOX)
- Dorzolamide (TRUSOPT)

OVERVIEW

Diuretics are used in the management of edema associated with cardiovascular, renal, and endocrine abnormalities, as well as in the treatment of hypertension, glaucoma, and several other clinical disorders (Table 13–1). The drugs act at various sites in the nephron to cause **diuresis** (an increase in urine production). Most diuretics inhibit the reabsorption of sodium from the nephron into the circulation and thereby cause an increase in **natriuresis** (the excretion of sodium in the urine). Several types of diuretics also cause an increase in **kaliuresis** (the excretion of potassium in the urine). Diuretics also affect the excretion of magnesium, calcium, chloride, and bicarbonate ions.

NEPHRON FUNCTION AND SITES OF DRUG ACTION

Sodium and other electrolytes are reabsorbed into the circulation at various sites throughout the nephron by active and passive processes that involve **ion channels, transport proteins,** and the **sodium pump** (Na^+,K^+-ATPase). Ion channels are unique membrane proteins through which a specific ion moves across the cell membrane in the direction that is determined by the electrochemical gradient for the ion. The transport proteins include **symporters,** which transport two or more ions in the same direction, and **antiporters,** which transport ions in opposite directions across cell membranes. Most diuretics act by blocking a specific ion channel or transporter in the tubular epithelial cells. The effects of diuretics on ion reabsorption and secretion in the nephron are illustrated in Box 13–1.

Glomerular Filtration

Urine formation begins with glomerular filtration, a process in which an ultrafiltrate of blood is forced out of the glomerular capillaries and into the nephron lumen by the hydrostatic pressure in these capillaries. In healthy individuals, this filtrate is essentially free of blood cells and plasma proteins. **Digitalis glycosides** and other cardiac stimulants can indirectly cause diuresis by increasing cardiac output, renal blood flow, and the glomerular filtration rate. The renal actions of these drugs are described in greater detail in Chapter 12. The diuretic drugs described in this chapter do not increase the glomerular filtration rate, and some of them

TABLE 13-1. Usefulness of Diuretics in the Management of Various Clinical Disorders*

Disorder	Thiazide and Related Diuretics	Loop Diuretics	Potassium Sparing Diuretics	Osmotic Diuretics	CarbonicThiazide Anhydrase Inhibitors
Cerebral edema	0	0	0	+	0
Cirrhosis	+	++	+	0	0
Congestive heart failure	+	++	+	0	0
Diabetes insipidus	++	0	0	0	0
Epilepsy	0	0	0	0	+
Glaucoma	0	0	0	+	++
High-altitude sickness	0	0	0	0	++
Hyperaldosteronism	0	0	+	0	0
Hypercalcemia	0	++	0	0	0
Hypertension	++	+	+	0	0
Hypokalemia	0	0	++	0	0
Nephrolithiasis	++	0	0	0	0
Nephrotic syndrome	+	++	+	0	0
Pulmonary edema	+	++	+	0	0
Renal impairment	+	++	0	+	0

*Ratings range from 0 (not useful) to ++ (highly useful).

may indirectly reduce it by decreasing plasma volume and renal blood flow.

Proximal Tubule

The proximal tubule is an important site of tubular reabsorption and secretion. Essentially all of the filtered glucose, amino acids, and other organic solutes are reabsorbed in the early portion of the proximal tubule. About 85% of filtered sodium bicarbonate is reabsorbed in the proximal tubule, and this reabsorption is inhibited by a class of diuretics known as **carbonic anhydrase inhibitors.** For reasons described later in this chapter, these drugs are relatively weak diuretics and are seldom used for this purpose, although their actions are useful in the treatment of glaucoma and other conditions.

About 40% of filtered sodium chloride is reabsorbed in the proximal tubule. This is a relatively unimportant site of diuretic action, however, because inhibition of sodium chloride reabsorption in the proximal tubule almost invariably leads to increased sodium chloride reabsorption in more distal segments of the nephron.

The proximal tubule is the major site of the active tubular secretion of organic acids and bases into the nephron lumen, including natural compounds (e.g., uric acid) and drugs (e.g., penicillins). The **loop diuretics** and **thiazide diuretics** are also secreted by proximal tubular cells, and then these drugs are carried in the tubular fluid to their site of action in the loop of Henle and the distal tubule, respectively.

Loop of Henle

The loop of Henle is responsible for the reabsorption of about 35% of the filtered sodium chloride. This segment also participates in the formation of a concentrated urine by transporting sodium chloride into the surrounding intersti-

tium, where a hypertonic interstitial fluid is formed. This fluid attracts water from the collecting duct under the influence of antidiuretic hormone. The reabsorption of sodium from the thick ascending limb is inhibited by **loop diuretics,** which produce a greater diuretic effect than any other class of diuretics.

Distal Tubule

The early distal tubule is responsible for the reabsorption of 5% to 10% of the filtered sodium chloride, and this reabsorption is inhibited by **thiazide and related diuretics.** Because a relatively small percentage of sodium reabsorption can be inhibited by these drugs, they have a more modest diuretic action than the loop diuretics.

Collecting Duct

The collecting duct serves to adjust the final composition and volume of urine to regulate extracellular fluid composition and pH and thereby maintain physiologic homeostasis. The collecting duct is the site of action of **aldosterone** and **antidiuretic hormone.** Aldosterone is a mineralocorticoid that increases sodium reabsorption, thereby promoting sodium retention by the body. Antidiuretic hormone increases the reabsorption of water from the collecting duct, which conserves body water and concentrates the urine. The actions of these hormones are partly responsible for maintaining plasma volume and osmolality in the normal range.

The collecting duct is responsible for the reabsorption of about 3% of the filtered sodium chloride. This reabsorption is coupled with potassium and hydrogen excretion. The **potassium-sparing diuretics** inhibit these processes and are used to reduce potassium excretion and prevent hypokalemia.

BOX 13-1. SITES AND MECHANISMS OF ACTION OF DIURETICS*

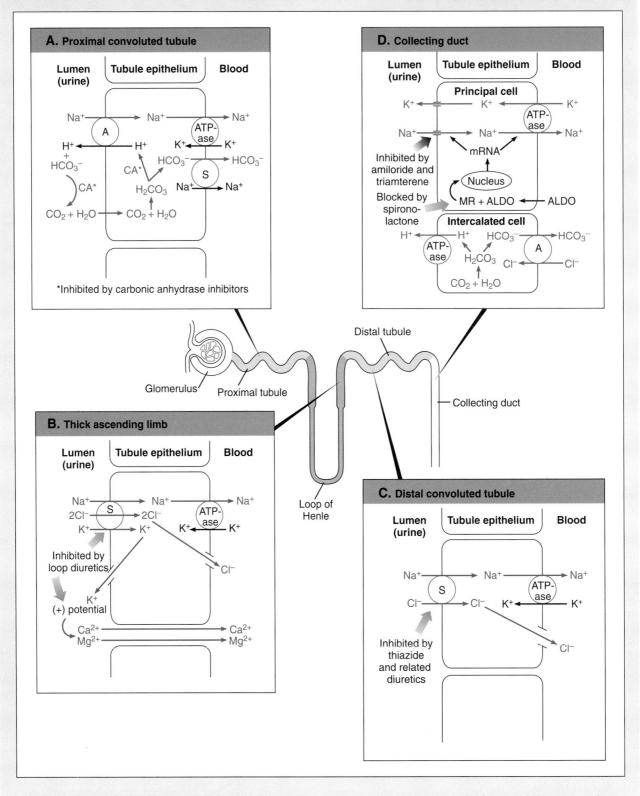

In the proximal tubule (**A**), carbonic anhydrase catalyzes the reversible conversion of hydrogen ion and bicarbonate to carbon dioxide and water, thereby enabling the reabsorption of sodium bicarbonate. This process is inhibited by **carbonic anhydrase inhibitors,** such as **acetazolamide.**

In the thick ascending limb of the loop of Henle (**B**), the $Na^+,K^+,2Cl^-$ symporter transports sodium, potassium, and

BOX 13–1. SITES AND MECHANISMS OF ACTION OF DIURETICS*—cont'd

chloride ions into the tubular cells, and then sodium is transferred to the interstitial fluid by the sodium pump. Potassium back-diffuses into the lumen and contributes to the positive transepithelial potential that drives paracellular calcium and magnesium reabsorption. By inhibiting the symporter, the **loop diuretics** reduce the back-diffusion of potassium and increase the excretion of calcium and magnesium.

In the distal tubule **(C),** sodium is transported into tubular epithelial cells by the Na^+,Cl^- symporter and then is transferred to interstitial fluid by the sodium pump. The Na^+,Cl^- symporter is inhibited by **thiazide and related diuretics.**

In the collecting duct **(D),** sodium enters the principal cells through sodium channels. Sodium is then transferred into the interstitial fluid by the sodium pump, while potassium is pumped in the opposite direction and then moves through potassium channels into the tubular fluid. Aldosterone stimulates these processes by increasing the synthesis of messenger RNA that encodes for sodium channel and sodium pump proteins. The **potassium-sparing diuretics** exert their effects via two mechanisms: **amiloride** and **triamterene** inhibit the entrance of sodium into the principal cells, whereas **spironolactone** blocks the mineralocorticoid receptor and thereby inhibits sodium reabsorption and potassium secretion.

*A = antiporter; ALDO = aldosterone; CA = carbonic anhydrase; MR = mineralocorticoid receptor; mRNA = messenger RNA; and S = symporter.

DIURETIC AGENTS

Thiazide and Related Diuretics

The thiazides and related diuretics are the most commonly used diuretics. They are orally efficacious, have a moderate natriuretic effect, and have few adverse effects in most patients.

Drug Properties

CHEMISTRY AND PHARMACOKINETICS. Thiazides are sulfonamide compounds that contain a benzothiadiazide (thiazide) moiety (Fig. 13–1A). They exhibit good oral bioavailability and were the first orally administered diuretics to be widely used for the treatment of hypertension and edema. Thiazides are actively secreted into the nephron by proximal tubular cells, and they travel through the nephron lumen to reach their site of action in the distal tubule. Some of the thiazides are partially metabolized before excretion in the urine (Table 13–2).

MECHANISMS AND PHARMACOLOGIC EFFECTS. Thiazide diuretics act primarily on the early portion of the distal tubule to inhibit the Na^+,Cl^- symporter that participates in the reabsorption of sodium and chloride from this segment of the nephron (see Box 13–1). This action leads to the delivery of a greater volume of sodium chloride-enriched tubular fluid to the late distal tubule and collecting duct, which in turn stimulates the exchange of sodium and potassium at these sites. In the process, a small amount of sodium is reabsorbed as potassium is secreted into urine in the tubules. By this mechanism, thiazides have a kaliuretic effect that leads to hypokalemia in some patients.

As shown in Table 13–3, thiazides increase magnesium excretion, but (unlike many diuretics) they decrease calcium excretion in the urine. The hypocalciuria induced by thiazides appears to result from decreased expression of calcium transport proteins, including the epithelial calcium channel, calbindin, and the sodium-calcium exchanger protein, in renal tubules. The ability of thiazides to reduce calcium excretion is the basis for their use in the treatment of kidney stones caused by excessive calcium in the urine.

ADVERSE EFFECTS AND INTERACTIONS. Table 13–4 lists the common adverse effects and interactions of thiazides and other diuretics.

Thiazide diuretics sometimes cause hypokalemia, particularly in patients whose dietary potassium intake is inadequate. Hypokalemia can eventually lead to hypokalemic metabolic alkalosis (Fig. 13–2). In this disorder, hydrogen ions enter body cells as potassium leaves these cells in an attempt to correct the plasma potassium deficiency. As the plasma potassium level falls, more hydrogen ions are secreted into urine in the tubules in exchange for sodium, and this further contributes to the development of metabolic alkalosis. In cases of hypokalemic metabolic alkalosis, potassium chloride is administered intravenously and orally. Correction of the serum potassium level then leads to correction of the acid-base disturbance as potassium displaces hydrogen ions from body cells and fewer hydrogen ions are secreted by the collecting duct.

In addition to causing electrolyte and acid-base disturbances, the thiazides can cause several metabolic abnormalities, including elevated blood glucose, uric acid, and lipid levels. An increase in blood glucose levels can be caused, in part, by diuretic-induced potassium deficiency, because hypokalemia reduces the secretion of insulin by pancreatic β-cells and thereby increases plasma glucose concentrations. Hyperuricemia, which is caused by inhibition of uric acid secretion from the proximal tubule, can lead to the development of gout. The effects of thiazide diuretics on serum lipid levels are discussed in greater detail in Chapter 10.

INDICATIONS. Thiazide diuretics are widely used in the management of cardiovascular and renal diseases (see Table 13–1). They are often prescribed for **hypertension** and can

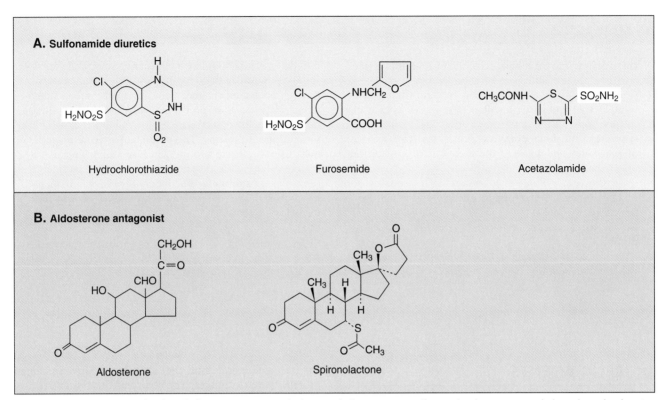

Figure 13-1. Structures of selected diuretics. (A) Several classes of diuretics are sulfonamide derivatives, including thiazide diuretics (hydrochlorothiazide), loop-acting diuretics (furosemide), and carbonic anhydrase inhibitors (acetazolamide). The sulfonamide moiety is unshaded. (B) Spironolactone, a potassium-sparing diuretic, is an aldosterone antagonist.

TABLE 13-2. Pharmacokinetic Properties of Diuretics*

Drug	Oral Bioavailability	Elimination Half-Life (Hours)	Route of Elimination	Duration of Action (Hours)
Thiazide and related diuretics				
Hydrochlorothiazide	70%	5	60% R and 40% M	12 fro oral
Indapamide	90%	16	70% R and 30% M	30 for oral
Metolazone	65%	8	80% R and 20 % M	18 for oral
Loop diuretics				
Bumetanide	85%	1.25	65% R and 35% M	5 for oral / 1 for IV
Ethacrynic acid	100%	1	65% R and 35% M	7 for oral / 2 for IV
Furosemide	60%	2	60% R and 40% M	7 for oral / 2 for IV
Torsemide	80%	3.5	30% R and 70% M	7 for oral / 7 for IV
Potassium-sparing diuretics				
Amiloride	20%	8	R	24 for oral
Spironolactone	65%	1.5	M	60 for oral
Triamterene	50%	4	M	14 for oral
Osmotic diuretics				
Glycerol	95%	.07	M	1 for oral
Mannitol	NA	1	R	7 for IV
Carbonic anhydrase inhibitors				
Acetazolamide	70%	7.5	R	10 for oral
Dorzolamide	NA	Biphasic†	R and M	8 for topical

*Values shown are the mean of values reported in the literature. IV = intravenous; M = metabolism; NA = not applicable (not administered orally); R = renal; and U = unknown.
†Dorzolamide is eliminated in a biphasic manner, with a rapid decline in serum levels followed by a much slower release from erythrocytes, and has a half-life of 4 months.

TABLE 13–3. Effects of Diuretics on Plasma pH and Urinary Excretion of Electrolytes*

Drug	Plasma pH	ELECTROLYTES EXCRETED				
		Ca²⁺	HCO₃⁻	K⁺	Mg²⁺	Na⁺
Thiazide and related diuretics	0 or +	−	0 or +	++	++	++
Loop diuretics	0 or +	++	0	++	++	+++
Potassium-sparing diuretics	0 or −	−	0	−	−	+
Osmotic diuretics	0	+	+	+	++	+++
Carbonic anhydrase inhibitors	−	0 or +	+++	+	−	+

*Acute effects are shown and are indicated as follows: decrease (–); no change or variable (0); and increase ranging from small (+) to large (+++).

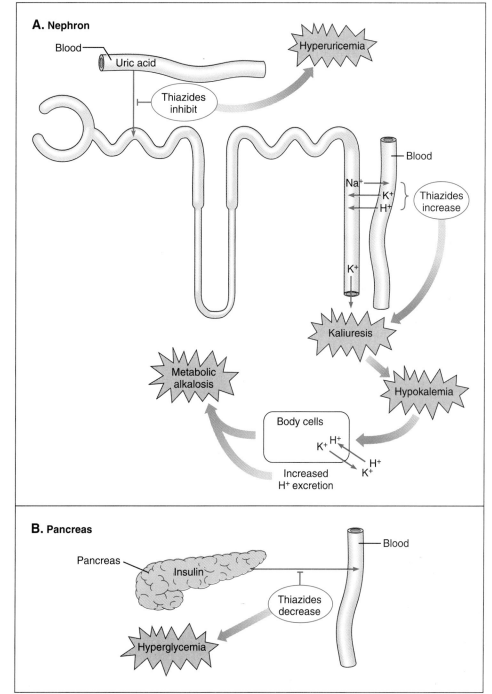

Figure 13-2. Adverse effects of thiazide diuretics. (A) Inhibition of uric acid secretion in the proximal tubule can lead to hyperuricemia and gout. Increased potassium secretion in the collecting duct can cause hypokalemia. Hypokalemia can lead to metabolic alkalosis by promoting the exchange of intracellular potassium for hydrogen ions and by increasing the excretion of hydrogen ions. The increased excretion is caused by lack of availability of potassium for exchange with sodium in the collecting duct. (B) In the presence of hypokalemia, the amount of insulin secreted by the pancreas can be reduced, thereby leading to hyperglycemia. Other mechanisms can also be involved in the development of hyperglycemia.

TABLE 13–4. **Adverse Effects, Contraindications, and Drug Interactions of Diuretics***

Drug	Common Adverse Effects	Common Drug Interactions
Thiazide and related diuretics		
Hydrochlorothiazide	Blood cell deficiencies; electrolyte imbalances; and increased blood cholesterol, glucose, or uric acid levels.	Potentiates the diuretic effect of loop diuretics.
Indapamide	Electrolyte imbalances and increased blood cholesterol, glucose, or uric acid levels.	Same as hydrochlorothiazide.
Metolazone	Blood cell deficiencies; electrolyte imbalances; and increased blood cholesterol or glucose levels.	Same as hydrochlorothiazide.
Loop diuretics		
Bumetanide	Blood cell deficiencies; electrolyte imbalances; hearing impairment; and hypersensitivity reactions.	Diuretic effect decreased by NSAIDs. Administration with ACE inhibitors may cause excessive hypotension.
Ethacrynic acid	Blood cell deficiencies; electrolyte imbalances; hearing impairment; and rash.	Diuretic effect decreased by NSAIDs.
Furosemide	Blood cell deficiencies; electrolyte imbalances; hearing impairment; hypersensitivity reactions; increased blood cholesterol, glucose, or uric acid levels; and photosensitivity.	Same as bumetanide.
Torsemie	Electrolyte imbalances and increased blood cholesterol, glucose, or uric acid levels.	Same as bumetanide.
Potassium-sparing diuretics		
Amiloride	Blood cell deficiencies; gastrointestinal distress; and hyperkalemia.	Administration with ACE inhibitors or potassium supplements may cause hyperkalemia. Administration with NSAIDs may cause renal failure.
Spironolactone	Gynecomastia; hyperkalemia; and impotence.	Administration with ACE inhibitors or potassium supplements may cause hyperkalemia.
Triamterene	Same as amiloride.	Same as amiloride.
Osmotic diuretics		
Glycerol	Heart failure; nausea and vomiting; and pulmonary congestion and edema.	Potentiates effects of other diuretics.
Mannitol	Same as glycerol.	Same as glycerol.
Carbonic anhydrase inhibitors		
Acetazolamide	Blood cell deficiencies; drowsiness; hepatic insufficiency; hyperglycemia; hypokalemia; metabolic acidosis; paresthesia, and uremia.	Serum levels of weak bases, such as amphetamine, ephedrine, and quinidine, are increased by CA inhibitors. Serum levels of CA inhibitors are increased by salicylates.
Dorzolamide	Bitter taste; blurred vision; and ocular discomfort and allergic reactions.	Unknown.

*ACE = angiotensin-converting enzyme; CA = carbonic anhydrase; and NSAIDs = nonsteroidal anti-inflammatory drugs.

be used to treat **edema** associated with **heart failure, cirrhosis, corticosteroid and estrogen therapy,** and **renal disorders** such as **nephrotic syndrome.** Because thiazides reduce calcium excretion and decrease urinary calcium levels, they are helpful in treating patients with **nephrolithiasis** (kidney stones) associated with **hypercalciuria.**

Thiazides are also used to treat nephrogenic **diabetes insipidus.** In this disorder, the kidneys are not responsive to circulating antidiuretic hormone, and patients may excrete from 10 to 20 L of urine per day. Thiazides exert a paradoxical antidiuretic effect in these patients and reduce the excessive urine volume dramatically. In cases of diabetes insipidus, the effectiveness of thiazides is believed to stem from a reduction in plasma volume caused by these drugs. The reduced plasma volume serves to increase sodium and water reabsorption from the proximal tubule, so that less water is delivered to the diluting segments of the nephron. As a result, the urine output falls.

Hydrochlorothiazide

The several thiazide compounds that are available have almost identical actions but differ in their potency and pharmacokinetic properties. Hydrochlorothiazide is the most frequently prescribed thiazide diuretic.

Thiazide-like Diuretics

Several thiazide-like diuretics exist whose structures are slightly different from those of the thiazide compounds but whose actions and uses are generally similar. One of them is **indapamide,** an agent primarily used to treat **hypertension** and **heart failure.** Another is **metolazone,** a diuretic that may be more effective than thiazide compounds in the treatment of patients with **impaired renal function.** Metolazone is sometimes combined with a loop diuretic to treat patients with **diuretic resistance.** Patients with diuretic resistance do not adequately respond to any single diuretic agent, but they may respond to the combination of a thiazide-like diuretic and a loop diuretic. The combined use of these diuretics produces **sequential nephron blockade,** in which the drugs inhibit the reabsorption of sodium in the ascending limb and the early distal tubule.

Loop Diuretics

Drug Properties

CHEMISTRY AND PHARMACOKINETICS. The structure of a loop diuretic, furosemide, is shown in Fig. 13–1A. The pharmacokinetic properties of loop diuretics are summarized in Table 13–2.

MECHANISMS AND PHARMACOLOGIC EFFECTS. Loop diuretics inhibit the $Na^+,K^+,2Cl^-$ symporter in the ascending limb of the loop of Henle and thereby exert a powerful natriuretic effect. In comparison with other diuretics, loop diuretics can inhibit the reabsorption of a greater percentage of filtered sodium. Loop diuretics are sometimes called **high-ceiling diuretics** because they produce a dose-dependent diuresis throughout their clinical dosage range. This property can be contrasted with the rather flat dose-response curve and limited diuretic efficacy of thiazides and other diuretic drugs (Fig. 13–3).

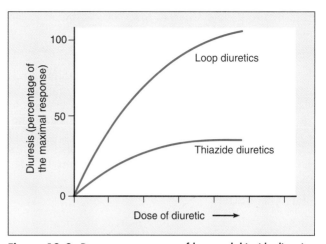

Figure 13–3. Dose-response curves of loop and thiazide diuretics. Loop diuretics produce dose-dependent diuresis throughout their therapeutic dosage range, whereas thiazide diuretics have a relatively flat dose-response curve and a limited maximal response.

In addition to their natriuretic effect, the loop diuretics produce kaliuresis by increasing the exchange of sodium and potassium in the late distal tubule and collecting duct via the same mechanisms as those described for the thiazide diuretics. Loop diuretics also increase magnesium and calcium excretion by reducing the reabsorption of these ions in the ascending limb (see Box 13–1). This action results from inhibition of the $Na^+,K^+,2Cl^-$ symporter, which reduces the back-diffusion of potassium into the nephron lumen. The reduction of potassium back-diffusion decreases the transepithelial electrical potential that normally drives the paracellular reabsorption of magnesium and calcium. Inhibition of this process thereby increases magnesium and calcium excretion.

ADVERSE EFFECTS AND INTERACTIONS. Loop diuretics can produce a variety of electrolyte abnormalities, including hypokalemia, hypocalcemia, hypomagnesemia, and metabolic alkalosis. These diuretics can also increase blood glucose and uric acid levels in the same manner as the thiazide diuretics. In some patients, use of loop diuretics causes ototoxicity with manifestations such as tinnitus, ear pain, vertigo, and hearing deficits. In most cases, the hearing loss is reversible. Other adverse effects and drug interactions are listed in Table 13–4.

INDICATIONS. Loop diuretics are used when intensive diuresis is required and cannot be achieved with other diuretics. Loop diuretics are highly effective in the treatment of pulmonary edema, partly because of the vasodilation that occurs when they are administered intravenously. They are the preferred diuretics in the treatment of persons with renal impairment, because (unlike thiazide and other diuretics) they are effective in patients whose creatinine clearance drops below 30 mL/min. Loop diuretics are often the drugs of choice for patients with edema caused by heart failure, cirrhosis, and other disorders. Although they are prescribed for patients with hypertension, the thiazide diuretics are usually preferred for this condition. Loop diuretics can be used to treat hypercalcemia, whereas the thiazide diuretics can increase serum calcium levels slightly.

Bumetanide, Furosemide, and Torsemide

Bumetanide, furosemide, and torsemide are sulfonamide derivatives with similar pharmacologic actions and effects. These drugs can be administered orally or intravenously. In comparison with other loop diuretics, torsemide has a somewhat longer half-life and a significantly longer duration of action after intravenous administration (see Table 13–2). All three of the drugs are partly metabolized before they are excreted in the urine.

Ethacrynic Acid

Ethacrynic acid is the only loop diuretic that is not a sulfonamide derivative. It is available for use when patients are hypersensitive to other drugs in this class. Otherwise, it is seldom used because it produces more ototoxicity than do the other loop diuretics.

Potassium-Sparing Diuretics

Two types of potassium-sparing diuretics exist: the epithelial sodium channel blockers and the aldosterone receptor antagonists.

Amiloride and Triamterene

Amiloride and triamterene are epithelial sodium channel antagonists. By blocking the entry of sodium into the principal tubular cells of the late distal tubule and collecting duct (see Box 13–1), these drugs prevent sodium reabsorption at this site and indirectly reduce the secretion of potassium into the tubular filtrate and urine. Through these actions, the potassium-sparing diuretics produce a modest amount of natriuresis while decreasing kaliuresis, and they are primarily used to prevent and treat **hypokalemia** induced by thiazide and loop diuretics. The properties, effects, and uses of amiloride, triamterene, and other potassium-sparing diuretics are outlined in Tables 13–1 to 13–4.

The most characteristic adverse effect of the potassium-sparing diuretics is hyperkalemia, but this is unlikely to occur unless the patient also ingests potassium supplements or other drugs that increase serum potassium levels (e.g., angiotensin antagonists) or unless the patient has a renal disorder that predisposes to hyperkalemia.

Spironolactone

Spironolactone, a steroid congener of aldosterone (see Fig. 13–1B), competitively blocks the binding of aldosterone to the mineralocorticoid receptor in tubular epithelial cells of the late distal convoluted tubule and collecting duct. Normally, the mineralocorticoid receptor is activated by aldosterone and then interacts with nuclear DNA to promote the transcription of genes that encode proteins of the epithelial sodium channels, sodium pump, and related compounds involved in the reabsorption of sodium and secretion of potassium in these tubular segments. By blocking these actions, spironolactone reduces sodium reabsorption and the coupled secretion of potassium.

Spironolactone is adequately absorbed from the gut and has a long duration of action, despite its short elimination half-life, indicating that its cellular actions persist longer

than its circulating drug levels (see Table 13–2). Spironolactone is used to prevent **hypokalemia** in the same manner as amiloride and triamterene, and it has a special role in the treatment of **primary hyperaldosteronism.** Clinical trials have shown that spironolactone reduces mortality in persons with heart failure, as described in Chapter 12. Its use in this condition, however, has been associated with an increased incidence of hyperkalemia. Because of its antiandrogenic effect, spironolactone is also used in the treatment of **polycystic ovary disease** and **hirsutism** in women.

The adverse effects of spironolactone include gynecomastia and impotence in men (caused by the drug's antiandrogenic effects) and hyperkalemia. Eplerenone is a new aldosterone antagonist that produces less endocrine side effects than does spironolactone. Eplerenone is used to counteract the effects of excessive aldosterone in persons with heart failure (see Chapter 12).

Osmotic Diuretics

Glycerol and **mannitol** are examples of osmotic diuretics. These diuretics increase the osmotic pressure of the plasma and thereby attract water from interstitial and transcellular fluids. Because of this action, mannitol is used to treat **cerebral edema** and reduce intracranial pressure. Glycerol and mannitol are both used in the treatment of **acute glaucoma.** By attracting water from ocular fluids into the circulation, the drugs reduce intraocular volume and pressure. Glycerol is administered orally for this purpose, whereas mannitol is administered intravenously.

Mannitol is also used as a diuretic. Following intravenous administration, it is filtered at the glomerulus but is not reabsorbed from the renal tubules. It osmotically attracts and retains water as it moves through the nephron and into the urine. This action reduces the tubular sodium concentration and the concentration gradient between the tubular fluid and cells and thereby retards the reabsorption of sodium. Hence, mannitol has both direct and indirect actions that promote diuresis. The diuretic effect of mannitol has been used to improve renal function in the oliguric phase of **acute renal failure**. Evidence for a renoprotective effect of mannitol has been obtained in studies of persons having renal transplantation.

Mannitol has also been administered along with intravenous fluids to maintain renal function and reduce the renal toxicity of antineoplastic platinum compounds (e.g., cisplatin), and mannitol is used to promote the renal excretion of toxic substances in cases of drug overdose or poisoning.

The primary adverse effect of mannitol is excessive plasma volume expansion, which is most likely to occur if the drug is administered too rapidly or with too large a volume of intravenous fluid. Excessive plasma volume can lead to heart failure and pulmonary congestion and edema in susceptible patients.

Carbonic Anhydrase Inhibitors

Drug Properties

The carbonic anhydrase (CA) inhibitors were the first sulfonamide derivatives to be used as diuretics, and their discovery eventually led to the development of the thiazide and loop diuretics (see Fig. 13–1A). **Acetazolamide, dorzolamide,** and other CA inhibitors, which are relatively weak diuretics, are seldom used to promote diuresis today. Instead, their ability to inhibit CA has led to their use in the treatment of disorders such as high-altitude sickness and glaucoma.

Specific Drugs

CHEMISTRY AND PHARMACOKINETICS. Acetazolamide is one of several orally administered CA inhibitors, whereas dorzolamide is used as an ophthalmic solution to treat glaucoma. Dorzolamide is partly absorbed from the eye into the circulation and undergoes some metabolic transformation before it is excreted in the urine. The drug is eliminated in a biphasic manner, with a rapid decline in serum levels followed by a much slower release from erythrocytes, and it has a half-life of 4 months. The pharmacokinetic properties of acetazolamide and dorzolamide are outlined in Table 13–2.

MECHANISMS, PHARMACOLOGIC EFFECTS, AND INDICATIONS. Acetazolamide and other drugs in this class inhibit CA throughout the body. This enzyme catalyzes the conversion of carbon dioxide and water to carbonic acid, which spontaneously decomposes to bicarbonate and hydrogen ions:

$$CO_2 + H_2O \rightleftharpoons H_2CO_3 \longrightarrow HCO_3^- + H^+$$

When the ciliary process forms aqueous humor, CA participates by catalyzing the formation of bicarbonate, which is secreted into the posterior chamber of the eye, along with water and other substances that make up the aqueous humor. In patients with **glaucoma,** inhibition of CA reduces aqueous humor secretion and intraocular pressure. The CA inhibitors are used in the treatment of both the acute and the chronic form of glaucoma, although they must be combined with other drugs to treat the acute form. Traditionally, the CA inhibitors have been administered orally to patients with glaucoma. Now some of these drugs, including dorzolamide, are available for topical ocular administration. Dorzolamide is administered every 8 hours in the treatment of **chronic ocular hypertension** and **open-angle glaucoma.**

Carbonic anhydrase is also required for the reabsorption of sodium bicarbonate from the proximal tubule and for the secretion of hydrogen ion in the collecting duct. In the reabsorption of sodium bicarbonate, bicarbonate must be converted to carbon dioxide and water by CA, because the apical cell membrane of the tubular epithelial cells is impermeable to bicarbonate. The carbon dioxide and water can diffuse into the tubular cells, where CA converts them back to bicarbonate, which is then transported into the interstitial fluid for diffusion into the circulation (see Box 13–1). Inhibition of this process by acetazolamide and other CA inhibitors causes a marked reduction in the reabsorption of sodium bicarbonate and a corresponding increase in its renal excretion. This leads to alkalinization of the urine and produces a mild form of hyperchloremic metabolic acidosis. The hyperchloremia results from the increased reabsorption of chloride as a compensation for reduced bicarbonate reabsorption.

Ccarbonic anhydrase inhibitors are seldom used as **diuretics,** although they are used occasionally to **alkalinize the urine.** They are effective in the prevention and treatment of **high-altitude sickness (mountain sickness),** in part because the metabolic acidosis produced by the drugs counteracts the respiratory alkalosis that can result from hyperventilation in this condition. By counteracting respiratory alkalosis, the drugs enhance ventilation acclimatization and maintain oxygenation during sleep at a high altitude. The drugs also counteract fluid retention and cause a decrease in cerebral spinal fluid (CSF) pressure, which can be elevated with acute high-altitude sickness. At the same time, CA inhibitors prevent the fall in CSF pH that occurs in this disorder.

Inhibition of CA in the central nervous system elevates the seizure threshold. For this reason, CA inhibitors have been used occasionally for the treatment of **epilepsy.**

ADVERSE EFFECTS AND INTERACTIONS. Acetazolamide and other orally administered CA inhibitors can cause drowsiness, paresthesia, and other central nervous system effects as well as hypokalemia and hyperglycemia. Less commonly, they are associated with various hypersensitivity reactions and blood cell deficiencies. By increasing the pH of the renal tubular fluid and alkalinizing the urine, the CA inhibitors decrease the excretion of weak bases, such as amphetamine, pseudoephedrine, and quinidine, and thereby increase their serum levels and cause drug toxicity.

MANAGEMENT OF EDEMA

Edema is a condition in which fluid accumulates in the interstitial space and body cavities, either because of increased hydrostatic pressure in the capillary beds or because of inadequate colloid osmotic pressure in the plasma. The plasma osmotic pressure is primarily influenced by the osmotic attraction of water by sodium and plasma proteins. Conditions that cause edema as a result of increased hydrostatic pressure include heart failure and certain renal diseases, all of which cause sodium and water retention. Conditions that cause edema as a result of inadequate colloid osmotic pressure include severe dietary protein deficiency and hepatic diseases (e.g., cirrhosis). In conditions such as cirrhosis, the liver is unable to synthesize adequate albumin and other plasma proteins to maintain plasma osmotic pressure. Hepatic cirrhosis can lead to ascites (accumulation of fluid within the peritoneal cavity) and portal hypertension. This disorder can be managed with dietary salt restriction and the use of diuretics (e.g., spironolactone and furosemide).

Nephrotic syndrome, a renal disease that leads to excessive protein excretion in the urine (proteinuria), can cause edema by this mechanism. Infection, neoplasms, and thromboembolism can also cause edema by various mechanisms that include inflammation, increased capillary fluid permeability, and increased hydrostatic pressure caused by obstruction of blood vessels.

The primary treatment of edema is to **correct the underlying disorder** and restore plasma osmotic pressure and hydrostatic pressure to normal values. In acute life-threatening situations (e.g., cerebral edema and pulmonary edema) **diuretics** and other drugs must be administered immediately to prevent tissue hypoxia, injury, and death. In milder forms of edema, diuretics can be used as short-term adjunct treatments that serve to mobilize edematous fluid while an attempt is made to correct the underlying cause. Most cases of mild peripheral edema, however, can be managed without pharmacologic therapy by correcting the underlying disorder or discontinuing a causative drug.

SUMMARY OF IMPORTANT POINTS

■ Diuretics are drugs that increase urine production. Most diuretics inhibit the reabsorption of sodium from various sites in the nephron.

■ Thiazide diuretics inhibit sodium chloride reabsorption from the distal tubule. They cause natriuresis and kaliuresis, but they decrease calcium excretion. They are primarily used to treat hypertension, edema, hypercalciuria, and nephrogenic diabetes insipidus.

■ Loop diuretics inhibit the $Na^+,K^+,2Cl^-$ symporter in the ascending limb and thereby increase sodium, potassium, calcium, and magnesium excretion. They are chiefly used to treat heart failure, renal failure, pulmonary edema, and hypercalcemia.

■ Thiazide and loop diuretics can cause hypokalemia and other electrolyte disturbances, as well as hyperglycemia and hyperuricemia.

■ Potassium-sparing diuretics, which inhibit potassium secretion in the collecting duct, are primarily used to prevent hypokalemia, which can be caused by thiazide and loop diuretics. Spironolactone is used to treat severe heart failure and hyperaldosteronism.

■ Osmotic diuretics increase the osmotic pressure of plasma and retain water in the nephron. They are used to treat cerebral edema, glaucoma, and the oliguria of acute renal failure.

■ Carbonic anhydrase inhibitors, which are weak diuretics that inhibit sodium bicarbonate reabsorption from the proximal tubule, can cause a mild form of metabolic acidosis. They reduce aqueous humor secretion and are primarily used to treat glaucoma.

Review Questions

For each numbered description of a diuretic, choose the corresponding drug from the choices provided.

1. Increases urine pH and decreases plasma pH

2. Reduces the excretion of calcium and used to prevent kidney stones

3. Large intravenous doses cause hearing impairment

4. More likely to cause hyperkalemia when combined with an angiotensin inhibitor or potassium supplements

   (A) furosemide
   (B) acetazolamide

   (C) mannitol
   (D) amiloride
   (E) hydrochlorothiazide

Select the single best answer from the lettered choices.

5. Which of the following is not an adverse metabolic effect of hydrochlorothiazide?
   (A) hyperglycemia
   (B) hyperuricemia
   (C) hypokalemia
   (D) metabolic alkalosis
   (E) decreased serum triglyceride levels

Answers and Explanations

1. The answer is B: acetazolamide. Acetazolamide and other carbonic anhydrase inhibitors decrease the reabsorpton of sodium bicarbonate from the nephron and thereby increase bicarbonate excretion, leading to an alkaline urine. By inhibiting bicarbonate reabsorption and thereby increasing chloride reabsorption, acetazolamide produces a mild hyperchloremic metabolic acidosis.

2. The answer is E: hydrochlorothiazide. Thiazide diuretics increase calcium reabsorption from the nephron, thereby reducing urinary calcium levels to decrease formation of calcium stones in the urinary tract.

3. The answer is A: furosemide. Loop-acting diuretics such as furosemide can cause reversible otic nerve toxicity manifested as both vesticular and cochlear (hearing) impairment. Of the loop-acting diuretics, ethacrynic acid is most likely to cause hearing deficits.

4. The answer is D: amiloride. Amiloride and other potassium-sparing diuretics, which reduce renal excretion of potassium, are used to prevent hypokalemia. They can cause hyperkalemia, however, and this effect is most likely to occur in persons receiving potassium supplements or other potassium-sparing drugs such as the angiotensin converting enzyme inhibitors and angiotensin receptor blockers.

5. The answer is E: decreased serum triglyceride levels. Thizide diuretics can increase plasma glucose levels in diabetic patients and cause hyperuricemia, hypokalemia, and metabolic alkalosis. Thiazides can also increase serum cholesterol and triglyceride levels.

SELECTED READINGS

Bartsch, P., D. M. Bailey, and M. M. Berger, et al. Acute mountain sickness: controversies and advancements. High Alt Med Biol 5:110–124, 2004.
Fuchs, F. D. Diuretics: drugs of choice for the initial management of patients with hypertension. Expert Rev Cardiovasc Ther 1:35–41, 2003.
Shah, S. U., S. Anjum, and W. A. Littler. Use of diuretics in cardiovascular disease: (1) heart failure. Postgrad Med J 80:201–205, 2004.

CHAPTER 14

Antiarrhythmic Drugs

CLASSIFICATION OF ANTIARRHYTHMIC DRUGS

Sodium Channel Blockers
Class IA Drugs
- Disopyramide (NORPACE)
- Procainamide (PRONESTYL)
- Quinidine

Class IB Drugs
- Lidocaine
- Mexiletine (MEXITIL)[a]

Class IC Drugs
- Flecainide (TAMBOCOR)
- Propafenone (RHYTHMOL)

Other Class I Drugs
- Moricizine

Other Antiarrhythmic Drugs
Class II Drugs
- Esmolol (BREVIBLOC)

- Metoprolol (LOPRESSOR)
- Propranolol (INDERAL)

Class III Drugs
- Amiodarone (CORDARONE)
- Ibutilide (CORVERT)
- Dofetilide (TIKOSYN)
- Sotalol (BETAPACE)

Class IV Drugs
- Diltiazem (CARDIZEM)
- Verapamil (CALAN, ISOPTIN)

Miscellaneous Drugs
- Adenosine
- Digoxin
- Magnesium sulfate

[a]also tocainide

OVERVIEW

In a healthy adult with a normal heart, each heartbeat originates in the sinoatrial (SA) node, the rhythm of heartbeats is regular, and the heart rate is about 70 beats per minute at rest. If the origin, rhythm, or rate of heartbeats is abnormal, the condition is called an **arrhythmia (dysrhythmia).** Arrhythmias occur primarily because of disturbances in cardiac impulse formation or conduction, and they can originate in any part of the heart. Those arising in the atria or atrioventricular (AV) node are called **supraventricular arrhythmias,** whereas those arising in the ventricles are called **ventricular arrhythmias.** Those in which the heart rate is too rapid are called **tachyarrhythmias,** and those in which the heart rate is too slow are called **bradyarrhythmias.**

Some arrhythmias are benign and do not necessarily require treatment. Others require treatment because they reduce cardiac output and blood pressure significantly or because they can precipitate more serious and even lethal rhythm disturbances. Both pharmacologic and electrophys-

iologic methods are used to terminate and prevent arrhythmias. This chapter describes the pathophysiology of arrhythmias and the mechanisms by which antiarrhythmic drugs work.

Cardiac Action Potentials and Electrocardiographic Findings

Fig. 14–1 depicts the relationships between ion currents, cardiac action potentials in phases 0 through 4, and findings on the surface electrocardiogram (ECG).

The SA node, located in the right atrium, is the site of origin of the normal heartbeat. The SA node spontaneously depolarizes to form an impulse that is conducted through the atrium to the AV node and then through the bundle of His, bundle branches, and Purkinje fibers to the ventricular muscle.

The spontaneous depolarization of the SA node is caused by the influx of sodium and calcium as the efflux of potassium subsides. When the threshold potential (TP) is reached at about −40 mV, the SA node is more rapidly depolarized

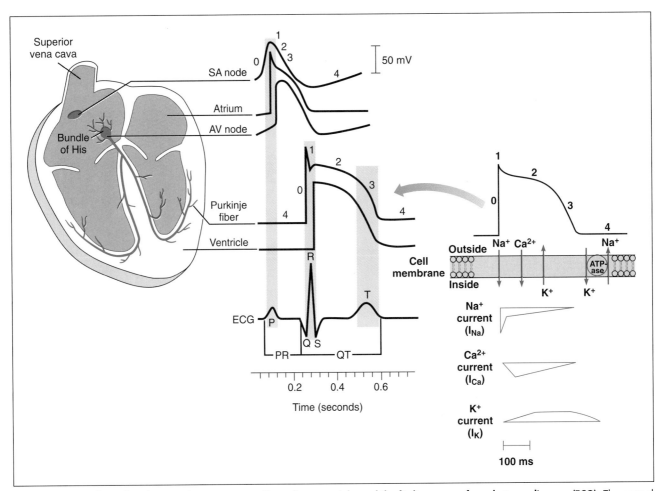

Figure 14–1. Relationships between ion currents, cardiac action potentials, and the findings on surface electrocardiogram (ECG). The normal heartbeat originates in the sinoatrial (SA) node. The impulse is conducted through internodal fibers to the atrioventricular (AV) node and then through the bundle of His, bundle branches, and Purkinje fibers to the ventricular muscle. On the ECG, the P wave represents atrial depolarization, the QRS complex represents ventricular depolarization, and the T wave represents ventricular repolarization. The PR interval is primarily related to the conduction time through the AV node, and the QT interval represents the time between ventricular depolarization and repolarization. In phase 0, ventricular depolarization is caused by sodium influx through the fast sodium channel. In phase 1, the membrane is transiently repolarized as a result of potassium efflux. In phase 2, the membrane potential is relatively stable because of the concurrent influx of calcium and efflux of potassium. In phase 3, repolarization is caused by continued potassium efflux as calcium influx declines. In phase 4, the ion balance is returned to normal by the action of the sodium pump (Na+,K+-adenosine triphosphatase [ATPase]). Calcium is removed from the cell by the sodium-calcium exchanger and the calcium ATPase (not shown).

by sodium and calcium influx to generate an impulse that can be conducted to the rest of the heart. As the impulse is conducted to atrial and ventricular muscle cells, these cells are rapidly depolarized by the influx of sodium through the fast sodium channel. As the cells depolarize to about −40 mV, the slow calcium channels open. The influx of calcium through these channels during phase 2 serves to activate muscle contraction. Cardiac tissues become repolarized during phase 3 as a result of the efflux of potassium through several types of rectifier potassium channels (I_K), an efflux that occurs when the influx of calcium declines.

As shown in Fig. 14–1, the surface ECG is a summation of action potentials generated by the heart during the cardiac cycle. The **P wave** represents atrial depolarization, whereas the **PR interval** corresponds to the time required to conduct the action potential through both the atria and the AV node. The **QRS complex** and the **T wave** represent ventricular depolarization and ventricular repolarization, respectively.

Hence, the **QT interval** represents the duration of the ventricular action potential.

Pathophysiology of Arrhythmias

Arrhythmias can be caused by the following: coronary ischemia and tissue hypoxia; electrolyte disturbances; overstimulation of the sympathetic nervous system; general anesthetics; and other conditions or drugs that perturb cardiac transmembrane potentials and lead to abnormal impulse formation or abnormal impulse conduction.

Abnormal Impulse Formation

Abnormal impulse formation can generate extrasystoles and result in tachycardia. The two mechanisms that are primarily responsible for abnormal impulse formation are increased automaticity and the occurrence of afterdepolarizations. These are depicted in Box 14–1.

BOX 14-1. THE ELECTROPHYSIOLOGIC BASIS OF ARRHYTHMIAS

Abnormal Impulse Formation

The two mechanisms primarily responsible for abnormal impulse formation are increased automaticity and afterdepolarizations.

Increased automaticity can be caused by any change that decreases the time required for depolarization from the maximal diastolic potential (MDP) to the threshold potential (TP). Increased automaticity occurs if the rate of diastolic depolarization (the slope of phase 4) in the sinoatrial node or in latent pacemakers is increased. It also occurs if a shift of the TP occurs to a more negative value or if a shift occurs of the MDP to a more positive value.

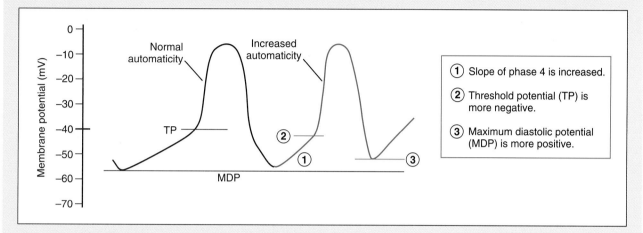

(1) Slope of phase 4 is increased.

(2) Threshold potential (TP) is more negative.

(3) Maximum diastolic potential (MDP) is more positive.

Afterdepolarizations are believed to result from abnormal calcium influx into cardiac cells during or immediately after phase 3 of the ventricular action potential. Afterdepolarizations can lead to extrasystoles and tachycardia.

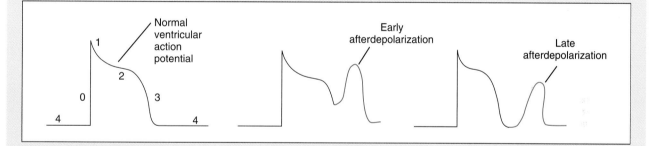

Abnormal Impulse Conduction

Reentry is characterized by the retrograde conduction of an impulse into previously depolarized tissue. It is usually caused by the presence of a unidirectional conduction block in a bifurcating conduction pathway. For reentry to occur, the conduction time through the retrograde pathway must exceed the refractory period of the reentered tissue.

In **ventricular tissue,** the unidirectional block is often caused by decremental conduction of the impulse in the anterograde direction, with normal conduction of the impulse in the retrograde direction.

Continued

BOX 14–1. THE ELECTROPHYSIOLOGIC BASIS OF ARRHYTHMIAS—cont'd

Reentry in the **atrioventricular (AV) node** is the most common electrophysiologic mechanism responsible for paroxysmal supraventricular tachycardia (PSVT). Reentry occurs when a premature atrial depolarization arrives at the AV node and finds that one pathway (β) is still refractory from the previous depolarization. The other pathway (α), however, is able to conduct the impulse to the ventricle. Ret-rograde conduction of the impulse through pathway β leads to reentry of the atrium and results in tachycardia. In the AV node, the unidirectional block results from the β pathway's longer refractory period, which blocks anterograde conduction but permits retrograde conduction after it has recovered its excitability.

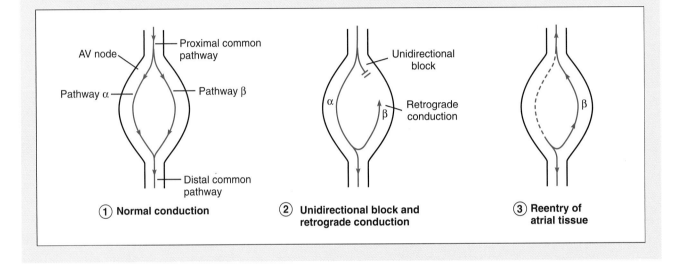

① **Normal conduction**

② **Unidirectional block and retrograde conduction**

③ **Reentry of atrial tissue**

INCREASED AUTOMATICITY. Spontaneous phase 4 depolarization generates an action potential that can be propagated to other parts of the heart. The SA node is the usual site of spontaneous impulse initiation (automaticity), but other cardiac tissues, including the AV node and the His-Purkinje system tissues, are also capable of spontaneous depolarization. Pathologic conditions or drugs can cause these tissues to depolarize more rapidly and thereby generate abnormal impulses. For example, overstimulation of the sympathetic nervous system or use of sympathomimetic drugs increases automaticity and can cause tachyarrhythmia.

The rate at which action potentials are generated in the SA node and elsewhere in the heart depends on the time required to depolarize the tissue from the maximal diastolic potential (MDP) to the TP. Automaticity is increased if the MDP becomes more positive or if the TP becomes more negative. Serum electrolyte abnormalities, hypoxia, and other pathologic changes can affect the MDP or TP in this manner and lead to arrhythmias.

AFTERDEPOLARIZATIONS. Afterdepolarizations are abnormal impulses resulting from the spontaneous generation of action potentials during or immediately after phase 3 repolarization. Depending on the time they occur, the abnormal impulses are designated as early afterdepolarizations or late afterdepolarizations. Afterdepolarizations are believed to be triggered by abnormal calcium influx and can be provoked by digitalis glycosides and by other drugs or pathologic events that prolong cardiac repolarization and the QT interval.

Abnormal Impulse Conduction

Abnormal impulse conduction is the basis for the formation of arrhythmias by the process of **reentry,** a process that involves reexcitation of a particular zone of cardiac tissue by the same impulse. Reentry is believed to be the most common mechanism responsible for the genesis of arrhythmias. It is usually caused by the presence of a **unidirectional conduction block** in a bifurcating conduction pathway (see Box 14–1).

REENTRY IN VENTRICULAR TISSUE. In ventricular tissue, ischemia and tissue hypoxia can cause a reduction in the resting membrane potential and a decrease in membrane responsiveness. Under these conditions, the cells do not depolarize as rapidly or completely during phase 0, and this reduces the rate at which the impulse is conducted to surrounding ventricular tissue. When a cardiac impulse is conducted through ischemic or infarcted tissue, the conduction velocity gradually slows until conduction ceases. This phenomenon, called **decremental conduction,** is the most common cause of a unidirectional block in ventricular tissue. If the unidirectional block occurs in one arm of a bifurcating pathway, the impulse can continue through the other arm in the normal (anterograde) direction and then reenter the ventricular tissue by retrograde conduction.

The reason that the impulse is blocked in the anterograde direction but is conducted in the retrograde direction is related to the characteristics of decremental conduction. In this type of conduction, the impulse encounters increasing resistance as it moves in the anterograde direction, and its velocity slows until the impulse is finally extinguished. The retrograde impulse has full velocity as it encounters the area of greatest resistance, and this enables it to jump across the ischemic area without being extinguished.

REENTRY IN THE ATRIOVENTRICULAR NODE. Reentry in the AV node is the most common electrophysiologic mechanism responsible for paroxysmal supraventricular tachycardia (PSVT). Of the several forms of PSVT, the form that occurs in patients with Wolff-Parkinson-White syndrome involves an accessory AV node conduction pathway through the bundle of Kent. In patients with the most common form of PSVT, however, the reentrant circuit is located entirely within the AV node. In the common form of PSVT, a premature atrial impulse is blocked in one pathway, is conducted through the AV node via the other pathway, and reenters the atrium by retrograde conduction. In AV node reentry, the unidirectional block does not result from decremental conduction but, instead, is caused by the difference in the refractory periods of the two pathways.

Drug-Induced Arrhythmias

Drugs can induce arrhythmias by several mechanisms.

Sympathomimetic drugs can increase the automaticity of the SA node, AV node, or His-Purkinje fibers and thereby produce tachyarrhythmias.

Digitalis glycosides sometimes evoke afterdepolarizations by increasing calcium influx into cardiac cells, and they can also impair AV node conduction and cause AV block.

Other drugs cause arrhythmias via their effects on ventricular conduction and repolarization. Drugs that slow ventricular repolarization and cause QT prolongation can evoke a form of polymorphic ventricular tachycardia called **torsade de pointes** (based on a French term meaning "fringe of pointed tips"). In this disorder, each QRS complex has a configuration that differs from the preceding one, and QT prolongation probably predisposes the ventricular tissue to afterdepolarizations that produce extrasystoles and tachycardia. Types of drugs that have been reported to induce torsade de pointes include **antiarrhythmic drugs** (e.g., quinidine and sotalol), **histamine antagonists** (e.g., astemizole and terfenadine), **psychotropic drugs** (e.g., phenothiazines), and other agents (e.g., cisapride).

Mechanisms and Classification of Antiarrhythmic Drugs

Antiarrhythmic drugs act primarily by suppressing or preventing abnormal impulse formation or conduction. Drugs that block sodium or calcium channels can reduce abnormal automaticity and slow conduction of the cardiac impulse. Drugs that block potassium channels can prolong repolarization and the action potential duration and thereby increase the refractory period of cardiac tissue. Drugs that block β-adrenergic receptors reduce the sympathetic stimulation of cardiac automaticity and conduction velocity and thereby prevent the overstimulation that contributes to some arrhythmias.

On the basis of these mechanisms, Vaughan-Williams has divided the antiarrhythmic drugs into four main classes,

with **class I** consisting of sodium channel blockers, **class II** consisting of β-adrenergic receptor antagonists (β-blockers), **class III** consisting of potassium channel blockers and other drugs that prolong the action potential duration, and **class IV** consisting of calcium channel blockers. Although this classification system is helpful, a few drugs (e.g, adenosine) do not fit into any of these categories, and some drugs (e.g., amiodarone) could be included in more than one category.

SODIUM CHANNEL BLOCKERS

Class I, the largest group of antiarrhythmic drugs, consists of sodium channel blockers. These drugs bind to sodium channels when the channels are in the open and inactivated states, and they dissociate from the channels during the resting state (Box 14–2). The sodium channel blockers have the most pronounced effect on cardiac tissue that is firing rapidly, because sodium channels in this tissue spend more time in the open and inactivated states than in the resting state. This is called **use-dependent blockade.** Because of use-dependent blockade, sodium channel blockers suppress cardiac conduction more in a patient with tachycardia than in a person with a normal heart rate.

The drugs in class I have been subdivided into three groups (IA, IB, and IC), based on whether they have greater affinity for the open state or the inactivated state and based on their rate of dissociation from sodium channels (rate of recovery). As shown in Box 14–2, **class IA drugs** have greater affinity for the open state and have a slow recovery; **class IB drugs** have greater affinity for the inactivated state and have a rapid recovery; and **class IC drugs** have greater affinity for the open state and a very slow recovery.

Class IB drugs have a more pronounced effect on ischemic tissue than on nonischemic tissue. In ischemic tissue, cells are partly depolarized because they lack the amount of adenosine triphosphate (ATP) needed to operate the sodium pump. As a result, these channels spend more time in the inactivated state than do channels in nonischemic tissue.

Class IC drugs have a greater effect on ventricular conduction than do class IA or IB drugs. This is because class IC drugs show an affinity for the open state and because they have the slowest recovery from blockade.

Class IA Drugs

Disopyramide, procainamide, and quinidine are class IA drugs. These drugs have similar electrophysiologic effects and clinical indications, but they differ in their pharmacokinetic properties and adverse effects.

Drug Properties

The class IA drugs block the fast sodium channel and also block potassium channels. Therefore, they slow phase 0 depolarization and phase 3 repolarization in ventricular tissue (Fig. 14–2). These actions decrease the ventricular conduction velocity and prolong the ventricular action potential duration and refractory period (Table 14–1). On the ECG, this increases the QRS duration and prolongs the QT interval. Class IA drugs suppress abnormal (ectopic)

BOX 14–2. ELECTROPHYSIOLOGIC PROPERTIES OF SODIUM CHANNEL BLOCKERS

During phase 0 of the ventricular action potential, the sodium channels open to depolarize the cell. The channels are then inactivated and no longer permit sodium entry during phases 1, 2, and 3. The channels must return to the resting state (phase 4) before they can open again during the next action potential.

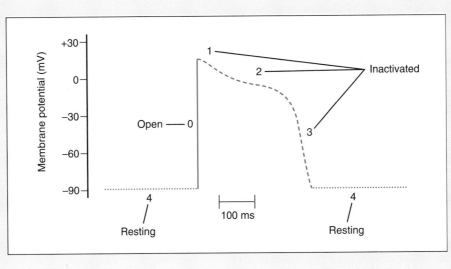

Drugs dissociate from the sodium channels at different rates (recovery). Drugs with a slow recovery have a greater effect on cardiac conduction velocity.

Drug Class	Example	Sodium Channel Affinity	Rate of Dissociation
Class IA	Quinidine	Open > inactivated	Slow
Class IB	Lidocaine	Inactivated > open	Rapid
Class IC	Flecainide	Open > inactivated	Very slow

TABLE 14–1. Electrophysiologic Properties of Antiarrhythmic Drugs*

Drug	Ectopic Auto-maticity	ATRIOVENTRICULAR (AV) NODE		HIS-PURKINJE SYSTEM AND VENTRICLE		ELECTROCARDIOGRAM			
		Conduction Velocity	Refractory Period	Conduction Velocity	Refractory Period	Heart Rate	PR Interval	QRS Duration	QT Interval
Class I drugs									
IA drugs	D	±	0/I	D	I	±	±	I	I
IB drugs	D	0	0	0/D†	±	0	0	0	0/D
IC drugs	D	D	0/I	D	I	0	I	I	0/I
Moricizine	D	D	0	D	0/I	0/I	I	I	0/D
Class II drugs	D	D	I	0	0	D	I	0	0/D
Class III drugs									
Amiodarone	D	D	I	D	I	D	I	I	I
Dofetilide	0	0/D	I	0	I	0	0	0	I
Ibutilide	U	0/D	I	0	I	0/D	0/I	0	I
Sotalol	D	D	I	0	I	D	I	0	I
Class IV drugs	D	D	I	0	0	D	I	0	0
Other drugs									
Adenosine	D	D	I	0	0	I	I	0	0
Digoxin	I	D	I	0	D	D	I	0	D
Magnesium sulfate	D	0	0	0	0	0	0	0	0

*Effects are indicated as follows: decrease (D); increase (I); variable increase or decrease (±); no change (0); and unknown (U).
†Slow conduction in ischemic tissue.

Figure 14–2. Effects of class I and class III antiarrhythmic drugs on the ventricular action potential duration and on the electrocardiogram (ECG). In each panel, the membrane potential scale is in millivolts (mV), and the time scale is in milliseconds (ms). Black tracings and black lines for the time scale depict normal findings; dashed lines and tracings depict the effects of drug administration. (A) Lightly shaded vertical bars show the relationship between the ventricular action potential duration and the findings on ECG in the normally functioning heart. (B) Class IA drugs slow phase 0 depolarization and phase 3 repolarization, thereby increasing the QRS duration and the QT interval. (C) Class IB drugs have little effect on normal cardiac tissue, but they can accelerate phase 3 repolarization and decrease the QT interval slightly. (D) Class IC drugs have the greatest effect on phase 0 depolarization and increase the QRS duration markedly, but they have little effect on phase 3 and the QT interval. (E) Class III drugs have no effect on phase 0, but they markedly prolong phase 3 and increase the QT interval.

automaticity, but they usually do not significantly affect SA node automaticity and the heart rate.

All of the class IA drugs have some degree of antimuscarinic (atropine-like) activity and may inhibit parasympathetic (vagal) effects on the SA and AV nodes. Disopyramide has the greatest antimuscarinic effect, procainamide has the least, and quinidine has an intermediate effect.

Quinidine

CHEMISTRY AND PHARMACOKINETICS. Quinidine is the dextrorotatory isomer of quinine, an alkaloid obtained from the bark of the cinchona tree that has been used to treat fever and malaria for centuries. The pharmacokinetic properties of quinidine and other antiarrhythmic drugs are summarized in Table 14–2. Quinidine is usually administered orally and is adequately absorbed from the gut. It undergoes considerable hepatic biotransformation and is excreted in the urine as the parent compound and metabolites. It has a moderately short half-life and can be given as a sustained-release preparation.

ADVERSE EFFECTS. The most common adverse effect of quinidine is diarrhea, which occurs in up to 30% of patients

TABLE 14-2. **Pharmacokinetic Properties of Antiarrhythmic Drugs***

Drug	Oral Bioavailability	Onset of Action	Duration of Action	Elimination Half-Life	Excreted Unchanged in Urine	Therapeutic Serum Concentration
Class IA drugs						
Disopyramide	90%	1 hour	6 hours	7 hours	50%	2–7 µg/mL
Procainamide	85%	1 hour	5 hours	3.5 hours	55%	4–8 µg/mL
Quinidine	75%	1 hour	7 hours	6 hours	30%	2–5 µg/mL
Class IB drugs						
Lidocaine	NA	See text	See text	1.5 hours	1%	1.5–6 µg/mL
Mexiletine	90%	1 hour	10 hours	11 hours	10%	0.5–2 µg/mL
Tocainide	92%	1 hour	12 hours	12 hours	40%	4–10 µg/mL
Class IC drugs						
Flecainide	75%	3 hours	21 hours	14 hours	30%	0.2–1 µg/mL
Propafenone	10%	3 hours	10 hours	6 hours	<1%	0.06–0.1 µg/mL
Other class I drugs						
Moricizine	35%	2 hours	16 hours	2.5 hours	<1%	0.2–3.6 µg/mL
Class II drugs						
Esmolol	NA	<5 minutes	20–30 minutes	0.15 hour	<2%	0.5–1 µg/mL
Metoprolol	35%	1 hour	15 hours	3.5 hours	7%	15–25 ng/mL
Propranolol	35%	0.5 hour	4 hours	4 hours	<0.5%	0.2–1 µg/mL
Class III drugs						
Amiodarone	45%	2 weeks	4 weeks	40 days	0%	0.5–2.5 µg/mL
Dofetilide	90%	1 hour	12 hours	10 hours	80%	NA
Ibutilide	NA	5 minutes	Unknonw	6 hours	<10%	NA
Sotalol	90%	2 hours	15 hours	12 hours	90%	1–4 µg/mL
Class IV drugs						
Diltiazem	55%	2 hours	8 hours	5 hours	3%	0.1–0.2 µg/mL
Verapamil	25%	2 hours	9 hours	5 hours	3%	0.1–0.3 µg/mL
Miscellaneous drugs						
Adenosine	NA	30 seconds	1.5 minutes	<10 seconds	0%	NA
Digoxin	75%	1 hour	24 hours	35 hours	60%	0.5–2 ng/mL
Magnesium sulfate	NA	<5 minutes	NA	NA	100%	NA

*Values shown are the mean of values reported in the literature. NA = not applicable (not administered orally).

taking the drug and is often responsible for their discontinuation of its use. A less common adverse effect is torsade de pointes, which can cause syncope secondary to a reduction in cardiac output and blood pressure. Thrombocytopenia has also been reported with quinidine use. Higher doses of quinidine can cause cinchonism, characterized by a constellation of neurologic symptoms that include tinnitus, dizziness, and blurred vision.

INDICATIONS. Although its use has declined, quinidine is occasionally used to suppress supraventricular and ventricular arrhythmias. It is seldom used parenterally, because intravenous administration can cause considerable hypotension owing to the drug's antagonism of α-adrenergic receptors. Because quinidine can increase the AV node conduction velocity and ventricular rate in patients with atrial fibrillation, these patients should be given a drug that decreases AV node conduction (e.g., digoxin) before they are given quinidine.

Procainamide

The electrophysiologic effects of procainamide are similar to those of quinidine.

CHEMISTRY AND PHARMACOKINETICS. Procainamide is the amide derivative of the local anesthetic procaine. It is well absorbed from the gut and is converted to an active metabolite, N-acetylprocainamide (NAPA), in the liver. NAPA exerts class III antiarrhythmic activity, which probably contributes to the overall antiarrhythmic effect of procainamide administration.

ADVERSE EFFECTS. Long-term use of procainamide often causes a syndrome that resembles lupus erythematous, presents with arthralgia and a butterfly rash on the face, and is reversible. This syndrome can be distinguished from idiopathic lupus on the basis of serologic tests for anti-DNA antibodies. It is often responsible for discontinuation of the drug.

INDICATIONS. Procainamide, which produces less hypotension after intravenous administration than does quinidine, is sometimes administered by this route to treat acute ventricular arrhythmias. Procainamide can be given orally for the suppression of supraventricular and ventricular arrhythmias. As with other class IA drugs, the clinical use of procainamide has declined in recent years owing to concerns about drug-induced arrhythmias and other adverse effects.

Disopyramide

Disopyramide, which is administered orally to prevent **ventricular arrhythmias**, is sometimes effective in patients who have not responded to other drugs. Disopyramide has electrophysiologic effects similar to those of quinidine. Because it has greater negative inotropic and antimuscarinic effects than do other class IA drugs, it should be used with caution in patients with heart failure and in elderly patients, who are often more susceptible to blurred vision, urinary retention, and other antimuscarinic side effects.

Class IB Drugs

Lidocaine, mexiletine, and tocainide are class IB drugs. Their electrophysiologic properties make them suitable for the treatment of ventricular arrhythmias.

Drug Properties

CHEMISTRY AND PHARMACOKINETICS. Lidocaine is a local anesthetic that also has antiarrhythmic activity. It undergoes extensive first-pass hepatic inactivation after oral administration and is not suitable for administration by this route. The other class IB drugs, mexiletine and tocainide, are lidocaine congeners that are not susceptible to first-pass inactivation and are intended for oral administration. Lidocaine is rapidly inactivated by hepatic enzymes, whereas mexiletine and tocainide are more slowly metabolized and have much longer half-lives (see Table 14–2).

MECHANISMS AND EFFECTS. Lidocaine has a strong affinity for sodium channels in depolarized ischemic tissue but a relative lack of effect on sodium channels in normal cardiac tissue. Therefore, in nonischemic tissue, it has little effect on electrophysiologic and electrocardiographic findings when given at therapeutic levels. Lidocaine is not very effective in the treatment of supraventricular arrhythmias, because these arrhythmias usually arise in nonischemic tissue. The lidocaine congeners, mexiletine and tocainide, have electrophysiologic properties similar to those of lidocaine, but they are less selective for inactivated sodium channels in ischemic tissue and can produce greater effects on normal cardiac tissue than does lidocaine.

Lidocaine

Lidocaine has been administered intravenously as a loading dose (bolus) followed by a continuous intravenous infusion in the treatment of **ventricular tachycardia and other acute ventricular arrhythmias.** Recent guidelines of the American College of Cardiology and American Heart Association, however, do not recommend lidocaine for treatment of recurrent sustained ventricular tachycardia or ventricular fibrillation (see below).

A high serum concentration of lidocaine can cause central nervous system side effects such as nervousness, tremor, and paresthesia. It can also slow the conduction velocity in normal cardiac tissue. Because lidocaine is extensively metabolized, concurrent use of a drug that inhibits cytochrome P450 enzymes (e.g., cimetidine) can increase the serum concentration of lidocaine and precipitate lidocaine toxicity.

Mexiletine and Tocainide

Mexiletine and tocainide are administered orally on a long-term basis for the suppression of **ventricular arrhythmias.**

Because use of tocainide can lead to agranulocytosis and other blood cell deficiencies, patients receiving this drug should have blood counts performed periodically. Mexiletine is less frequently associated with these adverse effects.

Class IC Drugs

Flecainide and propafenone, which are class IC drugs, are administered orally. Their properties are outlined in Table 14–1 and Table 14–2.

Class IC drugs block both fast sodium channels and the rate of rise of the action potential during phase 0 to a greater extent than do other class I drugs. By this mechanism, the class IC drugs slow conduction throughout the heart and especially in the His-Purkinje system. Flecainide and propafenone usually have less effect on the potassium rectifier current (I_K) and do not prolong the QT interval as much as do class IA drugs, such as quinidine.

Flecainide

Flecainide is indicated for the treatment of **supraventricular arrhythmias** and **documented life-threatening ventricular arrhythmias.** In the past, it was also routinely used to suppress ventricular arrhythmias in patients with cardiac disorders. This practice has changed, however, since a clinical study called the **Cardiac Arrhythmia Suppression Trial (CAST)** showed that flecainide actually increased the mortality rate in patients who were recovering from myocardial infarction.

Although flecainide does not cause afterdepolarizations and torsade de pointes, it is capable of increasing the ventricular rate and causing reentrant ventricular tachycardia. Other adverse effects of flecainide include bronchospasm, leukopenia, thrombocytopenia, and seizures.

Propafenone

The effect of propafenone on fast sodium channels and cardiac conduction is similar to that of flecainide. As with flecainide, propafenone prolongs the PR interval and QRS duration. Propafenone can also cause some degree of QT prolongation.

Propafenone is administered orally on a long-term basis to suppress **supraventricular tachycardia.** The drug is also used to treat life-threatening forms of ventricular arrhythmia, such as **sustained ventricular tachycardia.**

Propafenone has the potential to cause ventricular arrhythmias and several hematologic abnormalities, including agranulocytosis, anemia, and thrombocytopenia.

Other Class I Drugs

Moricizine is a class I drug whose unusual properties do not permit its assignment to one of the three main subgroups. Moricizine is a phenothiazine analogue that blocks sodium channels in a manner similar to flecainide. It slows both the

AV node conduction velocity and the ventricular conduction velocity, thereby increasing the QRS duration. It may shorten the ventricular action potential duration and QT interval in a manner similar to lidocaine, however.

In the CAST II study, long-term use of moricizine to suppress arrhythmias was found to increase the mortality rate in patients with a history of myocardial infarction. For this reason, the drug is approved only for the treatment of **documented life-threatening ventricular arrhythmias.**

OTHER ANTIARRHYTHMIC DRUGS

Tables 14–1 and 14–2 compare the electrophysiologic and pharmacokinetic properties of the various groups and subgroups of antiarrhythmic drugs.

Class II Drugs

Drug Properties

The class II antiarrhythmics include esmolol, metoprolol, and propranolol. These drugs are β-adrenergic receptor antagonists (β-blockers) used to prevent and treat supraventricular arrhythmias and to reduce ventricular ectopic depolarizations and sudden death in patients with myocardial infarction.

The β-blockers have antiarrhythmic effects because of their ability to inhibit sympathetic activation of cardiac automaticity and conduction. The β-blockers slow the heart rate, decrease the AV node conduction velocity, and increase the AV node refractory period (Fig. 14–3). They have little effect on ventricular conduction and repolarization. The general pharmacologic properties of β-blockers are discussed in Chapter 9.

Esmolol

Esmolol, a β-blocker given intravenously, is rapidly metabolized by plasma esterase, and has an extremely short half-life. Its pharmacologic properties make it ideally suited for the treatment of patients who suffer from **acute supraventricular tachycardia** or **hypertension** during or immediately after surgery, where its short duration of action enables continuous control of the patient's heart rate and blood pressure.

Metoprolol and Propranolol

Metoprolol and propranolol can be administered orally or intravenously to treat and suppress **supraventricular and ventricular arrhythmias.** In patients with **myocardial infarction,** metoprolol is often administered intravenously during the early phase of treatment, followed by oral maintenance therapy that can continue for several months. The β-blockers have been demonstrated to protect the heart against the damage caused by ischemia and free radicals that may be formed during reperfusion of the coronary arteries when fibrinolytic drugs are used.

Class III Drugs

Amiodarone, dofetilide, ibutilide, and sotalol are class III antiarrhythmics. The most common attribute of this heterogeneous group of drugs is the prolongation of the ventricular action potential duration and refractory period. Class III drugs act mostly by blocking potassium rectifier currents (I_K) that repolarize the heart during phase 3 of the action potential. Except for amiodarone, these drugs do not slow the ventricular conduction velocity or increase the QRS duration significantly.

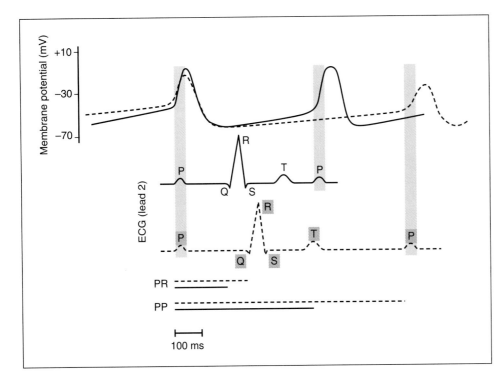

Figure 14–3. Effects of class II and class IV antiarrhythmic drugs on the sinoatrial (SA) node action potential duration and on the electrocardiogram (ECG). The membrane potential scale is in millivolts (mV), and the time scale is in milliseconds (ms). Black tracings and black lines for the time scale depict normal findings; dashed lines and tracings depict the effects of drug administration. Lightly shaded vertical bars show the relationship between the action potential duration and the findings on ECG. Class II drugs (ß-adrenergic receptor antagonists) and class IV drugs (calcium channel blockers) slow phase 4 depolarization in the SA node and increase the PP interval. They also slow the atrioventricular node conduction velocity and increase the PR interval.

Figure 14–4. Structures of amiodarone and thyroxine. The structure of amiodarone, which contains two iodine atoms, has some similarity to the structure of thyroid hormones such as thyroxine. Amiodarone can cause hypothyroidism and, less commonly, hyperthyroidism in some persons. The similar parts of the structures of amiodarone and thyroxine are shaded.

Amiodarone

CHEMISTRY AND PHARMACOKINETICS. Amiodarone is an organic iodine compound that is structurally related to thyroid hormones (Fig. 14–4). It can be administered orally or intravenously, and has unusual pharmacokinetic properties. After oral administration, amiodarone is slowly and variably absorbed and is primarily eliminated by biliary excretion. As shown in Table 14–2, the drug's action may not begin for about 2 weeks if loading doses are not given. In most cases, oral or intravenous administration of loading doses is used to accelerate the drug's onset of action. The half-life of amiodarone is extremely long (about 40 days with a range of 26 to 107 days).

MECHANISMS AND PHARMACOLOGIC EFFECTS. Although amiodarone has class III antiarrhythmic activity, it also blocks sodium channels, calcium channels, and β-adrenergic receptors. Hence, it is difficult to assign its antiarrhythmic activity to a specific mechanism.

As shown in Table 14–1, amiodarone decreases SA node automaticity, decreases AV node conduction velocity, and prolongs AV node and ventricular refractory periods. It increases the PR interval and the QT interval and causes a slight prolongation of the QRS duration. Amiodarone is a powerful inhibitor of ectopic pacemaker automaticity, and it prolongs repolarization and refractory periods throughout the heart. These actions probably account for much of its antiarrhythmic effects.

ADVERSE EFFECTS AND INTERACTIONS. Amiodarone can cause a number of adverse cardiovascular effects, including hypotension, AV block, and various arrhythmias. It is reported to cause drug-induced arrhythmias in only 2% of patients, however, and it is infrequently associated with torsade de pointes, despite its ability to cause QT prolongation. Although amiodarone has a mild negative inotropic effect, it has been successfully used to treat arrhythmias in patients with heart failure.

Amiodarone produces a constellation of other adverse effects, including blue-gray skin discoloration, thyroid abnormalities, and potentially fatal pulmonary fibrosis and pneumonitis. The thyroid abnormalities are caused by the iodine content of the drug and include both hypothyroidism and hyperthyroidism. Amiodarone can also cause corneal deposits, blurred vision, photosensitivity, and gastrointestinal disturbances. Low doses of the drug, however, are effective in many patients and are associated with fewer adverse effects.

Amiodarone inhibits the metabolism of a number of pharmacologic agents and significantly elevates the plasma concentrations of drugs such as digoxin, flecainide, phenytoin, procainamide, and warfarin. The dosage of these drugs should be decreased in patients receiving concurrent amiodarone therapy. Amiodarone also interacts with inhalational anesthetics and other central nervous system depressants to cause an increased incidence of adverse cardiovascular effects such as bradycardia.

INDICATIONS. Amiodarone is used orally on a long-term basis to suppress both supraventricular and ventricular arrhythmias, including atrial fibrillation, atrial flutter, supraventricular tachycardia, and life-threatening (sustained) ventricular tachycardia. Amiodarone is used intravenously to treat ventricular fibrillation or symptomatic, sustained ventricular tachycardia. In this setting, the drug can be given as a loading infusion followed by a maintenance infusion.

Ibutilide and Dofetilide

Ibutilide and dofetilide selectively block several types of outward potassium channels. These channels are called delayed rectifier channels (I_K) because they are responsible for repolarizing myocardial tissue during phase 3 of the action potential. By inhibiting these currents, dofetilide and ibutilide prolong ventricular repolarization and increase the QT interval of the ECG. Ibutilide also prolongs the action potential duration by promoting the influx of sodium through slow inward sodium channels. The sodium influx counteracts the outward potassium current and thereby prolongs repolarization.

Ibutilide is administered by intravenous infusion. It is rapidly biotransformed in the liver, and its metabolites are eliminated in the urine and feces, with an average half-life of 6 hours. The drug is indicated for the rapid conversion of **atrial fibrillation or flutter** to normal sinus rhythm. It does not significantly affect the heart rate, blood pressure, QRS duration, or PR interval. It can induce torsade de pointes, however, and should be avoided in patients with a history of this condition.

Dofetilide selectively blocks the rapidly activating delayed rectifier channel (I_{Kr}). The drug is administered orally to maintain sinus rhythm in patients with **atrial fibrillation**. Because of its potent ability to prolong the QT interval and induce torsade de pointes, the ECG must be closely monitored during dosage titration. When therapy is initiated, dosage adjustments are based on the degree of QT prolongation. The drug is primarily eliminated by renal excretion and doses must be reduced in persons with renal insufficiency.

Sotalol

Sotalol is a nonselective β-adrenergic receptor antagonist that prolongs the cardiac action potential duration and QT interval by blocking the delayed potassium rectifier current (I_K) during phase 3 of the ventricular action potential (see Fig. 14–2). The drug also decreases automaticity, slows the AV node conduction velocity, and increases the AV node refractory period without affecting the ventricular conduction and QRS duration.

Sotalol is approved for the treatment of **ventricular arrhythmias** and is also effective in the management of **atrial arrhythmias,** including **atrial fibrillation.** It produces a dose-dependent incidence of torsade de pointes, most likely because of QT prolongation. Some of its adverse effects (e.g., bronchospasm) are caused by β-adrenergic receptor blockade.

Class IV Drugs

Diltiazem and **verapamil** are calcium channel blockers that have significant effects on cardiac tissue. They primarily act to decrease the AV node conduction velocity and increase the AV node refractory period, and they have a smaller effect on the SA node and heart rate. As shown in Table 14–1, they have little effect on the ventricular conduction velocity and refractory period.

Diltiazem and verapamil can be administered intravenously to terminate **acute supraventricular tachycardia.** They are also used to reduce the ventricular rate in patients who have **atrial fibrillation** with a rapid ventricular response. These drugs can exacerbate ventricular tachycardia, so it is important that arrhythmias be correctly diagnosed before beginning treatment with diltiazem or verapamil. Other calcium channel blockers (including dihydropyridines such as amlodipine) have less effect on cardiac tissue and no role in the treatment of arrhythmias.

Miscellaneous Drugs

Adenosine

Adenosine is a naturally occurring nucleoside composed of adenine and ribose. When administered as a rapid intravenous bolus, it has an extremely short half-life of 10 seconds or less. In the body, adenosine is derived from ATP and activates specific G protein-coupled adenosine receptors. Stimulation of these receptors leads to activation of acetylcholine-sensitive potassium channels and blockade of calcium influx in the SA node, atrium, and AV node. It thereby causes cell hyperpolarization, slows the AV node conduction velocity, and increases the AV node refractory period. In fact, AV node conduction can be completely blocked for a few seconds, resulting in a brief period of asystole. These actions serve to terminate supraventricular tachycardia by preventing the retrograde conduction of reentrant impulses through the AV node. Because of its brief duration of action, adenosine has been termed a pharmacologic counterpart to electrical cardioversion.

Adenosine is primarily used to terminate **acute paroxysmal supraventricular tachycardia,** including the type associated with Wolff-Parkinson-White syndrome. It is not indicated for the treatment of atrial fibrillation or flutter. Dipyridamole, a vasodilator used to facilitate angiographic studies, inhibits the cellular uptake of adenosine and markedly increases its cardiac effects. Doses of adenosine, therefore, should be reduced in persons who have recently received dipyridamole. Adenosine can cause bronchospasm and should be used cautiously in persons with obstructive lung disease.

Digoxin

Digoxin, a digitalis glycoside discussed in Chapter 12, acts indirectly to increase vagal tone and thereby slow the AV node conduction velocity and increase the AV node refractory period. Digoxin has been used to slow the ventricular rate in patients with **atrial fibrillation**, although β-blockers and calcium channel blockers are usually preferred for this purpose because of their more rapid onset of action and greater degree of AV nodal blockade. Digoxin is sometimes used for this indication because it does not cause as much bradycardia as β-blockers and it does not reduce cardiac contractility as much as calcium channel blockers such as verapamil. In fact, digoxin has a positive inotropic effect and is also used to treat **heart failure** (see Chapter 12).

Magnesium Sulfate

The magnesium ion, the second most common intracellular cation, has a number of roles in normal cardiac function. Magnesium deficiency can be caused by use of drugs such as loop diuretics or by pathologic states, and this deficiency can contribute to the development of arrhythmias and congestive heart failure, as well as to gastrointestinal and renal disorders.

Magnesium sulfate is administered intravenously to suppress drug-induced torsade de pointes, to treat digitalis-induced ventricular arrhythmias, and to treat supraventricular arrhythmias associated with magnesium deficiency. Magnesium has been studied as a treatment for other arrhythmias, but its efficacy is not yet established.

MANAGEMENT OF SUPRAVENTRICULAR ARRHYTHMIAS

Atrial Fibrillation and Flutter

Atrial fibrillation is thought to be caused by a disorganized form of reentry in atrial tissue, a form in which atrial cells are continuously reexcited as soon as they have repolarized. Under these conditions, the AV node is continuously bombarded with atrial impulses, some of which are conducted to the ventricles, so that the ventricular rate is sometimes rapid and irregular.

The first objective of treatment is to control the rapid ventricular rate. This is accomplished by administering drugs that slow the conduction velocity and increase the refractory period of the AV node, so that fewer atrial impulses are transmitted to the ventricles. Drugs used for this purpose include β-blockers, calcium channel blockers, and digoxin. Although these drugs may slow the ventricular rate, they usually do not affect the underlying atrial fibrillation.

After controlling the ventricular rate, the atrial fibrillation can be converted to normal sinus rhythm by the use of direct current (DC) cardioversion (provided the arrhythmia is of less than 48 hours duration) or by the intravenous administration of ibutilide. Many patients whose condition is successfully converted will have relapse, however. Long-term suppression of atrial fibrillation with class I or class III drugs may be effective in some patients after conversion to normal sinus rhythm. These drugs, however, are not always efficacious and have numerous adverse effects. For this reason, many patients with chronic atrial fibrillation are treated with a drug to control the ventricular rate and with an anticoagulant to prevent thromboembolism, which is often associated with atrial fibrillation (see Chapter 16). Patients who have Wolff-Parkinson-White syndrome and develop atrial fibrillation should not be treated with digoxin or verapamil, because these drugs can decrease accessory pathway refractoriness and lead to ventricular tachycardia.

Atrial flutter is usually treated in the same manner as atrial fibrillation. Surgical ablation of the arrhythmogenic tissue can be effective in some patients with atrial flutter.

Supraventricular Tachycardia

Paroxysmal supraventricular tachycardia is caused most frequently by a reentrant circuit in the AV node. Acute PSVT is often treated with intravenous adenosine, which causes AV block and interrupts the reentrant pathway. Alternatively, AV block can be produced by a calcium channel blocker (e.g., verapamil) or by a β-blocker (e.g., esmolol). Esmolol is a short-acting drug whose use is often preferred in perioperative patients. Long-term suppression is usually accomplished by use of a calcium channel blocker, β-blocker, or digitalis glycoside. Surgical ablation of the arrhythmogenic tissue can also be effective.

Patients with Wolff-Parkinson-White syndrome exhibit an atypical form of PSVT caused by reentry through an accessory bypass conduction pathway between the atria and ventricles. This form of PSVT can also be terminated with drugs that cause AV block. Long-term treatment may consist of surgical ablation of arrhythmogenic tissue or use of a sodium or potassium channel blocker to suppress the arrhythmia.

MANAGEMENT OF VENTRICULAR ARRHYTHMIAS

Ventricular Tachycardia

Ventricular tachycardia is an arrhythmia that usually presents with a monomorphic, regular, wide QRS complex with a rate greater than 100 to 120 beats per minute. It is often associated with myocardial infarction and is thought to be caused by decremental conduction and reentry in ventricular tissue, phenomena that are described earlier in this chapter.

Sustained VT should be treated immediately because of its deleterious effect on cardiac output and myocardial ischemia, and because it can lead to ventricular fibrillation (see below).

If the patient with VT does not have a pulse or is hemodynamically unstable, electric (direct current, DC) cardioversion should be used to terminate the arrhythmia. If such persons do not respond to three shocks, they should be treated as if they had ventricular fibrillation (see below) and given epinephrine and amiodarone with continued attempts at cardioversion.

Persons with recurrent episodes of sustained VT not resulting from a reversible cause (e.g., hypokalemia) are usually treated with intravenous amiodarone administered as a series of bolus doses or as an intravenous infusion. Intravenous procainamide is an alternative to amiodarone. These treatments are given to prevent further episodes of VT and reduce the need for cardioversion. An implantable **cardioverter-defibrillator** (ICD) is usually inserted in patients with hemodynamically significant sustained VT that occurs more than 2 days after a myocardial infarction.

Clinical trials have shown that amiodarone is not as effective as an ICD for the long-term suppression of ventricular arrhythmias in patients with a history of syncope or aborted sudden cardiac death. Amiodarone, however, is sometimes used in conjunction with an ICD to reduce the number of shocks required to maintain normal sinus rhythm. Amiodarone or sotalol can also be used to control benign symptomatic arrhythmias such as nonsustained ventricular tachycardia and frequent premature ventricular beats.

The choice of drug therapy for long-term prophylaxis of ventricular arrhythmias is controversial. Clinical trials have found that amiodarone reduced arrhythmic deaths and arrhythmias requiring resuscitation in patients after myocardial infarction with frequent ventricular premature beats or a low ventricular ejection fraction, but amiodarone did not reduce total or cardiac mortality. The combination of β-blockers and amiodarone, however, significantly reduced both nonarrhythmic and arrhythmic death. In addition, adrenergic β-blockers are the only drugs currently recommended to prevent sudden death in persons who have had a myocardial infarction and do not have recurrent ventricular arrhythmias.

Patients who have taken an overdose of a tricyclic antidepressant drug (e.g., imipramine) can develop tachycardia that has a wide QRS complex and is believed to result from the blockade of cardiac sodium channels by the antidepressant. The treatment for this particular form of ventricular tachycardia is the intravenous administration of sodium bicarbonate, which increases the ratio of the nonionized form to the ionized form of imipramine and thereby causes dissociation of the drug from sodium channels.

Torsade de Pointes

Torsade de pointes is a polymorphic ventricular tachycardia that can be induced by drugs or electrolyte abnormalities that prolong the QT interval and predispose cardiac cells to afterdepolarizations. This arrhythmia can also result from a congenital, prolonged QT syndrome. Patients with a drug-induced arrhythmia can be treated by withdrawal of the causative agent, correction of any electrolyte abnormalities, intravenous administration of magnesium sulfate, cardiac overdrive pacing, or intravenous administration of isoproterenol (a β-adrenergic receptor agonist). These treatments act in part by shortening the QT interval.

Ventricular Fibrillation

Ventricular fibrillation (VF) is the most common cause of sudden cardiac death in persons with ischemic heart disease. In VF, the ECG shows rapid (300 to 400/min), irregular, shapeless depolarizations of variable amplitude and shape. VF is thought to be caused by a disorganized reentry circuit in the ventricles. Electrical defibrillation is the treatment of choice for patients with this disorder. If VF persists after three rapid shocks, intravenous epinephrine (or vasopressin) and amiodarone are administered followed by continued attempts at defibrillation. Lidocaine is no longer used routinely for this purpose, but some authorities suggest trying it if other measures fail.

Long-term therapy to prevent sudden cardiac death in patients who developed sustained VT or VF 24 to 48 hours after a myocardial infarction usually consists of an ICD and an adrenergic β-blocker.

SUMMARY OF IMPORTANT POINTS

- Antiarrhythmic drugs suppress the abnormal impulse formation or conduction that causes arrhythmias.

- Antiarrhythmic drugs are divided into four main classes, with class I consisting of sodium channel blockers, class II consisting of β-adrenergic receptor antagonists (β-blockers), class III consisting of potassium channel blockers and other drugs that prolong the action potential duration, and class IV consisting of calcium channel blockers.

- Class IA drugs (e.g., quinidine) slow conduction and prolong refractory periods, thereby increasing the QRS duration and the QT interval. They are primarily used for the long-term suppression of arrhythmias.

- Class IB drugs have little effect on normal cardiac tissue and electrocardiographic findings, but they can decrease the QT interval slightly. Lidocaine has been administered intravenously for the treatment of acute ventricular arrhythmias. Mexiletine and tocainide, oral congeners of lidocaine, have been used for long-term prophylaxis.

- Class IC drugs have a greater effect than other sodium channel blockers on cardiac conduction but have little effect on the action potential duration. Flecainide and propafenone are used to treat supraventricular arrhythmias and life-threatening ventricular arrhythmias.

- Class II drugs (β-blockers), which slow the AV node conduction velocity and prolong the AV node refractory period, are used to treat supraventricular arrhythmias. They also reduce the incidence of fatal ventricular arrhythmias in patients with myocardial infarction.

- Class III drugs (e.g., amiodarone, dofetilide, ibutilide, and sotalol) prolong the action potential duration, refractory periods, and QT interval.

- Amiodarone is given intravenously in the treatment of ventricular tachycardia and fibrillation, and can be given orally for chronic prophylaxis. Ibutilide and dofetilide are used for acute termination and chronic prophylaxis of atrial fibrillation, respectively. Sotalol is used for both acute and chronic treatment of supraventricular and ventricular arrhythmias.

- Class IV drugs (calcium channel blockers) slow the AV node conduction velocity, prolong the AV node refractory period, and thereby terminate the AV node reentry that is responsible for supraventricular tachycardia.

- Adenosine is administered as a rapid intravenous bolus to terminate acute supraventricular tachycardia.

Review Questions

For each numbered drug description, select the corresponding drug from the lettered choices.

1. Adverse effects include pulmonary fibrosis, hypothyroidism, and blue-gray skin discoloration.

2. Clinical trials show that it increases mortality in persons who have had a myocardial infarction.

3. Prolongs ventricular repolarization and increases the QT interval on the electrocardiogram, thereby predisposing patients to polymorphic ventricular tachycardia.

4. Ultra short-acting drug used to control hypertension and atrial (supraventricular) tachycardia in surgical patients.

(A) sotalol
(B) esmolol

(C) verapamil
(D) flecainide
(E) amiodarone

Choose the single best answer from the choices provided.

5. Which of the following drugs is often administered intravenously in persons with ventricular tachycardia or fibrillation to facilitate conversion to normal sinus rhythm?
(A) quinidine
(B) propranolol
(C) amiodarone
(D) adenosine
(E) verapamil

Answers and Explanations

1. The answer is E: amiodarone. Amiodarone is a thyroxine analogue that can cause hypothyroidism. Persons taking the drug should also be closely monitored for signs of pulmonary fibrosis.

2. The answer is D: flecainide. Class IC drugs such as flecainide have been shown to increase mortality in persons with ischemic heart disease. The class IC drugs, however, do not increase mortality in persons with nonischemic heart conditions and are used for chronic prevention of supraventricular tachycardia and atrial fibrillation.

3. The answer is A: sotalol. Sotalol and other class III drugs slow phase 3 ventricular repolarization and thereby prolong the QT interval. By slowing ventricular repolarization, the drugs predispose to afterdepolarizations leading to polymorphic ventricular tachycardia (torsade de pointes). Although amiodarone prolongs the QT interval, it causes less torsade de pointes than other drugs.

4. The answer is B: esmolol. Esmolol is an ultra short-acting adrenergic β-receptor antagonist that is often used during and after surgery to control hypertension and supraventricular tachycardia. The drug's short duration of action is an advantage in this setting should bradycardia or hypotension occur.

5. The answer is C: amiodarone. Amiodarone is often administered to persons with ventricular fibrillation or sustained ventricular tachycardia. Propranolol and other β-blockers have a role in the prevention of sudden death in persons with ischemic heart disease but are not useful in treating acute ventricular arrhythmias. Calcium channel blockers (e.g., verapamil) are contraindicated in persons with ventricular tachycardia but are used in suppressing and preventing supraventricular tachycardia. Adenosine is used in terminating acute supraventricular tachycardia but has no role in treating ventricular tachycardia.

SELECTED READINGS

Dorian, P., and I. Mangat. Role of amiodarone in the era of the implantable cardioverter defibrillator. J Cardiovasc Electrophys 14(Suppl):S78–S81, 2003.

Khan, M. H. Oral class III antiarrhythmics: what is new? Curr Opin Cardiol 19:47–51, 2004.

Kurnik, D., R. Loebstein, Z. Farfel, et al. Complex drug-drug-disease interactions between amiodarone, warfarin, and the thyroid gland. Medicine 83:107–113, 2004.

Tamariz, L. J., and E. B. Bass. Pharmacological rate control of atrial fibrillation. Cardiol Clin 22:35–45, 2004.

Trappe, H. J., B. Brandts, and P. Weismueller. Arrhythmias in the intensive care patient. Curr Opin Crit Care 9:345–355, 2003.

CHAPTER 15

Drugs for Hyperlipidemia

CLASSIFICATION OF DRUGS FOR HYPERLIPIDEMIA

HMG-CoA Reductase Inhibitors
- Atorvastatin (LIPITOR)
- Fluvastatin (LESCOL)
- Lovastatin (MEVACOR)
- Pravastatin (PRAVACHOL)
- Rosuvastatin (CRESTOR)
- Simvastatin (ZOCOR)

Bile Acid–binding Resins
- Cholestyramine
- Colestipol
- Colesevelam (WELCHOL)

Cholesterol Absorption Inhibitor
- Ezetimibe (ZETIA)

Fibric Acid Derivatives
- Fenofibrate (TRICOR)
- Gemfibrozil (LOPID)

Other Drugs
- Nicotinic acid (niacin)

OVERVIEW

Lipids are necessary molecules for human life. **Cholesterol,** which is an essential component of cell membranes, is the precursor to the sterol and steroid compounds that are synthesized in the body. **Triglycerides,** composed of three **fatty acids** and glycerol, are the main storage form of fuel used to generate high-energy compounds, such as adenosine triphosphate (ATP), that provide the energy for muscle contraction and metabolic reactions. Despite the vital functions of these and other lipids, elevated concentrations of cholesterol and triglycerides play an important role in the development of atherosclerotic heart disease and other disorders.

Whereas **hyperlipidemia** and **hyperlipoproteinemia** are general terms for elevated concentrations of lipids and lipoproteins in the blood, **hypercholesterolemia** and **hyper-triglyceridemia** refer specifically to high concentrations of cholesterol and triglycerides, respectively. Hypercholesterolemia contributes to the pathogenesis of **atherosclerosis** and has been causally associated with **coronary artery disease** and other atherosclerotic vascular diseases (Fig. 15–1). Hypertriglyceridemia is associated with **pancreatitis** and is also believed to have a role in the development of atherosclerosis and heart disease in some patients, although its role in cardiovascular disorders appears to be less significant than that of hypercholesterolemia.

Because **coronary heart disease** (CHD) is the main cause of premature death in industrialized countries, it is important to detect and eliminate **modifiable risk factors** associated with it. In addition to hyperlipidemia, these risk factors include hypertension, cigarette smoking, and a low high-density lipoprotein (HDL) cholesterol level (<40 mg/dL). Unmodifiable risk factors include male gender, family history of premature CHD (CHD in first-degree male relative under 55 years of age or first-degree female under 65 years of age), and advanced age (men >45 years; women >55 years). Diabetes mellitus and clinical manifestations of non-coronary forms of atherosclerotic disease (e.g., aortic aneurysm and carotid artery disease) are considered CHD risk equivalents when determining goals for treatment of hyperlipidemia. This means that persons with these conditions are considered to have the same risk for future occur-

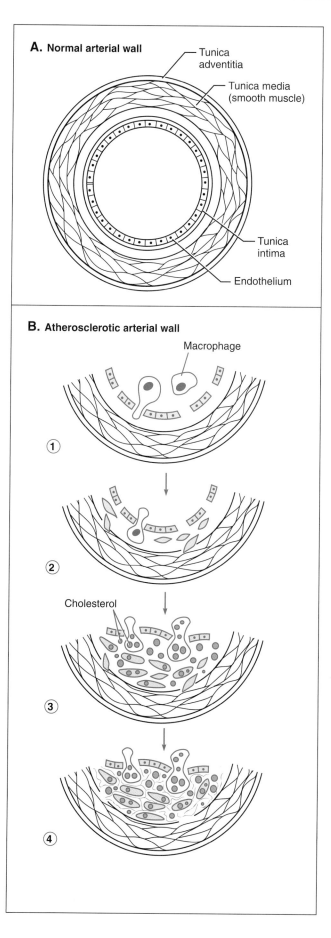

A. Normal arterial wall

Tunica adventitia

Tunica media (smooth muscle)

Tunica intima

Endothelium

B. Atherosclerotic arterial wall

Macrophage

① ② ③ ④

Cholesterol

rences of CHD as persons who already have some form of CHD (e.g., angina pectoris, myocardial infarction, or other types of clinically significant myocardial ischemia).

Women have a lower risk of heart disease until after menopause, and this lower risk may be partly owing to the favorable effect of estrogens on serum lipoprotein levels. Estrogens may also have beneficial effects on the microcirculation and energy metabolism.

After discussing lipoproteins, lipid transport, and the causes and types of hyperlipoproteinemia, this chapter describes how dietary restrictions, alone or in combination with drug treatment, can reduce serum lipoprotein levels and thereby reduce the risk of CHD.

Lipoproteins and Lipid Transport

Because lipids are insoluble in plasma, they must be transported in the circulation in the form of lipoproteins. There are numerous **types of lipoproteins,** including chylomicrons, very low-density lipoproteins (VLDL), low-density lipoproteins (LDL), intermediate-density lipoproteins (IDL), high-density lipoproteins (HDL), and lipoprotein(a). The various types are distinguished in terms of their buoyant density, lipid and protein composition, and role in lipid transport. Moreover, each type is associated with a unique group of **apoproteins.** Some of the apoproteins are exchanged between different types of lipoproteins as they transport lipids to various tissues. The composition and metabolism of lipoproteins is depicted in Box 15–1.

Chylomicrons

Chylomicrons are primarily involved in the transport of dietary lipids from the gut to the adipose tissue and liver. When cholesterol and triglycerides are ingested, they are emulsified in the intestines by the bile acids and other bile secretions, and the emulsified lipids are combined with proteins to form chylomicrons in the gut wall. After chylomicrons are secreted into the circulation, they deliver triglycerides to adipose tissue via the action of a **lipoprotein lipase** located in the vascular endothelial cells. By this process, chylomicrons are converted to a cholesterol-rich chylomicron remnant, which transports cholesterol to the liver.

Very Low-Density and Low-Density Lipoproteins

Golgi bodies in the liver form VLDL from triglycerides, cholesterol, and protein and then secrete the VLDL into the circulation. The VLDL deliver triglycerides to adipose tissue in the same manner as do the chylomicrons. During the process, the VLDL are transformed into IDL and LDL that contain a high percentage of cholesterol.

Figure 15–1. Comparison of normal (A) and atherosclerotic (B) arterial walls. Steps in the pathogenesis of atherosclerosis are as follows: (1) Damage to the endothelium is followed by invasion of macrophages. (2) Endothelial and macrophage growth factors stimulate smooth muscle cells to migrate into the tunica intima and to proliferate. (3) Oxidized cholesterol accumulates in and around macrophages (foam cells) and muscle cells. (4) Collagen and elastic fibers form a connective tissue matrix that results in a fibrous plaque.

BOX 15–1. LIPOPROTEIN METABOLISM AND ATHEROSCLEROSIS

The liver is the central processing site for lipoprotein metabolism. Cholesterol is derived from three sources: (1) biosynthesis from acetyl-CoA, (2) delivery of dietary cholesterol by chylomicron remnants, and (3) endocytosis of low-density lipoprotein (LDL) cholesterol by LDL receptors.

Triglycerides are formed in the liver from fatty acids, which are derived from lipolysis of triglycerides in adipose tissue. Triglycerides, cholesterol, and protein are packaged by Golgi bodies in the liver to form very low-density lipoproteins (VLDL), which are secreted into the circulation. The VLDL accept apoproteins C and E from high-density lipoproteins (HDL) and then return these apoproteins to HDL as they deliver triglycerides (as fatty acids) to adipose and other tissues via the action of lipoprotein lipase (LL) located in the capillary endothelium.

COMPOSITION OF LIPOPROTEINS

Lipoprotein	Core Lipids*	Apoproteins*
Chylomicron	Dietary triglycerides and cholesteryl esters	B-48, C, E, and A
VLDL	Endogenous triglycerides and cholesteryl esters	C, B-100, and E
LDL	Cholesteryl esters	B-100
HDL	Cholesteryl esters and phospholipids	A-I, A-II, C, E, and D

*Listed in order of quantitative importance.

With the removal of apoproteins and triglycerides, VLDL are transformed into LDL and intermediate-density lipoproteins (IDL). The LDL deliver cholesterol to various sites in the body, including peripheral tissues and the liver via endocytosis by LDL receptors. LDL cholesterol is also incorporated into atherosclerotic plaques.

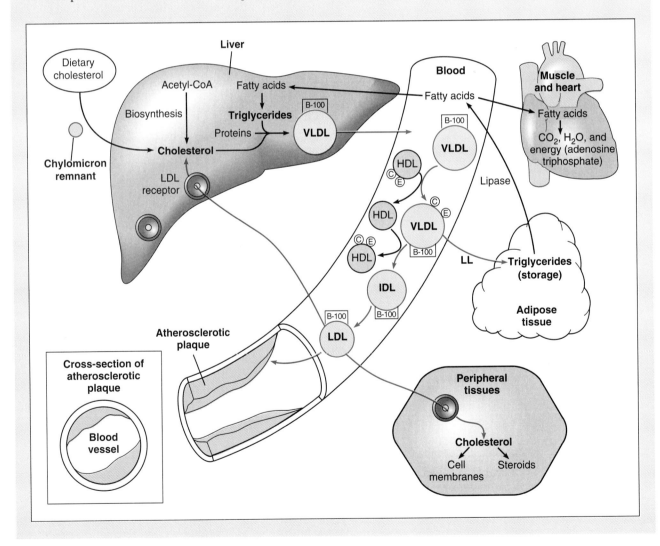

The LDL transport cholesterol to peripheral tissues for incorporation into cell membranes and steroids. In this process, the LDL bind to specific LDL receptors that are located in the plasma membrane of cells and recognize apoprotein B-100 on the surface of LDL molecules. After binding to their receptors, the LDL undergo endocytosis and are incorporated into lysosomes for further processing of cholesterol and protein.

The LDL can also deliver cholesterol to nascent atheromas and thereby contribute to the development of atherosclerosis (see Fig. 15–1). In atheromas, cholesterol is phagocytosed by macrophages, which are transformed into foam cells as they become filled with oxidized cholesterol.

High-Density Lipoproteins

The HDL are small lipoproteins that are secreted by the gut and liver. The nascent HDL contain protein and a small quantity of phospholipid, with relatively little cholesterol or triglycerides. Their high density is caused by the large ratio of protein to lipid in HDL molecules. As the HDL circulate in the blood, they exchange apoproteins C and E with VLDL, and they acquire cholesterol from peripheral tissues and atheromas. The exchange of apoproteins is related to the delivery of VLDL and triglycerides to adipose tissue via lipoprotein lipase.

The HDL also serve to transport cholesterol from atheromas and peripheral tissues to the liver. During this process of **reverse cholesterol transport,** the HDL acquire cholesterol from peripheral tissues and esterify the cholesterol with fatty acids via an enzyme called lecithin-cholesterol acyltransferase (LCAT). The cholesteryl esters either are transported by HDL to the liver or are transferred to LDL for transport to the liver. The contribution of reverse cholesterol transport to CHD has been supported by epidemiologic studies that show an inverse correlation between HDL cholesterol levels and the risk of this disease.

Lipoprotein(a)

Lipoprotein(a) is a unique lipoprotein whose physiologic function is unknown and whose occurrence is genetically determined. It is found in atherosclerotic plaques of some individuals, and plasma levels of lipoprotein(a) are highly correlated with angiographically demonstrable coronary artery disease.

Causes and Types of Hyperlipoproteinemia

Hyperlipoproteinemia occurs as a result of genetic or environmental factors that increase the formation of lipoproteins or reduce the clearance of lipoproteins from the circulation. These factors include biochemical defects in lipoprotein metabolism, excessive dietary intake of lipids, endocrine abnormalities, and use of drugs that perturb lipoprotein formation or catabolism. Table 15–1 provides information about the characteristics and types of hyperlipoproteinemia.

Primary hyperlipoproteinemias are relatively rare disorders, each of which is caused by a **monogenic defect** (a specific defect at a single gene). In some disorders, LDL cholesterol levels are severely elevated because of a deficiency of LDL receptors or a defect in the structure of apoprotein B. In the latter case, LDL receptors do not recognize LDL, so LDL removal from the circulation is markedly impaired. In another disorder, VLDL and triglyceride levels are severely elevated because of a lipoprotein lipase deficiency that prevents delivery of triglycerides to adipose tissue.

Most cases of hyperlipoproteinemia do not result from a single gene defect but instead result from the influence of several genes that predispose the patient to milder forms of hyperlipoproteinemia, particularly in the presence of excessive dietary intake of lipids. These milder forms, called **polygenic-environmental hyperlipoproteinemias**, which

TABLE 15–1.   Types and Characteristics of Hyperlipoproteinemia

Types	Incidence	Total Cholesterol Concentration (mg/dL)	Triglyceride Concentration (mg/dL)
Primary (monogenic) types			
Hypercholesterolemia	Rare	>300	<250
Hypertriglyceridemia	Rare	<250	>300
Mixed hyperlipidemia	Rare	>250	>300
Polygenic-environmental types			
Hypercholesterolemia	Common	200–270	<250
Mixed hyperlipidemia	Less common	>200	>300
Secondary types			
Hyperlipoproteinemia due to alcoholism, diabetes mellitus, uremia, or use of β-adrenergic receptor antagonists,[†] isotretinoin, oral contraceptives, or thiazide diuretics	Common	Usually normal*	Increased
Hyperlipoproteinemia due to hypothyroidism, nephrotic syndrome, or obstructive liver disease	Less common	Increased	Normal or slightly increased

*Use of thiazide diuretics may increase the total cholesterol concentration.
[†]Use of β-adrenergic receptor antagonists may decrease the high-density lipoprotein (HDL) cholesterol concentration.

are much more common than primary hyperlipoproteine-mias, are responsible for most cases of accelerated atherosclerosis.

Secondary hyperlipoproteinemias are commonly caused by the presence of alcoholism, diabetes mellitus, or uremia or by the use of drugs such as β-adrenergic receptor antagonists, isotretinoin, oral contraceptives, or thiazide diuretics. They are less commonly caused by hypothyroidism, nephrotic syndrome, or obstructive liver disease.

Guidelines for Management of Hypercholesterolemia

The Adult Treatment Panel III (ATP III) of the **National Cholesterol Education Program** (NCEP) issued evidence-based guidelines for the management of high blood cholesterol and related disorders in 2001. These recommendations were updated in 2004 based on evidence from five clinical trials published since the ATP III guidelines were issued. These trials confirmed the benefits of cholesterol-lowering therapy in high risk patients and encourage more aggressive reductions in low-density lipoprotein cholesterol (LDL-C) in very high risk patients.

The NCEP guidelines (Table 15–2) establish LDL-C goals and levels for initiating **therapeutic lifestyle changes** (TLC) and drug therapy for persons in different risk categories. For **high risk** patients (who already have CHD or have CHD risk equivalents), the basic goal is to achieve a LDL-C of less than 100 mg/dL, and TLC and drug therapy should be initiated if the patient's LDL-C is higher than 100 mg/dL. The updated guidelines suggest an optional LDL-C goal for *high risk* patients of less than 70 mg/dL, particularly for those whose LDL-C is less than 100 mg/dL at baseline. This optional goal is based on clinical trials that show that high risk patients benefit from LDL-C reduction regardless of their baseline level.

For **moderately high risk** patients (persons with two or more CHD risk factors and a 10% to 20% risk of develop-ing CHD in 10 years), the original guidelines suggest a LDL-C goal of less than 130 mg/dL, with TLC and drug therapy initiated if levels are higher 130 mg/dL. The updated guidelines recommend considering drug therapy for patients with LDL-C levels between 100 and 129 mg/dL. The 10-year risk of developing CHD can be estimated using calculators such as the one provided by the National Heart, Lung, and Blood Institute (see Table 15–2).

Patients with a **moderate risk** of CHD (two or more risk factors and <10% risk of developing CHD in 10 years) have the same LDL-C goal and TLC initiation level as moderately high risk patients, but drug therapy is recommended only at the start of therapy if LDL-C levels are above 160 mg/dL. If therapeutic lifestyle changes do not achieve the target level in 6 to 12 months, drug therapy should be considered for persons with a moderate risk of CHD.

For persons with a **lower risk** of CHD (zero to one risk factor), the target LDL-C level is less than 160 mg/dL and TLC should be initiated in persons exceeding this level. The original guidelines recommended drug therapy only at the start of treatment if LDL-C levels exceed 190 mg/dL, but the updated recommendations suggest considering drug therapy if levels are between 160 and 189 mg/dL.

The updated guidelines also suggest that high risk patients with high triglycerides or a low HDL-cholesterol level receive a fibrate drug or nicotinic acid (niacin) in combination with a LDL-cholesterol lowering drug to raise HDL-C levels and lower triglyceride levels.

Secondary causes of hyperlipidemia should be excluded before treatment is considered, because abnormal levels of cholesterol or triglycerides can often be corrected by proper management of the underlying condition or by replacing the offending drug with an alternative.

Therapeutic Lifestyle Changes

Therapeutic lifestyle changes (TLC) are an essential modality in the management of high cholesterol and triglyceride

---

TABLE 15–2.   **National Cholesterol Education Program Guidelines for Management of High Blood Cholesterol Levels for Persons in Different Risk Categories[1]**

Risk Category	LDL-C goal	Initiate TLC[2]	Consider Drug Therapy[2]
High risk: CHD or CHD equivalents[3] (10-year risk[4] of CHD >20%)	<100 mg/dL (optional: <70 mg/dL)	≥100 mg/dL	≥100 mg/dL (optional goal: <100 mg/dL)
Moderately high risk: 2+ risk factors[5] (10-year risk of CHD 10-20%)	<130 mg/dL (optional: <100 mg/dL)	≥130 mg/dL	≥130 mg/dL (optional: 100-129 mg/dL)
Moderate risk: 2+ risk factors (10-year risk of CHD <10%)	<130 mg/dL	≥130 mg/dL	≥160 mg/dL
Lower risk: 0–1 risk factor	<160 mg/dL	≥160 mg/dL	≥190 mg/dL (optional: 160-190 mg/dL)

[1]Adult Treatment Panel III (ATP III) Guidelines issued in 2001 and updated in 2004 (see Grundy et al.)
[2]LDL-C levels at which TLC or drug therapy initiated.
[3]Includes myocardial infarction, angina, myocardial ischemia, noncoronary forms of atherosclerosis, and diabetes mellitus.
[4]Electronic 10-year risk calculators available at www.nhlbi.nih.gov/guidelines/cholesterol.
[5]Risk factors include cigarette smoking, hypertension, low HDL-C, family history of premature CHD, and age (see text for details).
CHD, coronary heart disease; HDL-C = high-density lipoprotein cholesterol; LDL-C = low-density lipoprotein cholesterol:

levels, and may be effective by themselves in patients with mildly elevated cholesterol or triglyceride levels. The TLC include recommendations for diet, weight management, and physical activity. The diet of patients with hypercholesterolemia should be low in cholesterol, saturated fat, and calories. **Saturated fat** and **cholesterol** are restricted because each independently increases LDL-C, and **calories** are restricted to help the patient achieve or maintain an ideal body weight. The ATP III guidelines recommend the **American Heart Association (AHA) step II diet** as the initial diet for lowering cholesterol and triglyceride levels, and suggest adding **plant stanol or sterol esters**, also called phytosterols, (2 g/day) and soluble fiber (10 to 25 g/day) to enhance LDL-C reduction.

The AHA step II diet mandates that cholesterol intake should be under 200 mg/day, and total calories from fat should be limited to 25% to 35% of total calories, with saturated fat limited to less than 7% of total calories. Foods containing partially hydrogenated plant oils should be avoided because hydrogenation produces the *trans* isomers of fatty acids that acts to increase LDL-C levels, decrease HDL-C levels, increase systemic inflammation, and reduce the availability of fatty acid precursors to anticoagulant prostaglandins.

Dietary modulations are particularly useful in persons with multiple risk factors or angiographic evidence of coronary artery disease. Studies have shown that diets low in saturated and *trans* fatty acids and high in linoleic acid and **omega-3 (n-3) fatty acids** (lenolenic acid and those in **fish oils**) act to lower cholesterol levels, reverse the angiographic evidence of coronary atherosclerosis, and reduce the mortality rate in patients with CHD. In patients with hypertriglyceridemia, supplementing the diet with fish oils that contain **omega-3 fatty acids** often lowers triglyceride levels. These high–molecular-weight fatty acids contain a double bond between the third and fourth carbon from the end of the molecule.

DRUGS FOR HYPERCHOLESTEROLEMIA

The 3-hydroxy-3-methylglutaryl coenzyme A (HMG-CoA) reductase inhibitors, the bile acid-binding resins, and ezetimibe are primarily used to treat hypercholesterolemia, whereas the fibric acid derivatives and niacin are used primarily to reduce elevated triglyceride levels and to raise HDL-C levels. Tables 15–3, 15–4, and 15–5 outline the effects and pharmacokinetic properties of the drugs used to treat hypercholesterolemia and compare them with the effects and properties of other drugs discussed in this chapter.

HMG-CoA Reductase Inhibitors

Among the HMG-CoA reductase inhibitors are **atorvastatin, fluvastatin, lovastatin, pravastatin, rosuvastatin**, and **simvastatin.** These drugs have demonstrated a high degree of effectiveness in the treatment of hypercholesterolemia and have a good safety record. Their once-daily dosage regimen is highly convenient and fosters patient compliance.

Drug Properties

CHEMISTRY AND PHARMACOKINETICS. The reductase inhibitors are structurally related to HMG-CoA, which is the substrate for HMG-CoA reductase (Fig. 15–3). The drugs have a relatively low bioavailability, largely owing to extensive first-pass metabolism. Lovastatin and simvastatin are prodrugs that must be converted to an active metabolite in the liver, whereas the other reductase inhibitors are active compounds. All of the drugs, except atorvastatin, have a relatively short half-life (see Table 15–4). The reductase inhibitors are metabolized by two cytochrome P450 isozymes (CYP3A and CYP2C), and they can interact with other drugs metabolized by these isozymes (see below).

TABLE 15-3. **Effects of Diet and Drug Therapy on Serum Lipid Concentrations**

Therapy	Low-Density Lipoprotein (LDL) Cholesterol Concentration	High-Density Lipoprotein (HDL) Cholesterol Concentration	Total Triglyceride Concentration	Other Effects
Dietary modifications alone	↓ 10–15%	↑	↓ 10–20%	Reduction of weight and decrease in blood pressure.
Drug therapy				
HMG-CoA reductase inhibitors	↓ 20–50%	↑ 10%	↓ 10–40%	Increase in hepatic LDL receptors.
Bile acid–binding resins	↓ 10–20%	↑ 0–4%	↑ 0–5%	Increase in hepatic LDL receptors.
Fibric acid derivatives	↓ 10%*	↑ 10–20%	↓ 40–50%	Activation of lipoprotein lipase.
Other drugs				
Ezetimibe	↓ 18–22%	↑ 1–3%	↓ 8–12%	—
Niacin	↓ 10–20%	↑ 10–25%	↓ 20–80%	Decrease in lipolysis and lipoprotein(a) levels.

*Fenofibrate has a greater effect than gemfibrozil on the LDL cholesterol concentration.

TABLE 15–4. **Pharmacokinetic Properties of Drugs for Hyperlipidemia***

Drug	Oral Bioavailability	Elimination Half-Life (Hours)	Major Routes of Elimination	Other Properties
HMG-CoA reductase inhibitors				
Atorvastatin	12%	14	M and F	Does not cross the blood-brain barrier
Fluvastatin	25%	<1	M and F	Does not cross the blood-brain barrier
Lovastatin	5%	3.5	M and F	Is a prodrug; crosses the blood-brain barrier
Pravastatin	17%	1.8	M and F	Does not cross the blood-brain barrier
Rosuvastatin	20%	19	M and F	—
Simvastatin	<5%	3	M and F	Is a prodrug; crosses the blood-brain barrier
Bile acid–binding resins				
Cholestyramine	0%	NA	F	Is a high-molecular-weight polymer
Colestipol	0%	NA	F	Is a high-molecular-weight polymer
Fibric acid derivatives				
Fenofibrate	≈100%	23	M	Is a prodrug
Gemfibrozil	≈100%	2	M (98%)	Undergoes enterohepatic cycling
Other drugs				
Ezetimibe	Variable	22	M and F	Localizes in small intestine
Niacin	≈100%	0.5	M and R	—

*F = fecal; M = metabolism; NA = not applicable; and R = renal.
†The half-life of probucol is long (hours to days) and highly variable.

TABLE 15–5. **Adverse Effects, Contraindications, and Interactions of Drugs for Hyperlipidemia**

Drug	Common Adverse Effects	Common Drug Interactions
HMG-CoA reductase Inhibitors	Elevated serum levels of hepatic enzymes; hepatitis; and myalgia, rhabdomyolysis, and other myopathies.	Cause slight increase in serum levels of warfarin. Increase risk of myopathies when taken with erythromycin, gemfibrozil, or niacin*
Bile acid–binding resins	Constipation; fecal impaction; and rash.	Decrease absorption of digoxin, thyroxin, warfarin, and other drugs
Fibric acid derivatives	Allergic reactions; blood cell deficiencies; and myalgia, rhabdomyolysis, and other myopathies.	Increase risk of myopathy when taken with HMG-CoA reductase inhibitors or niacin
Other drugs		
Ezetimibe	Headache, myalgia	Absorption decreased by cholestyramine
Niacin	Gastric irritation; glucose intolerance; myalgia, rhabdomyolysis, and other myopathies; and vasodilation, flushing, and pruritus.	Increases risk of myopathy when taken with gemfibrozil or HMG-CoA reductase inhibitors*

*If niacin must be used in combination with an HMG-CoA reductase inhibitor, the safest combination is niacin plus fluvastatin and the combination that poses the greatest risk is niacin plus lovastatin.

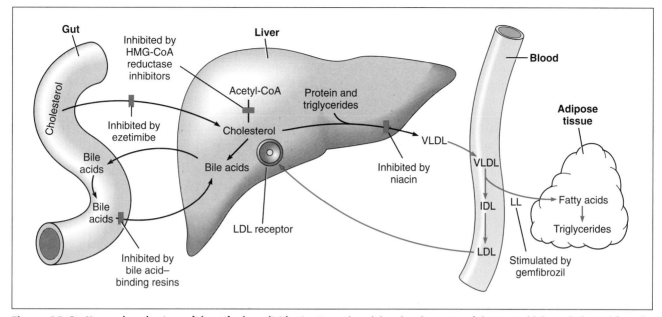

Figure 15–2. Sites and mechanisms of drugs for hyperlipidemia. Ezetimibe inhibits the absorption of dietary and biliary cholesterol from the intestines. The HMG-CoA reductase inhibitors block the rate-limiting step in cholesterol biosynthesis. The bile acid-binding resins inhibit the reabsorption of bile acids from the gut. Niacin inhibits the secretion of very low-density lipoproteins (VLDL) from the liver, while fibrates such as gemfibrozil stimulate lipoprotein lipase (LL) to increase the hydrolysis of VLDL triglycerides and the delivery of fatty acids to adipose and other tissues. IDL = intermediate-density lipoprotein.

MECHANISMS AND PHARMACOLOGIC EFFECTS. HMG-CoA reductase normally converts HMG-CoA to mevalonic acid and is the rate-limiting enzyme in cholesterol biosynthesis (Figs. 15–2 and 15–3). By competitively inhibiting HMG-CoA reductase, pravastatin and other drugs in this class reduce hepatic cholesterol biosynthesis. This increases the number of hepatic LDL receptors and enables more LDL to be delivered to the liver. As a result, a reduction occurs in the level of LDL-C in the serum and in the amount of cholesterol available for the formation of VLDL. In patients with hypercholesterolemia, these actions usually cause a decrease of 20% to 40% in serum LDL-C levels and an increase of 10% in serum HDL-C levels (see Table 15–3). The reductase inhibitors also reduce serum triglyceride levels.

Figure 15–3. Inhibition of cholesterol biosynthesis by HMG-CoA reductase inhibitors. HMG-CoA reductase catalyzes the conversion of 3-hydroxy-3-methylglutaryl-coenzyme A (HMG-CoA) to mevalonic acid, the rate-limiting enzyme in cholesterol biosynthesis. The reductase inhibitors contain a structure that is similar to the structure of HMG-CoA (the unshaded portions of pravastatin and HMG-CoA), and they compete with the substrate for the catalytic site of the enzyme.

ADVERSE EFFECTS AND INTERACTIONS. The HMG-CoA reductase inhibitors (statins) are well tolerated by most patients but may cause serious and life-threatening toxicity in a small percentage of persons. The most frequent adverse effects of statins consist of gastrointestinal problems, including abdominal cramps, constipation, diarrhea, and heartburn. Less frequently, statins elevate serum levels of hepatic enzymes and cause hepatitis (see Table 15–5). The most serious adverse effect of the statins is rhabdomyolysis, which is a potentially fatal form of statin-induced skeletal muscle toxicity (myopathy). Only about 0.2% of patients receiving statins develop myopathy, and only a few of these cases progress to rhabdomyolysis.

The precise mechanisms by which statins cause **myopathy** are still being elucidated. By inhibiting cholesterol synthesis, statins can alter muscle cell membrane composition and electrical properties (Rosenson, 2004). The earliest stage of statin-induced myopathy is **myalgia,** which consists of muscle ache or weakness without elevated creatine kinase (CK) levels. This stage is reversible on statin withdrawal and resolves in 2 to 3 weeks. Myalgia can be followed by **myositis** or muscle inflammation accompanied by muscle pain, leakage of muscle CK into the plasma, and elevated CK levels. Myositis can eventually lead to **rhabdomyolysis** in which muscle cells are destroyed, thereby releasing myoglobin into the circulation. Myoglobin can then accumulate in the kidneys and cause acute renal failure. CK levels in rhabdomyolysis are often greater than 10 times the upper limit of normal and persons with this affliction often report a dark urine resulting from **myoglobinuria.**

Patients taking a reductase inhibitor (statin) should be asked to report any sign of unusual, diffuse, or persistent muscle tenderness, pain, or weakness, especially if it is accompanied by malaise, fever, or dark urine. Factors that increase the risk of statin-induced myopathy include increasing age, female gender, renal or hepatic disease, hypothyroidism, and the use of drugs that inhibit statin metabolism. Use of the statin must be discontinued if myopathy is diagnosed or if levels of creatine phosphokinase are found to be significantly elevated. No specific treatment exists for rhabdomyolysis except drug withdrawal and fluid administration to maintain renal function.

Because fibric acid derivatives can also cause myopathies, the combination of these drugs and HMG-CoA reductase inhibitors should be avoided or used with great caution. Other drugs (e.g., erythromycin and itraconazole) can inhibit the metabolism of HMG-CoA reductase inhibitors and thereby increase the incidence of adverse effects such as myopathy.

The reductase inhibitors can interact with other drugs that are metabolized by cytochrome P450. For example, they increase warfarin levels slightly by inhibiting warfarin metabolism.

INDICATIONS. The reductase inhibitors (statins) are used to reduce blood cholesterol levels in persons with **hypercholesterolemia** to achieve the LDL-C goals recommended by the NCEP. The statins are capable of reducing serum cholesterol levels to a greater extent than any other type of drug that is currently available for this purpose. The NCEP guidelines recommend using a statin dose that can achieve a 30% to 40% reduction in LDL-C levels. The statins do not have equal potency with respect to reducing LDL-C levels. Rosuvastatin is the most potent statin currently available, followed by atorvastatin. Atorvastatin and rosuvastatin also have the greatest effect on triglyceride levels and can be useful in treating patients with **mixed hyperlipidemia.**

Clinical trials of reductase inhibitors have demonstrated that these drugs slow the progression of atherosclerosis, reduce the risk of CHD and other atherosclerotic vascular diseases, and reduce the cardiac mortality rate. A large prospective study of more than 4000 patients in Scandinavia showed that simvastatin reduced the cardiac disease-related mortality rate by 42% and the total mortality rate by 30% in men with a history of myocardial infarction. Some of these benefits may partly be caused by the ability of statins to improve vascular endothelial function and reduce inflammation. Clinical trials also indicate that statins may also protect against **osteoporosis** and certain forms of **cancer.**

Specific Drugs

Most of the reductase inhibitors are taken in the evening or at bedtime in order to inhibit nocturnal cholesterol biosynthesis. Lovastatin should be taken with the evening meal to facilitate its absorption, whereas the other drugs can be taken without regard to food. Atorvastatin and rosuvastatin have longer half-lives than the other drugs and can be taken at any time of day. Lovastatin and simvastatin cross the blood–brain barrier and can cause sleep disturbances in some patients, whereas the other drugs do not. Fluvastatin appears to be less likely to cause myopathy than other reductase inhibitors, especially when combined with niacin.

Bile Acid-Binding Resins

Drug Properties

Bile acid-binding resins are moderately effective drugs for hypercholesterolemia and have an excellent safety record. They are especially valuable for patients who cannot tolerate other drugs and for patients who are young and therefore may need to take drug therapy for a long time.

CHEMISTRY AND PHARMACOKINETICS. The bile acid-binding resins are large molecular-weight polymers containing a chloride ion that can be exchanged for bile acids in the gut. The resins are not absorbed from the gut and are excreted in the feces.

MECHANISMS AND PHARMACOLOGIC EFFECTS. After the resins bind to bile acids, the bile acid–resin complex is excreted. This action prevents the enterohepatic cycling of bile acids and obligates the liver to synthesize replacement bile acids from cholesterol. To obtain more cholesterol for this purpose, the liver increases the number of LDL receptors. Then the levels of LDL-C in the serum are reduced as more cholesterol is delivered to the liver. As shown in Table 15–3, the resins have relatively little effect on levels of HDL-C and triglycerides, which are usually increased slightly.

ADVERSE EFFECTS AND INTERACTIONS. The bile acid-binding resins have few adverse effects. They can cause constipation, fecal impaction, and other gastrointestinal side effects, some of which can be prevented by taking the drugs with a full glass of water. Occasionally, they cause irritation of the perianal area and a skin rash. In the gut, cholestyramine and colestipol can bind to digoxin, thyroxin, warfarin, and other drugs. For this reason, it is best to take these resins 2 hours before or after taking other medications. A newer resin, colesevelam, does not affect the oral bioavailability of digoxin, warfarin, or lovastatin, and, therefore, can be co-administered with most drugs, including HMG-CoA reductase inhibitors.

INDICATIONS. The resins are indicated for the treatment of **hypercholesterolemia** and are particularly useful in patients who cannot tolerate other drugs. Although the resins are less effective than the HMG-CoA reductase inhibitors, they do not cause hepatitis or myopathy, and they can be given in combination with other drugs to produce an additive effect on serum cholesterol levels. The resins have also been used to treat **diarrhea** and **pruritis** (itching) caused by excessive levels of bile acids.

Cholestyramine, Colestipol, and Colesevelam

Cholestyramine and colestipol are bile acid-binding resins that are available in powder (granular) form for mixing with water or juice just before administration. To obtain the maximal effect on serum cholesterol levels, these drugs must be taken before each meal and at bedtime. **Colesevelam** (WELCHOL) is a newer resin that is available as solid tablets that are usually taken twice daily with meals. It decreases LDL-C to a similar degree as the other resins and is more convenient and palatable.

Ezetimibe

Ezetimibe (ZETIA) is a unique drug that inhibits the absorption of dietary cholesterol. After oral administration, ezetimibe is absorbed from the intestines and then is mostly converted to pharmacologically active ezetimibe-glucuronide. This metabolite is distributed by the circulation to the small intestines where it localizes in the brush border and inhibits the absorption of both biliary and dietary cholesterol. Recent studies (Smart et al.) suggest that ezetimibe acts by disrupting a complex of two proteins, annexin 2 and caveolin 1, that mediate cholesterol transport in intestinal brush border cells. The half-lives of ezetimibe and ezetimibe-glucuronide are both 22 hours. The drugs are eliminated in the urine and feces.

Because of its unique mechanism of action, ezetimibe can be used alone or in combination with an HMG-CoA reductase inhibitor (statin) to treat hypercholesterolemia. A fixed-dose combination of ezetimibe and simvastatin (VYTORIN) is available for this purpose. When administered alone, ezetimibe lowers LDL-C 19% to 23%. An incremental reduction of LDL-C of about 22% was obtained when ezetimibe was added to statin therapy in one study. Hence, the co-administration of ezetimibe and a statin can achieve reductions in LDL-C similar to that obtained with the highest statin doses. This may permit the use of lower doses of statins to obtain desired LDL-C levels with correspondingly less risk of statin toxicity. This combination has been found to be effective in treating persons with homozygous familial hypercholesterolemia.

Ezetimibe has been well tolerated in clinical trials, although some persons complained of headache and myalgia.

OTHER DRUGS FOR HYPERLIPIDEMIA

Fibric acid derivatives and nicotinic acid (niacin) are the primary drugs used to treat hypertriglyceridemia and combined hypertriglyceridemia and hypercholesterolemia. These drugs are also used to increase HDL-C levels in persons with abnormally low levels of this lipoprotein. The effects and properties of these drugs are shown in Tables 15–3, 15–4, and 15–5.

Fibric Acid Derivatives

Drug Properties

Fibric acid derivatives are primarily used to treat hypertriglyceridemia or marked HDL deficiency.

CHEMISTRY AND PHARMACOKINETICS. The drugs are derivatives of a branched-chain carboxylic acid known as fibric acid or **fibrate**. The first drug in this class, clofibrate, is largely obsolete because of its high incidence of adverse effects. **Gemfibrozil** and **fenofibrate** are currently available in the United States.

MECHANISMS AND PHARMACOLOGIC EFFECTS. The fibrates reduce plasma levels of VLDL triglycerides and LDL-C, while raising levels of HDL-C. The fibrates are believed to produce these effects by binding to and activating a nuclear receptor that regulates gene transcription called the **peroxisome proliferator activated receptor-α** (PPARα). In the liver and elsewhere, PPARα increases the transcription of certain genes while inhibiting the transcription of other genes.

The effect of fibrates on plasma triglyceride levels can be partly attributed to PPARα–mediated expression of **lipoprotein lipase.** This enzyme is located in the vascular endothelium and catalyzes the hydrolysis and removal of triglycerides from VLDL, thereby lowering plasma triglyceride levels (see Fig. 15–2). PPARα activation also reduces expression of an inhibitor of lipoprotein lipase, **apolipoprotein C-III.** Other effects of PPARα activation include expression of enzymes that oxidize fatty acids. The effects of fibrates on HDL-C are primarily caused by PPARα-mediated expression of apoproteins A-I and A-II, which are important components of HDL. PPARα also increases expression of a cholesterol transport protein involved in reverse cholesterol transport (see *High-density Lipoproteins* above).

Fenofibrate reduces plasma LDL-C levels, in part, by increasing expression of hepatic LDL receptors via activation of PPARα. PPARα activation also results in changes in the triglyceride and cholesterol content of LDL that increase

LDL affinity for the LDL receptor. Together, these actions increase the uptake of LDL-C by the liver and reduce plasma LDL-C levels. Fenofibrate causes a greater reduction in LDL-C than does gemfibrozil.

ADVERSE EFFECTS AND INTERACTIONS. The fibrates can cause blood cell deficiencies and other hypersensitivity reactions. As with the HMG-CoA reductase inhibitors, the fibrates can also cause rhabdomyolysis and other myopathies (see Table 15–5). For this reason, the combination of reductase inhibitors and fibrates should be avoided or used with great caution. Fibrates can be given with cholestyramine and colestipol, but the doses must be separated by more than 2 hours, because these resins reduce fibrate absorption.

Gemfibrozil

Gemfibrozil is primarily indicated for the treatment of **hypertriglyceridemia.** It is also useful in patients with combined hypertriglyceridemia and hypercholesterolemia and can be administered to increase HDL-C in patients with an isolated **HDL deficiency.**

The Helsinki Heart Study, which involved 2000 men with hypercholesterolemia, found that gemfibrozil increased HDL-C levels and decreased LDL-C and triglyceride levels. It also reduced the CHD-related mortality rate, but the overall mortality rate was not affected because of an increase in deaths from other diseases, accidents, and violence.

Fenofibrate

Fenofibrate is indicated for the treatment of elevated triglyceride levels and mixed hyperlipidemia with elevated triglyceride and cholesterol levels.

Nicotinic acid (niacin)

Pharmacologic doses of nicotinic acid have profound effects on serum lipid levels. Although the drug is capable of causing a number of adverse effects, it nevertheless has a valuable role in the treatment of many patients with hyperlipidemia.

CHEMISTRY AND PHARMACOKINETICS. Nicotinic acid (niacin), is also known as vitamin B_3. The small amount of niacin that is ingested in food is converted in the body to enzyme cofactors required for oxidative reactions in intermediary metabolism. These cofactors are nicotinamide adenine dinucleotide (NAD) and its phosphate derivative (NADP). Niacin is well absorbed from the gut and is extensively metabolized before undergoing renal excretion.

MECHANISMS AND PHARMACOLOGIC EFFECTS. The quantity of niacin ingested in food does not have any measurable effect on serum lipid levels. The action of nicotinic acid on lipids is a pharmacologic effect that requires the administration of several grams of the compound each day. These large doses of nicotinic acid produce effects on plasma lipoproteins that are similar to those of fenofibrate. Nicotinic acid acts primarily by inhibiting the synthesis and secretion of hepatic VLDL, the major carrier of plasma triglycerides and the precursor to LDL (see Fig. 15–3). The effect on VLDL secretion is partly caused by inhibition of lipolysis in adipose tissue.

This action reduces the supply of circulating free fatty acids that the liver uses to synthesize triglycerides for incorporation into VLDL. The inhibition of lipolysis has been attributed to the binding of niacin to a G-protein coupled receptor in adipose tissue. Although nicotinic acid can decrease serum LDL-C levels, it significantly increases HDL-C levels (see Table 15–3).

ADVERSE EFFECTS AND INTERACTIONS. The large doses of nicotinic acid that are required to lower serum lipid levels sometimes produce marked vasodilation and flushing of the skin, accompanied by pruritus and a feeling of warmth and tingling. This effect can be significantly reduced by pretreatment with aspirin, and some tolerance to this effect develops with continued drug administration. These adverse effects are reduced with the use of sustained-release niacin preparations. Although nicotinic acid is effective and well tolerated by many patients, it has a number of more serious adverse effects that preclude its use by others. Nicotinic acid can elevate serum transaminase levels and cause hepatitis. It also produces gastric distress and may activate a peptic ulcer. Finally, nicotinic acid causes glucose intolerance in some patients and can aggravate diabetes mellitus. For these reasons, nicotinic acid use should usually be avoided in patients with hepatic disorders, peptic ulcers, or diabetes mellitus.

INDICATIONS. Nicotinic acid is an effective drug for the treatment of **mixed hyperlipidemia.** It favorably influences the serum levels of VLDL, LDL, and HDL, and it can be used in combination with bile acid-binding resins and other drugs to treat more severe cases of hyperlipidemia. Nicotinic acid can also be used in the treatment of patients with either **hypertriglyceridemia** or **hypercholesterolemia,** and it has been found to be effective in the treatment of patients who have lipoprotein(a) levels that put them at increased risk for heart disease.

DRUG COMBINATIONS

Drugs can be used in combination to treat high blood cholesterol in patients who do not respond to a single drug. The most useful combinations are those consisting of ezetimibe or a bile acid-binding resin in combination with a statin drug. Ezetimibe and simvastatin are available in a combination product (VYTORIN) which enables the use of a lower dose of the statin to achieve target LDL-C levels and reduce the risk of myopathy. Colesevelam (WELCHOL) is a newer resin that can be co-administered with statins.

Some drug combinations should be avoided or only used with great caution. The combination of gemfibrozil plus an HMG-CoA reductase inhibitor has a greater tendency to cause myopathy than does the use of either drug alone. For the same reason, lovastatin should not be used in combination with nicotinic acid, but other HMG-CoA reductase inhibitors appear to be safer with nicotinic acid.

SUMMARY OF IMPORTANT POINTS

■ Cholesterol and triglycerides are secreted by the liver in the form of very low-density lipoproteins (VLDL). After delivering triglycerides to adipose tissue, VLDL become low-density lipoproteins (LDL). The LDL deliver cholesterol to peripheral tissues, the liver, and atheromas. High-density lipoproteins (HDL) transport cholesterol from tissues and atheromas to the liver.

■ Hypercholesterolemia is a risk factor for atherosclerosis and coronary artery disease. Hypertriglyceridemia, which is associated with pancreatitis, is also believed to have a role in the development of heart disease in some patients.

■ Patients with high blood cholesterol levels should be managed with therapeutic lifestyle changes and drug therapy based on the guidelines of the National Cholesterol Education Program.

■ Ezetimibe inhibits the absorption of dietary and biliary cholesterol from the intestines, thereby causing a reduction in LDL-cholesterol levels.

■ Atorvastatin and other HMG-CoA reductase inhibitors block the rate-limiting enzyme in cholesterol biosynthesis and lead to a secondary increase in hepatic LDL receptors and cholesterol uptake, thereby causing a reduction in LDL-cholesterol levels.

■ Cholestyramine, colestipol, and colesevelam are bile acid-binding resins that prevent the enterohepatic cycling of bile acids and increase hepatic cholesterol conversion to replacement bile acids, thereby leading to a reduction in LDL-cholesterol levels.

■ Nicotinic acid (niacin) and the fibric acid derivatives (gemfibrozil and fenofibrate) reduce triglyceride levels and increase HDL-cholesterol levels. Nicotinic acid inhibits VLDL secretion. Fibrates increase VLDL clearance by increasing lipoprotein lipase activity via activation of the *perioxisome proliferator activated receptor-α*. Nicotinic acid and fenofibrate also reduce LDL-cholesterol levels.

Review Questions

For each numbered drug description, select the corresponding drug from the lettered choices.

1. Disrupts intestinal cholesterol transport protein complex

2. Inhibits enterohepatic cycling of bile acids

3. Inhibits the rate-limiting step in cholesterol biosynthesis

4. Activates peroxisome proliferator activated receptor-α

(A) simvastatin
(B) ezetimibe
(C) fenofibrate
(D) niacin
(E) colestipol

Choose the single best answer from the choices provided.

5. Concurrent administration of lovastatin and erythromycin is associated with an increased risk of which of the following conditions?
(A) hepatitis
(B) hyperglycemia
(C) peptic ulcer disease
(D) rhabdomyolysis
(E) gallstones

Answers and Explanations

1. The answer is B: ezetimibe. Ezetimibe inhibits the absorption of dietary and biliary cholesterol from the intestines. It appears to act by disrupting a cholesterol transport protein complex located in the brush border of the small intestines.

2. The answer is E: colestipol. Colestipol, cholestyramine, and colesevelam are bile acid-binding resins that prevent the reabsorption and enterohepatic cycling of bile acids secreted into the intestinal tract via the bile duct. This action leads to increased utilization of cholesterol to replace bile acids and thereby lowers plasma cholesterol levels.

3. The answer is A: simvastatin. The statin drugs inhibit HMG-CoA reductase, which is the rate-limiting enzyme in hepatic cholesterol synthesis and thereby increase the uptake of LDL-cholesterol by the liver, leading to a reduction in serum LDL-cholesterol levels.

4. The answer is C: fenofibrate. The fibrate drugs activate the peroxisome proliferator activated receptor-α, leading to expression of lipoprotein lipase and increased clearance of triglycerides from circulating very low-density lipoproteins.

5. The answer is D: rhabdomyolysis. Erythromycin inhibits the metabolism of lovastatin by cytochrome P450 3A4 and thereby elevates lovastatin plasma levels, leading to increased risk of adverse effects such as myositis and rhabdomyolysis.

SELECTED READINGS

Colhoun, H. M., D. J. Betteridger, and P. N. Durrington, et al. Primary prevention of cardiovascular disease with atorvastatin in type 2 diabetes in the Collaborative Atorvastatin Diabetes Study (CARDS): multicentre randomized placebo-controlled trial. Lancet 364:685–696, 2004.

Grundy, S. M., J. I. Cleeman, C. N. B. Merz, et al. Implications of recent clinical trials for the National Cholesterol Education Program adult treatment panel III guidelines. J Am Coll Cardiol 44:720–732, 2004.

Rosenson, R. S. Current overview of statin-induced myopathy. Am J Med 116:408–416, 2004.

Smart, E. J., R. A. De Rose, and S. A. Farber. Annexin 2-caveolin 1 complex is a target of ezetimibe and regulates intestinal cholesterol transport. Proc Natl Acad Sci USA 101:3450–3455, 2004.

CHAPTER 16

Anticoagulant, Antiplatelet, and Fibrinolytic Drugs

CLASSIFICATION OF ANTICOAGULANT, ANTIPLATELET, AND FIBRINOLYTIC DRUGS

Anticoagulant Drugs
Oral Anticoagulants
- Warfarin (COUMADIN)
- Dicumarol

Parenteral Anticoagulants
- Enoxaparin (LOVENOX)[a]
- Heparin
- Fondaparinux (ARIXTRA)
- Bivalirudin (ANGIOMAX)[b]

Antiplatelet Drugs
- Abciximab (REOPRO)

- Tirofiban (AGGRASTAT)
- Eptifibatide (INTEGRILIN)
- Aspirin
- Dipyridamole
- Clopidogrel (PLAVIX)[c]

Fibrinolytic Drugs
- Alteplase (ACTIVASE)[d]
- Streptokinase

[a]also dalteparin, danaparoid, tinzaparin
[b]also lepirudin
[c]also ticlopidine
[d]also reteplase (RETAVASE), tenecteplase (TNKASE)

BLOOD COAGULATION

Normal Hemostasis

When a small blood vessel is injured, hemorrhage is prevented by **vasospasm,** the formation of a **platelet plug** and a **fibrin clot** (Fig. 16–1). After the vessel is repaired, the clot is removed via the process of **fibrinolysis.**

Vasospasm reduces bleeding and blood flow and thereby facilitates platelet adhesion and coagulation. Exposure of the blood to extravascular collagen causes adherence of platelets to the injured vessel wall and initiates the sequential activation of numerous **coagulation factors,** or **blood clotting factors.** These factors and their synonyms are listed in Table 16–1, and the **coagulation pathways** are illustrated in Fig. 16–2. The **intrinsic pathway** may be activated by surface contact with a foreign body or extravascular tissue, whereas the **extrinsic pathway** is activated by a complex tissue factor. The pathways converge with the activation of **factor X,** which is the major rate-limiting step in the coagulation cascade. The activation of factor X leads to the formation of **thrombin,** and thrombin, in turn, catalyzes the conversion

of **fibrinogen** to **fibrin.** The fibrin meshwork traps erythrocytes and platelets to complete the formation of a hemostatic thrombus (clot).

Pathologic Thrombus Formation

The processes leading to **thrombosis** and **embolism** are complex and not completely understood.

Atherosclerosis and other abnormalities affecting the vascular endothelium can serve as a stimulus for platelet aggregation and blood coagulation in arteries. Venous pooling, sluggish blood flow, and inflammation of veins may permit inappropriate platelet adhesion and coagulation in vessels. Platelet aggregation appears to have a larger role in the formation of **arterial thrombi (white thrombi),** whereas coagulation predominates in the formation of **venous thrombi (red thrombi).** Platelet aggregation followed by coagulation, however, occurs both in arteries and in veins, and the processes differ only in the degree of contribution by platelets or coagulation to the thrombus.

An arterial or venous thrombus can become dislodged from the vessel wall and form an **embolus** that travels

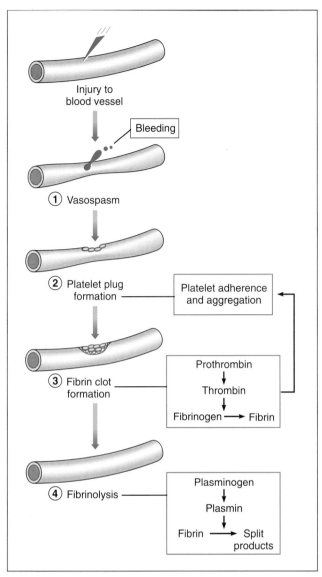

Figure 16–1. Normal hemostasis. (1) When a small blood vessel is injured, vasospasm reduces blood flow and facilitates platelet aggregation and coagulation. (2) The platelets, which adhere to extravascular collagen, are activated to release mediators that cause platelet aggregation and the formation of a platelet plug to arrest bleeding. (3) Exposure of the blood to tissue factors also activates coagulation and leads to the formation of a fibrin clot, which arrests bleeding until the vessel is repaired. (4) After the vessel is repaired, the clot is removed by the process of fibrinolysis.

FIGURE 16–2. Blood coagulation and sites of drug action. Blood coagulation involves the sequential activation of proteolytic clotting factors. The intrinsic pathway can be activated by surface contact with a foreign body, whereas the extrinsic pathway is activated by tissue factor. The pathways converge with the activation of factor X, which leads to the formation of thrombin and fibrin. Warfarin and other oral anticoagulants inhibit the synthesis of the vitamin K-dependent clotting factors. Heparin inactivates various clotting factors.

TABLE 16–1. **Coagulation Factors**

Factor*	Common Synonym	Dependent on Vitamin K[†]
I	Fibrinogen	No
II	Prothrombin	Yes
III	Tissue thromboplastin	No
IV	Calcium	No
V	Proaccelerin	No
VII	Proconvertin	Yes
VIII	Antihemophilic factor	No
IX	Plasma thromboplastin component	Yes
X	Stuart factor	Yes
XI	Plasma thromboplastin antecedent	No
XII	Hageman factor	No
XIII	Fibrin stabilizing factor	No

*Factor VI is no longer considered to be a coagulation factor.
[†]Proteins C and S, which are endogenous anticoagulants that inactivate factor Va and VIIIa and promote fibrinolysis, are also dependent on Vitamin K.

through the circulation and eventually occludes a smaller vessel in the lungs or brain, thereby causing pulmonary embolism or a cerebrovascular accident (stroke), respectively.

ANTICOAGULANT DRUGS

Oral Anticoagulants

Anticoagulants are drugs that retard coagulation and thereby prevent the occurrence or enlargement of a thrombus. Table 16–2 compares the properties of oral anticoagulants (e.g.,

warfarin) with those of parenteral anticoagulants (e.g., heparin).

Drug Properties

CHEMISTRY AND MECHANISMS. Coumarin compounds were originally discovered in spoiled clover hay and identified as substances that caused hemorrhage in cattle. Coumarin

A. Vitamin K and Warfarin

Phytonadione (vitamin K_1)

Warfarin sodium

B. Antithrombin-binding pentasaccharide of heparin

| Sulfated glucosamine | Glucuronic acid | Sulfated glucosamine | Sulfated iduronic acid | Sulfated glucosamine |

Figure 16–3. Structures of vitamin K and selected anticoagulants. (A) Warfarin is structurally similar to vitamin K (unshaded portions). If warfarin causes bleeding, phytonadione (vitamin K_1) can be given to accelerate the recovery of clotting factors. (B) Heparin is a naturally occurring mixture of sulfated mucopolysaccharides that binds to antithrombin III.

derivatives (e.g., warfarin and dicumarol) were subsequently developed as anticoagulants.

Warfarin and other coumarin derivatives are structurally related to vitamin K (Fig. 16–3A). These drugs work by inhibiting the synthesis of clotting factors II (prothrombin), VII, IX, and X, whose carboxylation is dependent on a reduced form of vitamin K. As shown in Fig. 16–4, warfarin blocks the reduction of oxidized vitamin K and thereby prevents the post-translational carboxylation of these four factors. Oral anticoagulants also inhibit the synthesis of proteins C and S, which are endogenous anticoagulants that inactivate factors V and VIII and promote fibrinolysis. It is possible that the inhibition of proteins C and S contributes to a transient procoagulant effect of the oral anticoagulants when they are first administered.

PHARMACOKINETIC AND PHARMACOLOGIC EFFECTS. Coumarin anticoagulants, which are absorbed from the gut, are extensively metabolized before being excreted in the urine. Unlike heparin and related anticoagulants, the coumarins cross the placenta and can cause fetal hemorrhage and malformations.

TABLE 16–2.	**Comparison of the Pharmacologic Properties of Warfarin and Heparin Anticoagulants**	
Property	**Warfarin Anticoagulants**	**Heparin Anticoagulants**
Active in vitro	No	Yes
Routes of administration	Oral	Parenteral
Onset of action	Delayed	Immediate
Mechanism of action	Inhibit synthesis of clotting factors	Inactive clotting factors
Safe to take during pregnancy	No	Yes
Antidote	Phytonadione (vitamin K_1)	Protamine sulfate

Figure 16–4. Mechanisms of action of warfarin and other oral anticoagulants. Oral anticoagulants block the reduction of oxidized vitamin K (vitamin K epoxide) and thereby prevent vitamin K-dependent carboxylation of clotting factors.

TABLE 16-3. **Adverse Effects, Contraindications, and Drug Interactions of Anticoagulant, Antiplatelet, and Fibrinolytic Drugs**

Drug	Common Adverse Effects	Common Drug Interactions
Oral anticoagulants		
Warfarin	Birth defects and bleeding	Serum levels altered by drugs that induce or inhibit cytochrome P450, by drugs that inhibit gut absorption, and by drugs that directly increase or decrease the anticoagulant effect (see text)
Parenteral anticoagulants		
Dalteparin	Bleeding and thrombocytopenia	Risk of bleeding increased by salicylates
Enoxaparin Heparin	Same as dalteparin	Same as dalteparin
	Bleeding, hyperkalemia, and thrombocytopenia	Same as dalteparin
Hirudin and related drugs	Bleeding	Same as dalteparin
Antiplatelet drugs		
Abciximab	Bleeding, bradycardia, hypotension, and thrombocytopenia	Unknown
Aspirin	Gastrointestinal irritation and bleeding, hypersensitivity reactions, and tinnitus	Increases hypoglycemic effect of sulfonylureas. Increases risk of gastrointestinal bleeding and ulceration associated with methotrexate, valproate, and other drugs. Inhibits uricosuric effect of probenecid
Dipyridamole	Gastrointestinal distress, headache, mild and transient dizziness, and rash	Decreases metabolism of adenosine. Increases risk of bradycardia associated with β-adrenergic receptor antagonists
Clopidogrel	Bleeding, diarrhea, gastrointestinal pain, increased cholesterol and triglyceride levels, nausea, and neutropenia	Increases levels of drugs metabolized by liver microsomal enzymes
Fibrinolytic drugs	Bleeding, hypersensitivity reactions, and reperfusion arrhythmias	Increases risk of bleeding associated with anticoagulant and antiplatelet drugs

The vitamin K antagonists have a delayed onset of action, owing to the time required to deplete the pool of circulating clotting factors after synthesis of new factors is inhibited. The half-life of circulating factors II, VII, IX, and X ranges from 6 hours (factor VII) to 50 hours (factor II). Therefore, the maximal effect of oral anticoagulants is not observed until 3 to 5 days after starting therapy with these drugs. Patients with acute thromboembolism are usually treated with a low molecular weight (LMW) heparin and warfarin, and the LMW heparin is then withdrawn after warfarin becomes effective. A period of several days is also required for coagulation factor levels to return to normal after coumarin anticoagulants are discontinued. The recovery of clotting factors can be accelerated by administration of phytonadione (vitamin K₁), as described later.

ADVERSE EFFECTS AND INTERACTIONS. The most common adverse effect of coumarin anticoagulants is bleeding (Table 16–3), which can range in severity from mild nosebleed to life-threatening hemorrhage. Patients should be instructed to report any signs of bleeding, including hematuria and bleeding into the skin (ecchymoses).

The coumarin anticoagulants are contraindicated in pregnancy because of their potential to cause fetal hemorrhage and various structural malformations that are collectively referred to as the fetal warfarin syndrome. These malformations are caused partly by antagonism of vitamin K-dependent maturation of bone proteins during a process in which certain proteins undergo carboxylation in the same manner as the nascent clotting factors. Warfarin and other oral anticoagulants block the process and can cause bone deformities and various birth defects that are listed in Table 4–6.

Most drug interactions with warfarin and other coumarin anticoagulants are caused by induction or inhibition of cytochrome P450 enzymes, but a few are caused by the antagonism or potentiation of the anticoagulant effect. The most serious interactions are with drugs that increase the anticoagulant effect and place the patient at risk for hemorrhage. Because the number of drugs that interact with warfarin is large, patients who are taking this drug should be instructed to consult their physician before starting or discontinuing any other medication.

Treatment with high doses of salicylates or with some third-generation cephalosporins has a direct hypoprothrombinemic effect and thereby increases the anticoagulant effect of warfarin and related drugs. In contrast, treatment with rifampin or barbiturates induces cytochrome P450 enzymes and thereby decreases the anticoagulant effect of warfarin. Cholestyramine inhibits the absorption of warfarin from the gut. Amiodarone, cimetidine, erythromycin, fluconazole, gemfibrozil, isoniazid, metronidazole, sulfinpyrazone, and other drugs inhibit the metabolism of warfarin and increase the risk of bleeding. The prothrombin time should be monitored when adding or deleting drugs with persons taking coumarin anticoagulants.

Phytonadione directly antagonizes the effect of coumarin anticoagulants on clotting factor synthesis and is used to treat hemorrhage caused by anticoagulant activity.

INDICATIONS. Warfarin and related anticoagulants are primarily used in the long-term treatment of patients who have a thromboembolic disorder such as **deep vein thrombosis** or **atrial fibrillation** and patients who have an **artificial heart valve** (Table 16–4). They are also used in conjunction with a heparin-type anticoagulant for the treatment of **myocardial infarction.** The goal of anticoagulant use is to inhibit embolization and thereby prevent the serious and potentially fatal sequelae of thrombosis. Anticoagulants can keep an established thrombus from extending, but they cannot dissolve one.

The dosage of oral anticoagulants to be given is based on the patient's **prothrombin time** (PT). This measurement is determined by drawing a blood sample, adding a tissue thromboplastin preparation to initiate coagulation in it, and comparing the in vitro clotting time in the sample with that in a standardized control preparation. As a general rule, the dosage of warfarin to be given should prolong the PT of the patient so that it is 1.3 to 1.5 times the PT of the control.

When the international reference thromboplastin preparation is used as the standardized control preparation, the ratio is expressed as the **international normalized ratio** (INR) and is calculated as follows:

$$INR = (PT_{observed} / PT_{control})^{ISI}$$

where the $PT_{observed}$ and $PT_{control}$ are the prothrombin times of the patient and control, respectively, and the ISI is the international sensitivity index of the thromboplastin reagent being used. For most indications, an INR of 2 to 3 is recommended. For patients with mechanical prosthetic heart valves and for those with recurrent systemic embolization, an INR of 3 to 4.5 is recommended.

The patient's PT should be monitored daily during the initiation of warfarin therapy and whenever another drug is added to or withdrawn from the treatment regimen. Concurrent heparin therapy can cause an increase of 10% to 20% in the patient's PT, so the target PT and INR levels should be increased by the same amount. Once the patient's PT has stabilized, it should be monitored every 4 to 6 weeks.

TREATMENT OF BLEEDING. If bleeding occurs, the coumarin anticoagulant should be withheld until the bleeding can be evaluated and the patient's PT can be determined. The treatment of bleeding can include a reduction in drug dosage and the administration of phytonadione (vitamin K_1). If bleeding is serious or if the INR is markedly elevated (>20), fresh frozen plasma or factor IX concentrate can be warmed and administered to rapidly replace clotting factors.

Specific Drugs

Warfarin is the most widely used orally administered anticoagulant. It is completely absorbed after oral administration. About 99% of the drug is bound to plasma proteins, and it is almost completely metabolized by cytochrome P450 enzymes. Warfarin is primarily metabolized by CYP 2C9, with smaller contributions from CYP1A2, 2C19, and 3A4. Drug interactions caused by induction or inhibition of these enzymes are described above. Other oral anticoagulants either have less favorable pharmacologic and pharmacokinetic properties or are more toxic and should be used only in cases in which the patient is intolerant of warfarin.

Dicumarol is a coumarin derivative that is incompletely absorbed from the gut and can cause considerable gastrointestinal distress. For these reasons, it is rarely used.

TABLE 16–4. **Clinical Uses of Antithrombotic Agents**

Clinical Use	Primary Drugs
Venous thromboembolism	
Acute	LMW heparin
Surgical prophylaxis	LMW heparin
Long-term prophylaxis	Warfarin or LMW heparin
Pulmonary embolism	Heparin, fibrinolytic drug
Acute coronary syndromes	
Unstable angina and non-STSE ACS*	Aspirin ± clopidogrel; eptifibatide or tirofiban; LMW heparin
STSE-MI†	Fibrinolytic drug and aspirin ± heparin
Percutaneous coronary interventions‡	Aspirin ± clopidogrel; abciximab or eptifibatide (alternative: bivalirudin)
Stroke, thrombotic	
Acute	Fibrinolytic drug or aspirin
Prophylaxis, including transient ischemic attacks (TIA)	Aspirin and dipyridamole combined, or clopidogrel
Atrial fibrillation	Heparin followed by warfarin
Artificial heart valve	Warfarin, aspirin

*Non-ST segment elevation acute coronary syndrome.
†ST segment elevation myocardial infarction.
‡Coronary angioplasty and stent placement.
LMW = low molecular weight.

Parenteral Anticoagulants

The parenteral anticoagulants include heparin, hirudin, and related compounds.

Heparin and Related Drugs

The heparin family of anticoagulants includes unfractionated heparin, low molecular weight heparins, a heparinoid drug, and fondaparinux. In its natural form, **heparin** contains fractions with high molecular weights ranging from 5000 to 30,000 and fractions with LMW ranging from 2000 to 9000. LMW fractions have been developed for specific clinical uses, including **enoxaparin, dalteparin,** and **tinzaparin.** Danaparoid, a so-called heparinoid anticoagulant, is a sulfated polysaccharide that is structurally distinct from heparin. Fondaparinux is a synthetic pentasaccharide whose mechanism and effects are similar to those of other heparin-like drugs.

CHEMISTRY AND MECHANISMS. Heparin is a naturally occurring mixture of sulfated mucopolysaccharides found in mast cells, basophils, and the vascular endothelium. For pharmaceutical use, it is obtained from porcine intestine or bovine lung.

As shown in Fig. 16–2, heparin inactivates clotting factors. Heparin accomplishes this by potentiating the activity of an endogenous anticoagulant called **antithrombin III** (AT-III), which is the most powerful endogenous inhibitor of thrombin (active factor II) and active factor X (Stuart factor). The structure of the heparin pentasaccharide that binds to and activates AT is shown in Fig. 16–3B and the activation of AT-III is depicted in Fig. 16–5.

In contrast to unfractionated heparin, LMW heparins (LMWH), such as enoxaparin and dalteparin, primarily inactivate active factor X because the LMWH–ATIII complex has less affinity for thrombin than does the heparin–AT-III complex. Fondaparinux is an even more selective active factor X inhibitor (Fig. 16–5).

PHARMACOKINETIC AND PHARMACOLOGIC EFFECTS. Heparin and related anticoagulants are not absorbed from the gut and must be given parenterally. Heparin is usually administered by continuous intravenous infusion. It is removed from the circulation by the reticuloendothelial system, is eliminated from the body by renal and hepatic mechanisms, and has a half-life of about 90 minutes. The dosage of heparin is generally determined by monitoring the **activated partial thromboplastin time** (aPTT). The dosage is considered adequate when the aPTT is 1.5 to 2 times normal.

Enoxaparin, dalteparin, tinzaparin, and danaparoid are administered subcutaneously, and their maximal effect occurs from 3 to 5 hours after injection. When they are used, the aPTT usually does not need to be monitored because the anticoagulant activity of LMW heparins and danaparoid is more predictable than is the activity of unfractionated heparin.

ADVERSE EFFECTS AND INTERACTIONS. Adverse effects and drug interactions are listed in Table 16–3. The most common serious adverse effect of fractionated and unfractionated heparin is bleeding caused by excessive anticoagulation.

Heparin can also cause two types of **heparin-induced thrombocytopenia** (HIT). Type I HIT, which occurs in about 25% of patients treated with heparin, is caused by a direct interaction between heparin and platelets, leading to platelet aggregation. Type I HIT is usually mild and is reversible within 4 days despite continued heparin treatment. Type II HIT is a much less common but more serious condition caused by immunoglobulin-mediated platelet inactivation, and has a high risk of thrombotic complications and mortality. Heparin must be discontinued if type II HIT occurs.

Heparin occasionally causes **hyperkalemia** because of the suppression of aldosterone secretion.

INDICATIONS. Heparin is indicated for the treatment of **acute thromboembolic disorders,** including peripheral and pulmonary embolism, venous thrombosis, and coagulopathies such as disseminated intravascular coagulation. It is used prophylactically to prevent clotting in **arterial and heart surgery,** during **blood transfusions,** and in **renal dialysis** and **blood sample collection.** Heparin is also used to prevent embolization of thrombi that might cause a cerebrovascular event in patients with **acute atrial fibrillation.** Low doses of heparin can be administered subcutaneously to prevent **deep vein thrombosis** and **pulmonary embolism** in high-risk patients.

Low molecular weight heparins (e.g., enoxaparin and dalteparin) are used to prevent **venous thromboembolism** associated with abdominal surgery and knee or hip replacement surgery. For this purpose, the drugs are administered once before surgery and for 5 to 10 days after surgery. Enoxaparin and dalteparin are also approved to prevent ischemic complications of **unstable angina** or non-ST segment elevation (non–Q-wave) myocardial infarction. Enoxaparin is approved for the treatment of deep vein thrombosis and to prevent thromboembolism caused by severely restricted mobility during acute illness.

Fondaparinux is administered subcutaneously for the prophylaxis of deep vein thrombosis in patients having hip fracture or hip replacement surgery, or knee replacement surgery.

TREATMENT OF BLEEDING. The treatment of bleeding caused by unfractionated or LMW heparins consists of administering protamine sulfate, which is a positively charged basic protein that physically combines with negatively charged heparin and thereby inactivates it. Protamine is administered intravenously for this purpose, and the dosage is based on the estimated amount of residual heparin in the body. Measurement of the aPTT 2 to 4 hours after protamine administration is used to guide the need for further protamine treatment. Severe bleeding may require the administration of fresh frozen plasma.

Hirudin Analogues

Hirudin is a mixture of homologous polypeptides produced by the salivary gland of *Hirudo medicinalis,* the medicinal leech. Hirudin and its analogues are direct thrombin inhibitors that do not require antithrombin III as a cofactor and have a more predictable anticoagulant effect than does heparin. **Lepirudin** is a recombinant hirudin obtained from

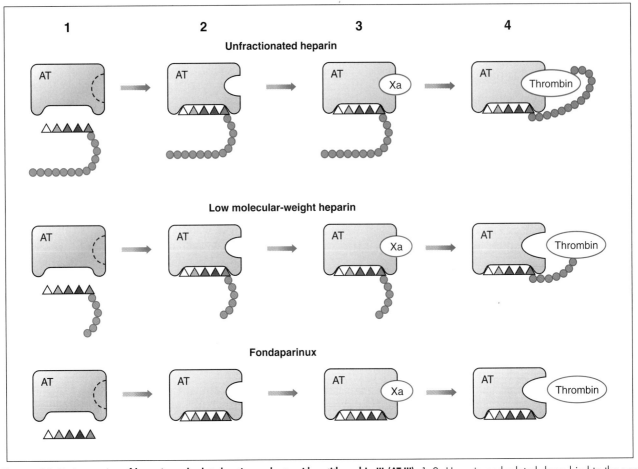

Figure 16–5. Interaction of heparin and related anticoagulants with antithrombin-III (AT-III). 1–2. Heparin and related drugs bind to the pentasaccharide-binding site on AT-III. 3. Anticoagulant–AT-III complexes inactivate factor Xa (active Stuart factor). 4. Unfractionated heparin–AT-III also inactivates thrombin, whereas low molecular-weight heparin–AT-III and fondaparinux–AT-III produce little or no inactivation of thrombin, respectively.

yeast cells, whereas **bivalirudin** is a synthetic derivative of hirudin. The hirudin compounds do not cause thrombocytopenia and lepirudin is indicated for management of thromboembolic disorders in persons who have experienced **heparin-induced thrombocytopenia.** Both lepirudin and bivalirudin have been used to prevent thrombosis in patients with **unstable angina** and **acute myocardial infarction,** including those having coronary angioplasty and stent insertion. Several clinical trials have established the efficacy and safety of these drugs in these settings.

The hirudin drugs are administered intravenously and their subcutaneous use is being studied. The most serious adverse effect of these drugs is bleeding. Orally administered direct thrombin inhibitors are currently being developed.

ANTIPLATELET DRUGS

The mechanisms of platelet aggregation and the sites of antiplatelet drug action are depicted in Fig. 16–6.

Platelets adhere to the damaged vascular endothelium via linkage of glycoprotein Ia receptors with exposed collagen and via linkage of Ib receptors with von Willebrand's factor, a circulating factor that is similar to clotting factor VIII. The

adherence of platelets to vascular endothelium activates the platelets and leads to the synthesis and release (degranulation) of various mediators of platelet aggregation, including thromboxane A_2 (TXA$_2$), adenosine diphosphate (ADP), and 5-hydroxytryptamine (5-HT, or serotonin). These mediators increase the expression of glycoprotein IIb/IIIa receptors that bind to fibrinogen and thereby cause platelet aggregation. Aspirin and ticlopidine act by inhibiting the synthesis or activity of specific mediators of platelet aggregation, whereas abciximab acts by binding to glycoprotein IIb/IIIa receptors.

Aspirin

Aspirin is a nonsteroidal anti-inflammatory drug (NSAID) that has analgesic, antipyretic, and anti-inflammatory effects. It also inhibits platelet aggregation and is used to prevent and treat arterial thromboembolic disorders.

MECHANISMS AND PHARMACOLOGIC EFFECTS. Aspirin and most other NSAID inhibit the synthesis of prostaglandins from arachidonic acid, as described in greater detail in Chapter 30. The most important prostaglandins affecting platelet aggregation are prostacyclin (also called prostaglandin I_2, or PGI$_2$) and TXA$_2$. Prostacyclin is synthe-

Figure 16-6. Platelet aggregation and sites of drug action. Platelets adhere to damaged endothelium via linkage of glycoprotein (GP) Ia receptors with exposed collagen and via linkage of GP Ib receptors with von Willebrand's factor (vWF). This activates the platelets and leads to the synthesis and release (degranulation) of various mediators of platelet aggregation, including thromboxane A2 (TXA$_2$), adenosine diphosphate (ADP), and 5-hydroxytryptamine (5-HT, or serotonin). These mediators increase the expression of GP receptors and promote platelet aggregation via the binding of fibrinogen to GP IIb/IIIa receptors.

sized by vascular endothelial cells and inhibits platelet aggregation, whereas TXA$_2$ is synthesized by platelets and promotes platelet aggregation. Under normal conditions, prostacyclin serves to prevent platelet aggregation and thrombosis, whereas TXA$_2$ becomes predominant during thrombus formation.

Low doses of aspirin have been found to selectively inhibit the synthesis of TXA$_2$ without having as much effect on prostacyclin, whereas higher doses inhibit the synthesis of both prostaglandins. Hence, the dosage of aspirin used to inhibit platelet aggregation is sometimes lower than that used to produce other pharmacologic effects. Unlike other NSAID, aspirin irreversibly inhibits cyclooxygenase, the enzyme that catalyzes an early step in TXA$_2$ synthesis. For this reason, aspirin inhibits platelet aggregation for the life of the platelet and effectively reduces platelet aggregation when administered once a day or every other day.

INDICATIONS. Aspirin is primarily used to prevent arterial thrombosis in patients with ischemic heart disease and stroke, but it has many other indications as well. In patients with unstable angina, it is used to prevent myocardial infarction. In patients with recent myocardial infarction, it is used to prevent enlargement of a coronary thrombus and potentially reduce the severity of cardiac damage. In patients with transient ischemic attacks (TIA), it can be used to prevent an initial or subsequent stroke. In patients who have artificial heart valves or are having percutaneous transluminal coronary angioplasty, it is used to prevent thrombosis. Aspirin is also used to treat persons with peripheral arterial occlusive disease and chronic limb ischemia.

ADVERSE EFFECTS AND INTERACTIONS. Aspirin can cause bleeding, especially in the gastrointestinal tract, where it inhibits the synthesis of prostaglandins that promote secretion of bicarbonate and mucus. These substances protect the gastric mucosa from the potentially damaging effects of stomach acid and pepsin. High doses of aspirin and other salicylates have a direct hypoprothrombinemic effect that can increase

the anticoagulant effect and thereby increase the likelihood of bleeding. Other adverse effects of aspirin are discussed in Chapter 30, and interactions are listed in Table 16-3.

Dipyridamole

Dipyridamole is a coronary vasodilator and a relatively weak antiplatelet drug.

As a vasodilator, dipyridamole is used during **myocardial perfusion imaging (thallium imaging)** to dilate and evaluate the arteries of patients with coronary artery disease.

As an antiplatelet drug, dipyridamole acts primarily by inhibiting platelet adhesion to the vessel wall. It can also inhibit platelet aggregation by increasing the formation of cyclic adenosine monophosphate (cAMP) and lowering the level of platelet calcium. Dipyridamole is used in combination with aspirin to prevent **ischemic (thrombotic) stroke** in persons who have previously had an atherothrombotic stroke and in persons experiencing TIA. Some authorities believe the combination of aspirin and dipyridamole is superior to aspirin alone, and to clopidogrel, for stroke prevention. A combination product containing aspirin and extended release dipyridamole is marketed as AGGRENOX.

Clopidogrel and Ticlopidine

Clopidogrel and ticlopidine are oral antiplatelet drugs unrelated to aspirin and dipyridamole. These drugs inhibit ADP-induced expression of platelet glycoprotein receptors and thereby reduce fibrinogen binding and platelet aggregation (Fig. 16-6). As with aspirin, clopidogrel and ticlopidine prolong bleeding time and irreversibly inhibit platelet function for the life of the platelet.

Clopidogrel and ticlopidine are well absorbed following oral administration. Clopidogrel is a prodrug that is rapidly metabolized to an active antiplatelet compound whose half-life is about 8 hours. The active metabolite is mostly excreted in the urine (50%) and feces (45%).

Because it can cause mild to severe neutropenia, patients who are treated with ticlopidine must have a complete blood count (CBC) with white cell differential every 2 weeks from the second week to the third month of treatment. After 3 months, a CBC is required only when patients exhibit signs or symptoms of an infection. Clopidogrel causes significantly less neutropenia than does ticlopidine and white blood cell counts are not required in persons taking clopidogrel. For this reason, clopidogrel has replaced ticlopidine for most purposes.

In patients who are intolerant of or unresponsive to aspirin, clopidogrel is used to prevent **thrombotic stroke,** and it is often used alone or with aspirin to treat acute coronary syndromes and in persons having percutaneous coronary interventions. Clopidogrel and ticlopidine have also been used in patients with intermittent claudication of blood vessels, chronic arterial occlusion, atrioventricular shunts or fistulas, open heart surgery, and sickle cell anemia.

Glycoprotein IIb/IIIa Antagonists

The final common pathway in platelet aggregation is the cross-linking of platelets by fibrinogen, which binds to an activated glycoprotein IIb/IIIa (GP IIb/IIIa) complex on the platelet surface (Fig. 16–6). The GP IIb/IIIa complex is a type of **integrin**. Integrins are cell surface transmembrane glycoproteins that function as adhesion receptors to structurally link the cell surface to the cytoskeleton.

Abciximab

Abciximab was the first platelet integrin GP IIb/IIIa inhibitor approved by the US Food and Drug Administration. It consists of the Fab fragment of a chimeric human-murine monoclonal antibody. The drug prevents platelet aggregation by binding to platelet glycoprotein IIb/IIIa (GP IIb/IIIa) receptors to prevent fibrinogen binding and cross-linking of platelets.

Abciximab is used to prevent platelet aggregation and thrombosis in patients having **percutaneous coronary interventions (PCI),** including coronary angioplasty and stent placement. In this setting, it is administered in combination with aspirin and heparin or LMW heparin. Abciximab has been shown to significantly prevent vessel restenosis, reinfarction, and death. It has also been used as an adjunct to thrombolysis with alteplase and similar drugs (see below).

The most common adverse effect of abciximab is bleeding. Other adverse reactions include thrombocytopenia, hypotension, and bradycardia.

Tirofiban and Eptifibatide

Tirofiban (AGGRASTAT) and eptifibatide (INTEGRILIN) also prevent platelet aggregation by preventing fibrinogen cross-linking of platelets. Unlike abciximab, tirofiban and eptifibatide are competitive, reversible inhibitors of fibrinogen binding to GP IIb/IIIa receptors. Eptifibatide is a cyclic heptapeptide from rattlesnake venom, whereas tirofiban is a tyrosine derivative. Both of these agents have short half-lives and are given as an intravenous loading dose followed by a maintenance infusion.

Tirofiban and eptifibatide are primarily used in persons with **acute coronary syndromes** (unstable angina and myocardial infarction). Eptifibatide is used in two ways: (1)

to prevent coronary thrombosis in persons with unstable angina or non-ST segment elevation (non–Q-wave) acute coronary syndrome, and (2) to prevent thrombosis in persons having coronary angioplasty or stent placement.

Bleeding is the major adverse effect of tirofiban and eptifibatide. The incidence of intracranial bleeding and gastrointestinal or genitourinary bleeding caused by tirofiban in one study was 0.1% and 0.2%, respectively.

FIBRINOLYTIC DRUGS

The fibrinolytic drugs, or **thrombolytic drugs,** include **alteplase** (ACTIVASE), **reteplase** (RETAVASE), **and tenecteplase** (TNKASE), which are recombinant forms of human tissue plasminogen activator (t-PA); **urokinase,** an enzyme obtained from human urine; **streptokinase,** a protein obtained from streptococci; and **anistreplase,** a complex of streptokinase and plasminogen. Unlike the anticoagulant and antiplatelet drugs, these drugs are administered intravenously to degrade an existing thrombus in patients having **myocardial infarction, thrombotic stroke,** or **pulmonary embolism.** Their use in patients with acute ischemic (thrombotic) stroke reduces the incidence of the neurologic sequelae of stroke.

CHEMISTRY AND PHARMACOLOGIC EFFECTS. The fibrinolytic drugs are enzymes that convert plasminogen to plasmin. Plasmin degrades fibrin and fibrinogen and thereby causes clot dissolution (Fig. 16–7). Streptokinase must first combine with plasminogen to form an activator complex that converts inactive plasminogen to plasmin. In anistreplase, streptokinase and plasminogen are already formed into a complex (the anisoylated plasminogen streptokinase activator complex [APSAC]).

ADVERSE EFFECTS AND INTERACTIONS. Table 16–3 lists adverse effects and drug interactions. The most common adverse effect is hemorrhage. Fibrinolytic drugs create a general lytic state that can lyse both normal and pathologic thrombi. Because t-PA selectively activates plasminogen that is bound to fibrin, the recombinant forms of t-PA can cause less bleeding than does streptokinase. Arrhythmias (e.g., bradycardia and tachycardia), which have been reported in patients treated with fibrinolytic drugs, are believed to be caused by free radicals that are generated during the reperfusion of the coronary artery after fibrinolysis. The administration of streptokinase can cause various types of hypersensitivity reactions, including fatal anaphylactic shock. For this reason, it should not be used repeatedly in the same patient.

TREATMENT OF BLEEDING. By competitively blocking plasminogen activation (see Fig. 16–7), aminocaproic acid inhibits fibrinolysis. This drug is used to stop the bleeding caused by fibrinolytic drugs. It is also used to prevent bleeding in patients who have hemophilia, patients who are recovering from gastrointestinal or prostate surgery, or patients who have cancer and are undergoing radiation therapy or chemotherapy. Aminocaproic acid can be administered orally or intravenously and is excreted by the kidneys. Its adverse effects include thrombosis, hypotension, and arrhythmias.

Figure 16–7. Fibrinolysis and sites of drug action. Alteplase, reteplase, and tenecteplase catalyze the conversion of plasminogen to plasmin. Streptokinase combines with plasminogen to form an active catalyst (activator complex) that converts inactive plasminogen to plasmin. In anistreplase, streptokinase and plasminogen are already formed into a complex. Plasmin is a protease that breaks down fibrinogen and fibrin to degradation (split) products. Aminocaproic acid inhibits the conversion of plasminogen to plasmin.

SUMMARY OF IMPORTANT POINTS

■ When a small blood vessel is injured, hemorrhage is prevented by the processes involved in normal hemostasis: vasospasm, platelet plug formation, and fibrin clot formation. After the vessel is repaired, the clot is removed via the process of fibrinolysis.

■ Orally administered coumarin anticoagulants (e.g., warfarin) inhibit vitamin K-dependent synthesis of clotting factors II, VII, IX, and X.

■ Parenteral anticoagulants, including heparin and hirudin derivatives, inactivate clotting factors. Unfractionated heparin primarily inactivates thrombin by activating antithrombin III, whereas low molecular-weight heparins and fondaparinux primarily inactivate factor Xa. These drugs are used to prevent and treat venous thromboembolism.

■ Bivalirudin is a direct thrombin inhibitor used in persons having coronary angioplasty, whereas lepirudin is indicated for treating thromboembolic disease in persons with heparin-induced thrombocytopenia.

■ Oral antiplatelet drugs act by interfering with the synthesis or activity of mediators of platelet aggregation. Aspirin inhibits thromboxane A_2 synthesis, and clopidogrel inhibits adenosine diphosphate activity. Abciximab, tirofiban, and eptifibatide are parenteral antiplatelet drugs that prevent the binding of fibrinogen to glycoprotein IIb/IIIa receptors and are primarily used in persons with acute coronary syndromes.

■ Fibrinolytic drugs (e.g., alteplase, reteplase, and tenecteplase) convert plasminogen to plasmin and thereby stimulate fibrin degradation. These drugs are used to lyse clots in patients having myocardial infarction, thrombotic stroke, or pulmonary embolism.

■ Any of the anticoagulant, antiplatelet, or fibrinolytic drugs can cause bleeding. Phytonadione (vitamin K_1) is used to counteract bleeding caused by oral anticoagulants. Protamine sulfate is used to neutralize heparins, and aminocaproic acid is used to inhibit fibrinolysis.

Review Questions

For each numbered drug description, select the corresponding drug from the lettered choices.

1. A selective inhibitor of active factor X

2. Preferentially inactivates thrombin (active factor II)

3. Prevents post-translational modification of prothrombin

4. Contains high- and low-molecular weight fractions
   (A) bivalirudin
   (B) heparin
   (C) eptifibatide
   (D) warfarin
   (E) fondaparinux

5. Which of the following drugs is a competitive antagonist of fibrinogen at GP IIb/IIIa platelet receptors?
   (A) clopidogrel
   (B) tirofiban
   (C) abciximab
   (D) aspirin
   (E) fondaparinux

Answers and Explanations

1. The answer is E: fondaparinux. Fondaparinux is a synthetic pentapeptide that selectively binds to active factor X (Stuart factor) and has much less affinity for thrombin (active factor II).

2. The answer is A: bivalirudin. Bivalirudin and other hirudin drugs act as direct thrombin inhibitors. Unlike heparin, they bind directly to thrombin and do not work by activating antithrombin III.

3. The answer is D: warfarin. Warfarin and other coumarin derivatives act by preventing vitamin K-mediated, post-translational carboxylation of glutamate residues of prothrombin (factor II) and factors VII, IX, and X. The anticoagulant effect of these drugs has a delayed onset of action caused by the long half-lives of circulating coagulation factors.

4. The answer is B: heparin. Unfractionated heparin acts primarily by binding to and activating an endogenous anticoagulant called antithrombin III (AT-III). AT-III is a serine protease that inactivates several active coagulation factors, including active factor II (thrombin) and active factor X (Stuart factor). Low molecular weight heparins more selectively inactivate active factor X.

5. The answer is B: tirofiban. Tirofiban and eptifibatide are competitive antagonists of fibrinogen at GPIIb/IIIa receptors. Abciximab is a noncompetitive monoclonal antibody that irreversibly binds to these receptors and, therefore, has a longer duration of action than tirofiban and eptifibatide.

SELECTED READINGS

Connors, J. J. Pharmacologic agents in stroke prevention, acute stroke therapy, and interventional procedures. J Vasc Interv Radiol 15(1 Pt2): S87–S101, 2004.

Greinacher, A. Lepirudin: a bivalent direct thrombin inhibitor for anticoagulation therapy. Expert Rev Cardiovasc Ther 2:339–357, 2004.

Kearon, C. Long-term management of patients after venous thromboembolism. Circulation 110 (Suppl):I2–I9, 2004.

Menon, V., R. A. Harrington, J. S. Hochman, et al. Thrombolysis and adjunctive therapy in acute myocardial infarction. Chest 126(3 Suppl): 549S–575S, 2004.

CHAPTER 17

Hematopoietic Drugs

OVERVIEW

Mature blood cells are continuously formed in the bone marrow and are removed from the circulation by reticuloendothelial cells in the liver and spleen. The process by which blood cells are replaced is called **hematopoiesis.** This process requires **minerals** and **vitamins** and is regulated by **hematopoietic growth factors** that promote the differentiation and maturation of marrow **stem cells** to form leukocytes, erythrocytes, and platelets.

Anemia, a subnormal concentration of erythrocytes or hemoglobin in the blood, can result from inadequate erythropoiesis, blood loss, or accelerated hemolysis. Erythropoiesis can be impaired by the lack of essential nutrients or by the myelosuppressive effects of certain drugs or irradiation. Infection, cancer, endocrine deficiencies, and chronic inflammation can also cause anemia. **Iron, folic acid, and vitamin B_{12} deficiencies** are the most common causes of **nutritional anemia.**

This chapter describes the pharmacologic properties and uses of minerals, vitamins, and hematopoietic growth factors in the treatment of anemia and other blood cell deficiencies.

DRUGS

Minerals

Iron, an essential dietary mineral, serves as an important component of hemoglobin, myoglobin, and a number of enzymes. The average dietary intake of iron is 18 to 20 mg/day, but people with normal iron stores absorb only about 10% of this amount. Absorption is enhanced twofold or threefold when stored iron is depleted or when erythropoiesis occurs at an accelerated rate. The absorption of iron is regulated by the amount of iron that is stored in the intestinal mucosa.

Iron is absorbed from the intestines into the circulation, where it is bound to **transferrin** and transported to various tissues, including the bone marrow and liver. In these tissues, iron is stored as **ferritin** (Fig. 17–1). In the marrow, iron is incorporated into heme and packaged in new erythrocytes. The erythrocytes circulate in the blood for about 120 days and then are taken up and degraded by reticuloendothelial cells. These cells later return most of the iron to the plasma so that it can be used again in erythropoiesis. Iron is highly conserved by the body, and only small amounts of it are excreted via the intestinal tract.

The dietary iron requirement per kilogram of body weight is highest in infants and pregnant women, somewhat lower in children and nonpregnant women, and lowest in men. Pregnant women have the greatest need for routine **iron supplementation** because their dietary iron often cannot meet the requirements for maternal and fetal erythropoiesis. Most multivitamin supplements contain iron, and many processed foods, including bread, are supplemented with iron.

If dietary iron intake is inadequate to support sufficient erythropoiesis and maintain a normal hemoglobin concentration in the blood, the body will utilize stored iron to maintain erythropoiesis until the stores are depleted. When iron stores are significantly depleted, the plasma iron level begins to fall and erythropoiesis is reduced. Over time, these

Figure 17–1. Iron metabolism. Ingested iron is absorbed from the intestinal mucosa into the circulation, where it is bound to transferrin. Iron is distributed to tissues for incorporation into hemoglobin, myoglobin, and enzymes, or it is stored as ferritin. After about 120 days, erythrocytes are degraded by reticuloendothelial cells, and the iron is returned to the plasma or stored.

changes lead to **hypochromic microcytic anemia,** a form of anemia in which the mean corpuscular hemoglobin concentration (MCHC) and the mean corpuscular volume (MCV) are decreased. The iron preparations described below are used to prevent and treat **iron deficiency anemia** in affected individuals.

Ferrous Sulfate and Related Compounds

Iron is administered orally in the form of **ferrous salts,** including **ferrous sulfate, ferrous gluconate,** and **ferrous fumarate.** Iron contained in these preparations is absorbed in the same manner as dietary iron. In patients with iron deficiency, the amount of iron absorbed increases progressively with larger doses, but the percentage absorbed decreases as the dosage increases. Food can retard iron absorption by 40% to 60%, but the gastric distress caused by iron often necessitates administering iron preparations with food. The percentage of iron absorbed from sustained-release preparations is lower than that absorbed from immediate-release preparations. This is because iron is primarily absorbed from the duodenum, and some of the sustained-release iron is transported to the lower intestinal tract before it is released for absorption.

In iron deficiency states, oral iron preparations are usually administered three times a day in doses that provide a total of 100 to 200 mg of elemental iron daily. The various iron salts contain different percentages of elemental iron. Ferrous sulfate contains about 20%, so that a 300-mg tablet contains approximately 60 mg of elemental iron. The duration of iron therapy depends on the cause and severity of the iron deficiency. In general, about 4 to 6 months of oral iron therapy is required to reverse uncomplicated iron deficiency anemia.

At therapeutic doses, iron salts have few adverse effects, but they sometimes cause epigastric pain, nausea, vomiting, diarrhea or constipation, and black stools. Liquid iron preparations can also stain the teeth. Bile acid-binding resins (e.g., cholestyramine) reduce the absorption of iron, whereas ascorbic acid increases iron absorption by maintaining iron in the reduced ferrous state. Ferrous iron is better absorbed than is ferric iron. Iron can reduce the absorption of tetracyclines, fluoroquinolones, levothyroxine, and vitamin E. The administration of these drugs should be separated from iron administration by at least 2 hours. The ingestion of large quantities of iron can cause serious and potentially lethal toxicity. Hence, iron preparations should be kept out of the reach of children.

Iron Dextran

Iron dextran is a mixture of ferric hydroxide and dextran. It is intended for intramuscular or intravenous treatment of iron deficiency anemia in patients who cannot tolerate oral iron preparations or fail to respond to oral iron therapy. The dosage of iron dextran required for each patient is calculated on the basis of the observed hemoglobin concentration and body weight.

Following administration, the iron dextran complex is removed from the circulation by the reticuloendothelial system, and the iron is transferred to the plasma for distribution to the bone marrow and other tissues.

Because treatment with iron dextran has been associated with fatal anaphylactic reactions, it should be limited to the indications described above. Intramuscular administration of iron dextran can cause several adverse reactions at the injection site, including pain, inflammation, sterile abscesses, and brown discoloration of skin. For this reason, the iron preparation must be given by deep intramuscular injection into the outer quadrant of the buttock. A Z-track technique, in which the skin is displaced laterally before injection, is used to avoid leakage into the subcutaneous tissue. Intravenous administration can cause peripheral flushing and hypotensive reactions.

Vitamins

Although many vitamins participate in the formation and function of erythrocytes, **folic acid** and **vitamin B$_{12}$** have a critical role in erythropoiesis, and a deficiency of either of them may cause **megaloblastic anemia.** The two vitamins serve as cofactors in biochemical reactions involving the addition of single-carbon units to various substrates, and the administration of one of the vitamins can partially compensate for a deficiency of the other. Therefore, it is critical that the specific vitamin deficiency be correctly identified before therapy is started.

Folic Acid

The structure of folic acid is shown in Fig. 17–2A. Active forms of this vitamin serve as enzyme cofactors that donate single-carbon atoms in the biosynthesis of amino acids and the purine and pyrimidine bases contained in DNA (Fig. 17–3A). Hence, folic acid plays a critical role in cell proliferation and erythropoiesis.

The requirement for folic acid increases markedly during pregnancy, and inadequate dietary intake of this vitamin can cause **neural tube birth defects** such as **spina bifida** as well as **megaloblastic anemia.** For this reason, folic acid supplementation is especially important before and during pregnancy. The standard US diet provides 50 to 500 µg of

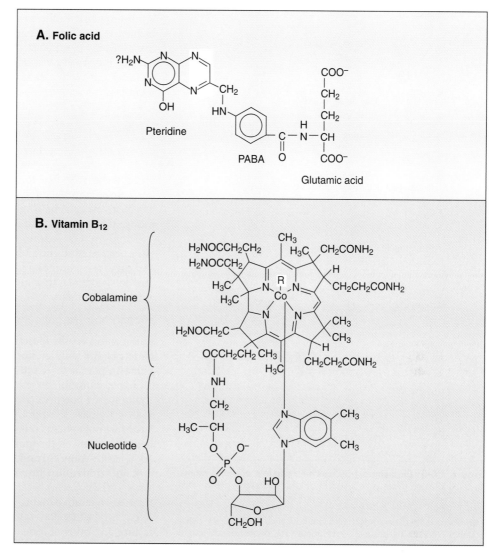

Figure 17–2. Structures of folic acid and vitamin B_{12}. (A) Folic acid consists of pteridine, p-aminobenzoic acid (PABA), and glutamic acid. The unshaded areas represent the bonds that are reduced by folate reductase to form tetrahydrofolic acid. (B) Vitamin B_{12} consists of a porphyrinlike ring with a central cobalt atom attached to a nucleotide. R = CN^- (cyanocobalamin) or OH^- (hydroxocobalamin).

absorbable folic acid daily. Women of child-bearing age should take an additional 400 µg/day of folic acid, the amount contained in most multivitamin preparations. Since 1998, the US Food and Drug Administration has required fortification of all enriched cereal grains sold in the United States of America (USA) with 140 µg of folic acid per 100 g of grain. The incidence of neural tube defects in the USA, which had been declining for decades, has fallen an additional 25% since fortification of cereals began.

Folic acid is well absorbed from the jejunum, and oral supplementation is effective both in preventing and in treating megaloblastic anemia associated with **folic acid deficiency.** This disorder often results from insufficient folic acid intake in the diet, but it can also result from impaired folic acid absorption, such as that seen in patients with alcoholism and certain malabsorption syndromes. In patients with megaloblastic anemia, vitamin B_{12} deficiency must be ruled out before treatment with folic acid is begun. This is because treatment with folic acid may partly correct the anemia caused by a vitamin B_{12} deficiency but will not correct other problems associated with it. Irreversible neurologic damage can occur if a B_{12} deficiency is incorrectly treated with folic acid.

Adequate intake of folic acid also appears to protect against **coronary artery disease** (CAD) by improving **endothelial cell function** and thereby reducing atherogenesis. Administration of high doses of folic acid (5 mg daily) can improve endothelial function in persons with CAD and may thereby reduce the risk of disease progression. The improved endothelial function can result from folate-stimulated regeneration of **tetrahydrobiopterin,** a cofactor required for formation of **nitric oxide,** which plays a critical role in normal endothelial function.

Several drugs can contribute to folate deficiency. These include chemotherapeutic **folate reductase inhibitors** such as trimethoprim, pyrimethamine, and methotrexate (see chapters 41, 44, and 45). Other drugs inhibit folate absorption, including cholestyramine and certain anticonvulsant drugs (e.g., phenytoin).

Vitamin B_{12}

Vitamin B_{12} consists of a porphyrinlike ring with a central cobalt atom attached to a nucleotide (see Fig. 17–2B). Exogenous vitamin B_{12} is available as **cyanocobalamin** and **hydroxocobalamin.** In the body, these forms of the vitamin

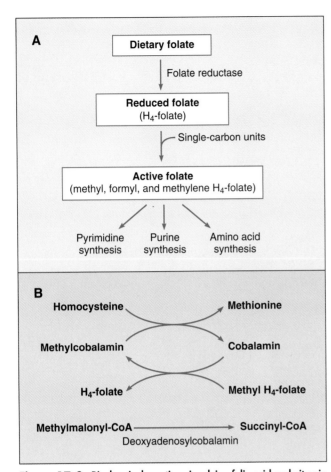

Figure 17–3. Biochemical reactions involving folic acid and vitamin B₁₂. (A) Dietary folate is reduced by folate reductase to tetrahydrofolate (H_4-folate). Single-carbon units are added to H_4-folate to form active folate, which donates single-carbon units in the synthesis of pyrimidine and purine bases and amino acids. (B) The two active forms of vitamin B_{12} are methylcobalamin and deoxyadenosylcobalamin. These forms are cofactors for methylation reactions, including the conversion of homocysteine to methionine and the conversion of methylmalonyl-CoA to succinyl-CoA. Methyl H_4-folate donates a methyl group to cobalamin to form methylcobalamin.

are converted to methylcobalamin or deoxyadenosylcobalamin, which are cofactors for biochemical reactions. Vitamin B_{12} serves as a cofactor for methylation reactions, including the conversion of homocysteine to methionine and the conversion of methylmalonyl CoA to succinyl CoA (see Fig. 17–3B).

Vitamin B_{12} is essential for growth, cell replication, hematopoiesis, and myelin synthesis. It is obtained from dietary meats, dairy products, and eggs, and it is absorbed from the gut in the presence of **intrinsic factor** (a glycoprotein secreted by gastric parietal cells) and calcium. An inadequate secretion of intrinsic factor leads to **vitamin B_{12} deficiency** and eventually results in **pernicious anemia.** Vitamin B_{12} deficiency is also seen in patients who have malabsorption disorders, in individuals who have had gastrectomy, and in strict vegetarians who have a low dietary intake of the vitamin.

Because vitamin B_{12} is not absorbed from the gut in the absence of intrinsic factor, the vitamin must be administered intramuscularly in the treatment of pernicious anemia, and treatment must be continued for life. At the start of therapy, injections are given daily for 5 to 10 days. Thereafter, maintenance doses are given once a month.

In patients with a dietary deficiency of vitamin B_{12}, treatment is given orally.

Hematopoietic Growth Factors

Colony-stimulating factors (CSF), **erythropoietin,** and other hematopoietic growth factors are endogenous glycoproteins that stimulate the differentiation and maturation of bone marrow progenitor cells. The growth factors bind to receptors on specific myeloid progenitor cells and thereby induce their differentiation and proliferation.

Some growth factors, including those discussed below, have been manufactured by recombinant DNA technology, and these are administered parenterally to treat hematopoietic deficiencies. Other growth factors are currently undergoing development.

Epoetin and Darbepoetin

Endogenous **erythropoietin** stimulates erythroid cell differentiation and proliferation and is secreted primarily by the kidney. Epoetin-α (EPOGEN, PROCRIT) was the first form of human erythropoietin to be produced by recombinant DNA technology. Epoetin-β (NEORECORMON) and darbepoetin-α (ARANESP) have been marketed more recently, and a pegylated form of epoetin-β is in phase III clinical trials. Recombinant human erythropoietin (r-HuEPO) is used to treat anemia caused by **chronic renal failure, cancer chemotherapy,** and **zidovudine therapy** for human immunodeficiency virus (HIV). Recombinant erythropoietin is also used to treat anemia in patients with **hematologic malignancies** (e.g., lymphoma) and to treat anemia in patients with **heart failure** and other chronic diseases.

In persons with cancer-related anemia, administration of r-HuEPO has been found to cause reticulocytosis, increase hemoglobin levels, reduce the need for blood transfusions, and improve the quality of life. The standard treatment has been to administer r-HuEPO intravenously or subcutaneously three times a week, but studies show that once weekly epoetin-β or darbepoetin-α is as effective as a three times weekly regimen. This is partly because darbepoetin-α has a threefold longer half-life than epoetin-α because of its increased sialic acid content. The dosage and duration of therapy are determined by the hematocrit response to epoetin treatment.

Recombinant erythropoietin is a safe and effective treatment for anemia in patients with chronic renal failure. The drug is usually well tolerated, and most of the adverse reactions that occur during therapy are attributable to the underlying disease state. The utilization of iron stores, however, is increased in patients treated with r-HuEPO. Therefore, patients should be given iron supplements to maintain transferrin saturation levels that will support epoetin-stimulated erythropoiesis.

Filgrastim, Pegfilgrastim, and Sargramostim

Filgrastim (NEUPOGEN) is recombinant human **granulocyte CSF** (G-CSF), and sargramostim (LEUKINE) is recombinant human **granulocyte-macrophage CSF** (GM-CSF). The endogenous forms of these growth factors are produced by various leukocytes, fibroblasts, and endothelial cells. Because filgrastim is produced in *Escherichia coli* by recombinant DNA technology, it is not glycosylated and differs in this manner from G-CSF isolated from human cells.

The addition of a **polyethylene glycol** (PEG) moiety to filgrastim has resulted in the development of pegfilgrastim (NEULASTA). Pegylation of filgrastim increases its molecular size so that it is too large for renal clearance, thereby increasing the half-life from about 3.5 hours for filgrastim to 42 hours for pegfilgrastim. Pegfilgrastim is primarily eliminated by neutrophil uptake and metabolism. The longer half-life of pegfilgrastim has enabled less frequent administration for treating cancer chemotherapy-induced neutropenia (see below).

Filgrastim, pegfilgrastim, and sargramostim are primarily used to treat **neutropenia associated with cancer chemotherapy and bone marrow transplantation.**

Filgrastim accelerates granulocyte recovery after myelosuppressive chemotherapy and thereby reduces the incidence of infections and shortens the period of hospitalization. Filgrastim is also used to mobilize hematopoietic progenitor cells into the peripheral blood when blood is being collected for leukapheresis. Studies indicate that filgrastim may be beneficial in the treatment of aplastic anemia, hairy cell leukemia, myelodysplasia, drug-induced and congenital agranulocytosis, and other forms of congenital or acquired neutropenia.

Sargramostim is used to accelerate myeloid cell recovery in patients who have **lymphoma,** acute lymphoblastic **leukemia,** or **Hodgkin's disease** and are having autologous **bone marrow transplantation** or chemotherapy. It has also been used to reduce the incidence of fever and infections in patients with severe chronic neutropenia. Although endogenous GM-CSF stimulates the production of several types of cells, sargramostim has little effect on erythrocytes or platelets in deficiency states and primarily serves to accelerate the development of neutrophils.

Filgrastim and sargramostim are administered subcutaneously or intravenously once a day for 2 weeks or until the absolute neutrophil count has reached 10,000/μL. Because of its longer half-life, pegfilgrastim requires administration only once during each cycle of cancer chemotherapy in order to manage chemotherapy-induced neutropenia.

SUMMARY OF IMPORTANT POINTS

■ Iron deficiency causes hypochromic microcytic anemia, whereas folic acid or vitamin B_{12} deficiency causes megaloblastic anemia.

■ Ferrous sulfate and other ferrous salts are administered orally for several months in the treatment of iron deficiency anemia.

■ Folic acid supplementation is used during pregnancy to prevent anemia and birth defects.

■ Folic acid treatment can partly mask the hematologic effect of vitamin B_{12} deficiency but does not prevent irreversible neurologic damage.

■ Pernicious anemia is caused by inadequate secretion of intrinsic factor and reduced vitamin B_{12} absorption. It is treated with intramuscular injections of cyanocobalamin or hydroxocobalamin.

■ Epoetin-α, epoetin-β, and darbepoetin-α are recombinant forms of human erythropoietin used to treat anemia caused by chronic renal failure, cancer-related anemia, and anemia caused by other conditions.

■ Filgrastim, pegfilgrastim, and sargramostim are recombinant forms of granulocyte colony-stimulating factor (G-CSF) or granulocyte-macrophage colony-stimulating factor (GM-CSF). They are used to treat neutropenia associated with cancer chemotherapy, bone marrow transplantation, and various disease states.

Review Questions

For each numbered patient, select the most appropriate drug therapy from the lettered choices provided.

1. A 19-year-old woman who complains of lethargy and fatigue is found to have a *blood hemoglobin concentration* of 9.8 g/dL (normal range 12–16 g/dL), a low *mean corpuscular volume,* and a low *mean corpuscular hemoglobin concentration.*

2. A 47-year-old woman exhibits severe neutropenia following a course of chemotherapy for breast cancer.

3. A 66-year-old man with progressive fatigability and anorexia is found to have a low *blood hemoglobin concentration,* an elevated *mean corpuscular volume,* and an elevated serum concentration of methylmalonic acid.

4. A 68-year-old man with diabetic nephropathy and end-stage renal disease exhibits peripheral reticulocytopenia and anemia.

    (A) cyanocobalamin
    (B) epoetin
    (C) ferrous gluconate
    (D) filgrastim
    (E) folic acid

Answers and Explanations

1. The answer is C: ferrous gluconate. Iron deficiency anemia is a hypochromic (low mean corpuscular hemoglobin concentration), microcytic (low mean corpuscular volume) anemia. Several months of treatment with oral ferrous sulfate or another ferrous salt may be required to correct the iron deficiency and restore hemoglobin concentrations to normal. Patients should also consume a diet containing adequate amounts of folic acid and vitamin B_{12} to ensure adequate erythropoiesis.

2. The answer is D: filgrastim. Filgramstim is a recombinant granulocyte colony-stimulating factor that is used to treat cancer chemotherapy-induced neutropenia in patients with neoplasms, such as breast cancer. Sargramostim has similar indications. Folic acid and vitamin B_{12} are required for normal leucopoiesis, but these vitamins will not by themselves accelerate leucopoiesis caused by drug-induced myelosuppression.

3. The answer is A: cyanocobalamin. Pernicious anemia usually results from inadequate vitamin B_{12} absorption because of decreased production of intrinsic factor by gastric parietal cells. Vitamin B_{12} deficiency causes a megaloblastic anemia characterized by an abnormally high *mean corpuscular volume.* Persons with pernicious anemia will also have a low serum level of vitamin B_{12} and a high serum concentration of methylmalonic acid, because B_{12} is required to convert methylmalonyl CoA to succinyl CoA.

4. The answer is B: epoetin. Epoetin is a recombinant form of erythropoietin. Patients with end-stage renal disease often require epoetin treatment to prevent anemia because their kidneys are unable to produce sufficient erythropoietin to maintain adequate erythrocyte production.

SELECTED READINGS

Biganzoli, L., M. Untch, T. Skacel, et al. Neulasta (pegfilgrastim): a once-per-cycle option for the management of chemotherapy-induced neutropenia. Semin Oncol 31(3 Suppl 8):27–34, 2004.

Cheer, S. M., and A. J. Wagstaff. Epoetin beta: a review of its clinical use in the treatment of anaemia in patients with cancer. Drugs 64:323–346, 2004.

Osterborg, A. New erythropoietic proteins: rationale and clinical data. Semin Oncol 31(3 Suppl 8):12–18, 2004.

CENTRAL NERVOUS SYSTEM PHARMACOLOGY

CHAPTER 18

Introduction to Central Nervous System Pharmacology

The central nervous system (CNS) consists of the brain and spinal cord. Sensory information arrives to the CNS from the special senses and peripheral nerves and is integrated with memories and internal drive states to generate cognitive, emotional, and motor responses.

This processing occurs because of the complex interplay of **neurotransmitters** and **neuromodulators** acting on their **receptors** to excite or inhibit CNS neurons. In persons with **brain disorders,** structural or functional disturbances of CNS processing produces aberrant cognitive, emotional, or motor responses. Brain disorders are seen in association with a variety of disease processes, including degenerative, ischemic, and psychologic disturbances.

Most CNS drugs correct an imbalance in neurotransmitters or their receptors. Drugs are used to relieve the symptoms of brain dysfunction, but they usually do not correct the underlying disorder. Although short-term drug treatment may be effective in relieving acute symptoms such as pain and insomnia, drug therapy for many brain disorders is a lifelong process.

After reviewing pertinent concepts of CNS function and neurotransmission, this chapter explains the general mechanisms by which drugs alter CNS activities and processes.

NEUROTRANSMISSION IN THE CENTRAL NERVOUS SYSTEM

Principles of Neurotransmission

In the last century, great debates raged about the nature of neuronal communication in the CNS. The early physiologists believed that neurons communicated by electrical signals directly passing from neuron to neuron in a **hard-wired** fashion much like wires in a telegraph relay. The early pharmacologists argued for chemical transmission, with substances released into the **synapse** between communicating neurons. Modern research shows that they were both right to some degree because most neuronal communication occurs by chemical **neurotransmitters** serving as messengers that enable neurons to communicate with one another. Evidence, however, also suggests the existence of a direct

voltage signaling between neurons at **electrotonic** or **gap junctions.**

The details of chemical neurotransmission undergo constant refinement as new mechanisms and neurotransmitters as discovered. An early statement by Sir Henry Dale, known as **Dale's principle,** suggested that each neuron contained only one type of neurotransmitter. This principle was revised with the finding that neurons may release more than one neurotransmitter, as is the case with co-transmitters (see below). It was also thought that neurotransmitter action was limited to the single synapse where released. The neuroanatomical demonstration of diffuse neuronal systems with fine, widespread projections throughout the CNS, such as norepinephrine and serotoninergic fibers arising from brainstem nuclei, led to the concept of the **chemical soup** or **chemical milieu** model of neurotransmission. Newer methods using in vitro brain slice preparations and other techniques show that neurotransmitters can diffuse far from the synapse and affect other neurons at other synapses. Identification of neuroactive substances both intrinsic and extrinsic to the CNS that exert generalized effects on neurons strengthened the concept of action at a distance. A **neuromodulator** is a general term for any substance that exerts an effect on neurotransmission among a set of neurons in the brain.

The action of drugs on the CNS is similar to the chemical soup model of neurotransmission, because drug molecules are widely distributed throughout the brain and can simultaneously interact with receptors on neurons in several different neuronal tracts. This lack of specificity can lead to therapeutic effects and adverse effects at the same time. For this reason, the development of agents that are more selective for specific receptor types and subtypes is a useful approach to improving the therapeutic index of CNS drugs.

Neurotransmitter Synthesis and Metabolism

Neurotransmitters are synthesized in neuronal cell bodies or terminals, and they are stored in neuronal vesicles until they are released into a synapse (Fig. 18–1). The release of neurotransmitters is activated by membrane depolarization and calcium influx into the cell. Calcium evokes the interaction of storage vesicle proteins (synaptobrevin and synaptotag-

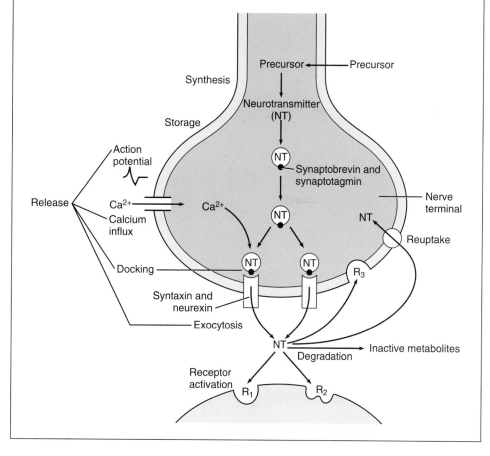

Figure 18–1. Central nervous system (CNS) neurotransmission and sites of drug action. CNS drugs act primarily by affecting the synthesis, storage, release, reuptake, or degradation of neurotransmitters (NT) or by activating receptors. NT are synthesized from precursors accumulated or synthesized in the neurons. The NT are stored in vesicles whose membranes contain proteins involved in NT release (synaptobrevin and synaptotagmin). The NT are released when an action potential-mediated calcium influx initiates interaction of synaptobrevin and synaptotagmin with neuronal membrane-docking proteins (syntaxin and neurexin). This leads to docking and exocytosis. Synaptic NT can activate presynaptic (R_3) or postsynaptic receptors (R_1, R_2). The action of NT is terminated by reuptake into the presynaptic neuron or by enzymatic degradation.

min) and membrane-docking proteins (syntaxin and neurexin) and leads to vesicle fusion with the membrane and exocytosis of the neurotransmitter.

Following exocytosis, the neurotransmitter may activate presynaptic and postsynaptic receptors. A neurotransmitter's action is then terminated either by its reuptake into the presynaptic neuron or by its degradation to inactive compounds, with degradation catalyzed by enzymes located on presynaptic and postsynaptic neuronal membranes or within the cytoplasm.

Neurotransmitters can also diffuse from the synapse of their origin to affect neurons in the surrounding vicinity. In this way, different neurotransmitters released from different types of neurons form a chemical soup or milieu, as described previously. The net influence of the chemical soup on neurotransmission depends on the concentrations of the excitatory and inhibitory neurotransmitters acting at a particular synapse.

Excitatory and Inhibitory Neurotransmission

Central nervous system neurotransmitters can evoke either an excitatory or an inhibitory synaptic membrane potential and trigger effects at presynaptic and postsynaptic sites on target neurons. If an **excitatory postsynaptic membrane potential** reaches firing threshold, an action potential is conducted along the dendritic and axonal membrane and evokes the release of a neurotransmitter from the nerve terminal. An **inhibitory postsynaptic membrane potential** hyperpo-

larizes the neuronal membrane and inhibits the firing of action potentials. Depending on whether a **presynaptic membrane potential** is excitatory or inhibitory, it will increase or decrease the release of a neurotransmitter from the neuron. Presynaptic receptors, also called **autoreceptors**, can also be coupled with cyclic adenosine monophosphate (cAMP) or other second messengers that modulate neurotransmitter release.

As shown in Box 18–1, the interaction of multiple neurotransmitters at a particular site in a neuronal tract enables the complex interplay of various neuronal systems and contributes to the wide range of functional expression exhibited in the CNS. For example, inhibition of the release of an inhibitory neurotransmitter will actually increase neurotransmission in the target neuron. Similarly, drugs can act in complex ways to affect neurotransmission. Ethanol (ethyl alcohol), for instance, can diminish the inhibitory influence of the cerebral cortex on certain human behaviors and thereby facilitate these behaviors. This phenomenon is called **disinhibition** (removal of inhibition).

Fast Versus Slow Signals

Neurotransmitters in the CNS can be characterized as slow or fast, depending on the receptors that are activated and the persistence of signal transduction pathways. The best examples of **fast neurotransmitters** are γ-aminobutyric acid (GABA) and glutamate acting at ion channels. Binding of these amino acid neurotransmitters directly to subunits of

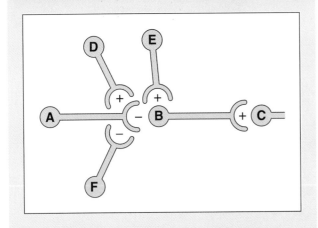

A, B, C, D, E, and F are neurons in a tract that projects from left to right. Neurons B, D, and E release excitatory neurotransmitters (+). Neurons A and F release inhibitory neurotransmitters (−). The net effect of neuronal interactions on neurotransmission from B to C is shown in the table below. Each interaction presupposes that the other neurons are quiescent at that time. Other, more complex interactions are possible.

Interaction	Effect on Neurotransmission (B → C)
A → B	Decreased
D → A → B	Greatly decreased
F → A → B	Increased
E → B	Increased

the ion channel protein directly initiates ion flow with a signal that lasts only for a few milliseconds. Examples of **slow neurotransmitters** are norepinephrine and serotonin acting at G-protein coupled receptors. These activated G-protein coupled receptor proteins initiate a slower, multi-step process with alterations in second messengers and membrane effects that can last from many milliseconds to as long as a second. A slow (long-acting) signal can influence the overall tone of a neuron because it can modulate the signals of several other fast neurotransmitters acting on the same neuron. For this reason, slow neurotransmitters can be called **neuromodulators.**

Neurotransmitters and Receptors

Important neurotransmitters in the CNS include acetylcholine and several amino acids, biogenic amines, and neuropeptides. Table 18–1 lists the names, receptors, mechanisms of signal transduction, and functions of the major neurotransmitters.

The receptors can be divided into two basic groups: **ionotropic receptors,** also called **ligand-gated ion channels,** which are directly associated with ion channels, and **metabotropic receptors,** which are typical **G-protein coupled receptors** (see Chapter 3). Although this terminology is most frequently applied to receptors for amino acid neurotransmitters (e.g., GABA and glutamate), it is equally appropriate for other classes of neurotransmitter receptors.

The **mechanisms of signal transduction** (effector mechanisms) for neurotransmitters in the CNS are similar to those for neurotransmitters in the autonomic nervous system. The activation of ionotropic receptors alters chloride, sodium, potassium, or calcium influx and thereby evokes excitatory or inhibitory membrane potentials. The linkage of metabotropic receptors with G proteins can lead to activation or inhibition of adenylyl cyclase and alteration in the levels of intracellular cAMP, or activation of phospholipase C and the formation of inositol triphosphate (IP_3) and diacylglycerol (DAG). Metabotropic receptor activity can also modulate ion channel activity via second messengers (most notably calcium) that activate protein kinases responsible for the phosphorylation of ion channels.

Acetylcholine

Acetylcholine, which is synthesized from acetyl CoA and choline, is degraded to acetate and choline by acetylcholinesterase (Fig. 18–2). Receptors for acetylcholine are called **cholinergic receptors,** and there are two types; **muscarinic receptors** and **nicotinic receptors.** The properties and mechanisms of these receptors are compared in Table 6–1.

Drugs can affect acetylcholine neurotransmission by activating or blocking cholinergic receptors or by inhibiting cholinesterase. The general pharmacologic properties of cholinergic receptor agonists and antagonists are described in Chapters 6 and 7, respectively.

In the CNS, acetylcholine acts as an excitatory or inhibitory neurotransmitter in a number of neuronal tracts, including those that innervate the hippocampus, cerebral cortex, and basal ganglia. These tracts participate in memory, sensory processing, and motor coordination, respectively.

Amino Acids

Several amino acids are important neurotransmitters in the brain and spinal cord. Some of them (e.g., GABA and glycine) are inhibitory. Others (e.g., aspartate and glutamate) are excitatory.

γ-AMINOBUTYRIC ACID. GABA, which is synthesized from glutamic acid, is the most ubiquitous inhibitory neurotransmitter in the brain and spinal cord. Its receptors are the ionotropic $GABA_A$ receptors and the metabotropic $GABA_B$ receptors. Most drugs affecting GABA neurotransmission primarily activate or inhibit the $GABA_A$-chloride ion channel complex. This ion channel complex contains receptors for several types of drugs, including the benzodiazepines and barbiturates (see Chapter 19), general anesthetics (Chapter 21), and alcohol (Chapter 25). Drugs acting at the $GABA_B$ receptor are used to control spasticity (Chapter 24). The functions of GABA include regulation of

TABLE 18-1. **Major Neurotransmitters and Their Receptors in the CNS**

Neurotransmitter	Receptors	Signal Transduction	Function
Acetylcholine	Muscarinic M_1, M_3, M_5	$\uparrow IP_3$, $\uparrow DAG$, $\uparrow iCa^{2+}$	Excitatory; role in arousal and consciousness, memory consolidation
	M_2, M_4	$\downarrow cAMP$, $\uparrow gK^+$, $\downarrow gCa^{2+}$	Inhibitory; autoreceptor and heteroreceptor, decreases NT release
	Nicotinic	$\uparrow gNa^+$, $\uparrow gCa^{2+}$	Excitatory; increases NT release, role in nicotine dependence
Amino Acids			
GABA	$GABA_A$	$\uparrow gCl^-$	Inhibitory (major); ligand-gated ion channel site of action of sedative-hypnotics, alcohol, general anesthetics
	$GABA_B$	$\downarrow cAMP$, $\uparrow gK^+$, $\downarrow gCa^{2+}$	Inhibitory; modulates motor neuron excitability
Glutamate	NMDA, AMPA, KA	$\uparrow gNa^+$, $\uparrow gCa^{2+}$	Excitatory (major); roles in LTP (memory), excitotoxicity of neurons
	$mGlu_1$, $mGlu_5$	$\uparrow IP_3$, $\uparrow DAG$, $\uparrow iCa^{2+}$	Excitatory; memory consolidation, neuronal excitation
	$mGlu_2$-$mGlu_4$, $mGlu_6$-$mGlu_8$	$\downarrow cAMP$, $\uparrow gK^+$, $\downarrow gCa^{2+}$	Inhibitory; role in thalamic sensory processing
Glycine	Strychnine-sensitive	$\uparrow gCl^-$	Inhibitory; highest levels in spinal cord
	Strychnine-insensitive	Co-agonist at NMDA receptor	Excitatory; obligate co-agonist for function of NMDA receptor
Biogenic Amines			
Dopamine	D_1, D_5	$\uparrow cAMP$, $\uparrow PKA$	Excitatory; basal ganglia function, memory and performance
	D_2, D_3, D_4	$\downarrow cAMP$, $\uparrow gK^+$, $\downarrow gCa^{2+}$	Inhibitory; decreases dopamine release, reduces firing of neurons
Norepinephrine	α_1	$\uparrow IP_3$, $\uparrow DAG$, $\uparrow iCa^{2+}$	Excitatory; autonomic nuclei in brainstem
	α_2	$\downarrow cAMP$, $\uparrow gK^+$, $\downarrow gCa^{2+}$	Inhibitory; sympathetic outflow from CNS; decreases pain transmission
	β_1, β_2	$\uparrow cAMP$, $\uparrow PKA$	Excitatory; cortex, limbic system, nucleus accumbens
Serotonin (5-HT)[a]	$5-HT_1$	$\downarrow cAMP$, $\uparrow gK^+$, $\downarrow gCa^{2+}$	Inhibitory; role in anxiety and depression
	$5-HT_2$	$\uparrow IP_3$, $\uparrow DAG$, $\uparrow iCa^{2+}$	Excitatory; widespread distribution, role in antipsychotic action
	$5-HT_3$	$\uparrow gNa^+$, $\uparrow gCa^{2+}$	Excitatory; mediate fast neuronal transmission in neocortex; presynaptic modulation of NT release.
	$5-HT_4$	$\uparrow cAMP$, $\uparrow PKA$	Excitatory; role in cognitive processes, anxiety
Histamine	H_1	$\uparrow IP_3$, $\uparrow DAG$, $\uparrow iCa^{2+}$	Excitatory; increases NT release, role in arousal, anxiety
	H_2	$\uparrow cAMP$, $\uparrow PKA$	Excitatory; located in hippocampus, amygdala and basal ganglia
	H_3	$\downarrow cAMP$, $\uparrow gK^+$, $\downarrow gCa^{2+}$	Inhibitory; autoreceptor and heteroreceptor, decreases NT release
Neuropeptides			
Opioid peptides	μ, δ, κ	$\downarrow cAMP$, $\uparrow gK^+$, $\downarrow gCa^{2+}$	Inhibitory; analgesic role in sensory processing, role in drug dependence for opioids and other substances
Tachykinins	NK_1, NK_2, NK_3	$\uparrow IP_3$, $\uparrow DAG$, $\uparrow iCa^{2+}$	Excitatory; role in pain processing, autonomic regulation

AMPA = α-amino-3-hydroxy-5-methyl-4-isoxazole propionate; cAMP = cyclic adenosine monophosphate; DAG = diacylglycerol; g = ion channel conductance; i = intracellular; KA = kainate; NK = neurokinin; NMDA = N-methyl-D-aspartate; NT = neurotransmitter; PKA = cAMP-dependent protein kinase; IP_3 = inositol triphosphate.
[a]Over a dozen types of serotonin receptors are cloned; the four given here are the main types.

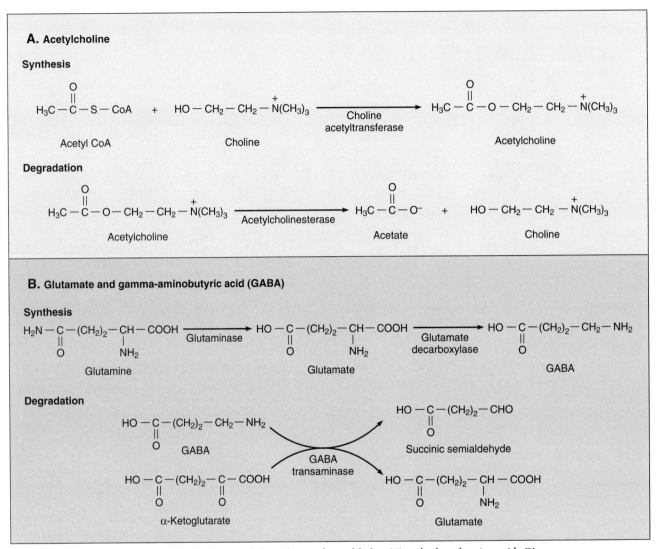

Figure 18–2. Synthesis and degradation of acetylcholine (A) and selected amino acids (B).

neuronal excitability throughout the CNS and motor coordination.

GLUTAMATE AND ASPARTATE. Glutamate and aspartate are acidic amino acids that function as excitatory neurotransmitters throughout the CNS. Their ionotropic receptors consist of three types that differ in their subunit composition and are named for drugs that show the most selectivity for each type: NMDA (*N*-methyl-D-aspartate), AMPA (α-amino-3-hydroxy-5-methyl-4-isoxazole propionate), and kainate (KA) receptors. These receptors are excitatory because their associated ion channels allow the flow of sodium or calcium ions into neurons causing depolarization. Metabotropic glutamate receptors consist of two main classes that are either coupled to phospholipase C and intracellular calcium signaling or are negatively coupled to adenylyl cyclase. Glutamate and aspartate participate in the long-term potentiation (LTP) needed for learning and memory and have a role in neuronal toxicity and apoptosis (cell death) evoked by trauma and ischemia. Antagonists of these excitatory amino acid receptors are used in the treatment of seizures (Chapter 20) and may find use in blocking the over-excitation of neurons that occurs following stroke and other disorders.

GLYCINE AND TAURINE. Glycine is a major inhibitory transmitter in the spinal cord. Its **strychnine-insensitive receptors** are coupled with the chloride ion channel, and activation of these receptors leads to membrane hyperpolarization. Its **strychnine-sensitive receptors** are associated with the glutamate NMDA receptor and serve to decrease glutamate excitation. Strychnine produces convulsive seizures by blocking the glycine site on the NMDA receptor.

Taurine is a sulfur-containing amino acid that is postulated to act as a neurotransmitter or neuromodulator in the CNS. Taurine is believed to activate both strychnine-insensitive and strychnine-sensitive types of glycine receptors. As with glycine, taurine can serve to counteract the excitotoxic effects of excessive glutamate on CNS neurons.

Biogenic Amines

The **biogenic amines** or **monoamines** that function as CNS neurotransmitters are the catecholamines, dopamine and norepinephrine; serotonin (5-hydroxytryptamine); and

TABLE 18–2. Sites of CNS Drug Action

Process	Mechanism	Drug example	Major uses
Neurotransmitter (NT) synthesis	Increase synthesis of NT by precursor loading	Levodopa	Parkinsonism
Neurotransmitter storage	Block transport of NT into vesicles	Reserpine	Hypertension
Neurotransmitter release	Increase NT release	Amphetamine	Attention-deficit disorder
Neurotransmitter reuptake	Block reuptake of NT	Fluoxetine	Depression
Neurotransmitter degradation	Block NT degradation enzyme	Donepezil	Alzheimer's disease
Receptor activation	Agonist activity at receptor	Diazepam	Anxiety
Receptor blockade	Antagonist activity at receptor	Clozapine	Schizophrenia
Signal transduction	Block formation of second messengers	Lithium	Bipolar disorder
Neuronal conduction	Block axonal action potentials	Lidocaine	Local anesthesia

histamine. These neurotransmitters, which are formed by decarboxylation of amino acids, are catabolized in part by the enzyme, monoamine oxidase.

DOPAMINE. Dopamine is a major CNS neurotransmitter that binds to five types of dopamine receptors. The D_1 and D_5 **receptors** activate adenylyl cyclase and thereby increase cAMP levels. In contrast, the D_2, D_3, and D_4 **receptors** inhibit adenylyl cyclase and decrease cAMP levels. As shown in Table 18–2, levodopa, clozapine, and other drugs have effects on various steps in the synthesis and metabolism of dopamine. Dopamine is found in several neuronal tracts originating from the ventral tegmental area (VTA), plays a significant role in behavioral and drug reinforcement, and regulates emesis (vomiting), prolactin release, mood states, motor coordination, and olfaction. Its degradation results in the formation of homovanillic acid (HVA), a metabolite that is subsequently excreted in the urine (Fig. 18–3).

NOREPINEPHRINE. Norepinephrine, which is formed from dopamine, is degraded by monoamine oxidase and catechol-O-methyltransferase to a number of metabolites. The major metabolite excreted in the urine is **3-methoxy-4-hydroxymandelic acid**, or **vanillylmandelic acid (VMA)**. The receptors for norepinephrine are **α-adrenergic receptors** and **β-adrenergic receptors**, and their subtypes and properties are described in detail in Chapter 8. Norepinephrine is associated with several neuronal tracts projecting from the locus ceruleus in the medulla (brainstem) to the thalamus, cerebral cortex, cerebellum, and spinal cord, and it is found in tracts projecting from the midbrain to the hypothalamus. This ubiquitous neurotransmitter participates in the regulation of anxiety, cerebellar function, learning, memory, mood, sensory processing (including pain), and sleep. Drugs can alter norepinephrine's neurotransmission by activating or blocking its receptors or by inhibiting its presynaptic neuronal uptake.

SEROTONIN. Serotonin, or 5-hydroxytryptamine (5-HT), is synthesized from tryptophan, is degraded to **5-hydroxyindoleacetic acid (5-HIAA)**, and functions as an excitatory and inhibitory neurotransmitter. Serotonin is found in neuronal tracts projecting from the raphe nuclei in the medulla to many other parts of the brain. These tracts are involved in emotional processing and pain processing, and have an effect on appetite, mood, sleep, and hallucinations. Serotonin or 5-HT acts on more than a dozen types of receptors;

all of them are metabotropic receptors, except for the 5-HT$_3$ receptor which is a ligand-gated ion channel protein. The main types and effector mechanisms of 5-HT receptors are outlined in Table 18–1. In most areas of the brain, serotonin has an inhibitory effect mediated by the 5-HT$_{1A}$ receptor decreasing cAMP levels and increasing potassium conductance causing membrane hyperpolarization. Drugs can affect serotonergic function by stimulating or blocking 5-HT receptors or by blocking serotonin reuptake.

HISTAMINE. Histamine is a neurotransmitter found in hypothalamic neurons that project to all the major parts of the brain, including the cerebral cortex. It is involved in the regulation of the sleep-wake cycle, cardiovascular control, regulation of the hypothalamic-pituitary-adrenal axis (HPA axis), learning and memory. Histamine acts on two types of receptors in the brain, H$_1$ and H$_3$, with action on a third type, H$_2$, in the periphery. All histamine receptors are metabotropic with H$_1$ receptors coupled to the phospholipase C pathway and H$_3$ receptors negatively coupled to adenylate cyclase. H$_3$ receptors were originally discovered as autoreceptors on histaminergic neurons but are now known to also inhibit the release of other neurotransmitters. CNS histamine receptors are not currently considered a major site of therapeutic drug action but antagonism of H$_1$ receptors is partly responsible for the drowsiness and sedation caused by some antihistamines.

Neuropeptides

A number of peptides function as slow neurotransmitters and neuromodulators in the CNS. Unlike other neurotransmitters, **neuropeptides** are synthesized in neuronal cell bodies and are then transported to nerve terminals for release. Once released, they are metabolized by various peptidases, but they do not undergo presynaptic reuptake. Some of the neuropeptides are released as **co-transmitters** with other, nonpeptide neurotransmitters. The co-transmitter neuropeptides usually serve to amplify or prolong the effects of these other neurotransmitters.

A growing list of neuropeptides are known to function as neurotransmitters in the CNS. One of the first classes of neuropeptides discovered contains the **endogenous opioid peptides (endorphins)** and includes **Met-enkephalin, dynorphin, and β-endorphin**. The opioid peptides inhibit pain transmission in the spinal cord and midbrain, among other CNS effects. A second important group consists of **tachykinins** and includes **neurokinins A and B** and

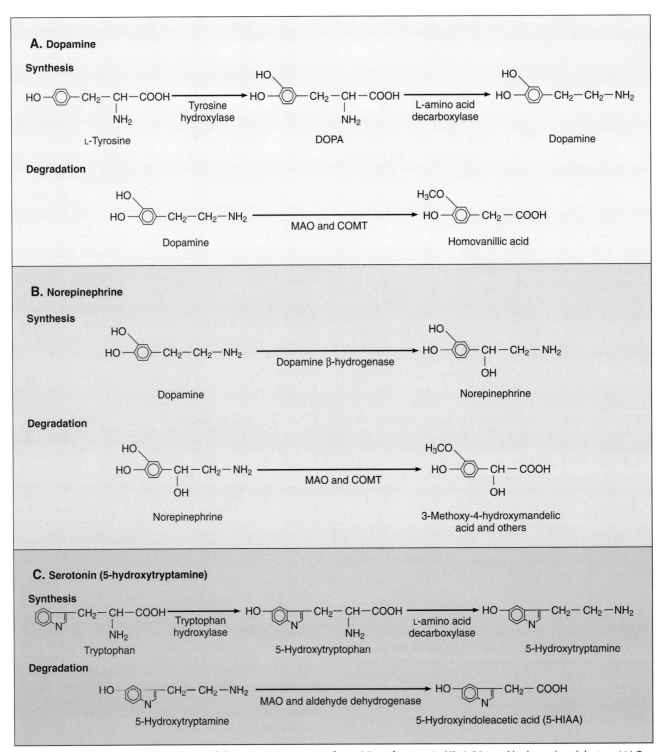

Figure 18–3. Synthesis and degradation of dopamine (A), norepinephrine (B), and serotonin (C). DOPA = dihydroxyphenylalanine; MAO = monoamine oxidase; and COMT = catechol-O-methyltransferase.

substance P. Neurokinins modulate cardiovascular and behavioral responses to stress, and substance P participates in pain processing, emesis, and anxiety.

Other peptides that were originally isolated from peripheral tissues are thought to function as neuromodulators in the CNS. These neuropeptides include **cholecystokinin, gastrin, somatostatin,** and **vasoactive intestinal polypeptide.**

Other Neurotransmitters

Several additional substances, including nitric oxide (NO), carbon monoxide, appetite-regulating peptides, and purines, may also serve as neurotransmitters or neuromodulators in the CNS.

Nitric oxide is a gas formed from arginine by calcium-calmodulin–stimulated NO synthase in CNS neurons.

Evidence suggests that NO acts as a **retrograde neurotransmitter** in that it is released by the postsynaptic neuron and diffuses to the presynaptic terminal, where it facilitates future neurotransmitter release by elevating levels of cyclic guanosine monophosphate (cyclic GMP, or cGMP). This action may contribute to LTP, which is a key process to establish memory. A similar function is postulated for **carbon monoxide (CO)** in the CNS.

Several recently discovered **appetite-regulating peptides** may function as neuromodulators or neurohormones in the CNS. These include **ghrelin**, a peptide synthesized in the stomach and hypothalamus, and **neuropeptide-Y** and **orexin**, contained in neurons in the lateral hypothalamus. All three peptides stimulate food intake and increase body weight in animal models. Conversely, **leptin** is a peptide hormone secreted from fat cells, which acts on the brain to reduce food intake and increase peripheral energy expenditure. As expected, the pharmaceutical industry has intense interest in developing drug therapies for the treatment of obesity based on these discoveries.

Purines that can serve as neurotransmitters include **adenosine** and **adenosine triphosphate (ATP)**. Adenosine activates specific receptors identified as A_1, A_2, and A_3 **receptors.** Activation of A_1 and A_3 receptors increases cAMP formation, whereas activation of A_2 receptors inhibits cAMP formation. The role of adenosine as a central neurotransmitter is not clearly established, but inhibition of A_2 receptors by methylxanthines (e.g., caffeine) causes CNS stimulation. ATP acts on both ionotropic receptors, called **P2X receptors**, and metabotropic **P2Y receptors**. Similarly, the role of ATP in neurotransmission is unclear, but some evidence indicates that ATP is a co-transmitter that is released with other neurotransmitters in the brain and serves to augment the effects of these neurotransmitters.

MECHANISMS OF DRUG ACTION

Table 18–2 lists the many processes by which drugs affect the CNS and provides examples of agents acting via each process.

Drugs that alter CNS neurotransmitter function generally do so by altering the synthesis, storage, or release of a neurotransmitter; blocking the reuptake of a neurotransmitter; inhibiting the degradation of a neurotransmitter; or activating or blocking neurotransmitter receptors. A few CNS drugs act by directly blocking membrane ion channels or by altering the physiochemical properties of neuronal membranes to inhibit neurotransmission. Although modulation of second-messenger signal transduction is an attractive target for novel pharmacologic agents, lithium is currently the only therapeutic drug shown to act by this mechanism.

Neurotransmitter Synthesis, Storage, and Release

Neurotransmitter synthesis can be increased by administering a precursor to a neurotransmitter, such as levodopa. Levodopa is taken up by dopamine neurons and is converted to dopamine, thereby increasing the amount of dopamine available for neurotransmission. The vesicular storage of norepinephrine is blocked by reserpine, a plant alkaloid first

used to treat hypertension. The side effect of severe depression in patients treated with reserpine provided an early clue that neurotransmitter levels may be inadequate in persons with this type of affective disorder. Drugs can cause non-exocytotic release of neurotransmitter by interacting with the presynaptic neurotransmitter transporter. For example, amphetamine increases the release of norepinephrine by this mechanism, and amantadine is used therapeutically to increase the release of dopamine in patients with parkinsonism.

Neurotransmitter Reuptake and Degradation

Presynaptic reuptake and enzymatic degradation are the two primary mechanisms for terminating the action of most CNS neurotransmitters, and drugs inhibit both of these processes. Cocaine and many of the antidepressant drugs act by blocking the reuptake of dopamine, norepinephrine, or serotonin. Donepezil and selegiline are examples of agents that inhibit the degradation of acetylcholine or dopamine and thereby elevate the synaptic concentration of these neurotransmitters.

Receptor Activation or Blockade

Postsynaptic receptors are activated or blocked by several types of CNS drugs. For example, bromocriptine, a drug used in the treatment of parkinsonism, acts as an agonist at dopamine receptors, whereas antipsychotic drugs act as antagonists at dopamine and serotonin receptors.

Presynaptic receptors are involved in feedback inhibition of neurotransmitter release. They are called **autoreceptors** when they are activated by the same neurotransmitter that is released by the neuron, and they are called **heteroreceptors** when they are activated by a different neurotransmitter. Activation of presynaptic receptors decreases the concentration of the released neurotransmitter found in synapses, whereas blockade of these receptors increases the concentration. For example, activation of 5-HT_{1D} autoreceptors inhibits the release of serotonin and decreases its concentration in synapses.

Receptor Alterations Caused by CNS Drug Treatment

As detailed in Chapter 3, receptor proteins not only regulate cell processes but are themselves regulated. Receptors undergo dynamic alteration in response to changes in synaptic neurotransmitter concentrations or in response to long-term drug administration. These alterations can affect the efficiency of receptor coupling to signal transduction pathways (desensitization or sensitization) or affect the number of receptor proteins expressed by the neuron (down-regulation or up-regulation). CNS drugs that act on metabotropic or G-protein coupled receptors are particularly noted for their alteration of receptor numbers. Receptor down-regulation may follow a sustained increase in neurotransmitter release, a sustained blockade of neurotransmitter reuptake, or long-term receptor activation by a drug. For example, long-term administration of an opioid

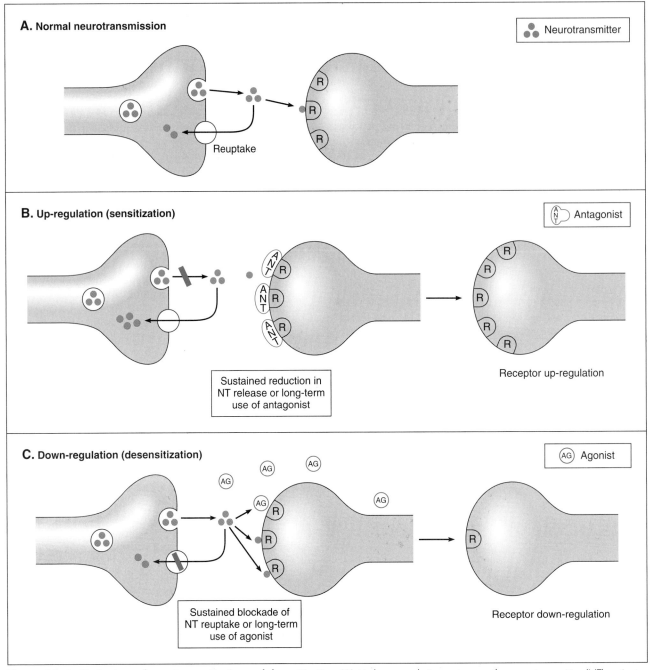

Figure 18–4. Mechanisms of receptor sensitization and desensitization. (A) Under normal circumstances, the neurotransmitter (NT) activates receptors and is removed from the synapse by neuronal reuptake. (B) The number of receptors can be increased (up-regulated) by a sustained reduction in NT release or by the long-term administration of a receptor antagonist (ANT). (C) The number of receptors can be decreased (down-regulated) by a sustained blockade of NT reuptake or by the long-term administration of a receptor agonist (AG).

agonist in a patient with chronic pain can cause down-regulation of opioid receptors in the brain and spinal cord (Fig. 18–4). Receptor down-regulation is one of the primary mechanisms of pharmacodynamic drug tolerance. Receptor up-regulation is a compensatory reaction to a sustained decrease in neurotransmission, a condition that can be caused either by a reduction in neurotransmitter release or by long-term receptor blockade. For example, daily administration of a dopamine receptor antagonist in a schizophrenic patient can lead to up-regulation of D_2 receptors.

NEURONAL SYSTEMS IN THE CENTRAL NERVOUS SYSTEM

Many CNS diseases and drug treatments affect cognitive processing, memory, motor coordination, and other complex brain functions discussed later. It is difficult to attribute these complex functions to specific neuronal tracts, because many of the functions are accomplished through the interaction of tracts that communicate with several brain regions and utilize various neurotransmitters. These six broad areas of functional processing, however, provide an introduction to the neuroanatomy and neuropharmacology of CNS agents.

Cognitive Processing

Cognitive processing occurs in **prefrontal cortical structures,** where sensory information is integrated with past experience and interpreted in a manner that can result in thoughts and behavioral action. The neuronal systems involved in cognitive processing include **association fibers** that arise from areas throughout the brain and converge on the anteromedial frontal, orbital frontal, and cingulate areas of the prefrontal cortex.

Cognitive processing utilizes memory and is influenced by emotions. At the same time, emotions are largely derived from past experience and cognition. Cognitive processing also encompasses abstract reasoning and forethought, which are processes that do not necessarily result in motor expression but can influence emotional processing and future acts.

Delirium is a general term that refers to disorders of cognitive processing, and one of manifestations of **schizophrenia** is impaired cognitive processing.

Drugs that affect cognitive processing include **antipsychotics, CNS stimulants, hallucinogens,** and **sedative-hypnotics.**

Memory

Memory is the ability to recall events and integrate them into cognitive processing, emotional processing, and ongoing motor activities. One form of memory, called **procedural memory,** is used to recall a set of practiced motor actions (e.g., riding a bicycle or typing on a keyboard) and it involves the interaction of **limbic structures,** the **cerebellum,** and the **basal ganglia.** Another form of memory, called **declarative memory,** involves thoughts and associations that may be used to determine future actions. For example, remembering that touching a hot stove is painful may keep a child from playing near the stove in the future, and remembering that a family member's birthday is approaching may trigger activities such as planning a dinner party. Declarative memory involves neuronal tracts in the **hippocampus, amygdala, thalamus,** and **neocortex.**

Dementia is a term used to describe a number of memory disorders, including **Alzheimer's disease.** The involvement of the basal ganglia in procedural memory may explain why some patients with **Parkinson's disease** have difficulties with practiced motor actions.

Drugs that affect memory include the cholinesterase inhibitors and CNS depressants such as the benzodiazepines.

Emotional Processing

Emotional processing is responsible for the generation of emotions such as anger, anxiety, fear, happiness, love, and sadness. These emotions represent the conscious perception of neuronal activity originating in the **limbic system,** including the hypothalamus, amygdala, septum, hippocampus, and mammillary bodies, as well as the cingulate and entorhinal portions of the frontal lobe cortex. Emotions contribute to a state of mental preparedness for anticipated future activities. For example, anxiety contributes to a state of heightened vigilance, which may amplify the response to a future stimulus or event.

Disorders in which emotional processing is defective include **anxiety states, mood disorders,** and **schizophrenia.**

Drugs that affect emotional processing in the limbic system include **anxiolytic (antianxiety) drugs, antidepressants, antipsychotics, CNS stimulants, opioids,** and **all drugs that produce drug dependence.** Hence, most CNS drugs have some effect on emotional processing.

Sensory Processing

Sensory processing involves neuronal tracts that perceive external stimuli and transmit that information to the brain. These include the sensory systems responsible for vision, hearing, olfaction, touch, and pain.

The spinothalamic tracts relay touch and pain sensations to the **thalamus,** which projects this information to the **cortex.** The brainstem region known as the **reticular formation** plays a significant role in filtering sensory information before it is relayed to the thalamus and hypothalamus and eventually to the cortex. The reticular formation includes the **locus ceruleus** and **raphe nuclei,** whose neurons release norepinephrine and serotonin, respectively, and play an important role in determining the level of consciousness, sleep, and wakefulness. The cortex of the parietal and occipital lobes and part of the temporal lobe is involved in the recognition and integration of sensory perceptions.

Disorders in which sensory processing is defective include **sleep disorders, chronic pain syndromes,** and **disorders of the special senses** such as blindness, deafness, and taste and olfactory dysfunction.

Among the drugs that affect sensory processing are **antidepressants, hallucinogens, local and general anesthetics, opioid analgesics,** and **sedative-hypnotics.**

Motor Processing

Motor processing refers to the neuronal activity that enables body movement. The structures involved in motor processing include the **cerebellum,** the motor strip of the **frontal lobe cortex,** the **basal ganglia,** and the suprasegmental nuclei that are found in the **brainstem** and are involved in the control of posture (e.g., the vestibular nuclei).

Disturbances in motor processing occur in Parkinson's disease, Huntington's disease, and a variety of degenerative and demyelinating neuron disorders.

Drugs that affect motor processing include antiparkinsonian drugs, antispasmodics, CNS stimulants, muscle relaxants, and sedative-hypnotics.

Autonomic Processing

Autonomic processing involves areas of the brain that integrate the activities of the **peripheral autonomic nervous system** (see Chapter 5). These areas include the **hypothalamus** and portions of the **brainstem,** such as the vasomotor center and the cranial nuclei of parasympathetic nerves.

Disorders of autonomic processing include orthostatic hypotension and postural tachycardia syndrome.

Some CNS drugs alter autonomic processing by affecting the actions of hypothalamic and brainstem nuclei, and others have a direct effect on peripheral autonomic neurotransmission. The drugs that affect autonomic processing include **antidepressants, antiparkinsonian drugs, antipsychotics,** and **drugs used to treat Alzheimer's disease.**

SUMMARY OF IMPORTANT POINTS

■ Central nervous system (CNS) drugs act primarily by affecting the synthesis, storage, release, reuptake, or degradation of neurotransmitters or by activating or blocking receptors.

■ Long-term administration of drugs sometimes causes up-regulation or down-regulation of receptors. Up-regulation is evoked by receptor antagonists, whereas down-regulation is evoked by receptor agonists or reuptake inhibitors.

■ Major CNS neurotransmitters include acetylcholine; amino acids (aspartate, γ-aminobutyric acid [GABA], glutamate, and glycine); biogenic amines (dopamine, histamine, norepinephrine, and serotonin); and neuropeptides such as the endogenous opioid peptides and the tachykinins.

■ Some CNS neurotransmitters (e.g., aspartate, glutamate, histamine, and tachykinins) are excitatory; others (e.g., dopamine, GABA, glycine, and opioid peptides) are inhibitory; and still others (e.g., acetylcholine, norepinephrine, and serotonin) are both excitatory and inhibitory, with these actions exerted via different receptors.

■ Neurotransmitters can be classified as fast or slow, depending on the type of receptor they activate and on the duration of the neuronal signal that they evoke. GABA and glutamate are fast, whereas norepinephrine, neuropeptides, and serotonin are slow.

■ Receptors for CNS neurotransmitters can be classified as ionotropic (directly coupled with ion channels) or metabotropic (coupled with G proteins and second messengers).

■ Many diseases of the CNS and the corresponding drugs used to treat these diseases have an effect on one or more of the following complex brain functions: cognitive processing, emotional processing, memory, motor processing, sensory processing, and autonomic processing.

Review Questions

1. Which of the following terms best describe receptors located on neuronal terminals that bind the same neurotransmitter released from the neuronal terminal, and decrease further release of the neurotransmitter?

(A) presynaptic receptors
(B) heteroreceptors
(C) postsynaptic receptors
(D) autoreceptors
(E) ionotropic receptors

2. Which of the following short statements best describes the characteristics of metabotropic receptors?
(A) associated directly with ion channels
(B) coupled to G proteins
(C) consists of numerous protein subunits
(D) located on presynaptic terminals
(E) mediate neurotransmitter reuptake

3. Which one of the following statements best describes the differences between classical neurotransmitters and neuropeptides?
(A) neuropeptides are synthesized in the cell body
(B) classical neurotransmitters have a longer duration of action
(C) neuropeptides undergo rapid reuptake into the presynaptic terminal
(D) classical neurotransmitters are packaged into vesicles
(E) neuropeptides are degraded by acetylcholinesterase in the synapse

4. A patient with terminal bone cancer has been treated for the last month with twice-daily doses of a long-acting morphine formulation. He complains that the drug is no longer working and he is in pain. Which one of the following statements best explains the onset of his apparent opioid tolerance?
(A) the metabolism of morphine is up-regulated
(B) pain intensity has greatly increased
(C) the efficiency of G-protein coupling is decreased
(D) opioid receptors are down-regulated
(E) the patient is a "drug-seeker" and addicted to opioid medications

5. Reserpine, a plant alkaloid used in the past to treat hypertension, has which site of action as a CNS drug?
(A) postsynaptic receptors
(B) vesicular storage
(C) vesicular release
(D) neurotransmitter reuptake
(E) neurotransmitter degradation

Answers to Review Questions

1. The best answer is D: autoreceptors. Autoreceptors are a type of presynaptic receptors in which the binding of the same neurotransmitter released from the neuronal terminal decreases further release of that neurotransmitter. Answer (A), presynaptic receptors, is a general term for any type of receptor located on the neuronal terminal. Answer (B), heteroreceptors, is a type of presynaptic receptor that is also located on the neuronal terminal but binds a different neurotransmitter than the one being released from the terminal. Answer (C), postsynaptic receptors, is incorrect because these receptors are located on the postsynaptic membrane. Answer (E), ionotropic receptors, is the term for a receptor associated with an ion

channel and could be located on either the presynaptic or postsynaptic membrane.

2. The best answer is B: coupled to G proteins. Metabotropic receptors are also known as G-protein coupled receptors or GPCR. Answer (A), associated directly with ion channels, describes the other main class of receptors called ionotropic receptors. Answer (C), consists of numerous protein subunits, is true for ionotropic receptors but not for metabotropic receptors, which consist of a single, polypeptide chain forming seven transmembrane domains as it weaves in and out of the cell membrane. Answer (D), located on presynaptic terminals, could be true of metabotropic receptors but is not a unique characteristic of metabotropic receptors. Answer (E), mediate neurotransmitter reuptake, does not describe a receptor but rather a transport protein located in the presynaptic terminal that limits the duration of neurotransmitter action in the synapse by pumping the neurotransmitter back into the terminal it was released from.

3. The best answer is A: neuropeptides are synthesized in the cell body. Unlike classical neurotransmitters that are synthesized in vesicles en route or at the neuronal terminal from precursor substances, neuropeptides arise from the transcription of a neuropeptide gene, processing of the neuropeptide messenger RNA (mRNA), and translation of the mRNA into a neuropeptide product in the endoplasmic reticulum in the cell body of a neuron. Answer (B), classical neurotransmitters have a longer duration of action, is not true in general and many studies show that neuropeptides act more as neuromodulators with longer duration of action than classical neurotransmitters. Answer (C), neuropeptides undergo rapid reuptake into the presynaptic terminal, is incorrect as there are no known transport proteins in presynaptic membranes to facilitate the reuptake of neuropeptides back into the terminal. Answer (D), classical neurotransmitters are packaged into vesicles, is true but does not differentiate between the two types of substances because neuropeptides are also packaged into vesicles for release, albeit into different types called dense-core vesicles. Answer (E), neuropeptides are degraded by acetylcholinesterase in the synapse, is incorrect because other enzymes called peptidases are responsible for the degradation of neuropeptides after release into the synapse.

4. The best answer is D: opioid receptors are down-regulated. Chronic administration of an agonist, such as the opioid agonist morphine, will cause a decrease in the number of receptor proteins expressed by the neuron in an attempt to decrease the signaling through that pathway and establish homeostasis. Answer (A), the metabolism of morphine is up-regulated, could be true because the metabolism of some CNS agents, most notably the barbiturates, self-induce metabolic enzymes but this mechanism is not known to occur to any great degree in opioid tolerance. Answer (B), pain intensity has greatly increased, could also be true but there is no information given in the question to assume that this might be the case. Answer (C), the efficiency of G-protein coupling is decreased, is a mechanism more noted for acute changes after agonist administration, whereas down-regulation is more likely with long-term or chronic administration of an agonist. Answer (E), the patient is a "drug-seeker" and addicted to opioid medications, is very unlikely because terminal bone cancer is a very painful condition and very few patients (<1%) receiving opioid analgesics for treatment of a clinical condition develop opioid addiction.

5. The best answer is B: vesicular storage. Reserpine disrupts the storage of norepinephrine into vesicles and results in less neurotransmitter available for release. Answers (A) and (C-E) describe other sites of CNS drug action but reserpine is not known for affecting those processes.

SELECTED READINGS

Barnes, G.N., and J.T. Slevin. Ionotropic glutamate receptor biology: effect on synaptic connectivity and function in neurological disease. Curr Med Chem 10(20):2059–2072, 2003.

Lynch J. W. Molecular structure and function of the glycine receptor chloride channel. Physiol Rev 84(4):1051–1095, 2004.

Miller, K. J., B. J. Murphy, and M. A. Pelleymounter. Central G-protein coupled receptors (GPCR)s as molecular targets for the treatment of obesity: assets, liabilities and development status. Curr Drug Targets CNS Neurol Disord 3(5):357–377, 2004.

Squire L. R. Memory systems of the brain: a brief history and current perspective. Neurobiol Learn Mem 82(3):171–177, 2004.

Strock, J., and M. A. Diverse-Pierluissi. Ca²⁺ channels as integrators of G protein-mediated signaling in neurons. Mol Pharmacol 66(5):1071–1076, 2004.

CHAPTER 19

Sedative-Hypnotic and Anxiolytic Drugs

CLASSIFICATION OF SEDATIVE-HYPNOTIC AND ANXIOLYTIC DRUGS

Benzodiazepines
- Alprazolam (XANAX)
- Chlordiazepoxide (LIBRIUM)
- Clonazepam (KLONOPIN)
- Diazepam (VALIUM)
- Lorazepam (ATIVAN)
- Midazolam (VERSED)
- Triazolam (HALCION)[a]
- Flumazemil (ROMAZICON)[b]

Barbiturates
- Amobarbital
- Pentobarbital
- Phenobarbital
- Thiopental

Antihistamines
- Diphenhydramine
- Hydroxyzine

Other Sedative-hypnotic Drugs
- Zolpidem (AMBIEN)
- Zaleplon (SONATA)
- Chloral hydrate
- Melatonin

Nonsedating Anxiolytic Drugs
- Buspirone (BUSPAR)
- Propranolol

[a]also estazolam, flurazepam, oxazepam, temazepam and others.
[b]benzodiazepine receptor antagonist.

OVERVIEW

Sedative-hypnotic drugs are among the most widely used pharmaceutical agents in the world. The **sedative** part of their name refers to the ability of these agents to calm or reduce anxiety, known as an **anxiolytic** effect. The **hypnotic** part of their name describes the ability of these agents to induce drowsiness and promote sleep. This latter action is caused by a greater depression of CNS activity and most sedative-hypnotic drugs will first cause sedation, then at higher doses, produce hypnosis or sleep. A few agents, however, exert anxiolytic effects without causing sedation or hypnosis.

This chapter describes the pharmacologic properties of benzodiazepines, barbiturates, and other sedative-hypnotic and anxiolytic drugs that are used in the treatment of anxiety and sleep disorders. Because of their greater safety, less adverse effects, and the availability of an antagonist, the benzodiazepines have largely replaced the older barbiturates for these indications. Although ethanol (ethyl alcohol) has sedative-hypnotic effects, it is not used therapeutically for these purposes, and its pharmacologic effects are described in Chapter 25.

ANXIETY DISORDERS

Anxiety is normally an **adaptive response** that prepares a person to react appropriately to a threatening event, such as a hurricane or tornado. Anxiety is characterized by changes in mood (apprehension and fear), sympathetic nervous system arousal, and hypervigilance. Chronic anxiety, however, is usually a **maladaptive response** to psychological stressors that can eventually impair a person's ability to perform the activities of daily living. Moreover, chronic anxiety often leads to visceral organ dysfunction and unpleasant symptoms. For example, patients with chronic anxiety may develop gastrointestinal, cardiovascular, and neurologic problems, including diarrhea, tachycardia, sweating, tremors, and dizziness. Ultimately, anxiety can contribute to heart disease and other disorders, including substance abuse.

Neurologic Basis of Anxiety

The neuronal pathways involved in anxiety disorders include the **sensory, cognitive, behavioral, motor, and autonomic pathways.** Sensory systems, cortical processing, and memory are involved in interpreting a stimulus to be dangerous and creating a state of heightened arousal. Motor systems and autonomic processing participate in the exaggerated responses to an anxiety state.

Growing evidence indicates that the **amygdala,** an almond-shaped structure in the temporal lobe, plays a central role in mediating most of the manifestations of anxiety, including the **conditioned avoidance reaction** (conditioned fear reaction) that underlies anxiety states. In experimental protocols, this reaction can be induced in animals by teaching them that a cue (e.g., a flashing light) will be followed by a noxious stimulus (e.g., a shock to the foot). During the anticipatory period, the animals conditioned in this manner will exhibit signs of anxiety, such as autonomic and behavioral arousal. Electrical stimulation of the amygdala induces signs of anxiety, whereas lesioning the amygdala or the administration of anxiolytic drugs prevents the behavioral and physiologic manifestations of anxiety during the anticipatory period. It is believed that long-term potentiation (LTP) in amygdala neurons establishes the memory of adverse events underlying anticipatory anxiety.

Classification and Treatment of Anxiety Disorders

The appropriate management of anxiety disorders requires an accurate diagnosis, may involve the use of pharmacologic agents, and for best results includes psychotherapy.

Acute Anxiety Disorders

Acute anxiety disorders, such as **adjustment disorder,** can result from illness, separation, or the anticipation of stressful events. Acute anxiety is often self-limiting and may resolve in a few weeks to a few months without drug treatment. A **benzodiazepine** might provide short-term relief from more severe acute anxiety conditions. **Propranolol** is useful in the prevention of **stage fright,** or **acute situational** or **performance anxiety.**

Panic Disorder

Panic disorder is characterized by acute episodes of severe anxiety with marked psychological and physiological symptoms. During a panic attack, an individual may feel an impending sense of doom that is often accompanied by sweating, tachycardia, tremor, and other visceral symptoms. Patients with panic disorder often respond to drug therapy with a **benzodiazepine** or an **antidepressant drug,** such as a **selective serotonin reuptake inhibitor** (SSRI, see Chapter 22). Benzodiazepines may provide immediate relief from panic attacks during the early phase of therapy, and **alprazolam** and **clonazepam** are benzodiazepines that have been particularly useful in this regard. For long-term treatment, an SSRI antidepressant such as **fluoxetine** is often prescribed.

Phobic Disorders

Phobias are conditions in which an individual is overly fearful about a particular situation or condition, such as traveling in an airplane. Panic disorder can co-exist with **agoraphobia,** an intense fear of open spaces or of being in a public place from which it might be difficult or embarrassing to cope with a panic attack. Patients with phobic disorders show the best outcomes when treated with a combination of psychotherapy and drug therapy. As with panic disorder, phobic disorders are treated with a **benzodiazepine** or an **antidepressant drug.** Benzodiazepines provide acute relief of symptoms and enable patients to more easily benefit from psychotherapy, whereas antidepressants are usually the most effective long-term drug therapy for these disorders.

Obsessive-Compulsive Disorder

Obsessive-compulsive disorder (OCD) has features similar to those of anxiety disorders and mood disorders. It is characterized by **obsessions** (i.e., recurring or persistent thoughts and impulses) and **compulsions** (i.e., repetitive behaviors in response to obsessions). OCD can be treated effectively with an **antidepressant drug** (see Chapter 22) and psychotherapy. Sedative-hypnotic drugs usually are not useful unless the patient concurrently suffers from another anxiety disorder.

Generalized Anxiety Disorder

Generalized anxiety disorder (GAD) is usually defined as a persistent state of fear and apprehension concerning future events. Short-term therapy with a **benzodiazepine** may relieve acute symptoms and provide a useful bridge to psychotherapy. The severity of the disorder often fluctuates over time, and benzodiazepines may be effectively used on an intermittent basis to help patients deal with exacerbations of the disorder. **Buspirone, a nonsedating anxiolytic,** provides a useful alternative to benzodiazepines for the treatment of chronic anxiety states, because it produces little sedation and is not associated with tolerance or dependence. It must be taken for 3 or 4 weeks, however, before its anxiolytic effects are felt.

SLEEP DISORDERS

Sleep is a reversible state of reduced consciousness that is accompanied by characteristic changes in the electroencephalogram (EEG). Five distinct patterns of brainwave activity occur during sleep, grouped into the four stages of **non-rapid eye movement sleep** (**NREM**), and a pattern characterized by paralysis of voluntary muscles and quick, saccadic movement of the eye called **rapid eye movement sleep** (**REM**).

As an individual falls asleep, the high frequency and low amplitude activity of the alert state gradually diminishes during stages 1 and 2 and is replaced by low frequency and high amplitude activity of **slow-wave sleep** (stages 3 and 4). Over time, the individual returns to stage 1 and eventually to the REM stage. REM sleep is also known as **paradoxical sleep** because the EEG pattern is similar to the awake state. A normal adult cycles through the sleep stages about every 90 minutes (Box 19–1).

Sleep patterns change with age and are altered by sedative-hypnotic and other central nervous system (CNS) drugs.

Neurologic Basis of Sleep

The neuronal systems involved in sleep include the **basal forebrain nuclei** and the **reticular formation.** Projecting from the basal forebrain to the cortex are cholinergic fibers that are believed to be involved in the induction of sleep. The basal forebrain is the only region of the brain that is active during slow-wave sleep and quiescent at other stages. The reticular formation facilitates the flow of sensory information from the thalamus to the cortex. When reticular nuclei are quiescent, the thalamus does not transfer information to the cortex, and this facilitates the onset of sleep.

Classification and Treatment of Sleep Disorders

Insomnia

Some patients with insomnia find it difficult to go to sleep or to stay asleep during the night, whereas others awaken too early in the morning. In general, the management of insomnia depends on whether the sleep disorder is caused by physiologic, psychologic, or medical conditions. As shown in Box 19–1, the patterns of sleep stages in patients with insomnia are irregular and include longer latency to fall asleep and frequent awakenings.

Insomnia caused by acute stress or a minor illness is usually self-limiting and may not require treatment. **Melatonin** is a useful drug to treat mild insomnia, and it is available without a prescription. Melatonin is particularly useful in relieving **jet lag,** a form of acute insomnia caused by travel across several time zones.

Insomnia caused by medical conditions whose symptoms interfere with sleep is effectively treated with **benzodiazepines** or other **sedative-hypnotic drugs,** such as **zolpidem** and **zaleplon,** whereas insomnia related to psychological and psychiatric disturbances is best managed with a combination of psychotherapy and sedative-hypnotic drugs. Benzodiazepines and most other hypnotic drugs decrease sleep latency (the time required to go to sleep) and increase sleep duration. Zolpidem and zaleplon have the advantages of not significantly affecting sleep architecture, and not causing as much tolerance and dependence as the older drugs. For these reasons, zolpidem and zaleplon have become the drugs of choice to treat most types of insomnia.

Other Sleep Disorders

Other sleep disorders include **hypersomnia** (difficulty in awakening), **narcolepsy** (sleep attacks), **enuresis** (bedwetting during sleep), **somnambulism** (sleepwalking), **sleep apnea** (episodes of hypoventilation during sleep), and **nightmares** and **night terrors.** Most of these disorders are managed with a combination of psychotherapy and **antidepressant drugs** or **CNS stimulants.** Sodium oxybate (XYREM) was recently approved for the treatment of cataplexy associated with narcoleptic attacks.

SEDATIVE-HYPNOTIC DRUGS

The sedative-hypnotic drugs include benzodiazepines, barbiturates, some antihistamines, and a few miscellaneous compounds, such as chloral hydrate, zolpidem and zaleplon. The properties of these drugs are summarized in Table 19–1, and their adverse effects, contraindications, and drug interactions are listed in Table 19–2.

Because the benzodiazepines have fewer adverse reactions and drug interactions and are safer in cases of overdose, they have largely replaced the barbiturates and other older drugs. Nevertheless, barbiturates are still used when benzodiazepines are ineffective or contraindicated. The sedating antihistamines are occasionally used to treat mild insomnia and anxiety and have less potential for abuse than do benzodiazepines and barbiturates. Many over-the-counter (nonprescription) sleep aids contain antihistamines as their effective ingredient.

Benzodiazepines

The benzodiazepines are a large group of drugs that have similar pharmacologic effects. They are so named because they share the common chemical structure of a benzene ring (*benzo*) joined to a seven-membered ring containing two nitrogen molecules (*diazepine*). The particular use of specific drugs is largely determined by their pharmacokinetic properties and route of administration. Some benzodiazepines have been developed and approved to treat anxiety, whereas others are approved for the management of insomnia or for other purposes.

Drug Properties

PHARMACOKINETICS. The pharmacokinetic properties of various benzodiazepines are compared in Table 19–1. The benzodiazepines are absorbed from the gut and distributed to the brain at rates that are proportional to their lipid solubility, which varies 50 times among individual drugs in the class. As the plasma concentration of a benzodiazepine declines, the drug is redistributed from the brain to the blood, and this mechanism contributes significantly to the termination of its effects on the CNS.

All benzodiazepines are extensively metabolized in the liver. Most benzodiazepines are converted to active metabolites in phase I oxidative reactions catalyzed by cytochrome P450 enzymes. The active metabolites of chlordiazepoxide, diazepam, and flurazepam are long acting and contribute to the long duration of action of these agents. The active metabolites of alprazolam, estazolam, midazolam, and triazolam are shorter acting. Each of these active metabolites is eventually conjugated with glucuronate to form an inactive polar metabolite that is excreted in the urine. Other drugs (e.g., lorazepam, oxazepam, and temazepam) bypass phase I oxidation and are metabolized only by phase II conjugation

BOX 19-1. EFFECT OF SEDATIVE-HYPNOTIC DRUGS ON SLEEP ARCHITECTURE TERMINOLOGY

Patterns on the electroencephalogram (EEG) vary with the stage of sleep. When a person falls asleep, the high-frequency and low-amplitude pattern of the **awake state** is gradually replaced by the progressively lower-frequency and higher-amplitude patterns of stages 1 through 4, which collectively are called **non-rapid eye movement sleep** (NREM sleep). Stages 3 and 4 are called **slow-wave sleep.** Another stage, called **REM sleep** for **rapid eye movement sleep**, is characterized by rapid, jerky eye movements. REM sleep is also called **paradoxical sleep** because it is during this stage that the pattern on EEG returns to the pattern seen during the awake state.

Normal and Abnormal Sleep Patterns

The normal sleep pattern in adults consists of about five cycles, each of which lasts approximately 90 minutes. During each cycle, an individual progresses from stage 1 to stage 4 and then returns to stage 1, followed by a period of REM sleep. As the cycles progress through the night, they become shorter, and the amount of slow-wave sleep decreases.

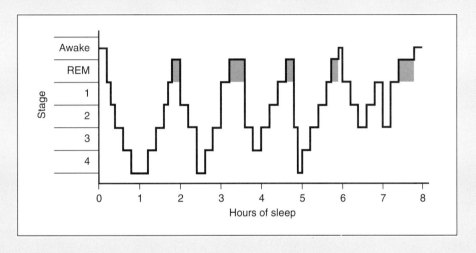

The sleep patterns of patients with insomnia vary widely but are often characterized by reduced amounts of slow-wave sleep and by one or more awakenings during the night. The time required to fall asleep (sleep latency) is usually pro-longed, and the total sleep time is decreased in most patients with insomnia. Elderly adults often have a similar sleep pattern.

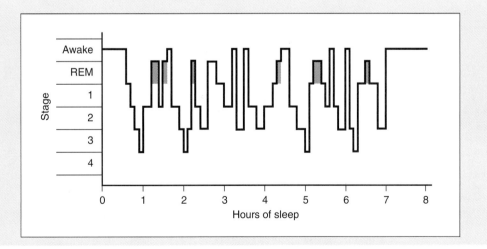

Continued

BOX 19-1. EFFECT OF SEDATIVE-HYPNOTIC DRUGS ON SLEEP ARCHITECTURE TERMINOLOGY—cont'd

Effects of Drugs on Sleep Architecture

Benzodiazepines and most other hypnotics suppress the stages of 3, slow-wave sleep and REM sleep. In contrast, zolpidem and zaleplon have little effect on sleep architecture. Therefore, use of zolpidem or zaleplon may restore the sleep pattern to normal.

State	Rapid Eye Movements	Pattern on EEG	Effect of Benzodiazepines	Effect of Zolpidem/Zaleplon
Awake	No	High-frequency, low-amplitude pattern	Induce sleep	Induces sleep
Stages 1 and 2 sleep	No	Lower-frequency, higher-amplitude pattern than awake state	Increase length of stages	Little change
Stages 3 and 4 sleep	No	Lower-frequency, higher-amplitude pattern than stages 1 and 2	Decrease length of stages	Little change
REM sleep	Yes	High-frequency, low-amplitude pattern	Decrease length of stage	Little change

TABLE 19-1. **Pharmacokinetic Properties and Clinical Uses of Sedative-Hypnotic and Anxiolytic Drugs**

Drug	Onset of Action*	Duration of Action*	Active Metabolites	Major Clinical Uses
Sedative-hypnotic drugs				
Benzodiazepines				
– Alprazolam	Fast	Medium	Yes	Anxiety, including panic disorder
– Chlordiazepoxide	Fast; very fast (IV)	Long	Yes	Alcohol detoxification; anxiety
– Clonazepam	Fast	Medium	No	Anxiety, including panic disorder; seizure disorders
– Diazepam	Fast; very fast (IV)	Long	Yes	Alcohol detoxification; anxiety; muscle spasm; seizure disorders; spasticity
– Estazolam	Fast	Medium	Yes	Insomnia
– Flurazepam	Fast	Long	Yes	Insomnia
– Lorazepam	Fast; very fast (IV)	Medium	No	Anxiety; seizure disorders
– Midazolam	Very fast (IV)	Short (IV)	Yes	Anesthesia
– Oxazepam	Fast	Short	No	Anxiety
– Temazepam	Fast	Medium	No	Insomnia
– Triazolam	Fast	Short	Yes	Insomnia
Barbiturates				
– Amobarbital	Fast	Medium	No	Insomnia
– Pentobarbital	Fast	Short	No	Insomnia
– Phenobarbital	Slow	Long	No	Seizure disorders
– Thiopental	Very fast (IV)	Short (IV)	No	Induction of anesthesia
Antihistamines				
– Diphenhydramine	Fast	Medium	No	Insomnia
– Hydroxyzine	Fast	Long	No	Anxiety; sedation
Other sedative-hypnotic drugs				
– Chloral hydrate	Fast	Medium	Yes	Insomnia; preanesthetic sedation
– Melatonin	Fast	Medium	No	Insomnia, including jet lag
– Zalelplon	Fast	Very short	No	Insomnia
– Zolpidem	Fast	Short	No	Insomnia
Nonsedating anxiolytic drugs				
– Buspirone	Very slow	Long	No	Chronic anxiety
– Propranolol	Fast	Medium	Yes	Situational or performance anxiety

*Unless onset and duration of action are specifically indicated for intravenous (IV) administration, they are for oral administration. Very fast = <15 minutes; fast = 15–59 minutes; slow = 1–4 hours; very slow = 3–4 weeks; short = 1–6 hours; medium = 7–12 hours; and long = >12 hours.

TABLE 19-2. **Adverse Effects, Contraindications, and Drug Interactions of Sedative-Hypnotic and Anxiolytic Drugs**

Drug	Common Adverse Effects	Common Drug Interactions
Sedative-hypnotic drugs		
Benzodiazepines		
– Alprazolam	Arrhythmia; central nervous system (CNS) depression; drug dependence; hypotension; and mild respiratory depression	Alcohol and other CNS depressants potentiate effects. Fluoxetine and fluvoxamine increase serum levels and effects
– Chlordiazepoxide	Same as alprazolam	Alcohol and other CNS depressants potentiate effects. Cimetidine increases and rifampin decreases serum levels
– Clonazepam	Same as alprazolam	Same as chlordiazepoxide
– Diazepam	Same as alprazolam	Same as chlordiazepoxide
– Estazolam	Same as alprazolam	Same as chlordiazepoxide
– Flurazepam	Same as alprazolam	Same as chlordiazepoxide
– Lorazepam	Same as alprazolam	Alcohol and other CNS depressants potentiate effects. Rifampin decreases serum levels
– Midazolam	Same as alprazolam	Alcohol and other CNS depressants potentiate effects. Calcium channel blockers, erythromycin, and ketoconazole increase serum levels
– Oxazepam	Same as alprazolam	Same as lorazepam
– Temazepam	Same as alprazolam	Same as chlordiazepoxide
– Triazolam	Amnesia; confusion; and delirium. Other adverse effects same as alprazolam	Alcohol and other CNS depressants potentiate effects. Cimetidine, erythromycin, ketoconazole, and oral contraceptives increase serum levels
Barbiturates		
– Amobarbital	CNS depression; drug dependence; and respiratory depression	Induces cytochrome P450 enzymes and increases metabolism of many drugs. Potentiates effects of other CNS depressants
– Pentobarbital	Same as amobarbital	Same as amobarbital
– Phenobarbital	Same as amobarbital	Same as amobarbital
– Thiopental	Same as amobarbital	Same as amobarbital
Antihistamines		
– Diphenhydramine	Anticholinergic effects, such as blurred vision, dry mouth, and urinary retention; dizziness; and drowsiness	Alcohol, barbiturates, and other CNS depressants potentiate CNS effects
– Hydroxyzine	Same as diphenhydramine	Same as diphenhydramine
Other sedative-hypnotic drugs		
– Chloral hydrate	Severe cardiac, hepatic, or renal disease; and severe gastritis	Alcohol and other CNS depressants potentiate effects
Melatonin	Drowsiness; fatigue; and lethargy	Alcohol and caffeine reduce melatonin secretion. Flumazenil and naloxone antagonize effects. Sedative-hypnotic drugs potentiate effects
– Zaleplon	Dizziness; drowsiness; and headache	Alcohol and other CNS depressants potentiate risk
– Zolpidem	Same as Zaleplon	Same as Zaleplon
Nonsedating anxiolytic drugs		
– Buspirone	Dizziness; headache; and nervousness	None
– Propranolol	Bradycardia; bronchoconstriction; depression; fatigue; hypersensitivity; hypotension; impaired glycogenolysis; and vivid dreams	Cardiac depression increased by calcium channel blockers

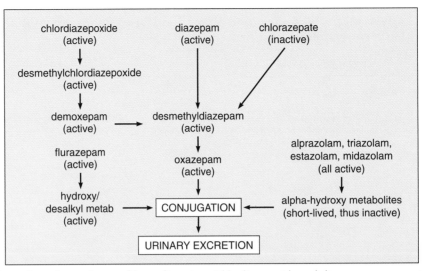

Figure 19–1. Major biotransformation pathways of benzodiazepines. Chlordiazepoxide and diazepam are converted to long-acting active metabolites. Alprazolam, midazolam, and triazolam are converted to a short-acting active metabolite. All benzodiazepines, including those with no active metabolites, are eventually converted to glucuronide compounds that are pharmacologically inactive and are excreted in the urine. The benzodiazepines that have no active metabolites include lorazepam, oxazepam, and temazepam, and these may be the safest benzodiazepines to use in treating elderly patients.

(Fig. 19–1). These three drugs may be safer for use by elderly patients, because the capacity to conjugate drugs does not decline with age as much as the capacity for oxidative biotransformation does. Hence, these three drugs are less likely to accumulate to toxic levels in elderly patients.

Benzodiazepines also undergo some degree of enterohepatic cycling that prolongs their duration of action. In fact, some patients who are taking a drug such as diazepam may notice an increased sedative effect after eating a fatty meal. The fatty meal causes the gallbladder to empty and thereby delivers bile containing diazepam to the intestines for reabsorption into the circulation.

MECHANISM OF ACTION. The **benzodiazepines** and **barbiturates** are believed to exert their effects on consciousness and sleep by facilitating the activity of γ-aminobutyric acid (GABA) at various sites in the neuraxis. GABA, the most ubiquitous inhibitory neurotransmitter in the CNS, regulates the excitability of neurons in almost every neuronal tract. As shown in Fig. 19–2, the **GABA$_A$ receptor-chloride ion channel** has binding sites for benzodiazepines and barbiturates, as well as alcohols, steroids, and inhalational anesthetics. Benzodiazepine increases the frequency with which the channel opens, whereas barbiturates increase the length of time that the channel remains open. By increasing chloride conductance, these drugs cause neuronal membrane hyperpolarization and this, in turn, counteracts the depolarizing effect of excitatory neurotransmitters. Barbiturates also increase chloride conductance independent of GABA, which is why they are capable of causing greater CNS depression and toxicity than the benzodiazepines.

The **benzodiazepine receptors** are also called **omega (ω) receptors**, and there are two types, designated ω$_1$ and ω$_2$. Benzodiazepines bind to both ω$_1$ and ω$_2$ receptor sites,

whereas the nonbenzodiazepine agents, zolpidem and zaleplon, are selective for the ω$_1$ receptor site. Activation of the ω$_1$ receptors increases the affinity of GABA for its binding site on the GABA$_A$ receptor-chloride ion channel. This is an example of an **allosteric binding site** and differs from drugs binding to iontropic or metabotropic receptors.

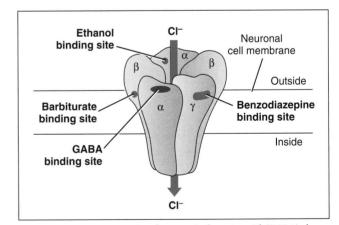

Figure 19–2. Receptor sites for γ-aminobutyric acid (GABA), benzodiazepines, barbiturates, and ethanol on the GABA$_A$ chloride ionophore. The GABA$_A$ chloride ionophore is a glycoprotein pentamer that has varying combinations of α, β, and γ subunits. GABA binds to a site on the α orβsubunit, and this causes conformational changes that open the chloride ion channel and lead to neuronal membrane hyperpolarization. Benzodiazepines bind to a site that is probably located on the γ subunit, and this facilitates GABA binding and increases the frequency of chloride channel opening. Barbiturates bind to another site and increase the duration of chloride channel opening, both in the presence and in the absence of GABA. Ethanol (ethyl alcohol) binds to a distinct site on the ionophore and enhances chloride influx. The ionophore also contains binding sites for steroids such as progesterone. These binding sites may mediate the behavioral effects of steroids.

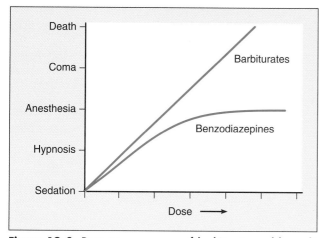

Figure 19–3. Dose-response curves of barbiturates and benzodiazepines. The barbiturates exhibit a linear dose-response effect, which progresses from sedation to respiratory depression, coma, and death. Benzodiazepines exhibit a ceiling effect, which precludes severe central nervous system depression following oral administration of these drugs. Intravenous administration of benzodiazepines can produce anesthesia and mild respiratory depression.

In addition to their effects on GABA, benzodiazepines also inhibit the neuronal reuptake of **adenosine.** This action increases the inhibitory effect of adenosine on neurons that release acetylcholine from the pedunculopontine nucleus of the reticular formation, which is a brain structure mediating arousal. The effect of benzodiazepines on adenosine may also explain why these drugs dilate coronary arteries and decrease total peripheral resistance.

PHARMACOLOGIC EFFECTS. The benzodiazepines produce a dose-dependent but limited depression of the CNS. Lower doses have a sedative and anxiolytic effect, whereas higher doses produce hypnosis (sleep) and anesthesia (Fig. 19–3). Benzodiazepines can relieve anxiety at doses that produce relatively little sedation. In contrast to the barbiturates, the orally administered benzodiazepines do not produce respiratory depression, coma, or death unless they are administered with another CNS depressant (e.g., alcohol). Because benzodiazepines only work in the presence of GABA released by neurons, the depth of CNS depression is limited. Barbiturates do not exhibit this ceiling effect and can produce severe respiratory depression and death after administration of an excessive amount.

In addition to producing sedative-hypnotic and anxiolytic effects, benzodiazepines can produce **anterograde amnesia,** which means that an individual will not remember what happens from the time that the drug is administered to the time that the drug effects dissipate. This is in contrast to retrograde amnesia, in which a person cannot remember what happened before a certain point in time. The benzodiazepines produce anterograde amnesia because they interfere with the formation of new memory; they do not affect the ability to recall past events. The amnesic property of benzodiazepines is often useful when patients are undergoing stressful procedures, such as endoscopy or surgery.

When these drugs are used on a long-term basis, such as in treating anxiety, the amnesic properties can have an adverse effect on the patient's ability to function. Triazolam, a widely used hypnotic, has been associated with problems caused by its amnesic effect.

The benzodiazepines have anticonvulsant effects and have been used in the treatment of seizure disorders (see Chapter 20). Although benzodiazepines cause muscle relaxation only at doses that produce considerable sedation, they are occasionally used to treat muscle spasm and spasticity. The muscle-relaxing effects of benzodiazepines are probably caused by the fact that these drugs potentiate the effects of GABA on interneurons in the spinal cord.

ADVERSE EFFECTS. The adverse effects of benzodiazepines are largely caused by CNS depression. The drugs frequently cause motor incoordination, dizziness, and excessive drowsiness. They impair cognitive processing and can affect concentration, judgment, and planning. They can also interfere with driving and other psychomotor skills. When longer-acting benzodiazepines (e.g., flurazepam) are used to treat insomnia, they can cause drowsiness and a drug hangover the next day. If this occurs, a shorter-acting drug (e.g., estazolam or zolpidem) should be substituted for the longer-acting drug.

Intravenous administration of benzodiazepines produces greater CNS depression than does oral administration, and intravenous administration can cause respiratory depression. Specific warnings of respiratory depression were issued by the US Food and Drug Administration (FDA) for **midazolam,** an agent indicated solely for intravenous administration. The greater effect produced by intravenous administration probably results from the more rapid uptake of the drug by brain tissue, which results in a greater potentiation of GABA before the self-limiting effect on GABA release has had time to develop.

The benzodiazepines have a mild euphoric effect and can reduce behavioral inhibitions in a manner similar to the disinhibitory effect of alcohol. The behavioral reinforcement produced by these drugs may contribute to their recreational abuse by polydrug abusers and to their inappropriate long-term use by patients. It appears that the reinforcing effects of benzodiazepines are less than the reinforcing effects of barbiturates but greater than the reinforcing effects of sedating antihistamines and possibly zolpidem and zaleplon.

Long-term use of the benzodiazepines can produce physical dependence, the severity of which is proportional to the dosage and duration of administration. After several months of continued use, most patients develop some degree of physical dependence. If their medication is abruptly discontinued, they will experience a withdrawal syndrome, characterized by rebound anxiety, insomnia, headache, irritability, and muscle twitches. The withdrawal syndrome is usually mild and not life-threatening. Abrupt withdrawal from **alprazolam** has been associated with seizures. Therefore, to prevent its occurrence, the dosage of benzodiazepines should be gradually tapered over a period of several weeks. Because the various drugs in the benzodiazepine class exhibit cross-tolerance, any of them can be substituted for another one to prevent or counteract the withdrawal reaction.

Pharmacodynamic tolerance also occurs during long-term use of benzodiazepines. Unlike barbiturates, however, the benzodiazepines do not induce their own metabolism or cause pharmacokinetic tolerance.

Although the overall safety of the benzodiazepines is high, their use has been associated with hypotension, arrhythmia (tachycardia or bradycardia), and a number of other less common effects. Rarely, a massive overdose of a benzodiazepine has been fatal, but is less likely than in the case of barbiturates because of the availability of a benzodiazepine antagonist, **flumazenil**.

The incidence of fetal malformations in the offspring of women who take benzodiazepines during pregnancy is very low. Nevertheless, chronic use of benzodiazepines during pregnancy is not recommended and they are included in pregnancy category D by the FDA. Zolpidem and zaleplon appear to be safer in pregnancy and are listed as pregnancy category B.

INTERACTIONS AND TREATMENT OF ADVERSE EFFECTS. Several drugs, including flumazenil and β-carboline derivatives, interact with benzodiazepine receptors.

Flumazenil is a competitive **benzodiazepine receptor antagonist.** In addition to blocking the effects of agonists, such as diazepam, it also blocks the effects of inverse agonists (see later text) at the benzodiazepine receptor. Flumazenil can be used to counteract the adverse effects of benzodiazepines, such as respiratory depression resulting from intravenous administration of these drugs or in the case of accidental or intentional overdose. Flumazenil is given intravenously and has a rapid onset and a short duration of action. Its potential adverse effects include seizures, arrhythmias, blurred vision, emotional lability, and dizziness.

The **β-carboline derivatives** act as **inverse agonists.** An inverse agonist is a drug that decreases the response of an effector system below the basal level (see Chapter 3). The β-carboline drugs act to decrease chloride conductance by the $GABA_A$ receptor-chloride ion channel, and this can cause anxiety and seizures. Some of the experimental inverse agonists enhance cognitive function and are being studied for the treatment of Alzheimer's disease.

Table 19–2 lists the individual benzodiazepines and outlines their interactions with various other drugs.

INDICATIONS. The benzodiazepines are effective in the treatment of anxiety disorders, insomnia, muscle spasm, seizure disorders, and spasticity. They are also used for the treatment of alcohol withdrawal. When possible, the use of benzodiazepines should be limited to the short-term treatment of these conditions. If long-term use is medically justified, the physician should carefully monitor drug usage to prevent dosage escalation.

Specific Agents

Alprazolam is converted to a short-acting α-hydroxyl metabolite before undergoing glucuronide formation. Alprazolam has a medium duration of action and is primarily used in the management of **anxiety.** Although it has special utility in the treatment of **panic disorder,** the larger doses usually required for controlling panic attacks can cause considerable sedation and contribute to drug dependence. Therefore, for many patients, the panic disorder can treated instead with antidepressants and behavioral therapy. Alprazolam is useful as a short-term measure to relieve acute symptoms while other therapies are instituted.

Chlordiazepoxide and diazepam are converted to long-acting metabolites, including desmethyldiazepam (also called nordiazepam). Desmethyldiazepam is converted to oxazepam, which is excreted as a polar glucuronide conjugate (see Fig. 19–1). Chlordiazepoxide and diazepam are effective in the treatment of **anxiety.** In patients undergoing **alcohol detoxification,** these drugs can be used to prevent seizures and other acute withdrawal reactions. The drug dosage is gradually tapered over several weeks.

Diazepam is also used to terminate **acute recurrent seizures** (see Chapter 20), to treat **severe muscle spasm,** and to treat **spasticity** associated with degenerative and demyelinating neurologic disorders.

Lorazepam, oxazepam, and temazepam do not form long-acting metabolites, so they have a short or medium duration of action. They are biotransformed to inactive glucuronide compounds. As mentioned, they may be preferable for elderly patients because glucuronide conjugation does not decline significantly with aging. Lorazepam can be administered orally or intravenously and is used to treat **anxiety** and to control **seizures.** Oxazepam is a short-acting drug that is administered to patients with **anxiety.** Temazepam is primarily used to treat **insomnia.**

Estazolam, flurazepam, and triazolam have active metabolites with varying durations of action. Estazolam has a medium duration of action, whereas flurazepam has a longer one and triazolam has a shorter one. All three drugs are used to treat **insomnia.** A short- or medium-acting drug may be preferred for patients whose primary problem is getting to sleep, whereas a medium- or long-acting drug may be preferred for patients who complain of waking up too early. The short-acting triazolam is more likely to cause rebound insomnia when it is discontinued. The long-acting flurazepam is less likely to cause rebound insomnia but is more likely to cause daytime drowsiness. Triazolam has been associated with a higher incidence of amnesia, confusion, and delirium, especially in elderly patients. The dosage of triazolam in formulations marketed in the United States of America has been reduced by the FDA, and triazolam has been banned in the United Kingdom.

Other Benzodiazepines

Clonazepam is used for the treatment of **panic disorder** and **other anxiety disorders,** as well as for the treatment of **seizure disorders** (see Chapter 20).

Midazolam is used intravenously as an **anesthetic** for patients undergoing endoscopy, other diagnostic procedures, or minor surgery.

Barbiturates

The barbiturates include **amobarbital, pentobarbital, phenobarbital,** and **thiopental.** The properties, adverse effects, contraindications, and interactions of these drugs are outlined in Tables 19–1 and 19–2.

Drug Properties

PHARMACOKINETICS. The onset and duration of action of barbiturates are determined by their lipid solubility and rate of metabolic inactivation. Highly lipid-soluble drugs (e.g., amobarbital, pentobarbital, and thiopental) are well absorbed from the gut, rapidly redistributed from the brain to peripheral tissues as plasma concentrations fall, and extensively metabolized to inactive compounds before they are excreted in the urine. Phenobarbital, a more polar drug, is more slowly absorbed from the gut and more slowly redistributed from the brain, and this contributes to its longer duration of action. Phenobarbital is partly converted to inactive metabolites, but a significant fraction of the parent compound is excreted unchanged in the urine.

MECHANISM OF ACTION. Barbiturates bind to a site on the $GABA_A$ receptor chloride ion channel that is distinct from the site to which benzodiazepines bind (see Fig. 19–2). The barbiturates increase the affinity of the receptor for GABA and the duration of time that the chloride channel remains open. In contrast to the benzodiazepines, the barbiturates also act to directly increase chloride influx in the absence of GABA. For this reason, barbiturates do not exhibit a ceiling effect. As shown in Fig. 19–3, they have a linear dose-response curve. The higher doses progressively depress the CNS, causing respiratory depression, coma, and death. This accounts for the fact that the barbiturates have greater toxicity and a lower margin of safety than do the benzodiazepines.

PHARMACOLOGIC EFFECTS. Unlike the anxiolytic effect of benzodiazepines, that of barbiturates is associated with considerable sedation. When used to treat insomnia, the barbiturates can cause hangover and daytime sedation. As with the benzodiazepines, the barbiturates suppress slow-wave and REM sleep. Barbiturates can also cause tolerance and physical dependence during continuous use, and a withdrawal syndrome occurs if the drugs are abruptly discontinued. Short-acting barbiturates (e.g., pentobarbital) have been extensively abused.

INTERACTIONS. The barbiturates induce cytochrome P450 enzymes in the liver and thereby accelerate their own metabolism as well as that of other drugs metabolized by these enzymes. Maximal enzyme induction is obtained by the daily administration of phenobarbital, a long-acting agent. Barbiturates also induce the rate-limiting enzyme in porphyrin biosynthesis, δ-aminolevulinate synthase, and may thereby exacerbate porphyria, a condition in which a hereditary defect causes excessive porphyrin synthesis and excretion, with attendant neurologic and cutaneous manifestations.

INDICATIONS. The barbiturates were extensively used to treat anxiety disorders and insomnia before the development of benzodiazepines, but they are seldom used for these purposes today. Unlike the benzodiazepines, the barbiturates do not produce significant muscle relaxation and are not used in treating muscle spasm or spasticity disorders.

Specific Agents

Amobarbital and **pentobarbital** have been primarily used to treat **insomnia. Phenobarbital** is used occasionally to treat **seizure disorders,** and **thiopental** is administered intravenously to induce **anesthesia.** Thiopental has a high degree of lipid solubility and a very fast onset of action. It is also rapidly redistributed from the brain to other tissues (muscle and fat), which accounts for its short duration of action.

Antihistamines

Some of the **histamine antagonists** (antihistamines) cross the blood–brain barrier and produce varying degrees of sedation, and these drugs have been used to treat **mild insomnia and anxiety disorders.** For example, **diphenhydramine** is the active ingredient in several nonprescription sleep preparations, and **hydroxyzine** has been used in the treatment of mild anxiety and is sometimes used as a **sedative** before surgery. The sedative action of these drugs is caused by their ability to bind to H_1 heteroreceptors and reduce acetylcholine released by neurons in the reticular activating system.

Drugs that block acetylcholine release, including the **antihistamines,** induce drowsiness and sleep via their effects on the cholinergic projections of the reticular nuclei as noted above. In contrast, **caffeine** and related **methylxanthines** can increase arousal by blocking presynaptic adenosine receptors and thereby increasing cholinergic activity in the reticular nuclei.

Some tolerance can occur during the long-term use of antihistamines, but these drugs are not associated with physical dependence or significant drug abuse. The pharmacologic properties of antihistamines are discussed in detail in Chapter 26.

Other Sedative-Hypnotic Drugs

Zolpidem and Zaleplon

Zolpidem, a unique imidazopyridine compound, is believed to selectively activate the ω_1 benzodiazepine receptor on the $GABA_A$ chloride ionophore. This selectivity may account for its relative lack of effects on normal sleep architecture, in that it does not significantly suppress REM or slow-wave sleep. Benzodiazepines also interact with ω2 binding sites that are linked to adverse effects on sleep, cognitive performance, and memory. Zolpidem appears to produce relatively little tolerance and dependence, and its short duration of action usually precludes daytime sedation and hangover. For these reasons, zolpidem has become the most widely used prescription drug for treating **insomnia.** Zaleplon has the advantage that its elimination half-life is even shorter and can be taken after patients awake in the middle of the night and have difficulty going back to sleep.

Chloral Hydrate

Chloral hydrate is an older hypnotic that is largely obsolete today. It is a prodrug that is converted to its active metabolite, trichloroethanol, by liver enzymes. Its effects are potentiated by alcohol, and the combination of alcohol and chloral hydrate gained fame under the monikers of "Mickey Finn" and "knock-out drops." Chloral hydrate is occasionally used for **preanesthetic sedation** in pediatric patients.

Melatonin

Melatonin is a neuroendocrine hormone synthesized in the pineal gland. The hormone interacts with specific receptors in the CNS and elsewhere, and it is believed to be the principal mediator of the biologic clock that determines circadian, seasonal, and reproductive rhythms in animal species. In humans, melatonin is released before the onset of sleep and produces drowsiness that facilitates sleep. Studies have shown that melatonin produces drowsiness even if administered during the daytime.

Melatonin is available without prescription and is sometimes effective in the treatment of **jet lag** in individuals who have rapidly traveled across several time zones and in the treatment of **insomnia in shift-change workers.** If melatonin is taken at bedtime for a few nights, it may accelerate the resetting of the biologic clock in these persons. Melatonin may also be effective in treating **insomnia in elderly patients** who do not secrete adequate melatonin, and it appears to be effective in treating **delayed sleep-phase syndrome** and **non-24-hour sleep-wake disorder.**

Melatonin has relatively few adverse effects when taken as a drug, but it can cause fatigue and lethargy. For this reason and also because some tolerance to its hypnotic effect can develop, the lowest effective dose should be used. Melatonin may potentiate the effects of benzodiazepines, and it has been used to prevent withdrawal syndrome in patients who are having treatment for benzodiazepine dependence. The effects of melatonin may be partly antagonized by flumazenil (a benzodiazepine receptor antagonist) or by naloxone (an opioid receptor antagonist).

NONSEDATING ANXIOLYTIC DRUGS

Buspirone

Buspirone is a unique anxiolytic agent that does not share structural similarity with the other agents. The drug is used in the treatment of **chronic anxiety** and produces an anxiolytic effect without causing marked sedation, amnesia, tolerance, dependence, or muscle relaxation. In some patients, it can cause headache, dizziness, and nervousness, but these side effects are usually mild and temporary.

Buspirone is a partial agonist at serotonin 5-HT$_{1A}$ receptors and may exert its anxiolytic effect by activating feedback inhibition of serotonin release. By this action, it can cause up-regulation of postsynaptic serotonin receptors. This effect takes time to develop and is consistent with the 3- to 4-week delay in the onset of the anxiolytic effect of buspirone.

Buspirone and other drugs affecting serotonin are discussed further in Chapter 26.

Propranolol

Propranolol, a β-adrenergic receptor antagonist (β-blocker), is sometimes used to prevent the physiologic manifestations of **stage fright,** or **acute situational or performance anxiety.** When taken an hour before the anticipated anxiety-provoking event, propranolol prevents tachycardia and other signs and symptoms of acute anxiety caused by sympathetic stimulation. The β-blockers also appear to have a role in preventing similar symptoms associated with other anxiety states, such as panic disorder.

The mechanisms and properties of β-blockers are discussed in detail in Chapter 9.

SUMMARY OF IMPORTANT POINTS

- Benzodiazepines, the most widely used sedative-hypnotic drugs, are indicated for the treatment of anxiety disorders, insomnia, muscle spasm, seizure disorders, and spasticity.

- Benzodiazepines bind to an allosteric receptor site on the GABA$_A$ receptor-chloride ion channel and thereby facilitate the binding of GABA and increase the frequency with which the chloride channel opens. Benzodiazepines also decrease the release of GABA, which limits the magnitude of central nervous system depression produced by these drugs.

- Some benzodiazepines (e.g., chlordiazepoxide and diazepam) have long-acting active metabolites. Others (e.g., alprazolam, midazolam, and triazolam) have shorter-acting active metabolites. All benzodiazepines, including those with no active metabolites, are eventually converted to inactive glucuronide compounds. The benzodiazepines that have no active metabolites (e.g., lorazepam, oxazepam, and temazepam) may be the safest ones to use in the treatment of elderly patients.

- Benzodiazepines and other hypnotic drugs reduce the time required to fall asleep (sleep latency), reduce early awakenings, and increase total sleep time. Benzodiazepines and barbiturates reduce slow-wave sleep and rapid eye movement (REM) sleep.

- Pentobarbital, phenobarbital, and other barbiturates bind to the GABA$_A$ receptor-chloride ion channel but do not exhibit a ceiling effect and can cause respiratory depression, coma, and death.

- Unlike benzodiazepines, barbiturates induce their own metabolism as well as that of many other drugs metabolized by cytochrome P450 enzymes.

- Long-term administration of benzodiazepines and barbiturates can lead to tolerance and physical dependence, and abrupt discontinuation of their use will cause symptoms of withdrawal.

- Zolpidem and zaleplon are effective short-acting sedative-hypnotic agents that have little effect on normal sleep architecture and produce few adverse effects.

■ Sedating antihistamines (e.g., diphenhydramine and hydroxyzine) have been used to treat mild insomnia and anxiety. Older hypnotics (e.g., chloral hydrate) are largely obsolete but are occasionally used for preanesthetic sedation.

■ Propranolol and other β-adrenergic receptor antagonists can be used to prevent the physiologic manifestations of situational or performance anxiety, including tachycardia.

■ Flumazenil is a benzodiazepine receptor antagonist that can be used to counteract respiratory depression and other reactions that are usually caused by excessive doses of intravenously administered benzodiazepines.

Review Questions

1. Which of the following molecular processes best describes the mechanism of action of benzodiazepines?
   (A) potentiating the effect of GABA at Cl⁻ ion channels
   (B) blocking glutamate excitation
   (C) blocking the inactivation of Na⁺ ion channels
   (D) binding to opioid receptors to produce sedation
   (E) potentiating the action of the inhibitory amino acid, glycine

2. Benzodiazepines are noted for altering which one of the following aspects of sleep?
   (A) increasing the time to sleep onset
   (B) decreasing stage 2 non-REM sleep
   (C) increasing slow-wave sleep
   (D) decreasing the REM stage of sleep
   (E) increasing sleep awakenings

3. Which one of the following statement best describes flumazenil?
   (A) does not produce withdrawal seizures
   (B) has the longest elimination half-life
   (C) is not metabolized into an active agent
   (D) is also used for the treatment of epilepsy
   (E) is a selective benzodiazepine antagonist

4. Zaleplon differs from zolpidem in which one of the following ways?
   (A) produces withdrawal seizures
   (B) has a shorter elimination half-life
   (C) has a different chemical structure than benzodiazepines
   (D) shows less tolerance to sedative effects
   (E) produces greater morning sedation

5. Which one of the following anxiolytic drugs is noted for its lack of sedation?
   (A) hydroxyzine
   (B) diazepam
   (C) oxazepam
   (D) alprazolam
   (E) buspirone

Answers to Review Questions

1. The correct answer is A: potentiating the effect of GABA at Cl⁻ ion channels. Benzodiazepines bind to an allosteric site on the GABA_A receptor-ion channel complex to increase the affinity of GABA. GABA action increases the conductance of Cl⁻ ion into the neuron, thereby hyperpolarizing the membrane and making it harder to reach depolarization threshold and fire action potentials. Answer (B), blocking glutamate excitation, is the mechanism of action of NMDA receptor antagonists. Answer (C), blocking the inactivation of Na⁺ ion channels, is the mechanism of action of certain antiepileptic agents. Answer (D), binding to opioid receptors to produce sedation, is the site of opioid analgesic action. Answer (E), potentiating the action of the inhibitory amino acid, glycine, is incorrect because benzodiazepines do not have significant binding affinity for the glycine receptor.

2. The correct choice is D: decreasing the REM stage of sleep. Benzodiazepines are noted for decreasing the time spent in REM sleep, an effect that is unmasked by REM rebound after the administration of the benzodiazepine is stopped. Answer (A), increasing the time to sleep onset, is the opposite effect of sedative-hypnotics, which decrease the latency to sleep. Answer (B), decreasing stage 2 non-REM sleep, is not correct, because studies do not show a consistent effect of benzodiazepines on stage 2 NREM sleep. Answer (C), increasing slow-wave sleep, may be beneficial to a restful sleep but no evidence suggests that benzodiazepines produce this effect. Choice (E), increasing sleep awakenings, occurs in patients with insomnia, a symptom that benzodiazepines and other sedative-hypnotic agents hope to treat.

3. The correct choice is E: is a selective benzodiazepine antagonist. Flumazenil is a competitive antagonist of the benzodiazepine receptor. The availability of flumanzenil to reverse benzodiazepine action is useful in cases of drug overdose or in outpatient procedures to bring patients back to normal wakefulness. Answer (A), does not produce withdrawal seizures, is certainly true; however, it is not the best statement describing flumazenil. Answer (B), has the longest elimination half-life, is not true because often flumazenil must be given in repeated administrations to reverse the effects of a longer-lasting benzodiazepine such as diazepam. Answer (C), is not metabolized into an active agent, is also true but is not the best choice. Answer (D), is also used for the treatment of epilepsy, is incorrect regarding the indicated uses of flumazenil.

4. The correct answer is B: has a shorter elimination half-life. Zaleplon, as with zolpidem, has a more selective action than true benzodiazepines. It has the advantage that it has a shorter half-life and therefore is approved for those patients who awaken in the middle of the night and cannot return to sleep. Answer (A), produces withdrawal seizures, is true for both zolpidem and zaleplon. Answer (C), has a different chemical structure than benzodiazepines, and answer (D), shows less tolerance to sedative

effects, are also true for both agents. Answer (E), produces greater morning sedation, is not true and both agents do not produce much sedation after their initial hypnotic effect.

5. The correct answer is E: buspirone. Buspirone is a unique, nonsedating anxiolytic agent mediating its effects by way of the 5-HT receptor. No sedative effects are associated with its action, although it differs in that it may take from 2 to 4 weeks of daily administration for clinical effectiveness. Answers (A) through (D) are all sedating drugs, including the antihistamine, hydroxyzine, and the benzodiazepines, diazepam, oxazepam, and alprazolam.

SELECTED READINGS

Bateson, A. N. The benzodiazepine site of the GABA$_A$ receptor: an old target with new potential? Sleep Med 5(Suppl 1):S9–S15, 2004.

Terzano, M. G., M. Rossi, V. Palomba, et al. New drugs for insomnia: comparative tolerability of zopiclone, zolpidem and zaleplon. Drug Saf 26(4):261–282, 2003.

Verster, J. C., D. S. Veldhuijzen, and E. R. Volkerts. Residual effects of sleep medication on driving ability. Sleep Med Rev 8(4):309–325, 2004.

Yaksh, T. L., and J. W. Allen. The use of intrathecal midazolam in humans: a case study of process. Anesth Analg 98(6):1536–1545, 2004.

Zhdanova, I. V. Advances in the management of insomnia. Expert Opin Pharmacother 5(7):1573–1579, 2004.

CHAPTER 20

Antiepileptic Drugs

OVERVIEW

Seizures are episodes of abnormal electrical activity in the brain that cause involuntary movements, sensations, or thoughts. Seizures can result from head trauma, stroke, brain tumors, hypoxia, hypoglycemia, fever, alcohol withdrawal, and other conditions that alter neuronal function. Recurrent seizures that cannot be attributed to any proximal cause are seen in patients with **epilepsy.** In some patients, epilepsy appears to have a genetic basis. Environmental perturbations (e.g., intrauterine or neonatal complications) have also been implicated in the development of epilepsy. In the United States of America, epilepsy affects 1% to 2% of the population and is the second most common neurologic disease after stroke.

Classification of Seizures

The two main categories of seizures are **partial (focal) seizures** and **generalized seizures** (Table 20–1). A partial seizure originates in one cerebral hemisphere, and the patient does not lose consciousness during the seizure. A generalized seizure arises in both cerebral hemispheres and involves loss of consciousness. Seizures are accompanied by characteristic changes in the electroencephalogram (EEG), as shown in Fig. 20–1. Most seizures are self-limited and last from about 10 seconds to 5 minutes. Some seizures are preceded by an **aura,** which is a sensation or mood that may help identify the anatomic location of the seizure focus.

About 60% of epileptic seizures are partial seizures. Electroencephalographic abnormalities are seen in one or more lobes of a cerebral hemisphere, and the patient may exhibit motor, sensory, and autonomic symptoms. In **simple partial seizures,** consciousness is not altered. In **complex partial seizures,** however, patients have an altered consciousness and exhibit repetitive behaviors (automatisms). Complex partial seizures often originate in the temporal lobe, in which case the disorder is called either **temporal lobe epilepsy** or **psychomotor epilepsy.** Some partial seizures progress along anatomic lines as the electrical discharges spread across the cortex. For example, the seizure first involves the fingers, then the hand, and finally the entire arm. This is characteristic of **jacksonian epilepsy,** or **jacksonian march.** Partial seizures can also evolve into generalized seizures.

The two main types of generalized seizures are **tonic–clonic seizures** and **absence seizures.** Generalized

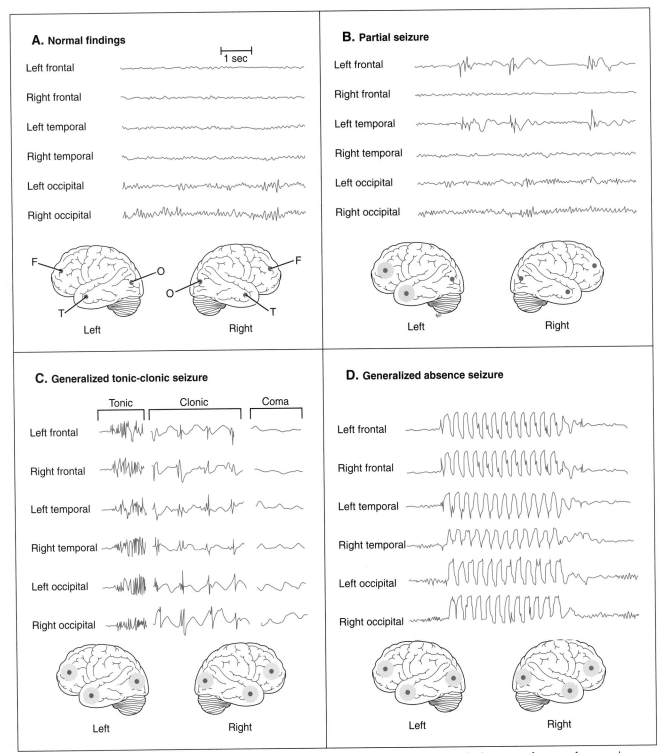

Figure 20–1. Patterns on electroencephalogram (EEG) in the normal state and during seizures. The locations of seizure foci are shown as shaded areas on the cerebral hemispheres. (A) In the normal state, the EEG shows asynchronous alpha (8 to 12 Hz) and beta (12 to 30 Hz) rhythms originating in the cortex of the frontal (F), temporal (T), and occipital (O) lobes. (B) During a partial seizure, synchronous discharges are observed in various areas of the brain. In this example, they are seen in the left frontal and left temporal lobes, but they are not seen in other lobes. (C) During a generalized tonic–clonic seizure, the tonic phase is characterized by low-frequency and high-amplitude waves, whereas the clonic phase shows synchronous oscillations. (D) During a generalized absence seizure, a synchronous 3-Hz spike-and-wave pattern is seen throughout the cortex.

TABLE 20-1. International Classification of Partial and Generalized Seizures

Classification	Characterization
Partial (focal) seizures	Arise in one cerebral hemisphere
Simple partial seizure	No alteration of consciousness
Complex partial seizure	Altered consciousness, automatisms, and behavioral changes
Secondarily generalized seizure	Focal seizure becomes generalized and is accompanied by loss of consciousness.
Generalized seizures	Arise in both cerebral hemispheres and are accompanied by loss of consciousness
Tonic-clonic (grand mal) seizure	Increased muscle tone is followed by spasms of muscle contraction and relaxation
Tonic seizure	Increased muscle tone
Clonic seizure	Spasms of muscle contraction and relaxation
Myoclonic seizure	Rhythmic, jerking spasms
Atonic seizure	Sudden loss of all muscle tone
Absence (petit mal) seizure	Brief loss of consciousness, with minor muscle twitches and eye blinking

tonic–clonic seizures, which were formerly called **grand mal seizures,** begin with a brief tonic phase that is followed by a clonic phase with muscle spasms lasting 3 to 5 minutes, and they conclude with a postictal period of drowsiness, confusion, and a glazed look in the eyes. **Status epilepticus** is a condition in which patients experience recurrent episodes of tonic–clonic seizures without regaining consciousness or normal muscle movement between episodes. Generalized **absence seizures,** or **petit mal seizures,** are characterized by abrupt loss of consciousness and decreased muscle tone, and they can include a mild clonic component, automatisms, and autonomic effects. On the EEG, generalized absence seizures exhibit a synchronous 3-Hz (three cycles per second) spike-and-dome pattern that usually lasts 10 to 15 seconds.

Less common types of generalized seizures include **myoclonic seizures** and **atonic seizures** (see Table 20–1).

Neurobiology of Seizures

Epileptic seizures are caused by synchronous neuronal discharges within a particular group of neurons, or **seizure focus,** which is often located in the cerebral cortex but can be found in other areas of the brain. Once initiated, the abnormal discharges spread to other parts of the brain and produce abnormal movements, sensations, or thoughts. The neuronal mechanisms that initiate a seizure are not fully understood, but growing evidence indicates the involvement of excessive excitatory neurotransmission mediated by **glutamate** (Fig. 20–2). Investigators believe that excessive activation by glumatate of N-methyl-D-aspartate (**NMDA**)

receptors displaces Mg^{2+} ions from the **NMDA-calcium ion channel** and thereby facilitates calcium entry into neurons. **Calcium** contributes to the long-term potentiation (LTP) of excitatory glutamate neurotransmission by activating the synthesis of nitric oxide (NO).

Nitric oxide is a gas that can diffuse backward to the presynaptic neuron, where it facilitates glutamate release via stimulation of a G protein that activates the synthesis of cyclic guanosine monophosphate (cGMP). These actions further increase NMDA receptor activation and calcium influx, which are believed to contribute to the **depolarization shift** that is observed in seizure foci. The depolarization shift consists of abnormally prolonged action potentials (depolarizations) that have spikelets. The shift recruits and synchronizes depolarizations by surrounding neurons and thereby initiates a seizure.

Several other mechanisms can be involved in seizures. One is the suppression of inhibitory neurotransmission of **γ-aminobutyric acid** (GABA), and another is an increase in calcium influx via T-type calcium channels in thalamic neurons.

Mechanisms of Antiepileptic Drugs

Antiepileptic drugs are believed to suppress the formation or spread of abnormal electrical discharges in the brain. As shown in Table 20–2, the currently available drugs accomplish these actions via three mechanisms: (1) inhibition of the sodium or calcium influx responsible for neuronal depolarization, (2) augmentation of inhibitory GABA neurotransmission, and (3) inhibition of excitatory glutamate neurotransmission.

Effects on Ion Channels

Under normal circumstances, **voltage-sensitive (voltage-gated) sodium channels** are rapidly opened when the neuronal membrane potential (voltage) reaches its threshold. This causes rapid depolarization of the membrane and the conduction of an action potential along the neuronal axon. When the action potential reaches the nerve terminal, it evokes the release of a neurotransmitter. After the neuronal membrane is depolarized, the sodium channel is inactivated by closure of the channel's inactivation gate. The inactivation gate must be opened before the next action potential can occur.

Many antiepileptic drugs, including carbamazepine, lamotrigine, phenytoin, and topiramate, prolong the time that the sodium channel's inactivation gate remains closed, and this delays the formation of the next action potential. These drugs bind to the channel when it is opened. Because rapidly firing neurons are opened a greater percentage of the time than are slowly firing neurons, the drugs exhibit use-dependent blockade. For this reason, the drugs suppress abnormal repetitive depolarizations in a seizure focus more than they suppress normal neuronal activity. By these actions, carbamazepine and other drugs prevent the spread of abnormal discharges in a seizure focus to other neurons.

A few drugs (e.g., ethosuximide and valproate) block **T-type (low-threshold) calcium channels** that are located in thalamic neurons and participate in the initiation of generalized absence seizures.

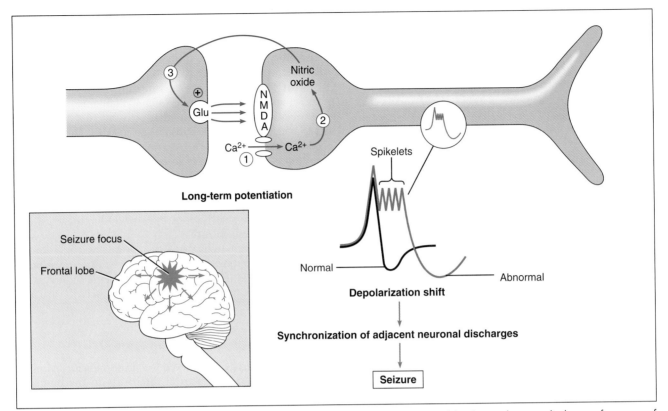

Figure 20–2. Neuronal mechanisms underlying seizures. In this example, a seizure is caused by the synchronous discharge of a group of neurons (focus) in the cortex. Activation of N-methyl-D-aspartate (NMDA) receptors increases calcium influx and nitric oxide synthesis. Nitric oxide then diffuses to the presynaptic neuron and increases the release of glutamate (Glu) via formation of cyclic guanosine monophosphate. Increased excitatory glutamate neurotransmission leads to long-term potentiation. Long-term potentiation is believed to facilitate a depolarization shift, characterized by prolonged depolarizations with spikelets. The depolarization shift can cause adjacent neurons to discharge synchronously and thereby precipitate a seizure.

TABLE 20–2. Mechanisms of Antiepileptic Drugs*

Drug	Effects on Ion Flux	Effects on GABA	Effects on Glutamate
Carbamazepine	Blocks voltage-sensitive sodium channels	—	—
Clonazepam	—	Enhances GABA-mediated chloride flux	—
Clorazepate	—	Enhances GABA-mediated chloride flux	—
Diazepam	—	Enhances GABA-mediated chloride flux	—
Ethosuximide	Blocks T-type calcium channels	—	—
Felbamate	—	—	Blocks glycine activation of NMDA receptors
Gabapentin	—	Increases GABA release	—
Lamotrigine	Blocks voltage-sensitive sodium channels	—	—
Lorazepam	—	Enhances GABA-mediated chloride flux	—
Phenobarbital	—	Enhances GABA-mediated chloride flux	—
Phenytoin	Blocks voltage-sensitive sodium channels	—	—
Primidone	Possibly blocks voltage-sensitive sodium channels	Enhances GABA-mediated chloride flux	—
Topiramate	Blocks voltage-sensitive sodium channels	Increases GABA activation of CABA$_A$ receptors	Blocks kainate and AMPA receptors
Valproate	Possibly blocks voltage-sensitive sodium channels and T-type calcium channels	Increases GABA synthesis and inhibits GABA degradation	Possibly decreases glutamate synthesis

*AMPA = α-amino-3-hydroxy-5-methyl-4-isoxazole propionic acid; GABA = gamma-aminobutyric acid; and NMDA = N-Methyl-D-aspartate.

Effects on GABAergic Systems

Antiepileptic drugs facilitate GABA neurotransmission by various means. Benzodiazepines (e.g., clonazepam) and barbiturates (e.g., phenobarbital) enhance GABA activation of the **GABA$_A$ receptor-chloride ion channel** (see Chapter 19). Topiramate is believed to enhance activation of the **GABA$_A$ receptor.** Gabapentin increases GABA release, whereas valproate inhibits GABA degradation. Drugs that augment GABA may serve to counteract the excessive excitatory neurotransmission responsible for initiating and spreading abnormal electrical discharges.

Effects on Glutaminergic Systems

A few antiepileptic drugs, including felbamate, topiramate, and valproate, inhibit glutamate neurotransmission, and other drugs that work via this mechanism are under development. This is an attractive mechanism of action because it may affect the formation of a seizure focus and thereby terminate a seizure at an early stage of its development.

TREATMENT OF SEIZURE DISORDERS

As indicated in the drugs listed in the box at the beginning of this chapter, some are active against only one or two types of seizures. In contrast, valproate has a broad spectrum of activity and is active against most types of seizures. Newer agents (e.g., lamotrigine and topiramate) are primarily used in combination with other drugs for the treatment of partial seizures. These newer agents are particularly useful because complex partial seizures are more resistant to treatment than are other types of seizures.

The pharmacologic properties of antiepileptic drugs are described below, whereas the mechanisms of action, adverse effects, contraindications, and drug interactions are given in Tables 20–2, 20–3, and 20–4.

Drugs for Partial and Generalized Tonic-Clonic Seizures

The first-line drugs for partial seizures and generalized tonic–clonic seizures are carbamazepine, phenytoin, and valproate. Carbamazepine and phenytoin have a similar mechanism of action and clinical effectiveness, and both drugs induce cytochrome P450 enzymes and increase drug metabolism. Valproate acts by a different mechanism and inhibits cytochrome P450 enzymes. Two other drugs that are effective against partial seizures as well as generalized tonic–clonic seizures are phenobarbital and primidone.

Carbamazepine

CHEMISTRY AND PHARMACOKINETICS. Carbamazepine has a tricyclic structure that resembles the structure of tricyclic antidepressants such as imipramine. Carbamazepine is adequately absorbed after oral administration, and it is biotransformed to an active metabolite, carbamazepine epoxide. Almost all the drug is excreted as metabolites in the urine and feces.

MECHANISMS AND EFFECTS. Carbamazepine blocks voltage-sensitive sodium channels in neuronal cell membranes. As described, blockade of these channels inhibits the spread of abnormal electrical discharges from the seizure focus to other neurons by preventing the release of excitatory neurotransmitters from nerve terminals. Carbamazepine has additional mechanisms of action, but their contributions to its antiepileptic effects are unknown. For example, carbamazepine blocks adenosine receptors in a way that leads to up-regulation of these receptors, and it blocks norepinephrine reuptake in the same way that tricyclic antidepressants block it. The latter action is probably responsible for the mood-elevating effect of carbamazepine.

Carbamazepine can cause drowsiness, ataxia, and other symptoms of central nervous system (CNS) depression, as well as gastrointestinal reactions. Rarely, its use has been associated with aplastic anemia. In general, carbamazepine usually produces fewer adverse effects than does phenytoin.

INTERACTIONS. Carbamazepine is a potent inducer of cytochrome P450 enzymes that metabolize a wide range of drugs. Carbamazepine accelerates its own metabolism as well as that of many other drugs, including lamotrigine, phenytoin, topiramate, and valproate. For this reason, it decreases the serum level and effects of these drugs. Carbamazepine can also increase lithium toxicity.

INDICATIONS. In addition to its use in treating partial seizures and generalized tonic–clonic seizures, carbamazepine is the drug of choice for trigeminal neuralgia (tic douloureux), a condition that can cause chronic and intense pain on one or both sides of the face. Carbamazepine is also effective as an alternative to lithium in the treatment of bipolar disorder, a mood disorder discussed in Chapter 22.

Phenytoin and Fosphenytoin

CHEMISTRY AND PHARMACOKINETICS. Phenytoin is a hydantoin derivative formerly called diphenylhydantoin. It is poorly soluble in water, and different pharmaceutical formulations of it may have different bioavailabilities. Hence, it is prudent to avoid switching from one formulation to another. If a switch must be made, serum drug levels should be monitored. A new formulation, called **fosphenytoin,** has become available for parenteral administration. Fosphenytoin is more soluble in water, and this prevents precipitation of the drug after intramuscular or intravenous administration.

Phenytoin is converted to an inactive hydroxylated metabolite by cytochrome P450 enzymes. The drug exhibits dose-dependent kinetics, whereby lower concentrations are eliminated by a first-order process but higher concentrations saturate biotransformation enzymes and exhibit zero-order kinetics. Phenytoin hydroxylation also exhibits genetic polymorphism. These factors are responsible for the considerable interpatient variation in the plasma drug concentrations produced by a given dose. Because of this variation, serum drug levels should be monitored at the start of therapy and whenever toxicity or therapeutic failure occurs.

MECHANISMS AND EFFECTS. As with carbamazepine, phenytoin blocks voltage-sensitive sodium channels by prolonging the inactivation state of these channels. This enables phenytoin to inhibit the repetitive firing of neurons in a seizure focus.

Phenytoin can cause a number of adverse effects. The drug interferes with folate metabolism, and this can lead to

TABLE 20–3. Adverse Effects, Contraindications, and Pregnancy Risk Data for Antiepileptic Drugs

Drug	Major Adverse Effects	Contraindications	Risk Category and Effects of Use During Pregnancy*
Carbamazepine	Aplastic anemia (rare); ataxia, drowsiness, and other symptoms of central nervous system (CNS) depression; gastrointestinal reactions; and nausea	Hypersensitivity	Category C; increased risk of birth defects; abnormal facial features; neural tube defects, such as spina bifida; reduced head size; and other anomalies
Clonazepam	Arrhythmia; CNS depression; drug dependence; hypotension; and mild respiratory depression	Acute angle-closure glaucoma; hypersensitivity; and severe liver disease	Category C; apnea in newborn; increased risk of birth defects
Clorazepate	Confusion; drowsiness; drug tolerance; and lethargy	Hypersensitivity	Category D; increased risk of birth defects
Diazepam	Same as clonazepam	Same as clonazepam	Category D; increased risk of birth defects
Ethosuximide	Dizziness; drowsiness; gastric distress; lethargy; and nausea	Hypersensitivity	Category C
Felbamate	Aplastic anemia; fatigue; gastrointestinal reactions; headache; hepatic toxicity; and insomnia	Bone marrow depression; hepatic disease; and hypersensitivity	Category C
Gabapentin	Ataxia; dizziness; drowsiness; nystagmus; and tremor	Hypersensitivity	Category C
Lamotrigine	Ataxia; diplopia; dizziness; drowsiness; headache; nausea; rash; and Stevens-Johnson syndrome	Hypersensitivity. Use cautiously in patients who are taking valproate or have hepatic or renal disease	Category C; may reduce folate levels
Levetiracetam	Somnolence, asthenia (weakness), infection and dizziness	Hypersensitivity	Category C; levetiracetam produced evidence of developmental toxicity at doses similar to or greater than human therapeutic doses
Lorazepam	Same as clonazepam	Same as clonazepam	Category D; increased risk of birth defects
Phenobarbital	Ataxia; cognitive impairment; dizziness; drowsiness; drug dependence; rash; and respiratory depression	Hypersensitivity; porphyria; respiratory depression; and severe liver disease	Category D; bleeding at birth; minor congenital defects
Phenytoin	Cerebellar symptoms; gastrointestinal disturbances; gingival hyperplasia; hirsutism; megaloblastic anemia and other blood cell deficiencies; osteomalacia; and psychiatric changes	Bradycardia; hypersensitivity; and severe atrioventricular block or sinoatrial dysfunction	Category D; may reduce folate levels; 2–3 times increased risk of birth defects; fetal hydantoin syndrome
Primidone	Same as phenobarbital	Hypersensitivity	Category D
Tiagabine	Dizziness, somnolence, nausea, nervousness, abdominal pain, and difficulty with concentration or attention	Hypersensitivity	Category C; adverse effects on embryo-fetal development, including teratogenic effects at doses greater than the human therapeutic dose
Topiramate	Ataxia; dizziness; drowsiness; nystagmus; paresthesia; and psychomotor impairment	Hypersensitivity. Use cautiously during pregnancy, during lactation, or in the presence of hepatic or renal disease	Category C
Valproate	Drowsiness; gastrointestinal disturbances; hepatic toxicity (rare); nausea; and weight gain	Hepatic disease and hypersensitivity	Category D; may reduce folate levels; teratogenic during the first trimester; neural tube defects, such as spina bifida
Vigabatrin	Amnesia; blurred visions; blue-yellow color blindness; decreased vision or other vision changes; eye pains; (rare) increase in seizures	Hypersensitivity	Category C; studies in rabbits have shown that vigabatrin causes birth defects
Zonisamide	Somnolence, anorexia, dizziness, headache, nausea, and agitation/irritability	Hypersensitivity	Category C; teratogenic in mice, rats, and dogs and embryolethal in monkeys when administered during the period of organogenesis at zonisamide dosage and maternal plasma levels similar to or lower than therapeutic levels in humans

*Pregnancy risk categories are defined by the Food Cand Drug Administration as follows: A = controlled studies show no risk; B = no evidence of risk in humans; C = risk cannot be ruled out; D = positive evidence of risk; and X = contraindicated in pregnancy.

TABLE 20-4. Interactions of Antiepileptic Drugs

Antiepileptic Drug	Interacting Drugs That Increase Serum Levels*	Interacting Drugs That Decrease Serum Levels†	Interactions That Cause Other Effects
Carbamazepine	Cimetidine, diltiazem, erythromycin, fluoxetine, isoniazid, and propoxyphene.	Carbamazepine.	Decreases serum levels of calcium channel blockers, clozapine, haloperidol, steroids, theophylline, thyroid, and warfarin. Increases lithium toxicity.
Clonazepam	Cimetidine and disulfiram.	Rifampin.	Increases central nervous system (CNS) depression if alcohol is ingested.
Clorazepate	Cimetidine and disulfiram.	Rifampin.	Increases CNS depression if alcohol is ingested.
Diazepam	Cimetidine.	Rifampin.	Increases CNS depression if alcohol is ingested.
Ethosuximide	Valproate.	—	May alter seizure pattern if taken in combination with haloperidol.
Felbamate	—	Carbamazepine and phenytoin.	Increases CNS depression if alcohol is ingested.
Gabapentin	—	Antacids.	—
Lamotrigine	Valproate.	Carbamazepine, phenobarbital, and phenytoin.	Decreases serum levels of valproate.
Lorazepam	—	Rifampin.	Increases CNS depression if alcohol is ingested.
Phenobarbital	Valproate.	Phenobarbital.	Decreases serum levels of many drugs. Increases meperidine toxicity.
Phenytoin	Chloramphenicol, cimetidine, isoniazid, and sulfonamides.	Carbamazepine.	Decreases serum levels of amiodarone, digoxin, quinidines, steroids, theophylline, vitamin K, and other agents.
Primidone	Valproate.	Phenobarbital.	—
Topiramate	—	Carbamazepine and phenytoin.	Decreases serum levels of oral contraceptives.
Valproate	Salicylates.	Carbamazepine, lamotrigine, and phenytoin.	May increase or decrease serum levels of carbamazepine and phenytoin.

*These drugs inhibit metabolism.
†Except for antacids (which reduce the absorption of gabapentin), these drugs induce metabolism.

megaloblastic anemia. Folate antagonism can also contribute to birth defects such as those seen in fetal hydantoin syndrome (a syndrome characterized by cardiac defects; malformation of ears, lips, palate, mouth, and nasal bridge; mental retardation; microcephaly; ptosis; strabismus; and other anomalies). By impairing cerebellar function, phenytoin can cause ataxia, diplopia, nystagmus, and slurred speech. By interfering with vitamin D metabolism and decreasing calcium absorption from the gut, phenytoin sometimes causes osteomalacia. Phenytoin adversely affects collagen metabolism and thereby contributes to gingival hyperplasia, a condition in which the gums can extend down over the teeth if good dental hygiene is not practiced. It can also cause hirsutism (excessive hair growth). Because of these effects, phenytoin use in children should generally be avoided.

INTERACTIONS. Phenytoin induces the CYP3A4 isozyme of cytochrome P450 and accelerates the metabolism of other antiepileptic agents, including felbamate, lamotrigine, topiramate, and valproate. It can also reduce levels of digoxin, steroids, vitamin K, and other drugs. In patients who are being treated with phenytoin, vitamin K supplements should be given to prevent hypoprothrombinemia and bleeding.

Carbamazepine induces the metabolism of phenytoin and decreases its serum levels, whereas cimetidine and other drugs inhibit the metabolism of phenytoin and increase its serum levels.

INDICATIONS. Despite its many adverse effects and drug interactions, phenytoin is widely used in the treatment of partial seizures and generalized tonic–clonic seizures. As with carbamazepine, it can worsen absence seizures and should not be used in patients with this type of seizures.

Phenobarbital and Primidone

Phenobarbital and primidone are both second-line drugs for **partial seizures** and **generalized tonic–clonic seizures.** Phenobarbital, a barbiturate, is the oldest of the currently used antiepileptic drugs. Its pharmacologic properties are discussed in Chapter 19. Primidone has two active metabolites, phenobarbital and phenylethylmalonamide (PEMA), and the parent drug and its active metabolites probably all contribute to its antiepileptic effects.

Phenobarbital enhances the GABA-mediated chloride flux that causes membrane hyperpolarization. Primidone probably acts primarily by blocking sodium channels and preventing membrane depolarization. It can also potentiate GABA via formation of phenobarbital. Both primidone and phenobarbital are well absorbed from the gut, but primidone has a shorter half-life and therefore reaches steady-state levels more rapidly. Both drugs can cause ataxia, dizziness, drowsiness, and cognitive impairment. In excessive doses, they can depress respiration. Hypersensitivity to these drugs develops in a few patients and most frequently presents as a rash.

Valproate

CHEMISTRY AND PHARMACOKINETICS. Valproate is a low molecular weight, branched-chain fatty acid. Several valproate formulations are available, including the free acid form (valproic acid), the sodium salt of valproic acid (valproate sodium), and a 1 : 1 mixture of valproic acid and valproate sodium (divalproex sodium). Divalproex sodium is absorbed more slowly than the other formulations, and it usually causes fewer adverse gastrointestinal and CNS side effects. Valproate is well absorbed from the gut and is metabolized to active metabolites and inactive conjugates before it is excreted.

MECHANISMS AND EFFECTS. Valproate has several mechanisms of action that probably contribute to its broad spectrum of antiepileptic effects. It inhibits voltage-sensitive sodium channels and T-type calcium channels; it increases GABA synthesis and decreases GABA degradation; and it may decrease glutamate synthesis. By these actions, valproate inhibits the repetitive firing of neurons and the spread of epileptic seizures.

Valproate produces relatively little sedation or drowsiness, but it occasionally causes nausea, gastrointestinal complaints, and weight gain. Mild hepatic toxicity sometimes occurs and is usually reversible. Rarely, the drug has been associated with fatal hepatic toxicity. To prevent liver damage, the hepatic function of patients should be monitored when they begin therapy with valproate. Patients under 2 years of age are at the greatest risk of liver failure.

Valproate has been associated with an increased incidence of spina bifida and other birth defects in the offspring of women treated with the drug during pregnancy.

INTERACTIONS. Valproate inhibits the metabolism of other drugs and can increase the serum levels of lamotrigine, phenobarbital, and primidone. It can either increase or decrease the levels of carbamazepine and phenytoin, whereas these drugs decrease the levels of valproate. Because of these interactions, serum levels should always be monitored when another drug is added to or removed from the treatment regimen of a patient with seizure disorders. Patients should be warned that salicylates can increase the serum levels of valproate.

INDICATIONS. Of the various antiepileptic drugs, valproate has the broadest spectrum of activity. It is effective in the treatment of partial seizures and all forms of generalized seizures, and it can be given in combination with other drugs when a single drug does not adequately control seizures (see below). Valproate is also used as an alternative to lithium to treat bipolar disorder (see Chapter 22).

Adjunct Drugs for Partial Seizures

The most difficult seizures to control with drug therapy are partial seizures and, especially, complex partial seizures. Efforts, therefore, have focused on developing new drugs for these seizures. Unlike clorazepate, the other drugs discussed below were recently introduced. Additional drugs recently approved for the adjunct treatment of partial seizures include tiagabine, vigabatrin, zonisamide, and levetiracetam.

Clorazepate

Clorazepate is a prodrug that is converted to diazepam in the body. Although it primarily has been used to treat patients with **anxiety disorders,** it also has been found useful as an adjunct drug for the treatment of **partial seizures.** It can cause drowsiness and lethargy, and tolerance can occur during long-term use of the drug.

Felbamate

Felbamate was a promising new drug for the treatment of partial seizures and other types of seizures until cases of fatal aplastic anemia and acute hepatic failure were reported. Since 1994, felbamate has been limited to the treatment of **partial seizures that are refractory to other drugs.** Felbamate has a unique mechanism of action in that it blocks glycine activation of NMDA receptors and thereby can inhibit processes responsible for the initiation of seizures. Efforts are under way to develop other drugs that act via this mechanism but exhibit less toxicity than felbamate.

Gabapentin

Gabapentin is a GABA analogue that appears to act by increasing the release of GABA from central neurons. It has no direct effect on GABA receptors itself. The absorption of gabapentin from the gut is inversely related to the dose. Because the drug has a relatively short half-life, it must be given several times a day. Gabapentin is effective when used in combination with other drugs to treat **all forms of partial seizures,** and studies indicate that for many patients it is also effective when used alone. Its adverse effects are minimal at usual therapeutic doses, but it can cause ataxia, dizziness, drowsiness, nystagmus, and tremor.

Lamotrigine

Lamotrigine blocks voltage-sensitive sodium channels and thereby interferes with neuronal membrane conduction and the release of excitatory neurotransmitters such as glutamate. It appears to be one of the more effective adjunct drugs for treating **partial seizures** in adults and children. It also appears to be useful in the treatment of **generalized tonic–clonic, atonic, and absence seizures** and in the treatment of **Lennox-Gastaut syndrome,** a syndrome characterized by multiple types of seizures in patients with mental retardation and other neurologic abnormalities.

Lamotrigine has excellent oral bioavailability. It is mostly conjugated with glucuronate in the liver and excreted by the kidneys. Serum levels of lamotrigine are decreased by carbamazepine and phenytoin and are increased by valproate. Serum levels of valproate are decreased by lamotrigine.

The primary side effects of lamotrigine include cerebellar dysfunction, drowsiness, and rash. Patients should be advised to report early signs of skin changes, because the rash can progress to Stevens-Johnson syndrome. This potentially fatal syndrome, a severe form of erythema multiforme, is characterized by mucocutaneous and systemic lesions, including ocular, gastrointestinal, cardiac, renal, and pulmonary inflammation and hemorrhage. The syndrome is more common in patients who are being treated with the combination of lamotrigine and valproate, possibly because valproate increases the serum level of lamotrigine. If children are treated with both drugs, the dosage of lamotrigine should be lower than that used in other patients. Dosage guidelines are provided in prescribing compendiums.

Topiramate

Topiramate is a monosaccharide derivative that has several mechanisms of action, including blockade of voltage-sensitive sodium channels; augmentation of GABA activation of $GABA_A$ receptors; and blockade of two types of glutamate receptors, namely, kainate receptors and α-amino-3-hydroxy-5-methyl-4-isoxazole propionic acid (AMPA) receptors.

Clinical studies indicate that about half of patients who have intractable partial seizures experience a 50% reduction in seizure frequency when topiramate is added to their treatment regimen. Therefore, topiramate is approved for adjunct use in the treatment of **partial seizures.** Because it has also demonstrated effectiveness as single-drug therapy (monotherapy) for partial seizures and as an adjunct in the treatment of generalized seizures, it may receive approval for these indications in the future.

Topiramate is adequately absorbed from the gut, is partly metabolized before excretion in the urine, and has a half-life of about 21 hours. Carbamazepine and phenytoin may induce the metabolism of topiramate and decrease its serum level. Topiramate may reduce the serum level of oral contraceptives. The side effects of topiramate include ataxia, dizziness, drowsiness, and other CNS effects listed in Table 20–3.

Tiagabine

Tiagabine binds to recognition sites associated with the GABA reuptake transport protein. By this action, tiagabine blocks GABA reuptake into presynaptic neurons, permitting greater levels of GABA in the synapse.

Vigabatrin

Vigabatrin is an irreversible inhibitor of γ-aminobutyric acid transaminase (GABA-T), the enzyme responsible for the breakdown of GABA in the brain. The inhibition of the GABA-T enzyme leads to increased levels of the inhibitory neurotransmitter, GABA.

Zonisamide

Zonisamide acts at sodium channels and voltage-dependent, transient inward currents (low-threshold, T-type Ca^{2+} currents). Zonisamide blocks Na+ channels in the inactivated state, and reduces the ion flow in Ca^{2+} channel proteins.

Levetiracetam

The mechanism of action for **levetiracetam** is not clearly delineated. In vitro and in vivo recordings of epileptiform activity from the hippocampus have shown that levetiracetam inhibits burst firing without affecting normal neuronal excitability, suggesting that levetiracetam selectively prevents hypersynchronization of burst firing and propagation of seizure activity. It does not appear to directly facilitate GABAergic neurotransmission, but has been shown to oppose the activity of negative modulators of GABA- and glycine-gated currents in neuronal cell culture. A saturable and stereoselective neuronal binding site in rat brain tissue has been described for levetiracetam; however, the identification and function of this binding site is currently unknown. It has shown exceptional promise as an adjunct drug in treating partial seizures in children.

Drugs for Generalized Absence, Myoclonic, or Atonic Seizures

Ethosuximide

CHEMISTRY AND PHARMACOKINETICS. Ethosuximide is the most effective and least toxic of the several succinimide derivatives that have been used to treat epilepsy over the past 50 years. It is well absorbed from the gut, widely distributed to tissues, and metabolized to inactive compounds before it is excreted in the urine. Ethosuximide has a relatively long half-life of about 30 hours in children and 55 hours in adults.

MECHANISMS AND EFFECTS. Ethosuximide inhibits T-type calcium channels in thalamic neurons. These low-threshold channels are believed to be responsible for the pacemaker current that generates the synchronous 3-Hz (three cycles per second) spike-and-wave depolarizations observed in the EEG during absence seizures (see Fig. 20–1). Ethosuximide produces little toxicity, but it can cause dizziness, drowsiness, gastric distress, and nausea, which can usually be minimized by starting treatment with lower doses and then gradually increasing doses to the desired level.

INTERACTIONS. Valproate inhibits the metabolism of ethosuximide and increases its serum levels. Haloperidol (an antipsychotic drug) can alter the seizure pattern in patients treated with ethosuximide. No other important interactions have been identified.

INDICATIONS. Ethosuximide is safe and highly effective in the treatment of generalized absence seizures in children and is the drug of choice for this particular group of patients. Ethosuximide is not very effective, however, in the treatment of adults with absence seizures or of patients with other types of seizures, so valproate (discussed above) is usually used instead.

Clonazepam and Other Drugs

Clonazepam is a benzodiazepine that is used to treat **absence, myoclonic, and atonic seizures.** It often produces more sedation than other antiepileptic drugs when used at doses that suppress seizures.

Because the efficacy of **valproate** is equal to or greater than that of clonazepam, it is frequently used instead to treat patients with **absence, myoclonic, and atonic seizures.**

Lamotrigine is sometimes used as an adjunct for the treatment of **absence and atonic seizures.**

The pharmacologic properties of valproate and lamotrigine are discussed earlier in this chapter, and those of clonazepam are discussed in Chapter 19.

Drugs for Status Epilepticus

Status epilepticus is a life-threatening emergency. Patients with this condition have recurrent episodes of tonic–clonic seizures without regaining consciousness or normal muscle movement between episodes. If their seizures are not controlled, prolonged hypoxia can lead to severe brain damage. Immediate attention must be given to cardiopulmonary support and to the administration of drugs that rapidly terminate the seizures. In fact, published reports indicate that seizures must be controlled within 60 minutes of the onset of an episode in order to have a favorable prognosis.

The drug of choice for status epilepticus is **diazepam** or **lorazepam.** Either drug is administered as a slow intravenous injection given every 10 to 15 minutes until seizures are controlled or a maximal dosage has been administered. The pharmacologic properties of these drugs are described in Chapter 19.

After diazepam or lorazepam is administered, **phenytoin** (or the newer form, **fosphenytoin**) is often administered intravenously to provide a longer duration of seizure control than is provided by a benzodiazepine. Large doses of **phenobarbital** may be effective if a benzodiazepine or phenytoin fails to control the seizures. In highly resistant cases, general anesthesia can be used to control the seizures.

THE MANAGEMENT OF SEIZURE DISORDERS

The effective management of patients with epilepsy requires an accurate diagnosis of the type of seizures that occur and also requires the rational selection and use of drugs.

First-Line Drugs

Table 20–5 lists the drugs of choice for treating the major types of seizures and also lists adjunct medications that can be used in combination with a drug of choice to improve seizure control. The drugs of choice are based on clinical studies of their relative efficacy and safety.

For **partial seizures** and **generalized tonic–clonic seizures,** carbamazepine, phenytoin, and valproate are first-line drugs, and phenobarbital and primidone are second-line drugs. Carbamazepine generally causes fewer adverse effects than phenytoin, although phenytoin can be slightly less sedating than carbamazepine at equally effective doses. Of the several drugs that have been recently developed as adjunct medications for partial seizures, lamotrigine and topiramate appear particularly attractive at this time. The relative safety and efficacy of these drugs are still being evaluated.

For **generalized absence seizures,** ethosuximide is clearly the first choice in treating children with this condition, which usually has its onset during childhood and often remits during adolescence. Valproate is generally more effective in treating adults with absence seizures and in treating patients with multiple types of seizures.

For **generalized myoclonic and atonic seizures,** valproate is the drug of choice.

TABLE 20-5. **Choice of Antiepileptic Drugs for Seizure Disorders***

| Drug | Partial Seizures | Generalized Seizures | | | | Status Epilepticus |
		Tonic-Clonic	Absence	Myoclonic	Atonic	
Carbamazepine	1	1	W	—	—	—
Clonazepam	—	W	3	2	1	—
Clorazepate	A	—	—	—	—	1
Diazepam	—	—	—	—	—	1
Ethosuximide	—	—	1†	—	—	—
Felbamate	A	—	—	—	—	—
Gabapentin	A	—	—	—	—	—
Lamotrigine	A	A	A	—	A	—
Levetiracetam	A	—	—	—	—	—
Lorazepam	—	—	—	—	—	1
Phenobarbital	2	2	—	—	—	3
Phenytoin	1	1	W	—	—	2
Primidone	2	2	—	—	—	—
Tiagabine	A	—	—	—	—	—
Topiramate	A	—	—	—	—	—
Valproate	2	1	2†	1	1	—
Vigabatrin	A	—	—	—	—	—
Zonisamide	A	—	—	—	—	—

*1 = drug of first choice; 2 = drug of second choice; 3 = drug of third choice; A = drug for adjunct use with other drugs; and W = drug may worsen the type of seizure shown.
†For absence seizures in children, ethosuximide is the drug of first choice and valproate is the drug of second choice. For absence seizures in adults, valproate is probably the drug of first choice.

For **status epilepticus,** intravenous treatment with diazepam or lorazepam can be followed by intravenous treatment with fosphenytoin or phenobarbital.

Principles of Drug Use

In most cases, an attempt should be made to control seizures with single-drug therapy (monotherapy) because this will minimize side effects, reduce costs, and increase patient compliance.

Unless the patient is experiencing frequent seizures, it is usually best to start with a single drug and give it in a low dose (one fourth to one third of the therapeutic dose). The dose can be gradually increased until effective serum concentrations are achieved or intolerable adverse effects occur. Starting with a low dose enables the patient to develop tolerance to the CNS side effects of antiepileptic drugs and improves compliance.

If a single drug has significantly reduced the occurrence of seizures but has not eliminated them, it is usually prudent to add another drug to the regimen, rather than to switch to a new drug. Two drugs acting by different mechanisms may control seizures when a single drug is not adequate. The second drug should be given initially in a low dose, and the dosage should be gradually increased until therapeutic concentrations are reached or adverse effects occur. Because of the many interactions between antiepileptic drugs (see Table 20–4), the doses that are both safe and effective for combination therapy may differ from the doses that are safe and effective for monotherapy. For example, lamotrigine causes a much higher incidence of serious dermatologic toxicity in children who are concurrently taking valproate, and lamotrigine should be started at much lower doses in these patients.

Once a satisfactory drug regimen is achieved, the patient should be monitored periodically for drug toxicity and efficacy. Serum drug levels should be determined if there is evidence or suspicion of adverse effects, therapeutic failure, or patient noncompliance.

The appropriate duration of antiepileptic drug therapy is a topic of considerable controversy. If a patient who is undergoing drug therapy has not had a seizure for several years, it seems prudent to consider slowly withdrawing the medication, because this will minimize long-term side effects and offer life-style benefits and cost savings. About 25% of patients who withdraw from medication will relapse within 1 year, however. Factors that increase the likelihood of relapse include onset of seizures during adolescence, occurrence of complex partial seizures or generalized seizures, and abnormal interictal findings on EEG. If antiepileptic medication is to be discontinued, the dosage should be tapered slowly over several weeks, because abrupt withdrawal from medication is associated with a higher incidence of rebound seizures.

SUMMARY OF IMPORTANT POINTS

■ Seizures are caused by episodic, synchronous neuronal discharges in the cerebral cortex or elsewhere in the brain. They are classified as partial or generalized seizures on the basis of their clinical characteristics and electroencephalographic pattern.

■ Some antiepileptic drugs work by blocking voltage-sensitive sodium channels or T-type calcium channels. Others augment inhibitory γ-aminobutyric acid (GABA) neurotransmission or block excitatory glutamate neurotransmission.

■ Carbamazepine, phenytoin, and valproate are the first-line drugs for partial seizures and generalized tonic–clonic seizures.

■ Ethosuximide is the drug of choice for generalized absence seizures in children. Valproate and clonazepam are effective in absence, myoclonic, and atonic seizures.

■ Gabapentin, lamotrigine, topiramate, and several other new drugs are used as adjuncts in the treatment of partial seizures, and some of these agents have activity against other types of seizures.

■ Status epilepticus is a medical emergency that requires intravenous administration of diazepam or lorazepam, sometimes followed by intravenous use of phenytoin (fosphenytoin) or phenobarbital.

■ Many antiepileptic drugs interact with other medications. Carbamazepine and phenytoin induce cytochrome P450 enzymes and decrease serum levels of the drugs with which they interact, whereas valproate inhibits the metabolism of the drugs with which it interacts.

■ Antiepileptic drugs frequently produce central nervous system and gastrointestinal side effects, and some drugs cause infrequent but severe hematologic or hepatic toxicity. Valproate and phenytoin are known to cause birth defects, and both of these drugs can reduce folate levels.

■ Except in urgent situations, antiepileptic therapy should begin with a low dose of a single drug, and the dosage should be increased until the desired serum concentration or full dosage is achieved. If a single drug is not effective, another drug can be added to the regimen or substituted. Drug use should be discontinued slowly. Serum levels should be monitored to verify adequate dosage and whenever toxicity, therapeutic failure, or noncompliance occurs or is suspected.

Review Questions

1. The molecular mechanism underlying the antiepileptic effects of carbamazepine and phenytoin is best described by which one of the following statements?
   (A) inhibiting low threshold Ca^{2+} ion channels
   (B) prolonging the inactivation of the Na^+ ion channel
   (C) potentiating the release of GABA by inhibiting GABA reuptake
   (D) increasing the release of GABA by vesicular fusion
   (E) blocking glutamate receptor excitation

2. Which antiepileptic agent gained wider therapeutic use also to treat trigeminal neuralgia and the manic phase of bipolar disorder?
   (A) ethosuximide
   (B) zonisamide
   (C) levetiracetam
   (D) carbamazepine
   (E) phenytoin

3. Which one of the following agents is considered the drug of choice for initial treatment of absence seizure ("*petit mal*") in children?
   (A) ethosuximide
   (B) zonisamide
   (C) levetiracetam
   (D) carbamazepine
   (E) phenytoin

4. Topiramate has which set of three mechanisms of action?
   (A) increases Na^+ channel inactivation, increases GABA, blocks glutamate
   (B) decreases Na^+ channel inactivation, decrease GABA, blocks glutamate
   (C) increases Ca^{2+} channel inactivation, increases GABA, blocks glutamate
   (D) decreases Ca^{2+} channel inactivation, increases GABA, blocks glutamate
   (E) decreases Ca^{2+} channel flow, increases GABA, blocks glutamate

5. Gabapentin has which mechanism of action?
   (A) inhibits monoamine oxidase
   (B) agonist effect at dopamine receptors
   (C) increases Na^+ channel inactivation
   (D) blocks reuptake of neurotransmitters
   (E) increases release of neurotransmitter

Answers and Explanations

1. The correct answer is B: prolonging the inactivation of the Na^+ ion channel. Both these agents bind to the Na^+ channel protein and prolong the state of inactivation. This leads to a decrease of repetitively firing neurons. Answer (A), inhibiting low threshold Ca^{2+} ion channels, is the mechanism of action of ethosuximide and valproic acid, particularly useful in controlling absence seizures.

Answer (C), potentiating the release of GABA by inhibiting GABA reuptake, is the mechanism of action of tiagabine. Answer (D), increasing the release of GABA by vesicular fusion, is the action of gabapentin, although the precise mechanisms are unknown. Answer (E), blocking glutamate receptor excitation, is part of the mechanism of action of topiramate.

2. The correct choice is D: carbamazepine. This agent has also gained approval for the use as an antimanic agent or mood-stabilizer, for treatment of bipolar disorder and for trigeminal neuralgia. Answer (A), ethosuximide, is the drug of choice for treating absence seizures in children. Answers (B), zonisamide, and (C), levetiracetam, are approved only for adjunct treatment of partial seizures. Answer (E), phenytoin, has gained some acclaim as a mood stabilizer but has not been mentioned for use in trigeminal neuralgia.

3. The correct answer is A: ethosuximide. Ethosuximide acts by inhibiting the low-threshold Ca^{2+} channels thought to be active during absence seizures. Answers (B), zonisamide, and (C), levetiracetam, are newer agents for the treatment of partial seizures. Answers (D), carbamazepine, and (E), phenytoin, are classic drugs used to treat partial seizures and generalized tonic–clonic seizures.

4. The correct answer is A: increases Na^+ channel inactivation, increases GABA, blocks glutamate. Topiramate is a newer agent with three known mechanisms of action. The other answers (B) through (E) contain at least one mechanism of action that would produce greater excitation of neurons, or is not a mechanism of topiramate.

5. The correct choice is E: increases release of neurotransmitter. Gabapentin is an analogue of GABA and is known to cause greater release of GABA from neurons but the precise mechanism is unknown. Answer (A), inhibits monoamine oxidase, is an action of certain types of antidepressant drugs. Answer (B), agonist effect at dopamine receptors, is an action of some antiparkinsonism agents. Answer (C), increases Na+ channel inactivation, and answer (D), blocks reuptake of neurotransmitters, describes the action of the newer antiepileptic agent, tiagabine.

SELECTED READINGS

Leppik, I. E., G. K. Bergey, R. E. Ramsay, et al. Advances in antiepileptic drug treatments. A rational basis for selecting drugs for older patients with epilepsy. Geriatrics 59(12):14–18, 22–24, 2004.
McCorry D., D. Chadwick, and A. Marson. Current drug treatment of epilepsy in adults. Lancet Neurol 3(12):729–735, 2004.
Tomson, T. Drug selection for the newly diagnosed patient: when is a new generation antiepileptic drug indicated? J Neurol 251(9):1043–1049, 2004.
Varelas, P. N., and M. A. Mirski. Management of seizures in critically ill patients. Curr Neurol Neurosci Rep 4(6):489–496, 2004.
Yogeeswari, P., J. V. Ragavendran, R. Thirumurugan, et al. Ion channels as important targets for antiepileptic drug design. Curr Drug Targets 5(7):589–602, 2004.

CHAPTER 21

Local and General Anesthetics

CLASSIFICATION OF LOCAL AND GENERAL ANESTHETICS

Local Anesthetics
Ester-Type Drugs
- Procaine (NOVOCAIN)
- Chloroprocaine (NEACAINE)[a]
- Benzocaine
- Cocaine

Amide-Type Drugs
- Lidocaine (XYLOCAINE)
- Bupivacaine (MARCAINE)[b]
- Etidocaine (DURANEST)
- Mepivacaine (CARBOCAINE)
- Prilocaine (CITANEST)
- Ropivacaine (NAROPIN)

General Anesthetics
Inhalational Anesthetics
Nonhalogenated Drugs
- Nitrous oxide

Halogenated Drugs
- Halothane (FLUOTHANE)
- Desflurane (SUPRANE)
- Enflurane (ETHRANE)
- Isoflurane (FORANE)
- Sevoflurane (ULTANE)[c]

Parenteral Anesthetics
- Fentanyl (SUBLIMAZE)[d]
- Ketamine (KETALAR)
- Midazolam (VERSED)
- Propofol
- Thiopental (PENTOTHAL)

[a]also tetracaine (PONTOCAINE)
[b]also levobupivacaine (CHIROCAINE)
[c]also methoxyflurane (METOFANE)
[d]also sufentanil (SUFENTA), alfentanil (ALFENTA), and remifentanil (ULTIVA).

OVERVIEW

Anesthesia is the loss of all sensation, whereas **analgesia** is the selective loss of pain sensation. **Local anesthetics** block the conduction of nerve impulses in the peripheral nerves or spinal cord. **General anesthetics** block cortical neuronal activity underlying consciousness and all sensation.

Local anesthetics, which are used to anesthetize a particular part or region of the body, are given to patients undergoing surgery on the skin and subcutaneous tissues, ears, eyes, joints, or pelvis. They are also used for anesthesia during labor and delivery and for diagnostic procedures such as gastrointestinal endoscopy. Occasionally, local anesthetics are used to relieve pain associated with pathologic conditions.

General anesthetics are used to prevent consciousness during major surgical procedures. Unlike local anesthetics, general anesthetics produce loss of consciousness and amnesia and thereby prevent the anesthetized patient from recalling the surgical procedure.

LOCAL ANESTHETICS

Drug Properties

Chemistry and Pharmacokinetics

Based on their chemical structure, local anesthetics can be divided into ester-type drugs and amide-type drugs. Each local anesthetic has a lipophilic (hydrophobic) portion and a hydrophilic portion (Fig. 21–1). The hydrophilic portion, an amine that is a weak base, exists in both ionized and nonionized forms. The ionized, protonated form predominates at lower pH levels, and the nonionized, unprotonated form predominates at higher pH levels. Only the nonionized form can penetrate neuronal membranes to reach binding sites on the internal surface of sodium channels. Inflammation and acidosis decrease the pH of tissues, thereby increasing the ionization of local anesthetics. For this reason, local anesthetics are less effective in the presence of these conditions, requiring larger doses.

Figure 21–1. Structures of selected local anesthetics.

Local anesthetics are formulated as hydrochloride salts with a pH less than 7 as the ionized molecule is more soluble and stable than the free base. Once injected, the local anesthetic solution is quickly buffered to the pH of the tissue.

The duration of action of local anesthetics can be short, medium, or long (Table 21–1). Because local anesthetics act directly at the site of administration, their duration of action is primarily determined by the rate of diffusion and absorption away from the site of administration. Diffusion and absorption, in turn, depend on the chemical properties of the anesthetics and on such factors as local pH and blood flow. In some formulations, epinephrine is added to prolong a local anesthetic's duration of action by producing vasoconstriction and slowing its rate of absorption. Because of the risk of ischemia and necrosis, however, local anesthetics with epinephrine are not used to anesthetize tissues with end arteries, such as tissues of the fingers, toes, ears, nose, and penis.

Following systemic absorption, **ester-type local anesthetics** are metabolized in the plasma by butyryl-cholinesterases to *p*-aminobenzoic acid (PABA) derivatives. **Amide-type local anesthetics** undergo metabolism by hepatic P450 enzymes to yield polar metabolites. In both cases, the metabolites are excreted in the urine.

Mechanism of Action

Local anesthetics cause a reversible inhibition of action potential conduction by binding to the sodium channel and decreasing the nerve membrane permeability to sodium. The nonpolar, lipophilic form of the anesthetic molecule passes through the neuronal membrane and switches to the polar, hydrophilic form in the cytoplasm of the neuron. This cationic form of the anesthetic binds to the cytoplasmic side of the sodium channel protein and prolongs the inactivation state of the sodium channel (Fig. 21–2). With sodium channels blocked, action potentials cannot propagate along the neuronal fiber and sensory input is lost.

Pharmacologic Effects

Local anesthetics have a greater affinity for sodium channels that are in the depolarized (open) configuration than for channels that are closed. Nerve fibers that are firing, therefore, are more susceptible to sodium channel blockade. This use-dependent blockade causes a selective inhibition of nerve fibers that are stimulated by the surgical procedure such as pain fibers during suturing. Size-dependent blockade refers to the finding that small diameter fibers are blocked more easily than larger fibers. Small unmyelinated

TABLE 21-1. **Properties of Selected Local Anesthetics**

Drug	Potency	Duration of Action*	Parenteral Uses	Topical Uses
Ester-type drugs				
Procaine	Low	Short	Infiltration, nerve block, and spinal anesthesia	None
Benzocaine	Low	Medium	None	Dermal, laryngeal, and oral
Chloroprocaine	Low	Short	Epidural, infiltration, and nerve block anesthesia	None
Cocaine	Low	Medium	None	Laryngeal, nasal, and urogenital
Amide-type drugs				
Lidocaine	Intermediate	Short	Epidural, infiltration, nerve block, and spinal anesthesia	Dermal, laryngeal, and oral
Bupivacaine	High	Medium	Epidural, infiltration, nerve block, and spinal anesthesia	None
Etidocaine	Intermediate	Long	Infiltration and nerve block anesthesia	None
Mepivacaine	Intermediate	Short	Epidural, infiltration, nerve block, and spinal anesthesia	None
Prilocaine	Intermediate	Short	Infiltration anesthesia	Dermal
Ropivacaine	High	Long	Epidural, infiltration, and nerve block anesthesia	None

*The duration varies with the dose and route of administration. Short = 0.25–1.5 hours; medium = >1.5–5 hours; and long = >5 hours.

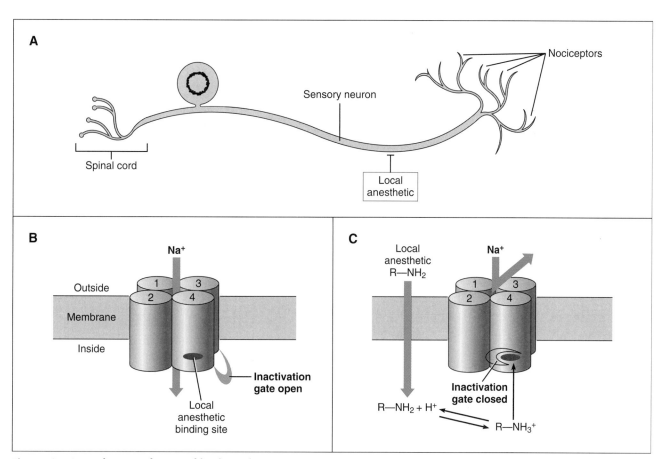

Figure 21-2. Mechanisms of action of local anesthetics. (A) The local anesthetic binds to sodium channels and blocks the generation and conduction of action potentials in peripheral neurons. (B) The sodium channel includes four transmembrane domains. The inactivation gate is a short, intracellular loop between domains 3 and 4. The local anesthetic binds to amino acid residues located on domain 4. (C) The non-ionized form of the local anesthetic (R-NH2) penetrates the axonal membrane and is then converted to the ionized form (R-NH3+). The ionized form binds to the sodium channel in the open state, and this prolongs the sodium channel inactivation state. Sodium entry is blocked during the inactivation state.

C and lightly myelinated Aδ pain fibers, therefore, are more easily anesthetized than are large myelinated touch fibers. Autonomic and sensory nerves are blocked more easily than are motor nerves. Nerves recover from blockade in the reverse order.

Adverse Effects and Interactions

The adverse effects of local anesthetics are primarily caused by their absorption into the systemic circulation and subsequent alteration of central nervous system (CNS), cardiovascular, and other organ system functions.

Local anesthetics often produce CNS stimulation (restlessness, tremor, and euphoria) followed by inhibition (drowsiness and sedation). Other symptoms of local anesthetic toxicity include headache, paresthesias, and nausea. Higher concentrations can cause seizures followed by coma. Death is usually caused by respiratory failure.

Adverse cardiovascular effects include hypotension and cardiac depression. Most local anesthetics are vasodilators, and they also block vasoconstriction induced by the sympathetic nervous system. Most local anesthetics have antiarrhythmic activity, but toxic levels of local anesthetics suppress cardiac conduction and can cause tachyarrhythmia characterized by a wide QRS complex.

Local anesthetic blockade of autonomic ganglia and neuromuscular transmission can lead to loss of visceral and skeletal muscle tone. For this reason, local anesthetics potentiate the effect of neuromuscular blocking drugs (e.g., tubocurarine) and local anesthetics must be used with great caution in patients with myasthenia gravis.

Allergic reactions to local anesthetics are fairly common. Patients who have repeated applications of topical anesthetics are particularly susceptible to sensitization. The ester-type anesthetics cause hypersensitivity reactions more frequently than do the amide-type anesthetics. This is because ester-type anesthetics (e.g., procaine) are metabolized to PABA. PABA causes allergic reactions in a small percentage of individuals. Patients who are allergic to an ester-type anesthetic will usually tolerate an amide-type anesthetic.

Indications

Local anesthetics are usually administered parenterally but are sometimes applied topically. The route of administration depends on factors such as the site of anesthesia.

TOPICAL ANESTHESIA. The topical application of local anesthetics is used to anesthetize the skin, mucous membranes, or cornea. A local anesthetic can be applied to the skin to treat pruritus (itching) caused by poison ivy, insect bites, eczema, or cutaneous manifestations of systemic diseases such as chickenpox (varicella). A eutectic mixture of local anesthetics (EMLA), consisting of two or more solid compounds that form a liquid when they are combined, is sometimes used to anesthetize the skin before venipuncture or minor surgery. The topical application of a local anesthetic to mucous membranes can relieve pain caused by oral, nasal, laryngeal, rectal disorders, or surgery. For example, an anesthetic ointment is used to relieve the discomfort of hemorrhoids. The topical ocular administration of local anesthetics is used to anesthetize the cornea before diagnostic or surgi-

cal procedures (e.g., radial keratotomy), the removal of foreign bodies, and cataract surgery.

INFILTRATION ANESTHESIA. Infiltration is probably the most common route used to administer local anesthetics. The process involves injecting an anesthetic directly into subcutaneous tissue just under the skin. Infiltration is primarily used for minor surgical procedures (e.g., suturing a wound) or for the removal of foreign bodies. It is also frequently used for dental procedures. When a local anesthetic is to be administered by infiltration, epinephrine can be added to it to decrease its dosage and prolong its duration of action. As mentioned earlier, however, epinephrine should not be used to anesthetize fingers, toes, and other tissues with end arteries.

IONTOPHORESIS. Local anesthetics can also be administered by iontophoresis. This technique uses a small electric current to force molecules of the anesthetic into the tissue. Iontophoresis is primarily used in dentistry. It eliminates the need to inject the anesthetic and is used by some dentists for this reason.

NERVE BLOCK AND FIELD BLOCK ANESTHESIA. Nerve block and field block anesthesia are forms of regional anesthesia, the goal of which is to anesthetize an area of the body by blocking the conductivity of sensory nerves from that area. In nerve block anesthesia, a local anesthetic is injected into or adjacent to a peripheral nerve or nerve plexus. For example, a radial nerve block can be used to anesthetize the structures innervated by the radial nerve, including portions of the forearm and hand. Intraorbital block is often used for ocular surgery. Other examples of nerve block anesthesia are brachial plexus and cervical plexus blocks. In field block anesthesia, a local anesthetic is administered in a series of injections to form a wall of anesthesia encircling the operative field.

SPINAL INTRATHECAL ANESTHESIA. Spinal anesthesia is used to block somatic sensory and motor fibers during procedures such as surgery on the lower limb or pelvic structures. A local anesthetic is injected into the subarachnoid, intrathecal space below the level at which the spinal cord terminates. The spread of the anesthetic along the neuroaxis is controlled by the horizontal tilt of the patient and by the specific gravity (baricity) of the local anesthetic solution. Hyperbaric solutions of local anesthetics are available for this purpose, and these spread along the neuroaxis for about 15 minutes. By this time, they have mixed with cerebrospinal fluid (CSF) to become isobaric and are said to be "fixed" at a certain level of the spinal cord. Spinal anesthesia can cause headaches associated with CSF leakage from the lumbar puncture, and respiratory depression can occur if the anesthetic ascends too high up the spinal cord. Entry into the CNS by spinal injection also carries a small risk of infection or meningitis.

EPIDURAL ANESTHESIA. Epidural anesthesia is produced by injecting a local anesthetic into the lumbar or caudal epidural (extradural) space. A local anesthetic (e.g., bupivacaine) is often administered by this route to provide anesthesia during labor and delivery. After epidural administration, the local anesthetic is absorbed into the systemic circulation. Therefore, doses must be carefully monitored to prevent cardiac depression and neurotoxicity in the mother and neonate.

SPECIFIC AGENTS

Ester-Type Local Anesthetics

Cocaine, a naturally occurring plant alkaloid, was the first local anesthetic to be discovered. It has both local anesthetic and CNS stimulant properties, and it is the only local anesthetic that causes significant vasoconstriction as a result of its sympathomimetic effect. Because of its CNS effects and potential for abuse (see Chapter 25), cocaine is seldom used as a local anesthetic. It is occasionally used, however, to anesthetize the internal structures of the nose, where its vasoconstrictive action helps prevent bleeding after nasal surgery. A cocaine solution is applied to gauze and inserted into the nose for this purpose.

Procaine, the first synthetic local anesthetic drug to be prepared after the discovery of cocaine, became the standard of comparison for many years. Procaine and **chloroprocaine** have a low potency and a relatively short duration of action. They are not effective after topical administration and must be administered parenterally. Both drugs are metabolized to PABA. For this reason, they are more likely to cause allergic reactions than are the amide-type local anesthetics. Tetracaine is another ester-type local anesthetic with a longer duration of action than procaine. It is used for infiltration anesthesia. It is also available in a topical spray and gel formulation in combination with butamben (butyl aminobenzoate) and benzocaine in a preparation called cetacaine.

Benzocaine, a frequently used topical anesthetic, is available in a number of nonprescription products for the treatment of sunburn, pruritus, and other skin conditions. In some patients, the drug causes hypersensitivity reactions, which can exacerbate preexisting dermatitis. Benzocaine is also used to anesthetize mucous membranes and is available in cough lozenges and sprays to relieve coughing.

Amide-Type Local Anesthetics

Lidocaine produces local anesthesia after topical or parenteral administration. The most widely used local anesthetic, it is available in a number of formulations. These include topical solutions and ointments, oral sprays, viscous gels for oral and laryngeal application, and various parenteral formulations. A eutectic mixture of lidocaine and prilocaine is available as a cream to anesthetize intact skin to a depth of 5 mm. In pediatric patients, this **EMLA** (eutectic mixture of local anesthetics) has been used for local anesthesia before venipuncture, intravenous cannulation, or circumcision. Lidocaine is also used for infiltration, nerve block, epidural, and spinal anesthesia.

Etidocaine has properties similar to those of lidocaine, but its duration of action is considerably longer. It is primarily used for infiltration and nerve block anesthesia.

Bupivacaine, mepivacaine, and **ropivacaine** have similar clinical uses but differ in their duration of action, as shown in Table 21–1. Bupivacaine has been the most widely used local anesthetic for obstetrical anesthesia, but it causes cardiac depression more frequently than do many other local anesthetics. Ropivacaine is a newer drug that may cause fewer cases of cardiac toxicity. **Levobupivacaine** is the isolated S(-)-stereoisomer of racemic bupivacaine, which is the active form of the chiral drug mixture. It is used in epidural anesthesia for labor and delivery.

Prilocaine is a congener of lidocaine. It is converted to O-toluidine, a toxic metabolite that can cause methemoglobinemia if it is allowed to accumulate. For this reason, prilocaine use is limited to topical and infiltration anesthesia.

GENERAL ANESTHETICS

The first demonstration of general anesthesia for surgery was performed by William Morton at the Massachusetts General Hospital in 1846. The anesthetic that Morton used was diethyl ether, and his demonstration had a profound impact on the field of surgery. Before that time, surgery was limited to rapid procedures such as limb amputations. General anesthesia and the subsequent development of aseptic techniques permitted the evolution of surgical procedures to the sophisticated level achieved today.

Diethyl ether is no longer used in developed countries, because it has a slow rate of induction, causes considerable postoperative nausea and vomiting, and is highly flammable. Use of another anesthetic gas, cyclopropane, has also been abandoned, because of its explosive nature and its tendency to cause cardiac arrhythmias. A variety of anesthetics are currently available for inhalational use, however. These include **nitric oxide** and a growing number of halogenated hydrocarbons. The pharmacologic properties and adverse effects of these drugs are listed in Tables 21–2 and 21–3, respectively.

INHALATIONAL ANESTHETICS

Drug Properties

Chemistry and Pharmacokinetics

The inhalational anesthetics are divided into nonhalogenated drugs and halogenated drugs. Structures of selected inhalational anesthetics are shown in Fig. 21–3A. These anesthetics are either gases or volatile liquids whose gaseous phase can be inhaled.

The **potency** of inhalational anesthetics is expressed in terms of the inspired concentration of the anesthetic required to produce anesthesia in half of the subjects. This is called the **minimal alveolar concentration (MAC).** The MAC value is used to compare potency among different inhalational agents similar to the median effective dose (ED_{50}) of other drugs.

The pharmacokinetics of inhalational anesthetics differ from those of other drugs because the gaseous anesthetics are absorbed and eliminated through the same organ, the lungs. Moreover, as the activity of inhalational agents is caused by anesthetic molecules in the gas phase, molecules that enter the liquid phase and become soluble in the blood decrease the onset of anesthesia. The movement of anesthetic molecules between the lungs and other tissues is

TABLE 21-2. **Properties of Inhalation Anesthetics**

Drug	Minimum Alveolar Concentration (% vol/vol)*	Blood: Gas Partition Coefficient	Rate of Induction	Amount Metabolized	Amount of Skeletal Muscle Relaxation
Nonhalogenated drugs					
Nitrous oxide	>100	0.47	Fast	0%	None
Halogenated drugs					
Desflurane	6.0	0.42	Fast	<2%	Medium
Enflurane	1.7	1.9	Medium	5% (fluoride)	Medium
Halothane	0.75	2.3	Slow	20%	Low
Isoflurane	1.2	1.4	Medium	<2% (fluoride)	Medium
Sevoflurane	1.9	0.63	Fast	<2%	Medium

*The minimum alveolar concentration (MAC) is the concentration needed to produce anesthesia in half of the subjects.

TABLE 21-3. **Adverse Effects of Inhalational Anesthetics**

Drug	Airway Irritation	Respiratory Depression	Bronchodilation	Hypotensive Effect	Arrhythmia Potential*
Nonhalogenated drugs					
Nitrous oxide	Low	None	None	None	None
Halogenated drugs					
Desflurane	Moderate	Low	None	Reduced systemic vascular resistance	Low
Enflurane	Low	Moderate	Moderate	Reduced cardiac output	Low
Halothane	Moderate	Low	Moderate	Reduced cardiac output	Moderate
Isoflurane	Moderate	Moderate	Moderate	Reduced systemic vascular resistance	Low
Sevoflurane	Low	Low	None	Reduced systemic vascular resistance	Low

*Anesthetics that sensitize the heart to catecholamines have the potential to cause epinephrine-induced arrhythmias.

determined by the partial pressure of the anesthetic and as the anesthetic's partial pressure in the blood increases, molecules of the anesthetic move across the blood–brain barrier into the brain and produce anesthesia.

The **induction rate** of anesthesia is determined by three primary factors: (1) the alveolar partial pressure of the anesthetic in the inspired air; (2) the ventilation rate; and (3) the rate at which the anesthetic's partial pressure in the blood increases as the anesthetic is administered. This third factor is largely dependent on the **blood:gas partition coefficient** (Box 21–1).

Because anesthetic molecules move from an area of higher partial pressure to an area of lower partial pressure, both the rate of induction and the depth of anesthesia can be rapidly adjusted by increasing or decreasing the partial pressure of the anesthetic in the patient's inspired air. After the concentration in inspired air is increased or decreased, the concentration in the blood and brain will increase or decrease. The ability to control rapidly the depth of anesthesia increases the safety of the inhalational anesthetics.

Mechanism of Action

It was thought that the action of inhalational anesthetics resulted from a nonspecific interaction of anesthetic molecules within the lipid bilayer of neuronal membranes causing a disruption of ion flow and inhibiting neuronal activity. This hypothesis was supported by the correlation of the anesthetic potency with its lipophilicity, known as the Meyer-Overton principle (see oil:gas partition coefficient, Box 21–2).

More recently, the molecular actions of inhalational anesthetics were elucidated. These agents bind to specific amino acid residues in the transmembrane portions of $GABA_A$ receptor-chloride ion channel. The inhalational anesthetics appear to increase chloride influx and potassium efflux from neurons. Both of these actions cause hyperpolarization of neuronal membranes and reduce membrane excitability. The effect of the anesthetics on chloride flux appears to be caused by potentiation of the action of γ-aminobutyric acid (GABA) at the $GABA_A$ receptor-chloride ion channel. Inhalational anesthetics also reduce sodium and calcium influx, and this prevents nerve firing and the release of neurotransmitters.

Pharmacologic Effects

The induction by general anesthetics is characterized by four stages. In stage I, neurons in the spinal cord are prevented from firing and analgesia and conscious sedation occurs. In

Figure 21-3. Structures of selected general anesthetics. (A) Inhalational anesthetics include nitrous oxide, which is a nonhalogenated gas; halothane, which is a halogenated hydrocarbon; and desflurane, enflurane, isoflurane, and sevoflurane, all of which are halogenated ethers. (B) Parenteral anesthetics include fentanyl (shown in Fig. 23–2B), ketamine, midazolam, propofol, and thiopental.

stage II, inhibition of firing in small inhibitory neurons can cause paradoxical excitation, although with modern balanced anesthesia this stage is often not observed. Stage III is the goal of surgical anesthesia with suppression of the reticular-activating system, loss of consciousness, and inhibition of spinal reflexes. The latter effect contributes to the muscle relaxation needed for surgery; however, adjunct muscle relaxant agents (see Chapter 7) are commonly used. Stage IV, which is to be avoided because it can lead to cardiovascular collapse, is noted by depression of the respiratory and vasomotor nuclei in the brainstem.

Adverse Effects

Table 21–3 compares the adverse effects of nonhalogenated and halogenated anesthetics. Of particular importance with the administration of halothane is toxicity of the liver, called halothane hepatitis, and a rare condition leading to muscle fiber breakdown and renal failure called malignant hyperthermia. Because of a reactive fluoride group incorporated as one of the halogens in methoxyflurane, this anesthetic has caused fluoride ion nephrotoxicity in some cases.

SPECIFIC AGENTS

NONHALOGENATED DRUGS

Nitrous oxide (N_2O) is the only anesthetic gas used today. It is the least potent of the inhalational anesthetics, and it does not reduce consciousness to the extent required for major surgical procedures. Nitrous oxide, however, produces more analgesia than do the other inhalational anesthetics, and it is often used for minor surgery and dental procedures that do not require loss of consciousness. Nitrous oxide is frequently used as a component of **balanced anesthesia** in combination with another anesthetic agent and other drugs (see below). The nitrous oxide in balanced anesthesia provides greater analgesia and enables the use of a lower concentration of the other anesthetic agent.

Because nitrous oxide has a low blood:gas partition coefficient, induction and recovery are rapid when it is used. The anesthetic produces virtually no cardiovascular or respiratory depression, and it is generally considered quite safe. It oxidizes the cobalt moiety of vitamin B_{12}, however, and thereby inhibits methylation of nucleic acids and proteins. Although

BOX 21-1. PHARMACOKINETICS OF INHALATIONAL ANESTHETICS RATE OF INDUCTION OF ANESTHESIA

The rate of induction of anesthesia is determined by three primary factors: (1) the alveolar concentration, or alveolar partial pressure, of the anesthetic; (2) the ventilation rate; and (3) the rate at which the anesthetic's partial pressure in the blood increases as the anesthetic is administered. This third factor, in turn, is influenced by the blood:gas partition coefficient.

The blood:gas partition coefficient is a measure of the anesthetic's solubility in the blood. In the example shown here, the coefficient of nitrous oxide is 0.47, whereas that of halothane is 2.3.

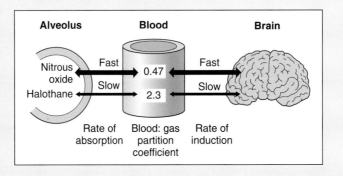

A high blood:gas partition coefficient corresponds with a high degree of solubility in the blood and with a low rate of rise in the anesthetic's partial pressure in the blood during induction. Anesthetics with a low coefficient (e.g., nitrous oxide) have a fast rate of induction because they saturate the blood quickly and their partial pressure rises quickly. Anesthetics with a higher coefficient (e.g., halothane) have a slow rate of induction because they dissolve slowly in the blood and it takes a long time for their partial pressure in the blood to rise.

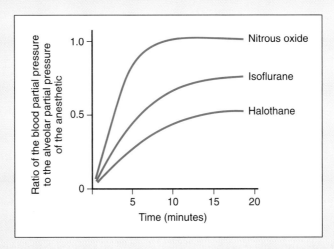

Adjusting the Rate or Depth of Anesthesia

The anesthetic's alveolar concentration and the ventilation rate can be altered by the anesthesiologist to accelerate or slow the rate of induction or recovery, to adjust the depth of anesthesia during surgery, or to maintain tissue oxygenation and eliminate carbon dioxide.

The anesthetic's alveolar concentration after induction is usually about half as high as during induction. In patients having mechanical ventilation, the rate of induction or depth of anesthesia can be adjusted by changing the respiratory rate or tidal volume.

BOX 21-2. MECHANISMS OF ACTION OF INHALATIONAL ANESTHETICS

The potency of an inhalational anesthetic, expressed in terms of the minimal alveolar concentration (MAC), is highly correlated with the lipid solubility (oil:gas partition coefficient) of the anesthetic. This correlation suggests that anesthetics interact with a hydrophobic component of neuronal membranes.

Because of their effects on neuronal membrane proteins, anesthetics disrupt neuronal firing and sensory processing in the thalamus and thereby cause loss of consciousness and analgesia. Anesthetics also inhibit neuronal output from layer V (the internal pyramidal layer) of the cortex, and this reduces motor activity.

Inhalational anesthetics are believed to bind stereoselectively to hydrophobic regions of neuronal membrane proteins that interface with membrane lipids. The anesthetics potentiate γ-aminobutyric acid (GABA) activity at the GABA$_A$ chloride ionophore and thereby increase chloride flux through the ionophore. They may also inhibit sodium and calcium influx through membrane channels. These actions hyperpolarize the neuronal membrane and inhibit neuron firing and the release of neurotransmitters.

---

these effects are minimal during acute exposure, chronic exposure to nitrous oxide can cause megaloblastic anemia.

Nitrous oxide, which is also called **"laughing gas,"** often produces mild euphoria when it is administered. For this reason, some recreational use of the drug occurs.

HALOGENATED ANESTHETICS

In most areas of the world, the halogenated anesthetics replaced older volatile liquid anesthetics (e.g., **diethyl ether**) because of several advantages. The halogenated drugs have a more rapid rate of induction and recovery, cause a much lower incidence of postoperative nausea and vomiting, and are not flammable. They, however, produce dose-dependent respiratory and cardiovascular depression. For this reason, respiratory and cardiovascular functions are monitored during the use of halogenated anesthetics, and artificial ventilation and circulatory support is often required. The halogenated anesthetics cause uterine relaxation, which usually limits their use in obstetrics to women having cesarean section. Because halogenated anesthetics produce relatively

little analgesia or skeletal muscle relaxation, they are often given in combination with nitrous oxide, opioids, muscle relaxants, and other adjunct drugs in what is called **balanced anesthesia.**

Halothane is the prototypical halogenated anesthetic, and **desflurane, enflurane, isoflurane,** and **sevoflurane** are newer halogenated anesthetics.

Halothane is the most potent inhalational agent, but it has several disadvantages. Because of its relatively high blood:gas partition coefficient, its rate of induction and recovery is slower than that of other halogenated anesthetics. Because it sensitizes the heart to catecholamines more than other anesthetics do, it places patients at greater risk for cardiac arrhythmias. Hence, the utilization of epinephrine for hemostasis must be strictly limited in patients receiving halothane. Halothane undergoes appreciable metabolism and is converted to substances that can produce a hypersensitivity reaction and hepatitis. For this reason, a patient who is anesthetized with halothane should not be reexposed to it for 6 to 12 months.

Enflurane and isoflurane exhibit more rapid induction and recovery than halothane exhibits. They undergo less metabolic degradation and produce little cardiac arrhythmia. Enflurane and isoflurane produce more muscle relaxation, so this reduces the need for muscle relaxants during surgery. They cause more respiratory depression, however, than the other halogenated drugs cause. At high concentrations, enflurane can produce CNS excitation, leading to seizures.

Desflurane and sevoflurane have a more rapid rate of induction and recovery than other halogenated anesthetics do, but desflurane is irritating to the respiratory tract, so this limits the concentrations of this agent that can be administered during induction. Sevoflurane is close to an ideal anesthetic. It exhibits a rapid and smooth induction and recovery, and it causes little cardiovascular or other organ system toxicity.

PARENTERAL ANESTHETICS

The parenteral anesthetics include barbiturates, benzodiazepines, opioids, and other compounds such as propofol. These drugs are used for a variety of purposes, including preanesthetic sedation, induction of anesthesia, perioperative analgesia, and anesthesia for minor surgical and diagnostic procedures. The structures and properties of several parenteral anesthetics are shown in Fig. 21–3B and Table 21–4.

Fentanyl is a strong opioid agonist used to treat moderate to severe pain (see Chapter 23). Because of its potent analgesic properties, it is also administered intravenously or epidurally in combination with other drugs for surgical or obstetric analgesia and anesthesia. For example, it is used to provide anesthesia during cardiac surgery (e.g., coronary artery bypass grafting), because it does not cause cardiovascular toxicity. Fentanyl does not produce amnesia or complete loss of consciousness, so it is often combined with a benzodiazepine (e.g., **diazepam**) to produce amnesia and increased sedation.

Fentanyl has been used in combination with **droperidol,** a member of the antipsychotic class of agents (previously called neuroleptics) that produces a condition called **neuroleptanesthesia.** Droperidol is a butyrophenone compound whose properties are similar to those of haloperidol (see Chapter 22). The advantage of neuroleptanesthesia is that it provides adequate analgesia and sedation during surgery while maintaining a sufficient level of consciousness to permit the patient to respond to questions during the surgical procedure. The disadvantages of neuroleptanesthesia include chest wall rigidity, which is caused by the effects of fentanyl and droperidol on the basal ganglia. Fentanyl has a much shorter half-life than does droperidol, and supplemental doses of fentanyl may be needed during long surgical procedures.

Fentanyl and **sufentanil,** a closely related opioid, are also used with or without a local anesthetic for epidural administration or by the spinal intrathecal route during labor or to provide postoperative analgesia. Other shorter-acting opioids (e.g., **alfentanil** and **remifentanil**) are used intravenously for induction or for ambulatory surgery. Remifentanil is unique as it is metabolized extremely rapidly by esterases in the blood and tissues.

Ketamine is chemically and pharmacologically related to phencyclidine (PCP), a street drug that is abused because of its pronounced effects on sensory perception (see Chapter 25). Both ketamine and PCP act by blocking the action of excitatory amino acids, primarily glutamate, at *N*-methyl-D-aspartate (NMDA) receptors. Ketamine produces less sensory distortion and euphoria than does PCP and, therefore, is more suitable for use as an anesthetic.

When administered intravenously, ketamine produces **dissociative anesthesia,** a mental state in which the individual appears to be dissociated from the environment without complete loss of consciousness. This type of anesthesia is characterized by analgesia, reduced sensory perception, immobility, and amnesia. Unlike many inhalational anesthetics, ketamine usually increases blood pressure, but it has little effect on respiration with typical doses. The main drawback of ketamine is its tendency to cause unpleasant effects during recovery, including delirium, hallucinations, and irrational behavior. Because children are less likely than adults to experience these adverse effects, ketamine is most often used in pediatric patients and is given in combination with a benzodiazepine for anesthesia during minor surgical or diagnostic procedures.

Midazolam is a short-acting benzodiazepine used for preoperative sedation as well as for endoscopy and other diagnostic procedures that do not require a high level of analgesia. Although its onset of action is slower than that of thiopental or propofol, it has the advantage of causing little cardiovascular or respiratory depression. If an overdose of midazolam occurs, the effects of the drug can be reversed by administration of flumazenil, a benzodiazepine antagonist.

TABLE 21–4. **Properties of Parenteral Anesthetics***

Drug	Duration of Action (Minutes)	Analgesia	Muscle Relaxation	Other Effects
Fentanyl	5–10 for IV 30–60 for IM	++++	0	Respiratory depression
Ketamine	5–10 for IV 12–25 for IM	+++	0	Postanesthetic delirium and hallucinations
Midazolam	5–20 for IV 20–40 for IM	0	+++	Amnesia
Propofol	5–10 for IV	0	0	Respiratory depression
Thiopental	5–10 for IV	0	0	Respiratory depression

*Values shown are the mean of values reported in the literature. IV = intravenous; and IM = intramuscular. Ratings range from none (0) to high (++++).

Propofol is a diisopropyl phenol compound, whereas **thiopental** is a thiobarbiturate. These drugs potentiate GABA activity at the GABA$_A$ receptor-chloride ion channel, and they are primarily used for induction of anesthesia. Their use is followed by the administration of an inhalational anesthetic to maintain anesthesia. Both drugs have a rapid onset of action, causing unconsciousness in about 20 seconds. Their duration of action is short (5 to 10 minutes) because they are redistributed from the brain to the peripheral tissues as their blood concentrations fall. Propofol has the advantages of being rapidly metabolized and eliminated from the body and causing little hangover. Thiopental is accumulated in fat and muscle. It is more slowly eliminated from the body, and some hangover can occur. Either drug can depress cardiovascular and respiratory function.

SUMMARY OF IMPORTANT POINTS

■ Local anesthetics produce use-dependent blockade of nerve conduction and thereby prevent pain associated with surgical and diagnostic procedures. Autonomic and sensory nerves are blocked more easily than are nerves affecting proprioception, muscle tone, and somatic motor activity.

■ Local anesthetics are weak bases. The nonionized form permeates neuronal membranes, and the ionized form binds to the internal surface of sodium channels.

■ Ester-type anesthetics (e.g., procaine and chloroprocaine) are converted to *p*-aminobenzoic acid (PABA) and may elicit hypersensitivity reactions.

■ Amide-type anesthetics (e.g., lidocaine and mepivacaine) produce fewer allergic reactions than do ester-type anesthetics.

■ All local anesthetics can cause central nervous system and cardiac toxicity, including seizures and cardiac arrhythmias.

■ General anesthetics include inhalational agents (e.g., nitrous oxide and halothane) and parenteral agents (e.g., ketamine and propofol).

■ The potency of inhalational anesthetics is expressed as the minimal alveolar concentration (MAC) required to produce anesthesia. The potency is proportional to the oil:gas partition coefficient.

■ The rate of induction of inhalational anesthetics is determined in part by the blood:gas partition coefficient. Nitrous oxide has a low coefficient and a rapid rate of induction. Halothane has a higher coefficient and a slower rate of induction.

■ All inhalational anesthetics, except nitrous oxide, suppress respiratory function and decrease blood pressure in a dose-dependent manner.

■ Parenteral anesthetics are used to induce anesthesia and to provide anesthesia during minor surgical and diagnostic procedures. They are also used in combination with other anesthetics during major surgical procedures.

Review Questions

1. Local anesthetics exert their effects by which one of the following mechanisms?
   (A) increasing K^+ conductance and hyperpolarizing nerves
   (B) blocking the Na^+ channels in nerves
   (C) inactivating the Na^+-K^+ adenosine triphosphatase (ATPase) pump
   (D) blocking excitation at postsynaptic receptors
   (E) blocking by a direct action only at the synapse

2. Epinephrine is sometimes added to commercial local anesthetic (LA) solutions for which purpose?
   (A) decrease the rate of absorption of LA
   (B) decrease the duration of action of the LA
   (C) block the metabolism of ester-type local anesthetics
   (D) enhance the distribution of LA
   (E) act synergistically with LA at the nerve ion channel

3. Which of the following characteristics is used to quantitate and compare the potency of gaseous general anesthetics?
   (A) blood:gas partition coefficient
   (B) minimal alveolar concentration
   (C) blood:brain partition coefficient
   (D) rate of uptake and elimination
   (E) relative analgesic potency

4. Which one of the following inhalational anesthetics is most likely to cause fluoride ion nephrotoxicity?
   (A) enflurane
   (B) nitrous oxide
   (C) halothane
   (D) methoxyflurane
   (E) isoflurane

5. Muscle rigidity can be a side effect of which intravenous anesthetic?
   (A) fentanyl
   (B) midazolam
   (C) ketamine
   (D) propofol
   (E) thiopental

Answers and Explanations

1. The correct choice is B: blocking the Na^+ channels in nerves. LA produce a block of voltage-gated sodium channels needed to conduct action potentials along nerve fibers. The unprotonated form of the LA molecule passes through the neuronal membrane and is changed to the protonated form in the cytoplasm. This form then binds to the inside of the sodium channel protein. Answer (A), increasing K^+ conductance and hyperpolarizing nerves, would cause inhibition of firing but not total blockade of action potentials because they are not dependent on potassium channels for nerve fiber conduction. Answer (C), inactivating the Na^+-K^+ ATPase pump, is the action of some cardiovascular agents used for congestive heart failure. Answer (D), blocking excitation at postsynaptic receptors, is the action of a receptor antagonist. Answer (E), blocking by a direct action only at the synapse, again,

is not the action of an LA, which can block all along the nerve fiber.

2. The correct answer is A: decrease the rate of absorption of LA. Epinephrine causes vasoconstriction acting at α_1 receptors and thus decreases the amount of systemic absorption of the LA. Answer (B), decrease the duration of action of the LA, is wrong because epinephrine actually prolongs the duration of action by reducing absorption away from the nerve fiber. Answer (C), block the metabolism of ester-type local anesthetics, and (E), act synergistically with LA at the nerve ion channel, are wrong because no evidence exists for epinephrine having this effect. Answer (D), enhance the distribution of LA, is incorrect because epinephrine affects the pharmacokinetic property of absorption directly.

3. The correct answer is B: minimal alveolar concentration. The MAC value, which is used for inhalational agents to determine potency, is defined as the percent concentration in the administered air that produces no response to surgical incision in 50% of the subjects. Answers (A), (C), and (D) are measures of the characteristics of anesthetics but do not give the potency. Answer (E), relative analgesic potency, is a term used when comparing analgesic agents.

4. The correct answer is D: methoxyflurane. The F element on the structure of halogenated anesthetics can produce toxic F metabolites, which has occurred in the case of methoxyflurane. This has not been reported for the other anesthetics given as answers (A) through (C) and (E).

5. The correct choice is A: fentanyl. Fentanyl is a potent opioid agonist given as part of balanced anesthesia. It can cause chest-wall (truncal) rigidity because of interactions in the striatum. This effect has not been noted for (B) midazolam, (C) ketamine, (D) propofol, or (E) thiopental.

SELECTED READINGS

Gupta, A., T. Stierer, R. Zuckerman, et al. Comparison of recovery profile after ambulatory anesthesia with propofol, isoflurane, sevoflurane and desflurane: a systematic review. Anesth Analg 98(3):632–641, 2004.

Miller, K. W. The nature of sites of general anaesthetic action. Br J Anaesth 89(1):17–31, 2002.

Patel, A. J., and E. Honore. 2P domain K$^+$ channels: novel pharmacological targets for volatile general anesthetics. Adv Exp Med Biol 536:9–23, 2003.

Raeder, J. Ketamine, revival of a versatile intravenous anaesthetic. Adv Exp Med Biol 523:269–277, 2003.

Rudolph, U., and B. Antkowiak. Molecular and neuronal substrates for general anaesthetics. Nat Rev Neurosci 5(9):709–720, 2004.

Sneyd, J. R. Recent advances in intravenous anaesthesia. Br J Anaesth 93(5):725–736, 2004.

CHAPTER 22

Psychotherapeutic Drugs

OVERVIEW

The major psychiatric disorders include psychoses, such as schizophrenia, and affective disorders, such as depression. **Psychoses** are disorders in which patients exhibit gross disturbances in their comprehension of reality, as evidenced by false perceptions (hallucinations) and false beliefs (delusions). In contrast, **affective disorders** are emotional disturbances in which the mood is excessively low (depression) or high (mania). During the past 50 years, tremendous advances have been made in the treatment of these disorders. The newer antipsychotic drugs used to treat schizophrenia and the newer antidepressant and mood-stabilizing drugs used to treat affective disorders cause fewer adverse reactions and are more effective than the older psychotherapeutic agents. Treatment-resistant disorders still pose a significant problem to clinicians, but some progress has been made in the treatment of refractory disease.

233

SCHIZOPHRENIA

Clinical Findings

Schizophrenia, the most common form of psychosis, affects about 1% of the world's population. Its hallmarks are delusions, hallucinations, disorganized thinking, and emotional abnormalities. Several forms of the disease, including paranoid, disorganized, and catatonic forms, are differentiated on the basis of symptomatology.

As shown in Table 22–1, the symptoms of schizophrenia can be divided into two groups. The **positive symptoms,** which include delusions and hallucinations, probably result from excessive neuronal activity in mesolimbic neuronal pathways. These symptoms are usually the primary manifestations of acute psychotic episodes. The **negative symptoms,** which include apathy, withdrawal, and lack of motivation and pleasure, probably result from insufficient activity in mesocortical neuronal pathways. The negative symptoms generally are more difficult to treat, often persist after positive symptoms resolve, and are associated with a poor prognosis.

Etiology and Pathogenesis

Schizophrenia is a complex and heterogeneous disease whose etiology and pathogenesis are incompletely understood.

Epidemiologic studies indicate that the children of two schizophrenic parents have about a 40% risk of developing the disease, so heredity appears to have a major role in determining susceptibility to schizophrenia. Adoption studies show that the risk is associated with the biologic parents and is not altered by the environment during childhood. At least one gene, which codes for a brain protein called *neuregulin 1,* is associated with schizophrenia discovered from linkage studies in Northern European populations. The role of this gene product in the etiology of schizophrenia is not known, however. In most patients, the clinical manifestations of schizophrenia do not appear until late adolescence, possibly because the brain dysfunction is not critical until brain maturation is completed.

Dopamine Hypothesis

Many hypotheses exist regarding the biological basis of schizophrenia. According to the **dopamine hypothesis,** schizophrenia results from abnormalities in dopamine neurotransmission in mesolimbic and mesocortical neuronal pathways (Box 22–1). Much of the evidence supporting this hypothesis is based on the clinical effects of agents that alter dopaminergic transmission.

Several observations support the dopamine hypothesis. First, most antipsychotic drugs block dopamine D_2 receptors, and an excellent correlation exists between the clinical potency of these drugs and their in vitro binding affinity for these receptors. Second, drugs that act by increasing the neuronal release of dopamine (amantadine) or by blocking the reuptake of dopamine (drugs such as amphetamines and cocaine) can induce psychotic behavior that resembles the behavior of schizophrenic patients.

Dopamine turnover in the brain, which reflects the neuronal release of dopamine, can be studied by measuring the concentration of the principal metabolite of dopamine, homovanillic acid, in the cerebrospinal fluid. Although elevated levels of homovanillic acid are not found in patients with chronic schizophrenia, they are found in some schizophrenic patients having acute psychotic episodes. Evidence also exists for a dopamine receptor defect in schizophrenic patients. Positive emission tomography (PET) scanning using D_2 receptor ligands has revealed that schizophrenic patients have decreased D_2 receptor densities in the prefrontal lobe cortex (but increased D_2 receptor densities in the caudate nucleus). These findings lend overall support to the dopamine hypothesis, although it is clear from the clinical effectiveness of atypical antipsychotics that 5-hydroxytryptamine ($5-HT_2$) and other types of dopamine receptors may be involved.

ANTIPSYCHOTIC DRUGS

Antipsychotic drugs are agents that reduce psychotic symptoms and improve the behavior of schizophrenic patients. Antipsychotic drugs were also called **neuroleptic drugs** because they suppress motor activity and emotional expression. The accidental discovery of the antipsychotic properties of chlorpromazine in the early 1950s began a new era in the treatment of schizophrenia and stimulated research concerning the neurobiology of mental illness and psychopharmacology. Nearly 40 years later, the introduction of clozapine had an equally important impact. Clozapine was the first agent to show greater activity against the negative symptoms of schizophrenia and to produce significantly fewer extrapyramidal side effects than the previous antipsychotic drugs. For this reason, the discovery of clozapine has stimulated the development of new antipsychotic drugs with improved pharmacologic properties.

Drug Properties

MECHANISM OF ACTION. The antipsychotic drugs interact with multiple neurotransmitter systems. Whereas the therapeutic effects of these drugs are believed to result from competitive blockade of **dopamine receptors** and **serotonin (5-hydroxytryptamine, or 5-HT) receptors,** the adverse effects are attributed to the blockade of a variety of receptors (Table 22–2).

Typical antipsychotic drugs have an equal or greater affinity for D_2 receptors than for $5-HT_2$ receptors. As shown in Fig. 22–1, an excellent correlation exists between the

TABLE 22–1.	Classification of Symptoms of Schizophrenia	
Positive Symptoms	**Negative Symptoms**	
Agitation	Apathy (avolition)	
Delusions	Affective flattening	
Disorganized speech	Lack of motivation	
Disorganized thinking	Lack of pleasure (anhedonia)	
Hallucinations	Poverty of speech (alogia)	
Insomnia	Social isolation	

BOX 22-1. NEUROBIOLOGY OF SCHIZOPHRENIA AND SITES OF DRUG ACTION

Postulated Neuronal Dysfunction in Schizophrenia

As shown in the accompanying figure, numerous dopamine pathways are found in the brain.

(1) **Mesolimbic pathway.** Dopamine travels from the midbrain tegmental area to the nucleus accumbens. Increased activity in this pathway may cause delusions, hallucinations, and other so-called positive symptoms of schizophrenia.

(2) **Mesocortical pathways.** There are several mesocortical pathways. Decreased activity in the pathway that goes from the midbrain to the prefrontal lobe cortex can cause apathy, withdrawal, lack of motivation and pleasure, and other so-called negative symptoms of schizophrenia. Mesocortical dysfunction also disinhibits the mesolimbic pathway.

(3) **Nigrostriatal pathway.** The pathway from the substantia nigra to the striatum is involved in the coordination of body movements. Inhibition of this pathway causes the extrapyramidal side effects of antipsychotic drugs.

(4) **Tuberoinfundibular pathway.** The pathway from the hypothalamus to the pituitary inhibits the release of prolactin. Inhibition of this pathway leads to elevated serum prolactin levels.

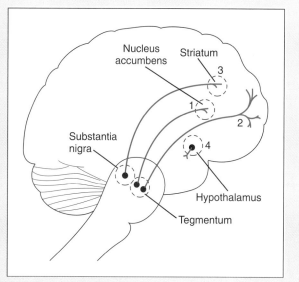

Sites of Drug Action

Some antipsychotic drugs (e.g., clozapine, olanzapine, and risperidone) block serotonin 5-HT$_2$ receptors in the mesocortical pathway to the prefrontal lobe cortex. This increases the release of dopamine (DA) and thereby alleviates the negative symptoms of schizophrenia. Most antipsychotic drugs (including those listed above) block dopamine D$_2$ receptors in the mesolimbic pathway to the nucleus accumbens, and this alleviates the positive symptoms of schizophrenia.

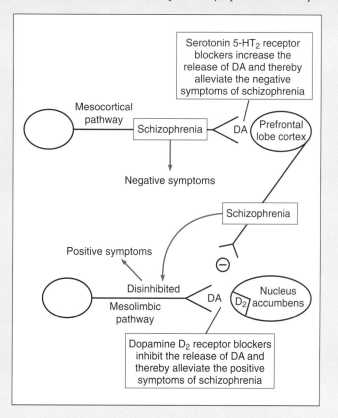

TABLE 22-2. **Mechanisms Responsible for the Therapeutic and Adverse Effects of Antipsychotic Drugs**

Mechanism	Therapeutic Effects	Adverse Effects
Blockade of α_1-adrenergic receptors	—	Dizziness, orthostatic hypotension, and reflex tachycardia
Blockade of dopamine D_2 receptors	Alleviation of positive symptoms of schizophrenia	Extrapyramidal effects (akathisia, dystonia, and pseudoparkinsonism) and elevated serum prolactin levels
Blockade of dopamine D_4 receptors	Alleviation of negative symptoms of schizophrenia and decrease in the incidence of extrapyramidal side effects	—
Blockade of histamine H_1 receptors	—	Drowsiness and increase in appetite and weight
Blockade of muscarinic receptors	—	Blurred vision, constipation, dry mouth, and urinary retention
Blockade of serotonin 5-HT_2 receptors	Alleviation of negative symptoms of schizophrenia and decrease in the incidence of extrapyramidal side effects	Anxiety and insomnia

clinical potency of these drugs and their in vitro affinity for D_2 receptors. Whereas antagonism of D_2 receptors in mesolimbic pathways is thought to repress the positive symptoms of schizophrenia, blockade of D_2 receptors in the basal ganglia is believed to be responsible for the parkinsonian and other extrapyramidal side effects that sometimes occur in patients taking antipsychotic drugs.

Atypical antipsychotic drugs (e.g., clozapine) have a greater affinity for 5-HT_2 receptors than for D_2 receptors, and some atypical drugs have increased the affinity for D_3 or D_4 receptors.

PHARMACOLOGIC EFFECTS. The mechanisms by which the blockade of dopamine and serotonin receptors alleviates the symptoms of schizophrenia are not completely understood. Whereas these receptors are blocked immediately when antipsychotic drugs are first administered, the therapeutic effects of the drugs usually require several weeks to fully develop. This is because antipsychotic drugs produce three time-dependent changes in dopamine neurotransmission. When first administered, the drugs cause an increase in dopamine synthesis, release, and metabolism. This probably represents a compensatory response to the acute blockade of postsynaptic dopamine receptors produced by antipsychotic drugs. Over time, continued dopamine receptor blockade leads to inactivation of dopaminergic neurons and produces what has been called **depolarization blockade.** Depolarization blockade results in reduced dopamine release from mesolimbic and nigrostriatal neurons. This action is believed to alleviate the positive symptoms of schizophrenia while causing extrapyramidal side effects. Eventually, the reduction in dopamine release caused by depolarization blockade leads to dopamine receptor up-regulation and supersensitivity to dopamine agonists. This supersensitivity may contribute to the development of a delayed type of extrapyramidal side effect called **tardive dyskinesia** (see later text).

In mesocortical and nigrostriatal pathways, 5-HT_2 receptors mediate presynaptic inhibition of dopamine release.

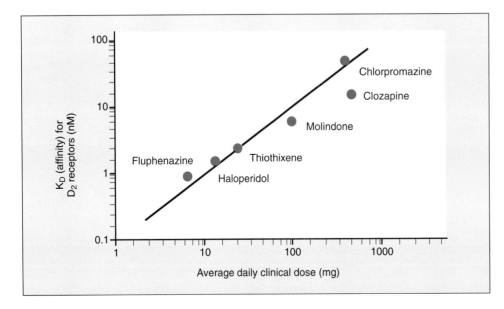

Figure 22-1. Correlation of antipsychotic drug potency and dopamine D_2 receptor binding. The clinical potency of the typical antipsychotic drugs is highly correlated with their in vitro affinity for D_2 (but not D_1) receptors.

TABLE 22-3. Adverse Effects of Antipsychotic Drugs*

Drug	Extrapyramidal Effects	Sedation	Anticholinergic Effects	Orthostatic Hypotension	Other Adverse Effects
Phenothiazines					
Chlorpromazine	+++	++++	+++	++++	Elevated serum prolactin levels and poikilothermy
Fluphenazine	+++++	++	++	++	Same as chlorpromazine
Thioridazine	++	++++	++++	++++	Cardiac arrhythmia, elevated serum prolactin levels, poikilothermy, and retinopathy
Trifluoperazine	++++	++	++	++	Same as chlorpromazine
Thioxanthenes					
Thiothixene	++++	++	++	++	Same as chlorpromazine
Butyrophenones					
Haloperidol	+++++	+	+	+	Same as chlorpromazine
Azepines					
Clozapine	+	+++++	+++++	++++	Agranulocytosis and cardiac arrhythmia
Loxapine	++++	+++	++	+++	Same as chlorpromazine
Olanzapine	+	++	+	+	Weight gain
Other antipsychotic drugs					
Molindone	+++	+	++	++	Same as chlorpromazine
Risperidone	++	+	+	++	Cardiac arrhythmia and elevated serum prolactin levels

*Ratings range from extremely low (+) to extremely high (+++++).

Blockade of these receptors by atypical antipsychotic drugs may increase dopamine release in these pathways. In the mesocortical pathway, this action may alleviate the negative symptoms of schizophrenia. In the nigrostriatal pathway, increased dopamine release counteracts the extrapyramidal side effects caused by D_2 receptor blockade.

ADVERSE EFFECTS. In the peripheral autonomic nervous system, antipsychotic drugs also block muscarinic receptors and α_1-adrenergic receptors, thereby causing adverse effects described in Tables 22–2 and 22–3. Antagonism at α_1-adrenergic receptors produces dizziness, orthostatic hypotension, and reflex tachycardia. Muscarinic receptor antagonism produces blurred vision, dry mouth, constipation, and urinary retention. Antagonism of brain H_1 receptors produces drowsiness and weight gain.

The most disturbing adverse effect is the development of motor abnormalities following the administration of high potency, typical antipsychotics. These and other adverse effects specific to particular agents are discussed below.

Neuroleptic malignant syndrome is a severe form of drug toxicity that occurs in 0.5% to 1% of patients treated with antipsychotic drugs. It is a life-threatening condition characterized by muscle rigidity, elevated temperature (>38°C), altered consciousness, and autonomic dysfunction (tachycardia, diaphoresis, tachypnea, and urinary and fecal incontinence). The syndrome resembles malignant hyperthermia in its rapid onset and mortality rate. Neuroleptic malignant syndrome is managed by providing supportive care and immediately discontinuing treatment with the offending antipsychotic drug. A dopamine receptor agonist (e.g., **bromocriptine**) may significantly reduce rigidity, fever, and other manifestations of the syndrome. If future antipsychotic therapy is required in patients who have experienced this syndrome, an atypical drug should be used because the atypical drugs are associated with a lower incidence of neuroleptic malignant syndrome.

INDICATIONS. Antipsychotic agents are primarily used to treat schizophrenia and other forms of psychosis, including drug-induced psychosis and psychosis associated with the manic phase of bipolar disorder. They are also used to treat severely agitated patients, including those with dementia and severe mental retardation. Because the phenothiazines have antiemetic activity, some of them are used in the management of nausea and vomiting (see Chapter 28).

Drug Classification

Antipsychotic drugs are usually classified on the basis of their chemical structure, but they can also be classified according to whether they display typical or atypical pharmacologic properties. The **typical antipsychotic drugs** include the phenothiazines, the thioxanthenes, the butyrophenones, and some azepines (e.g., loxapine). The **atypical antipsychotic drugs** include other azepines (e.g., clozapine and olanzapine) and a benzisoxazole drug called risperidone.

Phenothiazines

Numerous phenothiazines are available for the treatment of schizophrenia and related conditions. The four representative examples discussed here are chlorpromazine, fluphenazine, thioridazine, and trifluoperazine. These drugs have similar therapeutic effects but differ in their relative potency (Table 22–4) and in their side effect profiles (see Table 22–3).

CHEMISTRY AND PHARMACOKINETICS. Each phenothiazine drug is a tricyclic compound that contains a thiazine group and two benzene rings. An aliphatic, piperidine, or piperazine group is attached to the nitrogen atom of the thiazine ring, and this group influences the relative potency and side effects of the various phenothiazine drugs. Drugs with an aliphatic group (e.g., chlorpromazine) or a piperidine group (e.g., thioridazine) have a lower potency than do drugs with a piperazine group (e.g., fluphenazine). Low-potency drugs cause more autonomic side effects but fewer extrapyramidal side effects than do high-potency drugs.

The phenothiazines are adequately absorbed from the gut after oral administration. Several phenothiazines are also administered parenterally. The drugs are extensively metabolized to a large number of active and inactive metabolites before they are excreted in the urine, and they have elimination half-lives ranging from 20 to 30 hours (see Table 22–4).

MECHANISMS AND PHARMACOLOGIC EFFECTS. The phenothiazines are typical antipsychotic drugs whose therapeutic effects appear to be primarily caused by blockade of D_2 receptors. After therapy with a phenothiazine is initiated, the positive symptoms of schizophrenia usually subside in 1 to 3 weeks. Patients become less agitated and experience fewer auditory hallucinations. Grandiose or paranoid delusions subside and can disappear completely in some patients with continued treatment. At the same time, sleeping and eating patterns become normalized, and behavioral improvement occurs in the form of decreased hostility, combativeness, and aggression. Phenothiazines and other typical antipsychotic drugs can have some impact on negative symptoms, but it is usually less pronounced than the impact of atypical antipsychotic drugs.

ADVERSE EFFECTS. The most common adverse effects produced by phenothiazines and other antipsychotic drugs are shown in Table 22–3.

Blockade of dopamine receptors in the striatum can cause several forms of extrapyramidal side effects, including akathisia, pseudoparkinsonism, and dystonias. Patients with **akathisia,** or "motor restlessness," feel compelled to pace, shuffle their feet, or shift positions and are unable to sit quietly. **Pseudoparkinsonism** resembles idiopathic Parkinson's disease and is characterized by rigidity, bradykinesia, and tremor. **Dystonia** is a state of abnormal muscle tension that often affects the neck and facial muscles, including the tongue, pharynx, larynx, and eyes. Patients with dystonia can experience severe reactions, such as oculogyric crisis (a condition in which the eyeballs become fixed in one position, usually upward), glossospasm, tongue protrusion, and torticollis (a contracted state of the cervical muscles, producing twisting of the neck and an unnatural position of the head). Such reactions can be frightening and painful, and pharyngolaryngeal dystonias can even be life threatening. Young males who are given large doses of high-potency drugs are at great risk of developing dystonias.

Although akathisia, pseudoparkinsonism, and dystonias are acute extrapyramidal side effects that often occur early in the course of treatment with antipsychotic drugs, **tardive dyskinesia (TD)** is a disorder that usually develops after months or years of treatment. The disorder is characterized by abnormal oral and facial movements (e.g., tongue protrusion and lip smacking). In later stages, abnormal limb and truncal movements may also be observed. Investigators believe that TD results from supersensitivity to dopamine, which develops during long-term dopamine receptor blockade (see Chapter 18). This hypothesis is supported by the fact that the symptoms of TD temporarily subside if dopamine receptor blockade is increased by giving larger doses of an antipsychotic drug. This approach, however, eventually leads to further receptor supersensitivity and worsening of the manifestations of TD.

Phenothiazines can increase serum prolactin levels by blocking dopamine receptors in the tuberoinfundibular pathway (see Box 22–1) and thereby cause gynecomastia in men and menstrual irregularities in women. Via their effects on the hypothalamus, antipsychotic drugs sometimes impair thermoregulation and cause poikilothermy, a condition in which the body temperature tends to approach the ambient temperature. This can lead to hyperthermia (including heat stroke) or hypothermia. In addition, high doses of thioridazine can cause pigmentary retinopathy and cardiac toxicity.

TREATMENT OF ADVERSE EFFECTS. Acute extrapyramidal effects (akathisia, pseudoparkinsonism, and dystonias) that are caused by phenothiazines and other antipsychotic drugs can be managed by lowering the drug dosage, changing to an atypical antipsychotic drug, or administering an additional drug to counteract the adverse effects. Drugs that counteract the effects include **benztropine** (an anticholinergic drug), **diphenhydramine** (an antihistamine with significant anticholinergic activity), and **amantadine** (an agent that increases dopamine release in the basal ganglia and can be used in conjunction with an anticholinergic drug).

Tardive dyskinesia is not easily managed and does not necessarily subside if a causative drug is discontinued. Hence, prevention is important. To prevent TD, antipsychotic drugs should be used in the lowest doses for the shortest period of time required to control symptoms of schizophrenia. The drugs should be discontinued periodically to assess the need for continued treatment and possibly to reduce the development of dopamine supersensitivity. Patients should be evaluated regularly for early signs of TD, which are sometimes reversible. TD often becomes irreversible if it is not detected early or is allowed to persist.

Once detected, TD is best managed by reducing the dosage of antipsychotic medication. This results in significant improvement in many patients. No drugs are approved for the treatment of TD, but some success has been reported with the use of **amantadine, dopamine receptor agonists,** and **clozapine.** Other drugs that may be effective include **physostigmine** (an indirect-acting cholinergic agonist) and the **benzodiazepines.**

INTERACTIONS. The major drug interactions of phenothiazines, and other antipsychotics, are listed in Table 22–4.

TABLE 22–4. **Pharmacologic Properties of Antipsychotic Drugs***

Drug	Relative Potency[†]	Receptor Selectivity	Route of Administration	Elimination Half-Life and Route	Major Drug Interactions
Phenothiazines					
Chlorpromazine	Low	$D_2 > 5\text{-}HT_2$	Oral, IM, and IV	30 hours (M)	Additive effects with antiadrenergic, anticholinergic, and CNS depressants. Decreases serum levels of lithium. Concurrent use of a β-adrenergic receptor antagonist or an antidepressant may increase serum levels of both drugs.
Fluphenazine	High	$D_2 > 5\text{-}HT_2$	Oral and depot IM	20 hours (M)	Additive effects with anticholinergic and CNS depressants. Concurrent use of a β-adrenergic receptor antagonist or an antidepressant may increase serum levels of both drugs.
Thioridazine	Low	$D_2 > 5\text{-}HT_2$	Oral	30 hours (M)	Same as chlorpromazine
Trifluoperazine	High	$D_2 > 5\text{-}HT_2$	Oral and IM	24 hours (M)	Same as chlorpromazine
Thioxanthenes					
Thiothixene	High	$D_2 > 5\text{-}HT_2$	Oral and IM	35 hours (M)	Additive effects with anticholinergic and CNS depressants. Concurrent use of a β-adrenergic receptor antagonist may increase serum levels of both drugs.
Butyrophenones					
Haloperidol	High	$D_2 > 5\text{-}HT_2$	Oral and depot IM	24 hours (M)	Barbiturates and carbamazepine decrease serum levels. Quinidine increases serum levels.
Azepines					
Clozapine	Low	$5\text{-}HT_2 = D_4$ and $> D_2$	Oral	24 hours (M)	Not established; possible interaction with drugs that induce or inhibit cytochrome P450 isozyme CYP1A2.
Loxapine	Medium	$D_2 > 5\text{-}HT_2$	Oral and IM	20 hours (M)	Concurrent use of an antidepressant may increase serum levels of both drugs.
Olanzapine	High	$5\text{-}HT_2 > D_2$	Oral	30 hours (M)	Same as clozapine
Other antipsychotic drugs					
Molindone	Medium	$D_2 > 5\text{-}HT_2$	Oral	2 hours (M)	Additive effects with anticholinergic and CNS depressants. Concurrent use of a β-adrenergic receptor antagonist or an antidepressant may increase serum levels of both drugs.
Risperidone	High	$5\text{-}HT_2 > D_2$	Oral	24 hours (M)	Not established; possible interaction with drugs that induce or inhibit cytochrome P450 isozyme CYP2D6.

*Values shown are the mean of values reported in the literature. D_2 = dopamine D_2 receptor; $5\text{-}HT_2$ = serotonin $5\text{-}HT_2$ receptor; IM = intramuscular; IV = intravenous; depot = long-acting form; M = metabolized; and CNS = central nervous system.
[†]Low = 50–2000 mg/d; medium = 20–250 mg/d; and high = 1–100 mg/d.

The interactions include additive effects on central nervous system (CNS) depression when used with other CNS drugs and pharmacokinetic interactions caused by antipsychotics and other drugs existing as substrates for the same cytochrome P450 isozymes.

Chlorpromazine and Thioridazine

Chlorpromazine and thioridazine are low-potency phenothiazines with similar properties. Of the two agents, thioridazine produces greater anticholinergic effects, and this probably accounts for its tendency to cause fewer extrapyramidal side effects. High doses of thioridazine can cause pigmentary retinopathy and cardiac arrhythmia.

Fluphenazine and Trifluoperazine

Fluphenazine and trifluoperazine are high-potency phenothiazines that produce fewer autonomic side effects but more extrapyramidal side effects than do low-potency phenothiazines. Fluphenazine is available in a long-acting depot preparation that is intended for intramuscular injection every 1 to 3 weeks and is useful for treating patients who are not compliant with oral medication or are unable to take oral drugs.

Thioxanthenes

The chemical structure of the thioxanthenes is similar to that of the phenothiazines. In the thioxanthene structure, however, the nitrogen atom of the phenothiazine ring is replaced with a carbon atom.

Thiothixene is one of the most widely used thioxanthenes, and it has pharmacologic properties that are similar to those of trifluoperazine (see Tables 22–3 and 22–4). Thiothixene is primarily used to treat **schizophrenia.**

Butyrophenones

The first of the high-potency agents and the most widely used butyrophenone is **haloperidol.** Haloperidol, a high-potency drug that has properties similar to those of fluphenazine, can cause significant extrapyramidal side effects (see Tables 22–3 and 22–4). As with fluphenazine, haloperidol is available in a long-acting depot preparation for intramuscular administration. Haloperidol is extensively metabolized in the liver, and its metabolites are excreted in the urine and bile.

In addition to its use in treating psychoses (e.g., **schizophrenia**), haloperidol is used in the treatment of **Tourette's syndrome** (Gilles de la Tourette's syndrome). This syndrome is characterized by facial and vocal tics, coprolalia (compulsive use of obscene words, particularly those related to feces), and echolalia (repetition of another person's words or phrases).

Azepines

Loxapine, clozapine, and **olanzapine** are azepine derivatives. Whereas loxapine is a typical antipsychotic drug, clozapine and olanzapine are atypical drugs that produce fewer extrapyramidal side effects than do other antipsychotic drugs. Another member of this class, **quetiapine,** was recently approved for the treatment of schizophrenia and for acute manic episodes associated with bipolar disorder, as either monotherapy or adjunct therapy to lithium or valproate (see later text).

Loxapine

Loxapine, a dibenzoxazepine, is a typical antipsychotic drug whose properties are similar to those of the phenothiazines.

Clozapine

Clozapine has a tricyclic dibenzodiazepine structure and a unique profile of pharmacologic and clinical effects. It is the first of a new generation of atypical antipsychotic drugs that cause significantly fewer extrapyramidal side effects while exhibiting greater activity against the negative symptoms of schizophrenia.

Because clozapine is a potent antagonist of a large number of receptors, it has been difficult to attribute its effects to a particular mechanism of action. It seems likely that its therapeutic effects result from blockade of D_4 receptors and 5-HT_2 receptors. Both of these actions may contribute to its greater efficacy against the negative symptoms of schizophrenia and to its lower incidence of extrapyramidal side effects. The use of clozapine is associated with significant sedation and autonomic side effects. These adverse reactions are caused by blockade of histamine, muscarinic, and α_1-adrenergic receptors. The use of clozapine is also associated with a 1.3% first-year incidence of potentially fatal agranulocytosis. For this reason, the Food and Drug Administration has required weekly monitoring of leukocyte counts during the first 6 months of therapy, the period during which the risk of agranulocytosis is greatest. After 6 months, biweekly monitoring of leukocyte counts is required.

Olanzapine

Olanzapine is a thienobenzodiazepine analogue of clozapine. Its pharmacologic properties are similar to those of clozapine, but it causes fewer autonomic side effects and has not been reported to cause agranulocytosis. As with clozapine, olanzapine causes minimal extrapyramidal side effects.

Olanzapine has about twice the affinity for 5-HT_2 receptors as it does for D_2 receptors, and it can block dopamine D_3 and D_4 receptors. Although it also blocks histamine, muscarinic, and α_1-adrenergic receptors, it does so to a lesser extent than does clozapine.

Clinical trials indicate that olanzapine is as effective as haloperidol in alleviating the positive symptoms of schizophrenia, is superior to haloperidol in alleviating the negative symptoms, and it produces significantly fewer extrapyramidal side effects. The most common adverse reactions to olanzapine have been sedation and weight gain. At higher doses, olanzapine can cause akathisia, pseudoparkinsonism, and dystonias.

Other Antipsychotic Drugs

RISPERIDONE. Risperidone is a newer atypical antipsychotic drug that has a benzisoxazole structure. Its pharmacologic properties are similar to those of olanzapine, but it appears to cause less sedation, more orthostatic hypotension, and a higher incidence of extrapyramidal side effects than does olanzapine. Its effects on treating both the positive and negative symptoms of schizophrenia are caused by antagonism at both D_2 and serotonin (5-HT_2) receptors. In some patients, risperidone elevates levels of serum prolactin. It also lengthens the QT interval seen on the electrocardiogram and can predispose patients to cardiac arrhythmias, including torsade de pointes. Another agent sharing the pharmacologic profile of risperidone is **ziprasidone.** A newer agent, **aripiprazole,** differs slightly in that it is a partial agonist at dopamine receptors but a 5-HT receptor antagonist.

MOLINDONE. Molindone is a dihydroindolone derivative with a unique spectrum of pharmacologic activities. Some authorities classify it as an atypical drug, but others do not. It appears to cause a relatively low incidence of autonomic side effects and sedation. Although its incidence of extrapyramidal side effects also appears to be relatively low, it is probably higher than that of the newer atypical antipsychotic agents when they are given in equivalent doses. Molindone has a relatively short half-life but is metabolized to active and inactive compounds that have a longer half-life. Molindone is sometimes effective in patients who do not tolerate or respond to other drugs.

Treatment Considerations

All typical antipsychotic drugs appear to be equally effective when used in equipotent doses for the treatment of schizophrenia. The highly sedating drugs are no more effective than the less-sedating drugs in calming agitated patients, and the less-sedating drugs are no more effective than the highly sedating drugs in treating withdrawn patients. Hence, the choice of drug is primarily based on the need to minimize autonomic or extrapyramidal side effects. Several controlled trials indicate that low-dose regimens are as effective as high-dose regimens and produce fewer side effects.

The atypical antipsychotic drugs represent an appealing choice for the treatment of schizophrenia, and they may become the drugs of choice for treating most forms of psychosis. In comparison with the typical drugs, the atypical drugs produce a lower incidence of extrapyramidal side effects and appear to be more effective against the negative symptoms of schizophrenia. Data on the long-term effectiveness of atypical drugs in patients with chronic schizophrenia, however, have not yet been obtained.

During the first 2 weeks of treatment with an antipsychotic drug, many patients exhibit some alleviation of positive symptoms and an improvement in socialization, mood, and self-care habits. The maximal response to treatment, however, generally requires 6 weeks or longer, at which time it may be possible to reduce the dosage during maintenance therapy. Antipsychotic medication is usually continued for at least 12 months after the remission of acute psychotic symptoms. At that time, a low-dose regimen or gradual withdrawal of medication should be considered in order to reduce the probability of developing TD. Antipsychotic drugs should be tapered slowly before discontinuation, because abrupt discontinuation can cause withdrawal symptoms such as insomnia, nightmares, nausea, vomiting, diarrhea, restlessness, salivation, and sweating.

AFFECTIVE DISORDERS

Affective disorders are also called **mood disorders.** The two most common affective disorders are major depressive disorder and bipolar disorder. The primary drugs used in their treatment are antidepressant drugs and mood-stabilizing drugs.

Clinical Findings

Major Depressive Disorder

Major depressive disorder (unipolar depression) is characterized by depressed mood, loss of interest or pleasure in life, sleep disturbances, feelings of worthlessness, diminished ability to think or concentrate, and recurrent thoughts of suicide. Depressed patients can also be irritable or anxious.

Bipolar Disorder

Bipolar disorder (previously called manic-depressive disorder) is characterized by recurrent fluctuations in mood, energy, and behavior that encompass the extremes of human experience. This disorder differs from major depression in that periods of mania alternate or occur simultaneously with depressive symptoms. The clinical presentation varies widely. The manic phase is characterized by elevated mood, inflated self-esteem (grandiosity), increased talking (pressure of speech), racing thoughts (flight of ideas), increased social or work activity, and decreased need for sleep. Manic patients can become hostile and uncooperative. As the manic phase intensifies, some patients experience psychotic symptoms such as delusions.

Typically, the manic phase occurs just before or just after a depressive episode. In many patients, depressive and manic episodes last several weeks or months. In some patients, however, the episodes change within hours or days (rapid cycling bipolar disorder).

Etiology and Pathogenesis

According to the **biogenic amine hypothesis,** mood disorders result from abnormalities in serotonin, norepinephrine, or dopamine neurotransmission. Serotoninergic fibers projecting from the raphe nuclei in the midbrain to limbic structures are important in regulating mood, and these neuronal pathways are believed to be hypofunctional in depressed patients. The serotoninergic system is activated during behavioral arousal and increases cortical awareness of emotional reactions to environmental events. It is believed that impaired serotonin neurotransmission can decrease cortical responsiveness to emotional activation, leading to affective dysfunction and depression. Noradrenergic fibers that project from the locus ceruleus to the cerebral cortex can also play a role in depression, as can dopaminergic fibers innervating the nucleus accumbens.

Evidence links depression with abnormal circadian rhythms and melatonin regulation. Melatonin, the principal mediator of biologic rhythms, is known to suppress the activity of serotoninergic neurons. Investigators postulate that excess melatonin production contributes to the development of depression. This hypothesis is particularly relevant to **seasonal affective disorder (SAD),** which usually occurs during the winter months, when daylight is reduced and melatonin levels are increased. Other types of depression, however, can also be caused by abnormal melatonin regulation. Abnormalities in melatonin and serotonin metabolism can also contribute to the sleep disturbances seen in patients with affective disorders.

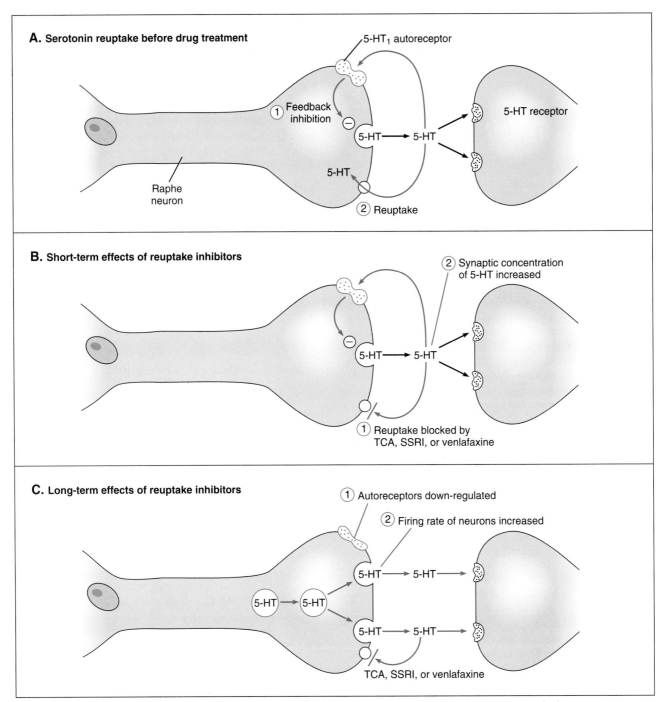

A. Serotonin reuptake before drug treatment

5-HT₁ autoreceptor

(1) Feedback inhibition

5-HT receptor

5-HT

Raphe neuron

5-HT

(2) Reuptake

B. Short-term effects of reuptake inhibitors

(2) Synaptic concentration of 5-HT increased

5-HT

(1) Reuptake blocked by TCA, SSRI, or venlafaxine

C. Long-term effects of reuptake inhibitors

(1) Autoreceptors down-regulated

(2) Firing rate of neurons increased

5-HT

TCA, SSRI, or venlafaxine

Figure 22–2. Mechanisms of neuronal reuptake inhibitors. (A) In the absence of a reuptake inhibitor, serotonin (5-hydroxytryptamine, or 5-HT) is released from raphe neurons that project to limbic structures. Serotonin activates postsynaptic and presynaptic 5-HT receptors and undergoes reuptake into the presynaptic neuron. (B) When a tricyclic antidepressant (TCA), a selective serotonin reuptake inhibitor (SSRI), or venlafaxine is initially given, the drug blocks the reuptake of 5-HT and increases its synaptic concentration. (C) With continued use of a TCA, SSRI, or venlafaxine, increased synaptic concentrations of 5-HT cause the down-regulation of presynaptic autoreceptors and an increase in the firing rate of raphe neurons.

The biogenic amine hypothesis is supported by the fact that all antidepressant drugs act to increase serotonin, norepinephrine, or dopamine neurotransmission in the brain. Most antidepressant drugs increase the synaptic concentration of serotonin, and this leads to down-regulation of presynaptic autoreceptors. Investigators believe that the down-regulation, in turn, increases the firing rate of

serotonergic neurons and thereby produces the delayed therapeutic effect of antidepressant drugs. These mechanisms are depicted in Figure 22–2.

Recent data demonstrating that antidepressant medications produce an increase in the rate of appearance of new neurons in the brain of nonhuman mammals suggest a novel mechanism of antidepressant drug action. Studies have yet to show the correlation between increased appearance of brain neurons and the clinical effectiveness of antidepressants but this interesting finding provides another view to the possible causes of depression and its treatment.

ANTIDEPRESSANT DRUGS

Depression can be treated with **tricyclic antidepressants (TCA), selective serotonin reuptake inhibitors (SSRI),** and a host of other antidepressants that have different structures and act by various mechanisms of action. If patients fail to respond to these drugs, **monoamine oxidase inhibitors (MAOI)** can be used.

Because depressed patients might attempt suicide, the safety of an antidepressant in overdose is an important consideration when selecting a drug for a particular patient.

Indications

Antidepressants have been used to treat all forms of **depression** and to treat several other conditions. The antidepressants are also effective in the treatment of certain **anxiety disorders,** such as panic disorder, phobic disorders, and obsessive-compulsive disorder. **Clomipramine** is particularly effective in treating patients with obsessive-compulsive behavior. Some antidepressants are beneficial in the management of certain **sleep disorders,** including somnambulism, night terrors, and enuresis. Antidepressants repress excessive rapid eye movement (REM) sleep and dreaming, which are conditions that contribute to somnambulism and night terrors. In patients with enuresis, antidepressants appear to increase the awareness of the need to urinate and thereby facilitate waking up for this purpose. Other antidepressants also have a role in the treatment of **chronic pain syndromes** because of their mood-elevating effect and analgesic activity.

The SSRI are used to treat **depression, eating disorders** (e.g., bulimia nervosa and anorexia nervosa), and **anxiety disorders** (e.g., panic disorder, phobic disorders, and obsessive-compulsive disorder). SSRI may be effective in the management of other conditions (e.g., **fibromyalgia, autism,** and **premenstrual syndrome [premenstrual dysphoric disorder]**).

Tricyclic Antidepressants

The tricyclic antidepressants include **amitriptyline, clomipramine, desipramine, imipramine,** and **nortriptyline.** These agents are highly effective in the treatment of depression and several other disorders, but they are associated with a high incidence of adverse effects. They also cause severe toxicity when taken in excessive doses.

Drug Properties

CHEMISTRY AND PHARMACOKINETICS. Each TCA contains a three-ring nucleus with an aliphatic side chain attached to the central ring (Fig. 22–3A). The side chain terminates in either a secondary or tertiary amine group. The type of amine group partly determines the drug's pharmacologic properties, as discussed later. The TCA are incompletely absorbed after oral administration and are extensively metabolized to active and inactive metabolites in the liver. The tertiary amines are deaminated to pharmacologically active secondary amines, and several of these metabolites are available as drugs. For example, amitriptyline is converted to nortriptyline, and imipramine is converted to desipramine. The TCA and their active metabolites have relatively long half-lives, ranging from 18 to 70 hours.

MECHANISM OF ACTION. All TCA block the neuronal reuptake of norepinephrine and serotonin, but they do so to differing degrees. The blockade occurs as soon as drug administration begins and causes an immediate increase in the synaptic concentration of serotonin. The blockade is also believed to trigger a series of adaptive changes in norepinephrine and serotonin neurotransmission.

PHARMACOLOGIC EFFECTS. TCA produce an antidepressant effect that becomes apparent about 2 to 4 weeks after drug therapy is started. Over time, the increased synaptic concentration of serotonin can cause down-regulation of presynaptic autoreceptors and thereby increase the firing rate of serotoninergic neurons. The short-term and long-term effects of TCA and other reuptake inhibitors on serotonin neurotransmission are illustrated in Fig. 22–2.

ADVERSE EFFECTS. As with many of the antipsychotic drugs, the TCA produce autonomic side effects by blocking muscarinic and α_1-adrenergic receptors. Some of the TCA also produce marked sedation (Table 22–5). In fact, TCA are often administered at bedtime, when their sedative effects can have the added benefit of promoting sleep. The TCA lower the seizure threshold and can induce seizures at therapeutic as well as toxic serum concentrations.

Taking an overdose of a TCA can cause life-threatening cardiac arrhythmia, which frequently presents as a wide QRS complex tachycardia; marked autonomic effects, including hypotension and sinus tachycardia; excessive sedation; and seizures.

TREATMENT OF ADVERSE EFFECTS. The type of arrhythmia that occurs with an overdose can be treated by the intravenous administration of sodium bicarbonate. Sodium bicarbonate increases the ratio of nonionized TCA to ionized TCA and thereby decreases the binding of the TCA to the sodium channel in cardiac membranes.

Specific Drugs

Nortriptyline and **desipramine** are secondary amines formed by the demethylation of amitriptyline and imipramine, respectively. Secondary amines block norepinephrine uptake more than they block serotonin reuptake, and this is especially true of desipramine.

Amitriptyline, clomipramine, and **imipramine** are tertiary amines. They block serotonin reuptake to a greater extent than do secondary amines. They also produce more sedation and autonomic side effects than do secondary amines.

Studies have shown that all TCA are equally effective in relieving depression, although some patients respond better to one drug than to another. The choice of a TCA is primarily based on the relative incidence of adverse effects produced by the different drugs. A drug that causes a higher

SECTION IV ■ Central Nervous System Pharmacology

Figure 22–3. Structures of selected antidepressant drugs. (A) Each tricyclic antidepressant contains a three-ring nucleus with an aliphatic side chain attached to the central ring. The side chain terminates in either a secondary or tertiary amine group. Amitriptyline and imipramine are tertiary amines that are deaminated to nortriptyline and desipramine, respectively. All four of these substances are pharmacologically active. (B) The selective serotonin reuptake inhibitors include fluoxetine, paroxetine, and sertraline. (C) Phenelzine and tranylcypromine are first-generation monoamine oxidase (MAO) inhibitors that block both MAO-A and MAO-B.

degree of sedation may be chosen for highly agitated or anxious patients with depression, whereas a drug that causes a lower degree of sedation may be preferred for patients who are more apathetic or withdrawn.

Selective Serotonin Reuptake Inhibitors

The **selective serotonin reuptake inhibitors** are a newer class of antidepressants that include **fluoxetine, fluvoxamine, paroxetine, sertraline, citalopram,** and **escitalopram.** The SSRI have become the most widely used drugs for the treatment of depression and certain anxiety disorders, such as panic disorder and obsessive-compulsive disorder. They

are as effective as the TCA but cause fewer autonomic side effects and less sedation. They are also much safer than the TCA following an overdose, in that the SSRI seldom cause cardiac arrhythmia and are less likely to induce seizures.

Reboxetine, an antidepressant used in Europe, is selective for norepinephrine uptake, thus increasing the amount of norepinephrine in the synapse. It may represent the first of a class of norepinephrine selective reuptake inhibitors (NSRI). As opposed to older TCA agents that also block both serotonin and norepinephrine reuptake but also interact with many other receptor types to produce adverse effects, new drugs that are selective for just the reuptake transporters are now available. Preclinical studies show that **duloxetine** is a potent and selective inhibitor of both neuronal serotonin

TABLE 22-5.   Adverse Effects of Antidepressant Drugs*

Drug	Sedation	Anticholinergic Effects	Orthostatic Hypotension	Cardiac Conduction Disturbances
Tricyclic antidepressants				
Amitriptyline	++++	++++	+++	+++
Clomipramine	++++	++++	++	+++
Desipramine	++	++	++	++
Imipramine	+++	+++	+++	+++
Nortriptyline	++	++	++	++
Selective serotonin reuptake inhibitors				
Fluoxetine	0	0	0	0
Fluvoxamine	+	0	0	0
Paroxetine	+	+	0	0
Sertraline	0	0	0	0
Monoamine oxidase inhibitors				
Phenelzine	++	++	++	+
Tranylcypromine	+	++	++	+
Other antidepressant drugs				
Bupropion	+	+	0	+
Hypericum	0	0	0	0
Mirtazapine	+	+	++	+
Nefazodone	+++	0	+++	+
Trazodone	++++	0	+++	+
Venlafaxine	+	+	0	+

*Ratings range from none (0) to high (++++).

and norepinephrine reuptake. It is indicated for major depressive disorder and is also used for chronic pain. It may be the first of a class of serotonin norepinephrine selective reuptake inhibitors (SNSRI).

Drug Properties

CHEMISTRY AND PHARMACOKINETICS. The SSRI are a structurally heterogeneous group of compounds (see Fig. 22–3B). They are well absorbed from the gut after oral administration and are extensively metabolized by cytochrome P450 isozymes. Fluoxetine, which has a longer half-life than the other drugs in this class, is converted to an active metabolite that has an even longer half-life. The metabolites of other SSRI have little or no pharmacologic activity.

MECHANISM OF ACTION AND PHARMACOLOGIC EFFECTS. The SSRI selectively block the neuronal reuptake of serotonin and have much less effect on the reuptake of norepinephrine. Their efficacy in the treatment of depression supports the hypothesis that serotonin dysfunction plays a significant role in the pathophysiology of depression. The short-term and long-term effects of serotonin reuptake inhibition are illustrated in Fig. 22–2.

ADVERSE EFFECTS. The SSRI produce fewer sedative, autonomic, and cardiovascular side effects than do the TCA. Unlike the TCA, the SSRI are usually administered in the morning, because they tend to increase alertness in patients. Their most common adverse effects are nervousness, dizziness, and insomnia. They occasionally cause male sexual dysfunction in the forms of priapism and impotence. Many of the side effects of SSRI subside with continued use. The SSRI

should be used with caution in patients with seizure disorders, hepatic disorders, diabetes, or bipolar disorder.

Fluoxetine

Fluoxetine, the first drug approved for the treatment of bulimia nervosa, may be effective in the management of anorexia nervosa. The drug is well absorbed orally and is converted to an active metabolite, norfluoxetine. The parent compound has a half-life of 2.5 days, but its active metabolite has a half-life of about 8 days. This long duration of action can be a disadvantage if severe adverse effects occur.

Fluoxetine causes more drug interactions than do other SSRI. It can impair the regulation of blood glucose levels in diabetic patients. It can also cause a syndrome of inappropriate antidiuretic hormone secretion (SIADH), characterized by persistent hyponatremia and elevated urine osmolality.

Fluvoxamine

Fluvoxamine is approved for the treatment of obsessive-compulsive disorder but has also been used to treat depression and panic disorder. Fluvoxamine has a half-life of about 15 hours and can be associated with sedative effects.

Paroxetine and Sertraline

Paroxetine and sertraline have half-lives of 21 hours and 26 hours, respectively. Paroxetine has a high bioavailability, whereas sertraline undergoes extensive first-pass elimination. Sertraline has relatively little effect on P450 isozymes and causes fewer drug interactions than does fluoxetine. Sertraline may be preferred in elderly patients because its elimination is not affected substantially by aging. Paroxetine is somewhat more sedating than fluoxetine and sertraline.

Citalopram and escitalopram

Citalopram has chemical structure unrelated to that of other SSRI or of tricyclic, tetracyclic, or other available antidepressant agents. It is a racemic mixture (contains both R and S enantiomers of the drug molecule) and highly selective for serotonin reuptake transporters in preclinical models. Escitalopram is the pure S-enantiomer (single isomer) of the racemic citalopram drug. Escitalopram (the S-form) is at least 100 times more potent than the R-enantiomer with respect to inhibition of 5-HT reuptake.

Monoamine Oxidase Inhibitors

Because the monoamine oxidase inhibitors have many potentially serious interactions with other drugs and with food, they are not considered drugs of choice in the treatment of depression. They are generally used as alternative therapy when patients have failed to respond adequately to other drugs.

Drug Properties

CHEMISTRY AND PHARMACOKINETICS. The chemical structures of MAOI are shown in Fig. 22–3C. The first-generation MAOI, phenelzine and tranylcypromine, are adequately absorbed from the gut and have relatively short half-lives. They irreversibly bind to and inhibit MAO, however, and their pharmacologic effects persist for many hours after their serum levels have declined. Phenelzine and tranylcypromine can increase serotonin levels more than they do norepinephrine levels in the brain, and their antidepressant effects are probably caused by down-regulation of presynaptic autoreceptors and subsequent increased firing of serotoninergic neurons. As with other antidepressants, the clinical effects of MAOI are delayed for several weeks after therapy begins.

MECHANISM OF ACTION. The MAOI bind irreversibly to an enzyme, monoamine oxidase, responsible for the degradation of the biogenic amine neurotransmitters, norepinephrine, dopamine and serotonin. The binding of MAOI prevents the substrate from reaching the active site on the enzyme.

The MAOI are classified according to their selectivity for the two main types of MAO. Type A (MAO-A) preferentially oxidizes serotonin but will also metabolize norepinephrine and dopamine. Type B (MAO-B) preferentially metabolizes dopamine. MAO-A is found in higher concentrations in the gut and other peripheral tissues than is MAO-B, and the inhibition of MAO-A is believed to be responsible for the antidepressant effects of the MAOI.

PHARMACOLOGIC EFFECTS. MAOI increases the concentration of dopamine, norepinephrine and serotonin in storage sites throughout the nervous system and, in theory, this increased concentration of monoamines in the brain is the basis for its antidepressant activity.

ADVERSE EFFECTS. The major adverse effect reported with MAOI is the occurrence of a **hypertensive crisis,** which is sometimes fatal. Such crises are characterized by some or all of the following symptoms: occipital headache which may radiate frontally, palpitation, neck stiffness or soreness, nausea or vomiting, sweating, and photophobia. Hypertensive crisis can occur with MAOI alone or, more commonly, following the administration of sympathomimetic amines or dining on foodstuffs containing **tyramine** (see Interactions, below).

Specific agents

The first-generation MAOI for treating depression include **phenelzine** and **tranylcypromine,** which are irreversible inhibitors of both MAO-A and MAO-B. The second-generation MAOI include **moclobemide** and are reversible inhibitors of MAO-A (RIMA). The RIMA are used in many countries to treat depression but are not yet available in the United States of America. **Selegiline** represents a third type of MAOI, which selectively inhibits MAO-B and is used in the treatment of Parkinson's disease (see Chapter 24).

Other Antidepressant Drugs

Several other drugs with diverse chemical structures (see Fig. 22–3D) and diverse mechanisms of action are available for the treatment of depression.

Bupropion

Bupropion is an aminoketone whose mechanism of action is not well understood. It is a relatively weak inhibitor of the neuronal reuptake of dopamine, norepinephrine, and serotonin. Bupropion produces few anticholinergic side effects, causes very little sedation, and rarely produces cardiovascular effects or sexual dysfunction. It can cause agitation, insomnia, nausea, and weight loss. A formulation of bupropion has been developed as adjunct therapy for patients who are attempting to quit smoking cigarettes (see Chapter 25).

Mirtazapine

Mirtazapine, a newer tetracyclic piperazinoazepine drug, is structurally different from other antidepressants and has both antidepressant and antianxiety effects. Mirtazapine blocks presynaptic α_2-adrenergic autoreceptors and heteroreceptors and thereby increases the neuronal release of norepinephrine and serotonin, respectively. It increases central norepinephrine concentrations to a greater degree than do the TCA, and it is also a potent antagonist of 5-HT$_2$ and 5-HT$_3$ receptors. Mirtazapine is better tolerated and causes fewer adverse reactions than do the TCA. It can significantly elevate hepatic enzyme levels, however, and it has been associated with a few cases of agranulocytosis.

Trazodone

Trazodone selectively inhibits the neuronal reuptake of serotonin. It causes considerable sedation and orthostatic hypotension, but it does not produce anticholinergic side effects and has minimal effects on cardiac conduction.

Venlafaxine

Venlafaxine is a structurally unique antidepressant that strongly blocks the reuptake of both norepinephrine and serotonin (see Fig. 22–2). It has a side effect profile similar to that of the SSRI. It does not inhibit muscarinic, adrenergic, or histamine receptors, and it produces few autonomic, sedative, or cardiovascular side effects.

Hypericin

Extracts of the plant called St. John's wort (*Hypericum perforatum*) exhibit antidepressant activity, and products containing these extracts are available in health food stores. The extracts contain a substance called **hypericin** and several flavones. Some of these compounds inhibit MAO, whereas others appear to block the neuronal reuptake of serotonin. *Hypericum* extracts appears to cause fewer adverse effects than do TCA. Clinical studies are being conducted to evaluate the clinical efficacy and safety of hypericin.

Interactions

The serum levels of TCA are elevated by concurrent administration of antipsychotic drugs, calcium channel blockers, cimetidine, and SSRI, which compete with TCA for metabolic enzymes in the liver. Barbiturates, carbamazepine, and phenytoin decrease the serum levels of TCA because of upregulation of hepatic metabolic enzymes. As with SSRI (see below), TCA should not be used with an MAOI.

Because of their ability to inhibit cytochrome P450 isozymes, the SSRI have significant interactions with a variety of drugs. Among the SSRI, fluoxetine has the greatest effect on the CYP2D isozyme and sertraline has the least effect. Inhibition of CYP2D can increase the serum levels of antipsychotic drugs, TCA, and dextromethorphan. Inhibition of CYP2C and CYP3A can increase serum levels of alprazolam, diazepam, carbamazepine, phenytoin, and other drugs. SSRI can also increase the hypoprothrombinemic effect of warfarin.

The SSRI should not be used concurrently with monoamine oxidase inhibitors, because both types of drugs increase the serotonin levels in the brain and their concurrent use can precipitate the **serotonin syndrome.** This syndrome is characterized by agitation, restlessness, confusion, insomnia, seizures, severe hypertension, and gastrointestinal symptoms. At least 2 weeks should elapse between the discontinuation of treatment with either an MAOI or an SSRI and the start of treatment with the other drug. The exception is that 5 weeks must elapse between the discontinuation of fluoxetine and the administration of an MAOI.

Monoamine oxidase inhibitors interact with SSRI, TCA, and other antidepressant drugs and have the potential to cause severe toxicity when administered with these drugs. Concurrent administration of MAOI and TCA or other antidepressants requires dosage reduction and careful monitoring.

Monoamine oxidase inhibitors can cause severe hypertension when administered with sympathomimetic amines or with foods containing **tyramines.** These foods include many types of cheese (especially aged cheeses), beer, some wines (especially Chianti), some meats and fish (especially canned meat, liver, sardines, and herring), some fruits and vegetables (especially raisins, broad beans, avocados, and canned figs), and some products when consumed in large quantities (especially chocolate and coffee).

Treatment Considerations

Depression is one of the most common mental illnesses. Because it tends to be underdiagnosed, it often goes untreated. The primary treatment for patients with depression is drug therapy, but psychotherapy enhances the response to pharmacologic treatment and increases patient compliance with medication. Electroconvulsive therapy is sometimes used as an alternative when antidepressants have been ineffective or are not tolerated. More than 80% of patients respond to treatment with drugs, psychotherapy, electroconvulsive therapy, or a combination of these modalities.

The initial drug used in the treatment of depression is usually either a TCA or an SSRI, depending on clinician preference. A growing body of evidence indicates that SSRI are better tolerated by patients, produce fewer adverse effects, and are safer in overdose than are TCA. The disadvantages of SSRI include their higher cost and the increased tendency of some SSRI to cause drug interactions. Sertraline causes fewer drug interactions than do other SSRI and may be preferred in the treatment of patients who are taking other drugs that can interact with SSRI.

If TCA or SSRI are not effective or well tolerated, the clinician has a growing choice of other antidepressants (e.g., mirtazapine, nefazodone, and venlafaxine). Mirtazapine and venlafaxine are attractive because of their low incidence of sedation, autonomic side effects, and cardiac toxicity (see Table 22–5). In comparison with other antidepressants, nefazodone has demonstrated a lower incidence of activating side effects, such as nervousness, agitation, and insomnia, and it does not cause sexual dysfunction.

It usually takes 2 to 4 weeks for antidepressants to elevate the mood of depressed patients, and some patients do not respond until after 6 weeks or longer. Some authorities believe that many cases of treatment-resistant depression are caused by inadequate drug dosage, inadequate duration of therapy, or patient noncompliance. Moreover, studies indicate that many patients who failed to respond to treatment in the past will respond to adequate doses of SSRI or other new antidepressants.

To prevent relapse, antidepressants are usually continued for 4 to 9 months after remission of depressive symptoms.

MOOD-STABILIZING DRUGS

Indications

Mood-stabilizing drugs act to normalize the swings of affect in bipolar disorder. Although the element lithium is the standard agent in this class, a number of other agents are being tested and used for this indication. Lithium has been called a mood stabilizer because it reduces both manic and depressive symptoms and thereby tends to normalize the mood in patients with bipolar disorder. Lithium, as with other mood-stablizers, however, has greater activity against manic symptoms than it does against depression, and it is primarily used to treat or prevent the manic phase of bipolar disorder.

Lithium

Lithium, the lightest of the alkali metal elements, was accidentally discovered to have a calming effect in patients with mania.

Drug Properties

PHARMACOKINETICS. Lithium, which is administered orally in the form of lithium carbonate or lithium citrate, is available in immediate-release and sustained-release preparations. About 95% to 100% of the administered dose is absorbed from the gut. Lithium is widely distributed throughout the body, with the highest concentrations found in the thyroid gland, bone, and some areas of the brain. The drug is not metabolized. It has a half-life of about 24 hours and is excreted in the urine. Lithium is extensively reabsorbed from the renal tubules, and the renal clearance of lithium is about 20% of the glomerular filtration rate. Lithium clearance increases during pregnancy. Sodium competes with lithium for renal tubular reabsorption and, thereby, can increase the excretion of lithium.

MECHANISM OF ACTION. The mechanisms by which lithium produces its mood-stabilizing effects are not well understood. The drug appears to act by suppressing the formation of second messengers involved in neurotransmitter signal transduction, but the relationship between this action and the drug's clinical effect is unclear. Lithium reduces the formation of inositol triphosphate (IP_3) by inhibiting *myo*-inositol-1-phosphatase, an enzyme in the inositol phosphate pathway. This enzyme participates in the regeneration of inositol and the inositol phosphate precursors to IP_3. By reducing IP_3 formation, lithium reduces the neuronal response to serotonin and norepinephrine, whose effects are partly mediated by IP_3 (see Table 18–1). Lithium also interferes with the formation of cyclic adenosine monophosphate.

PHARMACOLOGIC EFFECTS. Lithium produces a calming effect in manic patients, but the maximal response to lithium often requires several days or weeks of treatment. For this reason, other drugs may need to be used during the early phase of treatment while awaiting the full response to lithium (see below). The serum concentration of lithium should be monitored after initiating therapy and at periodic intervals thereafter. Although the concentration should be between 0.6 and 1.2 mEq/L, a concentration of 0.8 to 1.0 mEq/L is considered optimal for most patients. Monitoring the concentration serves to verify the adequacy of dosage and may warn of potential toxicity.

ADVERSE EFFECTS. Lithium has a relatively low margin of safety. Elevated lithium levels can cause neurotoxicity and cardiac toxicity leading to arrhythmia. Nausea with vomiting can be one of the earliest signs of lithium overdose. It is important for the clinician and patient to distinguish the signs of lithium toxicity from the adverse effects of lithium that often occur with therapeutic serum levels.

Lithium is fairly well tolerated by most patients, but it produces a number of unpleasant side effects that decrease patient compliance. Common side effects include drowsiness, weight gain, a fine hand tremor, and polyuria. The hand tremor can usually be controlled by the administration of a β-adrenergic receptor antagonist. Lithium causes polyuria because it interferes with the action of antidiuretic hormone and thereby inhibits the kidney's ability to concentrate the urine. In some patients, lithium causes hypothyroidism by blocking thyroid hormone synthesis and release.

INTERACTIONS. Nonsteroidal anti-inflammatory drugs (NSAID) and diuretics decrease lithium clearance by about 25% and increase lithium levels. Other drugs can increase lithium neurotoxicity.

Other Mood-Stabilizing Drugs

Although lithium is the primary drug used to treat and prevent manic symptoms in bipolar disorder, other drugs have been found to have equal or greater efficacy and may be better tolerated by some patients. These include **carbamazepine** and **valproate**, antiepileptic drugs whose pharmacologic properties are described in Chapter 20.

Treatment Considerations

Treatment of bipolar disorder must be individualized on the basis of symptoms, response to drug therapy and other treatment modalities, and the minimization of adverse effects. Drug treatment with **lithium** is often the cornerstone of therapy, because lithium can abort an acute manic episode, can prevent future manic episodes, and also appears to exert a mild antidepressive effect. Because of the dynamic nature of the disorder, however, therapy must be frequently reevaluated and modified.

Lithium usually controls an acute manic episode within 1 or 2 weeks after initiating therapy. Other drugs may be required to control acute symptoms while awaiting the full effect of lithium to develop. **Benzodiazepines** can relieve manic symptoms and promote sleep. An antipsychotic drug may be required to suppress delusions and other psychotic symptoms accompanying mania. **Risperidone** and **olanzapine** are effective in patients with bipolar disorder and cause fewer adverse effects than do typical antipsychotic drugs (e.g., haloperidol).

Lithium is usually continued for 9 to 12 months after the initial manic episode, and then its use can be slowly tapered, with continued monitoring of symptoms. Many patients experience hypomanic symptoms for several days or longer before developing a full manic episode, and lithium therapy can be reinstituted in these patients in an attempt to abort a full manic episode. Long-term prophylactic therapy can be given to patients who have had two or three episodes and to those whose symptoms develop rapidly. Long-term patient compliance with lithium, however, is often poor.

Depression that persists after lithium therapy is instituted may respond to **antidepressant drugs**. The use of antidepressants in patients who have bipolar disorder and are not taking lithium or another mood-stabilizing drug will evoke a manic response (switch phenomenon) in many patients.

A growing list of alternatives to lithium for bipolar disorder includes several antiepileptic drugs. **Carbamazepine** exhibits antimanic, antidepressant, and prophylactic effects that are equivalent to those of lithium, and it causes fewer adverse effects in many patients. Moreover, about 60% of manic patients who do not respond to lithium will respond to carbamazepine within the first several days of treatment. Evidence also suggests that lithium and carbamazepine can be synergistic in their antimanic activity in patients with refractory bipolar disorder. **Valproate** is another drug that is approved for the treatment of mania in bipolar disorder. It appears to be especially useful in patients with rapid cycling of manic and depressive episodes and in patients with coexisting substance abuse. Other antiepileptic drugs have demonstrated antimanic activity in clinical studies and may be approved for treating bipolar disorder in the future.

SUMMARY OF IMPORTANT POINTS

■ Schizophrenia can result from abnormal function of the dopaminergic pathways in the brain. According to the dopamine hypothesis, this abnormality leads to dysfunctional dopamine neurotransmission in the prefrontal lobe cortex.

■ Delusions, hallucinations, and other positive symptoms of schizophrenia can result from excessive dopamine neurotransmission in mesolimbic pathways. Apathy, withdrawal, lack of motivation and pleasure, and other negative symptoms can result from impaired dopamine neurotransmission in mesocortical pathways.

■ The typical antipsychotic drugs include the phenothiazines, the thioxanthenes, the butyrophenones, and some azepines (e.g., loxapine). The atypical antipsychotic drugs include other azepines (e.g., clozapine and olanzapine) and a benzisoxazole drug called risperidone.

■ Typical antipsychotic drugs are believed to act by blocking dopamine D_2 receptors in mesolimbic pathways. Atypical antipsychotic drugs act by blocking serotonin 5-HT_2 and D_2 receptors. Both classes of drugs alleviate the positive symptoms of schizophrenia, but the typical drugs cause a higher incidence of extrapyramidal side effects (akathisia, pseudoparkinsonism, dystonia, and tardive dyskinesia) and are less effective against the negative symptoms of schizophrenia.

■ Low-potency antipsychotics (chlorpromazine and thioridazine) produce more autonomic side effects and sedation than do high-potency drugs (fluphenazine and haloperidol), but the high-potency drugs cause more extrapyramidal side effects. Clozapine sometimes causes agranulocytosis, so leukocyte counts must be monitored.

■ Depression is believed to result from inadequate serotoninergic and noradrenergic neurotransmission in limbic structures and elsewhere in the brain.

■ The tricyclic antidepressants (TCA) block serotonin and norepinephrine reuptake. They effectively treat depression, but they have significant autonomic and cardiovascular side effects. When taken in an overdose, they can cause seizures and cardiac arrhythmia.

■ The selective serotonin reuptake inhibitors (SSRI) are antidepressants that have fewer autonomic and cardiovascular side effects and cause less sedation than do the TCA. In comparison with other SSRI, fluoxetine has a longer half-life and causes more drug interactions. Sertraline causes fewer drug interactions.

■ Other antidepressants (e.g., bupropion, mirtazapine, nefazodone, trazodone, and venlafaxine) have different pharmacologic profiles that lead to increased biogenic amines in the brain.

■ Nonselective monoamine oxidase (MAO) inhibitors (e.g., phenelzine and tranylcypromine) bind to and inhibit MAO type A and type B. These drugs prevent the breakdown of serotonin, norepinephrine, dopamine, sympathomimetic drugs, and amines contained in certain foods. To prevent a hypertensive crisis in patients who are taking MAO inhibitors, the use of interacting drugs and foods must be avoided.

■ Lithium is a mood-stabilizing drug that is primarily used to treat and prevent the manic phase of bipolar disorder. It has a narrow therapeutic range, so its serum concentrations must be carefully monitored. Overdose can result in neurotoxicity and cardiac toxicity. Lithium produces many side effects, including tremor, weight gain, and polydipsia. Alternatives to lithium include carbamazepine and valproate.

Review Questions

1. Clinical antipsychotic of potency for "typical" antipsychotics correlate with actions at which receptor?
   (A) dopamine D_2
   (B) α_2-adrenergic
   (C) muscarinic
   (D) histamine
   (E) serotonin

2. Which agent listed below is an antipsychotic that can improve BOTH positive and negative symptoms of schizophrenia?
   (A) chlorpromazine
   (B) haloperidol
   (C) thiothixene
   (D) risperidone
   (E) thioridazine

3. Which one of the following is NOT a class of antidepressant medications?
   (A) heterocyclic antidepressants
   (B) tricyclic antidepressants
   (C) monoamine oxidase inhibitor
   (D) acetylcholinesterase inhibitors
   (E) selective serotonin reuptake inhibitors

4. The older tricyclic antidepressants (TCA) share all of the following adverse effects EXCEPT which one?
   (A) orthostatic hypotension
   (B) sedation
   (C) seizures
   (D) weight gain
   (E) sexual dysfunction

5. Foodstuffs containing tyramine should be avoided when taken with which class of medications?
(A) tricyclic antidepressants
(B) monoamine oxidase inhibitors
(C) selective serotonin reuptake inhibitors
(D) atypical antidepressants
(E) antihypertensive medications

Answers and Explanations

1. The correct choice is A: dopamine D_2 receptors. Antipsychotic agents are classified as typical, generally the older agents with actions at dopamine receptors, and the atypical antipsychotics, which can have multiple receptor action but primarily interact at 5-HT receptors. Answers (B), α_2-adrenergic receptors, and (C), muscarinic receptors, mediate some of the adverse effects of typical antipsychotic agents. No evidence for answer (D), histamine receptors, in the clinical effects of typical antipsychotics, but they can be involved in sedative effects of the older, less-selective agents. Answer (E), serotonin receptors, is correlated to the efficacy of the atypical agents and not the typical ones as discussed above.

2. The correct answer is D: risperidone. Risperidone is a unique dual-acting antipsychotic agent that is an antagonist at both D_2 receptors and 5-HT$_2$ receptors and is effective in treating both positive and negative symptoms of schizophrenia. Answers (A), chlorpromazine, (B), haloperidol, (C), thiothixene, and (E), thioridazine, are all older, typical antipsychotics that block dopamine receptors (among other receptors) but with no appreciable affinity for 5-HT receptors.

3. The correct answer is D: acetylcholinesterase inhibitors. Acetylcholinesterase inhibitors, also known as indirect-acting cholinergic agonists, increase the synaptic concentration of acetylcholine. This has utility in the treatment of the dementia of Alzheimer's disease, but does not have antidepressant activity. The other answers are types of antidepressants.

4. The correct answer is E: sexual dysfunction. Whereas the older TCA antidepressants can cause all of the adverse effects listed from (A) through (D), it is the newer SSRI, such as fluoxetine, that are noted for sometimes causing sexual dysfunction including priapism and impotency.

5. The correct choice is B: monoamine oxidase inhibitors. The MAOI irreversibly inhibit, monoamine oxidase, the enzyme that degrades biogenic amines neurotransmitters. This elevates the levels of the amine neurotransmitter available for synaptic releases. Tyramine in food is not degraded because the MAO enzyme is blocked and a hypertensive crisis might ensue. Answers (A) and (C) through (E) are agents that do not interfere with the catabolism of dietary amines.

SELECTED READINGS

Bowden, C. L. Making optimal use of combination pharmacotherapy in bipolar disorder. J Clin Psychiatry 65(Suppl 15):21–24, 2004.
Duman, R. S. Depression: a case of neuronal life and death? Biol Psychiatry 56(3):140–145, 2004.
Sink, K. M, K. F. Holden, and K. Yaffe. Pharmacological treatment of neuropsychiatric symptoms of dementia: a review of the evidence. JAMA 293(5):596–608, 2005.
Shelton, C. I. Long-term management of major depressive disorder: are differences among antidepressant treatments meaningful? J Clin Psychiatry 65(Suppl 17):29–33, 2004.
Shelton, R. C. St John's wort for the treatment of depression. Lancet Neurol 1(5):275, 2002.
Silverstone, P. H. Qualitative review of SNRIs in anxiety. J Clin Psychiatry 65(Suppl 17):19–28, 2004.
Wirshing, D. A. Schizophrenia and obesity: impact of antipsychotic medications. J Clin Psychiatry 65(Suppl 18):13–26, 2004.

CHAPTER 23

Opioid Analgesics and Antagonists

CLASSIFICATION OF OPIOID ANALGESICS AND ANTAGONISTS

Strong Opioid Agonists
- Morphine
- Meperidine (DEMEROL)
- Methadone
- Oxycodone (OXYCONTIN)
- Hydromorphone (DILAUDID)
- Fentanyl (SUBLIMAZE)
- Sufentanil (SUFENTA)

Moderate Opioid Agonists
- Codeine
- Hydrocodone (VICODIN, LORTAB)
- Propoxyphene (DARVON)

Other Opioid Agonists
- Dextromethorphan
- Diphenoxylate (LOMOTIL)
- Loperamide (IMODIUM)
- Tramadol (ULTRAM)

Mixed Opioid Agonist-antagonists
- Buprenorphine (BUPRENEX)
- Butorphanol (STADOL)
- Nalbuphine (NUBAIN)
- Pentazocine (TALWIN)

Opioid Antagonists
- Naloxone (NARCAN)
- Naltrexone (TREXAN, REVIA)

OVERVIEW

PAIN AND ANALGESIC AGENTS

Pain is an unpleasant sensory and emotional experience that serves to alert an individual to actual or potential tissue damage. This damage can be caused by exposure to noxious chemical, mechanical, or thermal stimuli (e.g., acids, pressure, percussion, and extreme heat) or by the presence of a pathologic process (e.g., a tumor, muscle spasm, inflammation, nerve damage, organ distention, or other mechanism that activates nociceptors on sensory neurons). Although pain serves a protective function by alerting a person to the presence of a health problem, its unbridled expression often leads to considerable morbidity and suffering. For this reason, **analgesics** or drugs that relieve pain are used for symptomatic treatment of pain from a wide variety of disease states, ranging from acute and chronic physical injuries to terminal cancer.

Based on their mechanisms of action, analgesics can be classified as **opioid analgesics** or **non-opioid analgesics.** Opioid analgesics act primarily in the spinal cord and brain to inhibit the neurotransmission of pain. In contrast, nonopioid analgesics act primarily in peripheral tissues to inhibit the formation of **algogenic** or pain-producing substances such as prostaglandins. Because most of the nonopioid analgesics also exhibit significant anti-inflammatory activity, they are called **nonsteroidal anti-inflammatory drugs (NSAID).** The NSAID are described in greater detail in Chapter 30.

To facilitate the selection of an appropriate analgesic or anesthetic medication, patients are usually asked to describe their pain in terms of its intensity, duration, and location. In some cases, patients complain of an **intense, sharp,** or **stinging pain.** In other cases, they describe a **dull, burning,** or **aching pain.** These two types of pain are transmitted by different types of neurons and their primary afferent fibers (Box 23–1). Pain can be further distinguished on the basis

BOX 23-1. PAIN PATHWAYS AND SITES OF DRUG ACTION

Pain activates primary afferent neurons that enter the spinal cord, where they synapse with interneurons directly onto spinothalamic tract neurons (SST). The neospinothalamic tract projects to the primary sensory cortex, which alerts the individual to the presence and location of pain, the **sensory-discriminative** component. The paleospinothalamic tract projects to limbic structures, which mediate the **motivational-affective** response to pain. Descending neuronal tracts from the periaqueductal gray matter activate neurons that release norepinephrine (NE), serotonin (5-hydroxytryptamine, or 5-HT), and enkephalin (Enk) in the spinal cord and thereby block ascending pain transmission. Opioid analgesics activate the descending pathways and directly activate opioid receptors on afferent nerve terminals and on SST neurons in the spinal cord. Nonopioid analgesics reduce the activation of primary afferent neurons via inhibition of prostaglandin synthesis. NMR = nucleus magnus raphae; LC = locus ceruleus; SP = substance P; and Glu = glutamate.

Primary Afferent Neuron	Ascending Pathway	Projections	Type of Pain	Functions
Aδ (fast)	Neospinothalamic	Reticular formation, thalamus, and sensory cortex	Intense, sharp, stinging pain	Pain localization and withdrawal reflexes
C (slow)	Paleospinothalamic	Thalamus, periaqueductal gray matter, and limbic structures	Dull, burning, aching pain	Autonomic reflexes, pain memory, and pain discomfort

of whether it is somatic, visceral, or neuropathic in origin. **Somatic pain** is often well localized to specific dermal, subcutaneous, or musculoskeletal tissue. **Visceral pain** originating in thoracic or abdominal structures is often poorly localized and may be referred to somatic structures. For example, cardiac pain is often referred to the chin, neck, shoulder, or arm. **Neuropathic pain** is usually caused by nerve damage, such as that resulting from nerve compression or inflammation, or from diabetes. Neuropathic pain is characteristic, for example, of trigeminal neuralgia (*tic douloureux*), postherpetic neuralgia, and certain types of back and limb injuries.

PAIN PATHWAYS

Exposure to a noxious stimulus activates **nociceptors** on the peripheral free nerve endings of **primary afferent neurons.** The cell bodies of these neurons sit alongside the spinal cord in the dorsal root ganglia and send one axon to the periphery and one to the dorsal horn of the spinal cord. With noxious stimulation, substance P, glutamate, and other excitatory neurotransmitters are released from the central terminations of the primary afferent fibers onto neurons of the spinal cord. Many of these terminals synapse directly on **spinothalamic tract neurons** in the dorsal horn, which send long fibers up the contralateral side of the spinal cord to transmit pain impulses via **ascending pain pathways** to the medulla, midbrain, thalamus, limbic structures, and cortex.

As shown in Box 23–1, the primary afferent fibers transmitting nociceptive information are **Aδ fibers** and **C fibers,** which are responsible for sharp pain and dull pain, respectively. Spinal reflexes activated by these fibers can lead to withdrawal from a noxious stimulus before pain is perceived by higher structures. Ascending pain pathways consist of two main anatomical-functional projections; the **sensory-discriminative** component to the cerebral cortex and the **motivational-affective** component, to the limbic cortex. Projections to the sensory cortex alert an individual to the presence and anatomic location of pain, whereas projections to limbic structures (e.g., the amygdala) enable the individual to experience discomfort, suffering, and other emotional reactions to pain.

The activation of spinothalamic neurons in the spinal cord can be blocked by **descending inhibitory pathways** from the midbrain and by sensory **Aβ fibers** arising in peripheral tissues. These two systems constitute the neurologic basis of the **gate-control hypothesis.** According to this hypothesis, pain transmission by spinothalamic neurons can be modulated, or gated, by the inhibitory activity of other types of large fibers impinging on them. The activation of spinothalamic neurons is also inhibited by peripheral Aβ sensory fibers that stimulate the release of enkephalins from spinal cord interneurons. The Aβ fibers also mediate the analgesic effect produced by several types of tissue stimulation, including **acupuncture** and **transcutaneous electrical nerve stimulation (TENS).** These mechanisms also explain the pain relief that may be produced by simply rubbing or massaging an injured tissue.

The descending inhibitory pathways arise from periaqueductal gray (PAG) in the midbrain and they project to medullary nuclei that transmit impulses to the spinal cord

(see Box 23–1). The medullary neurons include serotonergic nerves arising in the nucleus magnus raphae (NMR) and noradrenergic nerves arising in the locus ceruleus (LC). When these nerves release **serotonin** and **norepinephrine** in the spinal cord, they inhibit dorsal spinal neurons that transmit pain impulses to supraspinal sites. Nerve fibers from the PAG also activate spinal interneurons that release an endogenous opioid peptide, met-enkephalin. The enkephalins act presynaptically to decrease the release of pain transmitters from the central terminations of primary afferent neurons. They also act on postsynaptic receptors on spinothalamic tract neurons in the spinal cord to decrease the rostral transmission of the pain signal. Opioid analgesics activate the descending PAG, NMR, and LC neurons, and they also directly activate opioid receptors in the spinal cord.

OPIOID PEPTIDES AND RECEPTORS

Since ancient times, **opium**, the raw extract of the poppy plant, *Papaver somniferum*, has been used for the treatment of pain and diarrhea. During the 19th century, **morphine** was isolated from opium, and its pharmacologic effects were characterized. Later, specific sites in central nervous system (CNS) tissue were discovered that bound morphine and other opioid agonists. The presence of stereoselective receptors for morphine in brain tissue indicated the likelihood of an endogenous ligand for these receptors, and this eventually led to the discovery of the three major families of endogenous opioid peptides: **enkephalins, endorphins,** and **dynorphins.**

The opioid peptides are derived from larger precursor proteins that are widely distributed in the brain. Endorphins and dynorphins are large peptides, whereas the two types of enkephalins are small pentapeptides containing Tyr-Gly-Gly-Phe-Met/Leu. Hence, the two types of enkephalins are called **Met-enkephalin** and **Leu-enkephalin.**

The enkephalins are released from neurons throughout the pain axis, including those in the PAG, medulla, and spinal cord. Enkephalins activate opioid receptors in these areas and thereby block the transmission of pain impulses. The enkephalins appear to act as neuromodulators in that they exert a long-acting inhibitory effect on the release of excitatory neurotransmitters by several neurons.

The three opioid receptor types are μ (*mu*) receptors, δ (*delta*) receptors, or κ (*kappa*) receptors. Most of the clinically useful opioid analgesics, however, have preferential or strong selectivity for μ receptors. Some of the mixed opioid agonist-antagonist agents have κ receptor selectivity, but attempts to develop useful opioid analgesics selective for δ receptors have not been successful.

OPIOID DRUGS

Classification

The opioid drugs can be classified as full agonists, mixed agonist-antagonists, or pure antagonists.

Based on their maximal clinical effectiveness, the **full agonists** can be characterized as strong or moderate agonists. In experimental pain models, all of the full agonists exert a maximal analgesic effect. In humans, the **strong opioid** agonists are well-tolerated when they are given in a dosage sufficient to relieve severe pain. The **moderate opioid agonists**, however, will cause intolerable adverse effects if they are given in a dosage sufficient to alleviate severe pain. For this reason, the moderate opioid agonists are administered in submaximal doses to treat moderate to mild pain, and they are usually formulated in combination with NSAID to enhance their clinical effectiveness.

The **mixed opioid agonist-antagonists** are analgesic drugs that have varying combinations of agonist, partial agonist, and antagonist activity and varying degrees of affinity for the different opioid receptor types.

The **opioid antagonists** have no analgesic effects. They are used to counteract the adverse effects of opioids taken in overdose and for the treatment of drug dependence.

Drug Properties

Mechanism of Action

The opioid receptors are members of the G-protein coupled receptor family. Activation of opioid receptors leads to inhibition of adenylyl cyclase and a decrease in the concentration of cyclic adenosine monophosphate (cAMP), an increase in K^+ conductance, and a decrease in Ca^{2+} conductance (Fig. 23–1). The activated $G\alpha_i$ subunit of the G protein directly inhibits the adenylyl cyclase enzyme and the $G\beta\gamma$ subunits are thought to mediate the changes at the Ca^{2+} and K^+ channels. These actions cause both presynaptic inhibition of neurotransmitter release and postsynaptic inhibition of membrane depolarization.

Pharmacologic Effects

CENTRAL NERVOUS SYSTEM. Morphine acts in the CNS to produce analgesia, sedation, euphoria or dysphoria, miosis, nausea, vomiting, respiratory depression, and inhibition of the cough reflex (Table 23–1).

Analgesia is produced by activation of opioid receptors in the spinal cord and at several supraspinal levels, as illustrated in Box 23–1. Sedation and euphoria can be caused by effects on midbrain dopaminergic, serotoninergic, and noradrenergic nuclei. Surprisingly, many patients experience **dysphoria** after administration of opioids. **Miosis** or constricted pupils is produced by the direct stimulation of the Edinger-Westphal nucleus of the oculomotor nerve (cranial nerve III), which activates parasympathetic stimulation of the iris sphincter muscle. Because little or no tolerance develops to the miosis, this sign can be diagnostic of an opioid overdose.

Codeine and other opioids inhibit the cough reflex at sites in the medulla where this reflex is integrated. The antitussive actions of opioids are discussed in greater detail in Chapter 27.

CARDIOVASCULAR SYSTEM. The most prominent cardiovascular effect of morphine and many other opioids is vasodilation, which is partly caused by histamine release from mast cells in peripheral tissues. Morphine can cause orthostatic hypotension from decreased peripheral resistance and a reduction in baroreceptor reflex activity. In patients with coronary artery disease, the decreased peripheral resistance leads to a reduction of cardiac work and myocardial oxygen demand.

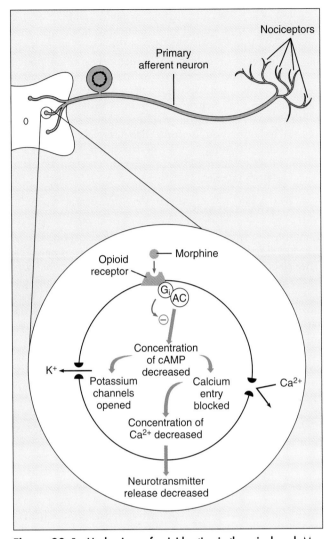

Figure 23–1. Mechanisms of opioid action in the spinal cord. Morphine and other opioid agonists activate presynaptic μ (*mu*) δ (*delta*) or κ (*kappa*) opioid receptors on primary afferent neurons. These receptors are coupled negatively to adenylyl cyclase (AC) via G proteins (G_i). Inhibition of cyclic adenosine monophosphate (cAMP) formation leads to opening of potassium channels and closing of calcium channels. Potassium efflux causes membrane hyperpolarization. The closing of calcium channels inhibits the release of neurotransmitters, such as substance P.

GASTROINTESTINAL, BILIARY, AND GENITOURINARY SYSTEM. Morphine and most other opioids act to increase smooth muscle tone in the gastrointestinal, biliary, and genitourinary systems.

In the gastrointestinal tract, increased muscle tone leads to inhibition of peristalsis and causes constipation. For this reason, the opioids are the oldest and most widely used medication for the treatment of diarrhea (see Chapter 28).

Morphine and other opioids increase the tone of the biliary sphincter (sphincter of Oddi), and can cause an exacerbation of pain in patients with biliary dysfunction or a gall bladder attack. Opioids also increase the tone of the bladder sphincter and can cause urinary retention in some patients. Because the opioid agonist, **meperidine**, has less

TABLE 23–1. Major Pharmacologic Effects of Opioid Agonists

Central nervous system (CNS) effects

Analgesia
Dysphoria or euphoria
Inhibition of cough reflex
Miosis
Physical dependence
Respiratory depression
Sedation

Cardiovascular effects

Decreased myocardial oxygen demand
Vasodilation and hypotension

Gastrointestinal and biliary effects

Constipation (increased intestinal smooth muscle tone)
Increased biliary sphincter tone and pressure
Nausea and vomiting (via CNS action)

Genitourinary effects

Increased bladder sphincter tone
Prolongation of labor
Urinary retention

Neuroendocrine system effects

Inhibition of release of luteinizing hormone
Stimulation of release of antidiuretic hormone and prolactin

Immune system effects

Suppression of function of natural killer cells

Dermal effects

Flushing
Pruritus
Urticaria (hives) or other rash

---

pronounced action on smooth muscle, it is the drug of choice for these patients and for the pain associated with labor.

OTHER EFFECTS. Opioids have an effect on neuroendocrine and immunologic function. In the hypothalamus, they stimulate the release of antidiuretic hormone and prolactin and inhibit the release of luteinizing hormone. Opioids also suppress the activity of certain types of lymphocytes, including natural killer cells, and this action may contribute to the high rate of infectious diseases in heroin addicts.

Adverse Effects

The major adverse effect of morphine and other opioids is **respiratory depression,** which is usually the cause of death in severe overdoses. Opioids reduce the hypercapnic drive (the stimulation of respiratory centers by increased carbon dioxide levels) while producing relatively little effect on the hypoxic drive. Opioids reduce the respiratory tidal volume and rate, causing the rate to fall to three or four breaths per minute after an opioid overdose. As the cerebral circulation is exquisitely sensitive to CO_2 levels and responds with an increase in cerebral blood flow, which leads to increased intracranial pressure, opioids should not be used in the case of a closed-head injury. The respiratory depressant effects of opioids are rapidly reversed by the intravenous administration of an opioid antagonist such as naloxone (see later text).

By stimulating the chemoreceptor trigger zone in the medulla, the opioids also cause **nausea and vomiting**. This is seen most often in ambulatory patients as opioids increase the sensitivity of the vestibular organ of the inner ear.

Opioids cause mast cells throughout the body to release histamine, which can cause itching, or **pruritis**. A flushing reaction, noted by redness and a feeling of warmth over the upper torso, may also occur from histamine release.

Allergic reactions to opioid analgesics are not uncommon. In most cases, however, a patient who is allergic to a particular opioid can use an opioid from a different chemical class. For example, someone who is allergic to codeine will probably not be allergic to propoxyphene or fentanyl.

Tolerance and Physical Dependence

Tolerance is defined as a decrease in initial pharmacologic effect observed following chronic or long-term administration. Repeated administration of an opioid agonist will lead to pharmacodynamic tolerance for both the administered opioid and other opioid analgesics. Tolerance primarily results from down-regulation of opioid receptors. Interestingly, in animal models, the magnitude of tolerance is inversely proportional to the efficacy of the opioid analgesic. This is because at equi-analgesic doses, a more efficacious opioid will occupy a lesser fraction of available opioid receptors than a less efficacious agent. Tolerance develops to most of the effects of opioids but not to miosis and constipation. Although considerable tolerance to respiratory depression occurs, a sufficiently high dose of an opioid can still be fatal to highly tolerant individuals.

Opioid tolerance is usually accompanied by a similar degree of **physical dependence.** Physical dependence is defined as a physiologic state in which a person's continued use of a drug is required for his or her well-being. Tolerance and physical dependence appear to represent the establishment of a new equilibrium between the neuron and its environment, wherein the neuron becomes less responsive to the opioid while requiring continued opioid inhibition to maintain cellular homeostasis. If the opioid drug is abruptly withdrawn, the equilibrium is disturbed and a rebound hyperexcitability occurs owing to the loss of the inhibitory influence of the drug. This produces a withdrawal reaction, the manifestations of which depend on the particular type of drug (see Chapter 25).

Because opioids demonstrate cross-tolerance, one opioid drug can substitute for another opioid drug and prevent symptoms of withdrawal in a physically dependent person. This is the basis for outpatient treatment of opioid dependence by the use of **methadone** or **buprenorphine** (see Chapter 25).

SPECIFIC AGENTS

STRONG OPIOID AGONISTS

The strong opioid agonists include naturally occurring drugs (e.g., morphine) and a number of synthetic drugs, including fentanyl, meperidine, and methadone. These drugs have equivalent analgesic effects but differ in their pharmacokinetic properties (Table 23–2), adverse effects, and uses.

TABLE 23–2. **Pharmacokinetic Properties of Opioid Drugs***

Drug	Route of Administration	Duration of Action (Hours)	Elimination Half-Life (Hours)	Active Metabolite
Strong opioid agonists				
Fentanyl	Parenteral, transdermal, and transmucosal[†]	1	4	No
Meperidine	Oral and parenteral	3	3	Yes
Methadone	Oral and parenteral	8	24	No
Morphine	Oral and parenteral	4	3	Yes
Oxycodone	Oral	4	Unknown	No
Sufentanil	Parenteral	1	2	No
Moderate opioid agonists				
Codeine	Oral	4	3	Yes
Hydrocodone	Oral	4	4	No
Propoxyphene	Oral	4	9	Yes
Other opioid agonists				
Dextromethorphan	Oral	6	11	No
Diphenoxylate	Oral	6	12	Yes
Loperamide	Oral	6	10	No
Tramadol	Oral	4	6	Yes
Mixed opioid agonist-antagonists				
Buprenorphine	Parenteral	5	5	No
Butorphanol	Intranasal and parenteral	3	3	No
Nalbuphine	Parenteral	4	5	No
Pentazocine	Oral and parenteral	4	4	No
Opioid antagonists				
Naloxone	Parenteral	2	4	No
Naltrexone	Oral	24	12	Yes

*Values shown are the mean of values reported in the literature.
[†]Fentanyl lozenges are available for pediatric preanesthetic use.

Morphine

The isolation of morphine from opium is illustrated in Fig. 1–2, and the structure of morphine is shown in Fig. 23–2A. Morphine is the principal alkaloid of the opium poppy, *Papaver somniferum*. A phenanthrene alkaloid, it constitutes about 10% of dried opium. Opium also contains papaverine and other benzylisoquinoline alkaloids that do not have analgesic properties. The diacetic acid ester of morphine is heroin, a drug that is frequently abused (see Chapter 25).

Morphine is well absorbed from the gut, but it undergoes considerable first-pass metabolism in the liver, where a significant fraction of the drug is converted to glucuronides. For this reason, larger doses are required when the drug is administered orally than when it is administered parenterally. The principal metabolite of morphine is the 3-glucuronide, which is pharmacologically inactive. A significant amount of the 6-glucuronide is also formed, which is more active than morphine and has a longer half-life. Hence, the 6-glucuronide contributes significantly to the analgesic effectiveness of morphine. Morphine is primarily excreted in the urine in the form of glucuronides. A small amount is excreted in the bile and undergoes enterohepatic cycling.

Morphine remains the standard of comparison for opioid analgesic drugs. It is primarily used to treat **severe pain associated with trauma, myocardial infarction, and cancer.** In patients with myocardial infarction, it relieves pain and anxiety while also dilating coronary arteries and reducing the myocardial oxygen demand. Morphine is available in both parenteral and oral formulations, including a long-acting oral formulation that is useful in patients with severe chronic pain.

Fentanyl and Its Derivatives

Fentanyl is a synthetic opioid agonist whose structure is shown in Fig. 23–2B. Fentanyl and its derivatives, including **sufentanil,** are the most potent opioid agonists available. Because of its high potency and lipid solubility, fentanyl has been formulated in a long-acting transdermal skin patch to provide continuous pain relief for patients with **severe or chronic pain.** It is also available for parenteral administration preoperatively and postoperatively and as an **adjunct to general anesthesia.** Fentanyl produces less nausea than does morphine, but is often associated with truncal rigidity when used as an adjunct parenteral anesthesia.

Meperidine

Meperidine is a synthetic opioid agonist with an unusual profile of pharmacologic properties. It has no antitussive activity and has variable effects on pupil size. Because its effect on gastrointestinal, biliary, and uterine smooth muscle is less pronounced than that of morphine, it is less likely than morphine to cause constipation or an increase in biliary pressure. Meperidine does not prolong labor as much as morphine does, so it can be used for analgesia in obstetrics.

A. Morphine and its derivatives

Morphine

Substitution on Morphine Structure

Drug	3 Position	6 Position	17 Position	Other Changes*
Agonists				
Morphine	—OH	—OH	—CH₃	–
Codeine	—OCH₃	—OH	—CH₃	–
Heroin	—OCOCH₃	—OCOCH₃	—CH₃	–
Hydrocodone	—OCH₃	=O	—CH₃	(1)
Oxycodone	—OCH₃	=O	—CH₃	(1), (2)
Agonist-antagonists				
Butorphanol	—OH	—H	—CH₂—◇	(2), (3)
Nalbuphine	—OH	—OH	—CH₂—◇	(1), (2)
Antagonists				
Naloxone	—OH	=O	—CH₂CH=CH₂	(1), (2)
Naltrexone	—OH	=O	—CH₂—◁	(1), (2)

*Other changes in the morphine molecule are as follows: (1) Single bond between C7 and C8. (2) OH added to C14. (3) No oxygen between C4 and C5.

B. Other opioid drugs

Fentanyl   Meperidine   Methadone

Figure 23–2. Structures of morphine and its derivatives (A) and of other selected opioid drugs (B).

The parenteral formulation of meperidine is often used as an **obstetric or postsurgical analgesic.** The oral formulation is used to treat **moderate to severe pain** in the outpatient setting. The drug is converted to a toxic metabolite, normeperidine, which can cause CNS excitation, convulsions, and tremors when meperidine is administered in large doses or for a prolonged period. Hence, the drug is usually used for the **short-term treatment of acute pain syndromes.**

Methadone

Methadone is a long-acting synthetic opioid agonist. Although it is available in parenteral formulations, it is most often administered orally to ambulatory patients to treat **opioid dependence** or **chronic pain.** Use of the oral formulation by opioid-dependent patients can prevent their craving for heroin or other opioids, but it does not cause significant euphoria or other reinforcing effects. Because of its long duration of action, it can be administered once a day for this purpose. The treatment for opioid-dependent patients in this fashion is called a **methadone maintenance program.**

Oxycodone

Oxycodone is one of several semisynthetic morphine derivatives (see Fig. 23–2A) that are available as analgesics. Oxycodone is usually administered orally in combination with a nonopioid analgesic (e.g., acetaminophen) to treat **moderate or severe pain.** A sustained-release oral form of oxycodone (OXYCONTIN) is available for long-term treatment of pain syndromes. It has been noted to cause several deaths by dependent persons crushing and dissolving the pills for intravenous administration.

MODERATE OPIOID AGONISTS

The moderate opioid agonists are less potent than the strong opioid agonists. Because they do not produce maximal analgesia at doses that are well tolerated by patients, the moderate agonists are used at submaximal doses, almost always in combination with an NSAID analgesic. Fixed-dose combination products containing one of the moderate opioid agonists and **acetaminophen, aspirin,** or **ibuprofen** are available for the treatment of moderate pain.

Codeine and Hydrocodone

Codeine is a naturally occurring opioid obtained from the opium poppy. Structurally, it is the 3-*O*-methyl derivative of morphine. Because codeine contains a methyl group at the 3 position, the principal site of morphine metabolism, codeine undergoes a lesser degree of first-pass metabolism. Codeine is converted to morphine by cytochrome P450 isozyme CYP2D6, and persons lacking this isozyme obtain little pain relief from the drug.

Codeine is a less potent analgesic than morphine, and the doses required to obtain maximal analgesia produce intolerable side effects, such as constipation. For this reason, codeine is usually given in lower doses in combination with an NSAID agent to treat **mild to moderate pain.** Codeine also produces a significant antitussive effect and is included in many cough syrups to alleviate or prevent **coughing.**

The properties and uses of hydrocodone are similar to those of codeine.

Propoxyphene

Propoxyphene, a chemical analogue of methadone, has much weaker opioid agonist properties. Propoxyphene has about half the analgesic activity of codeine when administered in usual therapeutic doses. It is most frequently used in combination with acetaminophen to treat **mild to moderate somatic and visceral pain.** Propoxyphene is usually well tolerated, but prolonged administration can lead to the accumulation of a toxic metabolite.

OTHER OPIOID AGONISTS

Tramadol is a dual-action analgesic. It is an agonist at μ receptors and inhibits the neuronal reuptake of serotonin and norepinephrine. The relationship between neuronal reuptake inhibition and analgesia is not certain. Reuptake inhibition, however, may potentiate the inhibitory effects of serotonin and norepinephrine on pain transmission in the spinal cord (see Box 23–1). Tricyclic antidepressants and other neuronal reuptake inhibitors also have analgesic effects, and some antidepressants are used to treat chronic pain syndromes. For this reason, investigators believe that neuronal reuptake inhibition by tramadol contributes to the drug's analgesic activity. Accordingly, the analgesic effect of tramadol is only partly inhibited by opioid antagonists (e.g., naloxone).

Tramadol is administered orally to treat **moderate pain.** It has a definite but limited drug dependence liability. Nevertheless, it has been used successfully in the treatment of **chronic pain syndromes** and produces minimal cardiovascular and respiratory depression. The drug lowers the seizure threshold, and the risk of seizures is increased if tramadol is used concurrently with antidepressants.

Several other opioid agents are available but have little analgesic activity. These include **dextromethorphan,** which has significant antitussive activity and is used in the treatment of **cough** (see Chapter 27), and **diphenoxylate** and **loperamide,** which activate opioid receptors in gastrointestinal smooth muscle and are used in the treatment of **diarrhea** (see Chapter 28).

MIXED OPIOID AGONIST-ANTAGONISTS AND PARTIAL AGONISTS

The mixed opioid agonist-antagonists are drugs that exhibit partial agonist or antagonist activity at μ receptors and show agonist or antagonist activity at κ receptors. Examples are **buprenorphine, butorphanol, nalbuphine,** and **pentazocine.**

Drug Properties

Chemistry and Pharmacokinetics

The opioid agonist-antagonists have a large chemical substituent on the nitrogen atom (see Fig. 23–2A), which is probably responsible for their partial agonist or antagonist activity at opioid receptors. Their pharmacokinetic and pharmacologic properties are shown in Table 23–2. All of the agonist-antagonists can be given parenterally. In addition, pentazocine is available for oral use and butorphanol is available as a nasal spray. Butorphanol is rapidly absorbed from the nasal mucosa, which thereby enables the use of the drug on an outpatient basis.

MECHANISMS AND EFFECTS. The most important pharmacologic property of these drugs with respect to their clinical activity is the lack of full agonist effects at μ receptors.

The opioid agonist-antagonists produce less respiratory depression as the doses are increased than do strong opioid agonists (e.g., morphine). Hence, the agonist-antagonists are safer in overdose. They also appear to have a lower liability for drug dependence and abuse than do full opioid agonists. The agonist-antagonists produce less constipation than do most of the full agonists. The agonist-antagonists, however, sometimes cause anxiety, nightmares, and psychotomimetic effects, including hallucinations, as a result of the activation of κ receptors. They can also precipitate withdrawal in a person dependent on a full opioid agonist.

Indications

The parenterally administered agonist-antagonist drugs are primarily used for **preoperative and postoperative analgesia** and for **obstetric analgesia during labor and delivery.** The orally and nasally administered drugs are used to alleviate **moderate to severe pain.**

Specific Drugs

Buprenorphine, which is a partial agonist at μ receptors, is noted for a slow dissociation from the μ receptor after binding. It is somewhat longer acting than most parenterally administered opioid analgesics and can be administered intramuscularly or intravenously. It was recently approved for outpatient treatment of opioid dependence. It is available in an oral and sublingual formulation combined with naloxone to prevent intravenous abuse.

Butorphanol and nalbuphine, which are κ receptor agonists, have partial agonist or antagonist activity at μ receptors. Both drugs are administered parenterally, and butorphanol is also available as a nasal spray.

Pentazocine is a κ receptor agonist with additional activity at *sigma (σ) receptors*. Sigma receptors were once considered a type of opioid receptor; it is now known that they are a distinct class of G-protein coupled receptor (GPCR) mediating the psychotomimetic effects of phencyclidine (PCP) and ketamine (see Chapter 25). It is available for parenteral and oral use. The parenteral formulation is primarily used as a preanesthetic medication and as a supplement to surgical anesthesia. The oral formulations are used to treat moderate to severe pain, and one of them contains naloxone (an antagonist) to discourage parenteral abuse of the drug. Parenteral use of an oral pentazocine formulation can cause severe cardiopulmonary reactions. Pentazocine is also available in combination with aspirin or acetaminophen for oral administration.

OPIOID ANTAGONISTS

Naloxone and **naltrexone** are competitive opioid receptor antagonists that can rapidly reverse the effects of morphine and other opioid agonists. The antagonists have two primary clinical uses: the treatment of opioid overdose and the treatment of opioid dependence.

Naloxone and naltrexone are chemical analogues of morphine. They have a large structural substitution on the nitrogen atom (see Fig. 23–2B), and this modification allows the molecule to occupy the opioid receptor but prevents the conformation change in the receptor required for agonist activity.

In cases of **opioid overdose,** naloxone is administered intravenously to rapidly terminate respiratory depression and other toxic effects of opioid agonists. Because naloxone has a relatively short half-life (see Table 23–2), repeated doses of the drug may be needed to counteract the effects of the longer-lasting opioid agonists. Naloxone is also formulated with opioid agonists in oral medications to

prevent crushing of the pill and intravenous abuse. Because naloxone has low bioavailability and is not effective when given orally, it does not block the effects of the oral opioid but would block opioid effects or even precipitate withdrawal if used by the intravenous route.

Naltrexone, in both oral and transdermal formulations, is used to treat **opioid dependence.** In contrast to naloxone, naltrexone has high oral bioavailability and can be used on a long-term basis by opioid addicts who have undergone detoxification and are no longer using opioids. Naltrexone is also effective in the treatment of alcohol dependence (see Chapter 25).

THE TREATMENT OF PAIN

CHOICE OF ANALGESIC

The location, cause, and severity of pain and the risk of producing drug dependence are all factors that influence the way in which pain is managed.

Acute pain caused by trauma, surgery, or short-term medical conditions can be effectively managed with an analgesic and appropriate treatment of the underlying condition. In patients with acute pain, the risk of producing drug dependence is extremely low. Hence, physicians and other health care professionals should not hesitate to administer adequate doses of a sufficiently strong analgesic to control pain.

Pain associated with arthritis, neuropathy, and other chronic but nonterminal conditions is more difficult to treat and is often managed with a combination of analgesics, coanalgesics, psychotherapy, physical therapy, and other treatment modalities. Use of opioid analgesics in the treatment of chronic pain is associated with a risk of opioid tolerance and physical dependence, so care must be exercised to prevent dosage escalation, drug dependence, and drug abuse. Strict guidelines for prescription refills should be in place, and a prescription refill flowchart can be used to monitor drug usage and prevent dosage escalation. In some clinics, patients are asked to sign an "opioid contract" in which they agree to procedures that will ensure proper utilization of opioid drugs, including random drug testing.

Patients with terminal illnesses (e.g., cancer) should receive sufficient doses of analgesics to control their pain, irrespective of the development of tolerance and dependence.

As a general rule, patients with acute or chronic pain should be treated with the least potent analgesic that will control their pain. Mild pain usually responds to a nonopioid analgesic, usually a NSAID. Moderate to severe pain is often treated with **codeine, hydrocodone,** or **oxycodone** in combination with a nonopioid analgesic. Severe pain usually requires the use of a strong opioid agonist (e.g., **fentanyl, meperidine, methadone,** or **morphine**). Although meperidine can be used for acute postsurgical pain and in other situations in which the duration of treatment is limited to a few days, it should not be used for longer durations, because of the possible accumulation of a toxic metabolite (normeperidine).

ACUTE PAIN

Giving analgesics on an as-needed basis sometimes produces wide swings in pain and sedation during the early phase of treatment. Therefore, in the initial stages of acute pain, analgesics should be given around the clock at regular intervals. The dosage should be titrated to control pain while minimizing sedation and other side effects. As the pain subsides over time and the need for analgesia decreases, the patient can be transferred to an as-needed schedule of medication.

Patient-controlled analgesia (PCA) is a method of intravenous administration that permits the patient to self-administer preset amounts of an analgesic (e.g., fentanyl) via a syringe pump that is interfaced with a timing device. The method enables the patient to balance pain control with sedation. Its use depends on the patient's ability to activate the device, so it may not be suitable for elderly patients or for patients immediately after surgery or trauma.

CHRONIC PAIN

Treatment of chronic pain varies greatly with the underlying cause. Although the discussion of specific chronic pain syndromes is beyond the scope of this text, a few general guidelines and comments will be offered.

Both **opioid analgesics** and **nonopioid analgesics** are useful in the management of chronic pain syndromes. If pain is associated with inflammation, nonopioid drugs with anti-inflammatory activity can be especially useful. If pain is associated with peripheral nerve or nerve root sensitization, treatment with **transcutaneous nerve stimulation** or a **local anesthetic** may help. In some cases, cream containing **capsaicin** is effective. Capsaicin activates peripheral nociceptors on primary sensory neurons, thereby leading to increased release of substance P and eventually to the depletion of substance P in the CNS. Capsaicin produces a burning sensation for the first few days of application, but this is gradually replaced by an analgesic effect.

Chronic pain is frequently seen in association with systemic disorders (e.g., diabetes). When pain has been present for a period of time, the responsiveness of dynamic wide-range nociceptive neurons in the spinal cord increases in a way that increases pain perception and memory. As these neurons become "wound up," their receptive fields increase so that pain is felt over a larger area. These changes appear to contribute to the maintenance of chronic neuropathic pain. Patients with this type of pain may benefit from a combination of nonpharmacologic therapies (e.g., TENS, acupuncture, and physical therapy), analgesic medications, and coanalgesic drugs. The most widely used **coanalgesics** are the **antiepileptic drugs** and the **antidepressant drugs.** These drugs provide pain relief in chronic pain syndromes and may potentiate the effects of opioid and nonopioid analgesics.

Antiepileptic drugs (e.g., **carbamazepine, gabapentin, phenytoin,** and **valproate**) are particularly effective in treating pain syndromes with an intermittent lancinating quality, such as trigeminal neuralgia and postherpetic neuralgia. They are also useful in syndromes characterized by continuous, burning neuropathic pain. They probably act by inhibiting the conduction of pain impulses in the CNS, but their exact mechanism is unknown. The general properties of these drugs are described in Chapter 20.

The **tricyclic antidepressants** (TCA) are the most widely used antidepressants for the treatment of chronic pain, and they may be more effective than the selective serotonin reuptake inhibitors (SSRI) in this respect. TCA (e.g., **amitriptyline** and **desipramine**) are particularly effective in the management of postherpetic neuralgia, diabetic neuropathy, migraine headache, and neuropathic pain syndromes. They can also be beneficial in the management of pain associated with chronic fatigue syndrome. The properties of these drugs are described in Chapter 22.

Tramadol is a dual-action analgesic that combines opioid receptor activation with inhibition of neuronal reuptake of neurotransmitters in a manner similar to TCA. As discussed, tramadol is effective in many chronic pain syndromes and causes little constipation, respiratory depression, or drug dependence.

CANCER PAIN

Pain is the most common symptom of cancer, and it can be acute, chronic, or intermittent. Cancer-related pain is frequently undertreated. Most patients can be managed with oral medications, including opioid and NSAID analgesics, antidepressant drugs, and antiepileptic drugs. Acupuncture, TENS, and other modalities are also useful. Severe cancer pain usually requires the administration of a strong opioid agonist (e.g., fentanyl, methadone, or morphine). To maintain stable serum drug levels and prevent breakthrough pain, it may be helpful to use a long-acting preparation (e.g., sustained-release morphine tablets or transdermal fentanyl skin patches), either alone or in combination with a rapid-acting preparation (e.g., morphine oral solution).

SUMMARY OF IMPORTANT POINTS

- Pain impulses are transmitted by primary afferent neurons to the spinal cord, where ascending connections from the spinothalamic tract neurons project to limbic structures and the cortex.

- Descending inhibitory fibers from the periaqueductal gray matter activate midbrain and spinal cord neurons that release enkephalins, serotonin, and norepinephrine. Opioids activate these pathways and thereby inhibit ascending pain impulses.

- Opioid drugs include strong and moderate agonists, mixed agonist-antagonists, and pure antagonists.

- In addition to analgesia, opioid agonists can cause sedation, euphoria, miosis, respiratory depression, peripheral vasodilation, constipation, and drug dependence.

- Opioid receptors can be divided into three types: μ (*mu*), δ (*delta*) or κ (*kappa*) receptors. All types mediate analgesia, but μ receptors are primarily responsible for analgesic effects, as well as respiratory depression and opioid dependence.

■ The strong opioid agonists include morphine, fentanyl, meperidine, and methadone, which act primarily at μ receptors. The first three of these agents are used to alleviate severe or moderate pain. Methadone is usually used in the treatment of opioid addiction (methadone maintenance programs).

■ The moderate agonists produce maximal analgesia at doses that cannot be tolerated, so they are usually combined with a nonopioid analgesic. The moderate agonists, codeine, hydrocodone, and propoxyphene, are used to treat moderate or mild pain.

■ Other agonists include tramadol, a dual-action analgesic that activates opioid receptors and blocks neuronal reuptake of serotonin and norepinephrine.

■ Buprenorphine, butorphanol, nalbuphine, and pentazocine are mixed opioid agonist-antagonists. These drugs exhibit partial agonist or antagonist activity at κ receptors and exhibit agonist or antagonist activity at μ receptors. They produce less respiratory depression and are associated with a lower risk of drug dependence than are full opioid agonists.

■ Naloxone and naltrexone are opioid antagonists. These antagonists are used to counteract the adverse effects of opioids in overdose or to prevent and treat opioid dependence.

Review Questions

1. Most clinically used opioid analgesics are selective for which type of opioid receptor?
   (A) kappa (κ)
   (B) alpha (α)
   (C) beta (β)
   (D) mu (μ)
   (E) delta (δ)

2. Codeine has a greater oral bioavailability compared with morphine because of which reason?
   (A) codeine undergoes less first-pass metabolism
   (B) morphine is conjugated more quickly
   (C) morphine directly passes into systemic circulation
   (D) codeine is only available in liquid formulation
   (E) codeine is metabolized more by hepatic enzymes

3. Which of the following statements best explains the observation that morphine is more likely to cause nausea and vomiting in ambulatory patients?
   (A) morphine inhibits "chemoceptor trigger zone" neurons
   (B) morphine sensitizes medulla cough center neurons
   (C) opioids cause sedation, which makes walking more difficult
   (D) patients on opioids eat more
   (E) opioids increase vestibular sensitivity

4. Which of the following opioids is so lipophilic that it is marketed in a skin patch used to treat chronic pain?
   (A) morphine
   (B) naltrexone
   (C) scopolamine
   (D) methadone
   (E) fentanyl

5. In a case of an opioid overdose, naloxone can be given in repeated doses because of which property of naloxone?
   (A) may have a shorter half-life than the opioid agonist
   (B) is only effective at high cumulative doses
   (C) is needed to stimulate the respiratory center
   (D) is safe only in extremely small doses
   (E) is only a partial opioid agonist

Answers and Explanations

1. The correct choice is D: μ receptors. Although there are three homologous opioid receptor proteins, most clinical opioid analgesics are agonists at the μ receptors. Answer (A), *kappa* (κ), is also a type of opioid receptor that can mediate analgesia, but only plays a minor role with the action of some mixed agonist-antagonist opioids. Answer (B), *alpha* (α), is part of the adrenergic receptor family. Answer (C), *beta* (β), is a type of adrenergic receptor. Answer (E), *delta* (δ), is also a type of opioid receptor and does mediate analgesic in preclinical models but δ-selective agents have not surfaced in the clinic.

2. The correct answer is A: codeine undergoes less first-pass metabolism. Codeine is methylmorphine with the methyl group at the 3 position. As this is the principal site of glucuronide metabolism of morphine, the codeine molecule is somewhat protected from the first-pass effect of hepatic metabolism. Answer (B), morphine is conjugated more quickly, is true but is not the best answer because codeine is not conjugated initially but first metabolized to morphine. Answers (C), morphine directly passes into systemic circulation, (D), codeine is only available in liquid formulation, and (E), codeine is metabolized more by hepatic enzymes, are not accurate statements.

3. The correct answer is E: opioids increase vestibular sensitivity. Ambulatory patients report more instances of nausea and vomiting than recumbent patients administered morphine. In vitro studies show that opioids modulate the inner ear vestibular complex to increase its sensitivity. Answers (A), morphine inhibits "chemoceptor trigger zone" neurons, and (B), morphine sensitizes medulla cough center neurons, are both wrong because morphine has the opposite effects and stimulates the chemoreceptor trigger zone neurons in the medulla and inhibits cough center neurons. Answer (C), opioids cause sedation that makes walking more difficult, may be true but does not affect the onset of nausea and vomiting. Answer (D), patients on opioids eat more, has no support from the literature although fasting does appear to increase endogenous opioid peptides in the CNS and has been implicated in the pathology of the eating disorder, anorexia nervosa.

4. The correct answer is E: fentanyl. This potent opioid is available as a transdermal patch for the treatment of

chronic pain. Answer (A), morphine, is not that lipophilic to allow transdermal administration. Answer (B), naltrexone, is an opioid antagonist that does come in a patch formulation but would not help with chronic pain. It is used to treat opioid and alcohol dependence. Answer (C), scopolamine, does also come in a patch but is used for motion sickness. Answer (D), methadone, is a long-acting opioid agonist but not available in a patch.

5. The correct choice is naloxone A: may have a shorter half-life than the opioid agonist. Treatment of opioid overdose often requires repeated doses of naloxone or continuous infusion to compete with the agonist at the receptor. Answer (B) naloxone is only effective at high cumulative doses, is not true and even the first dose of naloxone may provide miraculous reversal of opioid overdose. Answers (C) through (E) are not true.

SELECTED READINGS

Craft, R. M. Sex differences in opioid analgesia: "from mouse to man." Clin J Pain 19(3):175–186, 2003.

Evans, C. J. Secrets of the opium poppy revealed. Neuropharmacology 47(Suppl 1):293–299, 2004.

Herndon, C. M., D. A. Kalauokalani, A. J. Cunningham, et al. Anticipating and treating opioid-associated adverse effects. Expert Opin Drug Saf 2(3):305–319, 2003.

Moynihan, T. J. Use of opioids in the treatment of severe pain in terminally ill patients–dying should not be painful. Mayo Clin Proc 78(11):1397–1401, 2003.

Ossipov, M. H., J. Lai, T. King, et al. Antinociceptive and nociceptive actions of opioids. J Neurobiol 61(1):126–148, 2004.

Skaer, T. L. Practice guidelines for transdermal opioids in malignant pain. Drugs 64(23):2629–2638, 2004.

CHAPTER 24

Drugs for Neurodegenerative Diseases

CLASSIFICATION OF DRUGS FOR NEURODEGENERATIVE DISEASES*

Drugs for Parkinson's Disease
Drugs That Increase Fopamine Levels
- Levodopa (L-DOPA, LARODOPA)
- Carbidopa (with L-DOPA in SINEMET)
- Amantadine (SYMMETREL)
- Selegiline (ELDERYL)
- Tolcapone (TASMAR)
- Entacapone (COMTAN)

Dopamine Receptor Agonists
- Bromocriptine (PARLODEL)
- Pergolide (PERMAX)
- Pramipexole (MIRAPEX)
- Ropinirole (REQUIP)
- Apomorphine (APOKYN)

Acetylcholine Receptor Antagonists
- Benztropine (COGENTIN)
- Trihexyphenidyl (ARTANE)

Drugs for Huntington's Disease
- Diazepam (VALIUM)
- Haloperidol (HALDOL)

Drugs for Alzheimer's Disease
- Donepezil (ARICEPT)
- Tacrine (COGNEX)
- Rivastigmine (EXELON)
- Galantamine (REMINYL)
- Memantine (NAMENDA)

Drugs for Multiple Sclerosis
- Baclofen
- Tizanidine (ZANAFLEX)
- Prednisone
- Interferon beta-1b (BETASERON)
- Interferon beta-1a (AVONEX)
- Natalizumab (TYSABRI)
- Mitoxantrone (NOVANTRONE)
- Glatiramer acetate (COPAXONE)

Drugs for Amyotrophic Lateral Sclerosis
- Baclofen
- Gabapentin (NEURONTIN)
- Riluzole (RILUTEK)

*Note that baclofen is listed more than once.

OVERVIEW

Parkinson's disease, Huntington's disease, Alzheimer's disease, multiple sclerosis, and amyotrophic lateral sclerosis (ALS, or Lou Gehrig's disease) are neurodegenerative diseases characterized by the progressive loss of neuronal function in a particular part of the central nervous system (CNS). The signs and symptoms of neurodegenerative diseases do not reflect a normal age-related loss of brain neurons. Instead, these progressive disease states are the result of an underlying pathologic process.

Although the cause of these diseases in particular cases is usually unknown, evidence suggests the involvement of heredity, autoimmunity, and environmental factors. Although substantial progress is noted for the treatment of Parkinson's disease, drug therapy for the other neurodegenerative diseases shows limited success. New information concerning the pathogenesis of these diseases will enable the development of more successful drugs in the near future.

PARKINSON'S DISEASE

Parkinson's disease, or **paralysis agitans,** is characterized by a **resting tremor** (involuntary trembling when a limb is at rest), **rigidity** (inability to initiate movements), and **bradykinesia** (slowness of movement). The disease results from the degeneration of **dopaminergic neurons** that arise in the substantia nigra and project to other structures in the basal ganglia.

ETIOLOGY AND PATHOGENESIS

The causes of neuron degeneration in Parkinson's disease remain largely unknown. In most cases, heredity appears to have a limited role. Scientists, however, have identified a defective gene responsible for a rare condition called **autosomal recessive juvenile parkinsonism,** which usually affects people in their teens and 20s.

One of the better-known theories for an environmental origin of Parkinson's disease is called the **oxidative stress theory.** According to this theory, oxidation of **dopamine** in the basal ganglia yields highly reactive **free radicals** that are toxic to dopaminergic neurons and lead to their degeneration. Free radicals are molecules that lack an electron in their outer orbits and are capable of extracting an electron from other biomolecules and thereby causing molecular and cellular damage.

The **basal ganglia** are a group of interconnected subcortical nuclei that include the striatum (caudate and putamen), substantia nigra, globus pallidus, and subthalamus. In healthy individuals, the basal ganglia receive input from the entire cerebral cortex, process this information, and send feedback to the motor area of the cortex in a way that leads to the smooth coordination of body movements. Even simple movements, such as walking, involve a complex sequence of motor acts whose smooth execution requires the continuous interplay of the cortex and basal ganglia. In patients with Parkinson's disease, neuron degeneration interrupts this interplay. Because the basal ganglia also participate in procedural memory and other cognitive functions, patients with Parkinson's disease may have difficulty remembering how to perform learned motor skills, such as driving a car.

The basal ganglia function via a series of reciprocal innervations among themselves and the cortex (Fig. 24–1). The striatum receives input from the cerebral cortex and substantia nigra, and then sends output to the thalamus via the globus pallidus. The thalamus then feeds information back to the motor area of the cortex. Two pathways connect the striatum and the thalamus: a **direct pathway,** which is excitatory, and an **indirect pathway,** which is inhibitory. In patients with Parkinson's disease, the degeneration of dopaminergic neurons results in decreased activity in the direct pathway and increased activity in the indirect pathway. As a result, thalamic feedback to the cortex is reduced, and patients exhibit bradykinesia and rigidity.

Excitatory **cholinergic neurons** also participate in the interconnections between structures in the basal ganglia. In Parkinson's disease, the degeneration of inhibitory dopaminergic neurons leads to a relative excess of choliner-

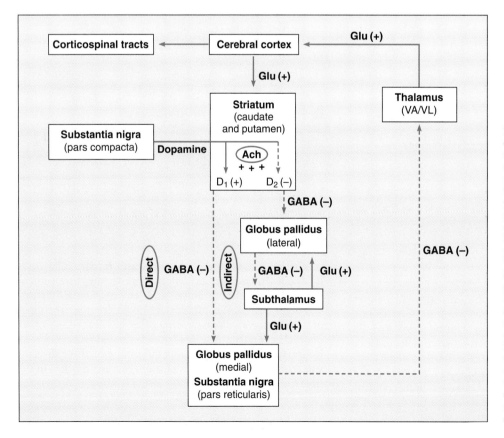

Figure 24–1. Pathophysiology of Parkinson's disease. The striatum receives input from the entire cerebral cortex and the substantia nigra and sends projections to the thalamus via direct and indirect pathways through the globus pallidus, substantia nigra, and subthalamus. Striatal dopamine D_1 receptors excite the direct pathway, whereas D_2 receptors inhibit the indirect pathway. In Parkinson's disease, the degeneration of dopaminergic neurons leads to decreased activity in the direct pathway and increased activity in the indirect pathway. As a result of these changes, thalamic input to the motor area of the cortex is reduced, and the patient exhibits rigidity and bradykinesia. GABA = γ-aminobutyric acid; Glu = glutamate; VA/VL = ventral anterior and ventral lateral nuclei; (+) = excitatory; and (-) = inhibitory.

gic activity in these pathways. For this reason, patients with Parkinson's disease can be treated effectively with drugs that inhibit cholinergic activity in the basal ganglia or with drugs that increase dopamine levels and dopaminergic activity in the basal ganglia.

DRUGS THAT INCREASE DOPAMINE LEVELS

Dopamine levels in the basal ganglia can be increased by various drugs in various ways. **Levodopa** increases dopamine levels by increasing dopamine synthesis; **selegiline** does so by inhibiting dopamine breakdown; and **amantadine** does so by increasing dopamine release from neurons. **Carbidopa** and **tolcapone** increase the amount of levodopa that enters the brain and thereby enhance dopamine synthesis. The sites of action of these drugs are illustrated in Fig. 24–2.

Levodopa

Chemistry and Pharmacokinetics. Levodopa, also called L-dopa or **dihydroxyphenylalanine,** is the biosynthetic precursor of **dopamine.** Levodopa increases the concentration of dopamine in the brain and is the main treatment used to alleviate motor dysfunction in patients with Parkinson's

disease. Dopamine itself is not effective in the treatment of Parkinson's disease when administered systemically, because it does not cross the blood–brain barrier.

Levodopa is absorbed from the proximal duodenum by the same process that absorbs large neutral amino acids (see Fig. 24–2). **Dietary amino acids** compete with levodopa for transport into the circulation, and amino acids can also reduce the transport of levodopa into the brain. For these reasons, the ingestion of high-protein foods can decrease the effectiveness of levodopa, and a protein-restricted diet may improve the response to levodopa in some patients.

Levodopa is metabolized by two pathways in peripheral tissues. It is converted to **dopamine** by L-aromatic amino acid decarboxylase **(LAAD)**, and it is metabolized to **3-O-methyldopa** (3OMD) by **catechol-O-methyltransferase (COMT)**. A drug that inhibits LAAD (e.g., carbidopa) or inhibits COMT (e.g., tolcapone) is used in combination with levodopa to increase the amount of levodopa that enters brain tissue. LAAD requires **vitamin B$_6$ (pyridoxine)** as a cofactor. For this reason, vitamin B$_6$ supplements may enhance the peripheral decarboxylation of levodopa and should not be coadministered with levodopa.

Levodopa exhibits a large first-pass effect, and about 95% of an administered dose is metabolized in the gut wall and liver before it reaches the systemic circulation. Additional

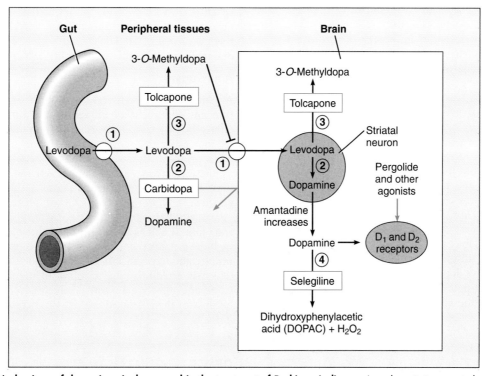

Figure 24–2. Mechanisms of dopaminergic drugs used in the treatment of Parkinson's disease. Levodopa is transported across the gut wall and the blood–brain barrier and is converted to dopamine in striatal neurons. Carbidopa inhibits the peripheral decarboxylation of levodopa and thereby increases the amount of levodopa that enters the brain. Carbidopa does not cross the blood–brain barrier and does not inhibit dopamine synthesis in the brain. Tolcapone inhibits the methylation of levodopa in both peripheral tissues and the brain. Tolcapone increases levodopa bioavailability and increases brain uptake of levodopa. Selegiline inhibits the degradation of dopamine to dihydroxyphenylacetic acid (DOPAC) and hydrogen peroxide (H$_2$O$_2$). By this action, selegiline increases dopamine levels in the striatum, and it may reduce the formation of free radicals that are derived from H$_2$O$_2$. Amantadine increases the release of dopamine from striatal neurons. Pergolide and other dopamine receptor agonists activate dopamine receptors in the striatum. Numbered structures and enzymes are as follows: 1 = pump that transports large neutral amino acids; 2 = L-aromatic amino acid decarboxylase (LAAD); 3 = catechol-O-methyltransferase (COMT); and 4 = monoamine oxidase type B (MAO-B).

amounts of levodopa are converted to dopamine and 3OMD before the drug enters the CNS. Therefore, only about 1% of the administered dose of levodopa reaches brain tissue.

MECHANISMS AND PHARMACOLOGIC EFFECTS. In the brain, levodopa is taken up by dopaminergic neurons in the striatum and is converted to dopamine by LAAD. Levodopa thereby increases the amount of dopamine released by these neurons in patients with Parkinson's disease, and it serves as a form of replacement therapy. Levodopa can counteract all of the signs of parkinsonism, although the degree and duration of its effectiveness usually are not optimal. As the disease progresses and more dopaminergic neurons are lost, the conversion of levodopa to dopamine declines.

About 60% to 70% of nigrostriatal dopaminergic neurons are lost before the clinical symptoms of Parkinson's disease are first observed, and the degeneration of these neurons continues throughout the course of the disease. Over time, patients begin to experience two types of fluctuation in the effectiveness of levodopa, both of which are probably related to a reduced concentration of dopamine in the striatum. The first type, a **"wearing off" effect,** occurs toward the end of a dosage interval. The second type, the **"on-off" phenomenon,** is characterized by severe motor fluctuations that occur randomly.

ADVERSE EFFECTS. When levodopa is used alone, nausea and vomiting occur in about 80% of patients, orthostatic hypotension is reported in 25%, and cardiac arrhythmias occur in 10%. These effects, which are caused by the action of dopamine on β-receptors in the case of cardiac arrhythmias, are substantially reduced when carbidopa is administered with levodopa to block the peripheral formation of dopamine.

About 30% of patients who are treated with levodopa on a long-term basis eventually develop involuntary movements, or dyskinesias, as a result of excessive dopamine concentrations in the striatum. Dyskinesias most often occur when levodopa concentrations are highest, in which case they are called **peak-dose dyskinesias.** The dyskinesias often involve the oral and facial musculature, and patients can appear as if they are chewing on large pieces of food while protruding their lips. Other common dyskinesias involve writhing and flinging movements of the arms and legs. Less commonly, levodopa causes psychotic effects, including hallucinations and distorted thinking, which are probably caused by excessive dopamine concentrations in mesolimbic and mesocortical pathways that utilize dopamine as a neurotransmitter. Although dyskinesias and psychotic effects could be managed by reducing the levodopa dosage, the therapeutic efficacy of the drug would be reduced as well.

Some patients treated with levodopa complain of sedative effects, agitation, delirium, vivid dreams, or nightmares. Others, however, report a pleasant euphoria after taking the drug.

INTERACTIONS. Levodopa has important interactions with a number of medications. Drugs that delay gastric emptying (e.g., anticholinergic drugs) can slow levodopa absorption and reduce its peak serum concentration. Drugs that promote gastric emptying (e.g., antacids and cisapride) can increase levodopa bioavailability. Nonselective monoamine oxidase (MAO) inhibitors (e.g., phenelzine) inhibit the breakdown of dopamine and sometimes cause a hypertensive crisis in patients receiving levodopa. Antipsychotic drugs block dopamine receptors and can reduce the effectiveness of levodopa and exacerbate motor dysfunction. Because clozapine is much less likely to do this than other antipsychotic drugs, it is often used to manage psychotic reactions in patients receiving levodopa (see Chapter 22).

INDICATIONS. Levodopa is effective in the management of patients with **idiopathic Parkinson's disease** and in the treatment of patients with **postencephalitic parkinsonism** (a disorder portrayed in the movie *Awakenings*). It is also used to treat **parkinsonian symptoms caused by carbon monoxide poisoning, manganese intoxication, or cerebral arteriosclerosis.**

Carbidopa

Carbidopa, a structural analogue of levodopa, inhibits the conversion of levodopa to dopamine in peripheral tissues and thereby increases the amount of levodopa that enters the brain (see Fig. 24–2). Carbidopa is highly ionized at physiologic pH, and it does not cross the blood–brain barrier. For this reason, it does not inhibit the formation of dopamine in the CNS.

Carbidopa substantially reduces the gastrointestinal and cardiovascular side effects of levodopa, enabling about a 75% reduction in the dosage of levodopa. A **levodopa-carbidopa combination** is available in immediate-release and sustained-release formulations that contain different ratios of the two drugs. The sustained-release formulations are designed to reduce the "wearing off" effect described above.

Amantadine

Amantadine is an antiviral drug that is used in the prevention and treatment of influenza but also has a beneficial effect on Parkinson's disease. Amantadine probably works by increasing the release of dopamine from nigrostriatal neurons, but it may also inhibit the reuptake of dopamine by these neurons. Amantadine is generally better tolerated than levodopa or dopamine agonists, but it is also less effective.

Amantadine is used to treat early or mild cases of Parkinson's disease and as an adjunct to levodopa. Its adverse effects include sedation, restlessness, vivid dreams, nausea, dry mouth, and hypotension. It can also cause livedo reticularis, which is a reddish-blue mottling of the skin with edema. CNS side effects are more likely to occur in the elderly because of their reduced capacity to excrete the drug by the kidneys.

Selegiline

CHEMISTRY AND PHARMACOKINETICS. Selegiline, also known as **deprenyl,** is a modified phenylethylamine compound. The drug is well absorbed from the gut and is partly metabolized to amphetamine.

MECHANISMS AND PHARMACOLOGIC EFFECTS. Selegiline inhibits MOA type B (MAO-B) and thereby prevents the oxidation of dopamine to **dihydroxyphenylacetic acid** (DOPAC) and **hydrogen peroxide,** as shown in Fig. 24–2. By this action, selegiline increases dopamine levels in the basal ganglia and decreases the formation of hydrogen peroxide. In the presence of iron, hydrogen peroxide is converted to **hydroxyl and hydroxide radicals** that may participate in the degeneration of nigrostriatal neurons in patients with Parkinson's disease.

Some investigators believe that selegiline inhibits the progression of Parkinson's disease either by inhibiting the formation of free radicals or by inhibiting the formation of an active metabolite of an environmental toxin. The ability of selegiline to inhibit disease progression is controversial. It was initially suggested by studies showing that selegiline could prevent a form of parkinsonism that is induced by **1-methyl-4-phenyl-1,2,3,6-tetrahydropyridine** (MPTP). MPTP is a toxic byproduct of the synthesis of "designer" street drugs, and people who took drugs contaminated with MPTP in the 1980s developed classic signs of parkinsonism. MPTP must be converted to 1-methyl-4-phenylpyridium (MPP$^+$) by MAO-B before it can damage dopaminergic neurons, and studies demonstrated that selegiline blocked this reaction. The results of these studies have led some investigators to postulate that idiopathic Parkinson's disease is caused by an environmental toxin whose action resembles that of MPTP.

ADVERSE EFFECTS AND INTERACTIONS. Adverse effects are listed in Table 24–1. Unlike the nonselective MAO inhibitors used in treating mood disorders, selegiline does not inhibit MAO-A, an enzyme that catalyzes the degradation of catecholamines. For this reason, selegiline is much less likely to cause hypertension when it is administered in combination with sympathomimetic amines or when it is taken with foods that contain tyramine. The drug's selectivity for MAO-B, however, is lost when it is given in higher doses, so the drug's potential for interactions of this type still exists. Selegiline can cause adverse effects if it is administered with meperidine or with selective serotonin reuptake inhibitors (e.g., fluoxetine).

INDICATIONS. Selegiline can be used as a single drug for the treatment of **early or mild Parkinson's disease,** and it is used as an adjunct with levodopa-carbidopa for **advanced disease.** Selegiline reduces the dosage requirement for levodopa, and it may improve motor function in patients who experience "wearing off" and "on-off" difficulties with levodopa.

The most controversial role of selegiline is its use as a **neuroprotective agent.** Although some clinical studies have indicated that selegiline slows the progression of Parkinson's disease, others have indicated that it does not.

Tolcapone

Tolcapone is a drug used to enhance the effectiveness of levodopa in the treatment of Parkinson's disease. It inhibits COMT, the enzyme that converts levodopa to 3OMD in the gut and liver. By this action, tolcapone produces a twofold increase in the oral bioavailability and half-life of levodopa. Because 3OMD competes with levodopa for transport into brain tissue, it may contribute to the "wearing off" and "on-off" effects that occur during long-term levodopa therapy. By inhibiting 3OMD formation, tolcapone may stabilize dopamine levels in the striatum and contribute to a more sustained improvement in motor function.

In clinical studies, tolcapone was found to increase the efficacy of levodopa while reducing the dosage requirement for it. Tolcapone was well tolerated, and most of the side effects were similar in frequency to those reported with use of a placebo. Although tolcapone caused diarrhea and nausea in some patients, these side effects tended to decrease over time. A few reports have been made of rare, but fatal hepatitis following administration of tolcapone.

Entacapone

Entacapone has the same mechanism of action as tolcapone but does not gain entry into the CNS. It may be safer to administer than tolcapone because of no reports of hepatic toxicity.

Dopamine Receptor Agonists

The dopamine receptor agonists directly activate dopamine receptors in the striatum. Because they do not require a functional dopaminergic neuron to produce their effects, they are sometimes helpful in advanced cases of Parkinson's disease, in which few dopaminergic neurons remain functional. The drugs work primarily by activating D_2 receptors. As shown in Fig. 24–1, activation of these receptors leads to inhibition of the indirect neuronal pathway from the striatum to the thalamus and increases thalamic stimulation of the motor area of the cortex.

Bromocriptine and Pergolide

Bromocriptine and pergolide are both **ergot alkaloids.** (Other ergot alkaloids are discussed in Chapter 29.) Bromocriptine is a D_2 receptor agonist and a D_1 receptor antagonist. In contrast, pergolide acts as both a D_1 and D_2 receptor agonist. Pergolide is much more potent than bromocriptine, has a higher affinity for D_2 receptors, and has a longer duration of action. Either drug can serve as a useful adjunct to levodopa in patients who have advanced Parkinson's disease and experience "wearing off" effects and "on-off" motor fluctuations.

Dopamine receptor agonists produce adverse effects that are similar to those of levodopa. Nausea, which occurs in as many as 50% of patients when they are first treated with a receptor agonist, primarily results from stimulation of dopamine receptors in the vomiting center located in the medulla. Dose-related CNS effects of the receptor agonists include confusion, dyskinesias, sedation, vivid dreams, and hallucinations. Other adverse effects include orthostatic hypotension, dry mouth, and decreased prolactin levels. Nausea and many other adverse effects subside over time. To enable patients to develop tolerance to the effects, treatment should begin with a low dose, and the dosage should be increased gradually.

Pramipexole and Ropinirole

In contrast to the older dopamine receptor agonists, pramipexole and ropinirole are not ergot alkaloids. Both act as selective D_2 receptor agonists. In addition, pramipexole activates D_3 receptors, and this may contribute to its effectiveness in Parkinson's disease. The adverse effects, contraindications, and drug interactions of pramipexole and ropinirole are summarized in Table 24–1.

TABLE 24-1. **Adverse Effects, Contraindications, and Interactions of Drugs for Neurodegenerative Diseases**

Drug	Major Adverse Effects	Major Drug Interactions
Drugs for Parkinson's disease		
Drugs that increase dopamine levels		
– Amantadine	Dry mouth; hypotension; livedo reticularis; nausea; restlessness; sedation; and vivid dreams.	Benztropine and trihexyphenidyl potentiate central nervous system (CNS) side effects
– Levodopa-carbidopa	Agitation; arrhythmias; delirium; distorted thinking, hallucinations, and other psychotic effects; dyskinesias; hypotension; nausea and vomiting; nightmares or vivid dreams; and sedation.	Antacids and cisapride may increase bioavailability. Anticholinergic drugs may reduce peak serum level. Antipsychotic drugs, such as haloperidol, may decrease effects. Nonselective monoamine oxidase (MAO) inhibitors, such as phenelzine, may cause a hypertensive crisis.
– Selegiline	Confusion; dyskinesias; hallucinations; hypotension; insomnia; and nausea.	Severe reactions may result if taken with meperidine or with fluoxetine or other selective serotonin reuptake inhibitor (SSRI).
– Tolcapone	Diarrhea and nausea	Unknown
Dopamine receptor agonists		
– Bromocriptine	Confusion; decreased prolactin levels; dry mouth; dyskinesias; hallucinations; nausea; orthostatic hypotension; sedation; and vivid dreams.	Dopamine antagonists may reduce effects.
– Pergolide	Same as bromocriptine	Same as bromocriptine
– Pramipexole	Dizziness; hallucinations; insomnia; nausea and vomiting; and sedation.	Cimetidine inhibits renal excretion and increases serum levels.
– Ropinirole	Same as pramipexole	Ciprofloxacin increases serum levels.
Acetylcholine receptor antagonists		
– Benztropine	Agitation; confusion; constipation; delirium; dry mouth; memory loss; urinary retention; and tachycardia.	Additive anticholinergic effect with antihistamines and phenothiazines
– Trihexyphenidyl	Same as benztropine	Same as benztropine
Drugs for Huntington's disease		
– Diazepam	Arrhythmias; CNS depression; drug dependence; hypotension; and mild respiratory depression.	Alcohol and other CNS depressants potentiate effects. Cimetidine increases and rifampin decreases serum levels.
– Haloperidol	Extrapyramidal side effects and increased prolactin levels	Barbiturates and carbamazepine decrease and quinidine increases serum levels.
Drugs for Alzheimer's disease		
– Donepezil	Bradycardia; diarrhea; gastrointestinal bleeding; and nausea and vomiting.	Anticholinergic drugs inhibit effects.
– Tacrine	Bradycardia; diarrhea; gastrointestinal bleeding; hepatotoxicity; nausea and vomiting; and urinary incontinence.	Anticholinergic drugs inhibit effects. Cimetidine increases serum levels. Smoking decreases serum levels. Tacrine increases effects of succinylcholine and theophylline.
Drugs for multiple sclerosis		
– Baclofen	Dizziness; fatigue; and weakness.	Unknown
– Interferon beta-1b	Chills; diarrhea; fever; headache; hypertension; myalgia; pain; and vomiting.	Increases serum levels of zidovudine
– Prednisone	Aggravation of diabetes mellitus; gastrointestinal bleeding; mood changes; pancreatitis; and seizures.	Barbiturates, carbamazepine, phenytoin, and rifampin decrease serum levels.
Drugs for amyotrophic lateral sclerosis		
– Baclofen	Dizziness; fatigue; and weakness.	Unknown
– Gabapentin	Ataxia; dizziness; drowsiness; nystagmus; and tremor.	Antacids decrease serum levels.
– Riluzole	Asthenia; diarrhea; dizziness; drowsiness; increased hepatic enzyme levels; nausea and vomiting; paresthesias; and vertigo.	Quinolones and theophylline can increase serum levels. Omeprazole, rifampin, and smoking can decrease serum levels.

Clinical studies have shown that pramipexole or ropinirole can delay the need for levodopa when used in early stages of Parkinson's disease. In advanced stages, pramipexole can reduce the "off" period and decrease the levodopa dosage requirement. Thus, although the older agonists (bromocriptine and pergolide) are primarily used as adjunct therapy in advanced Parkinson's disease, the newer agonists may prove effective as monotherapy in both early and advanced disease.

Apomorphine

Apomorphine, which is chemically related to morphine, does not bind to opioid receptors but rather is a dopamine receptor agonist. It is actually an old drug put to new use and was recently approved for the treatment of acute, intermittent **hypomobility** ("freezing") episodes associated with advanced Parkinson's disease. It is available for injection only and produces a rapid (within 5 to 10 min) reversal of the hypomobility state.

Acetylcholine Receptor Antagonists

Several centrally acting acetylcholine receptor antagonists, or **anticholinergic drugs,** are used in the management of Parkinson's disease. Two examples are **benztropine** and **trihexyphenidyl.** The anticholinergic drugs are generally less effective than the dopaminergic drugs, but they may be helpful as adjunct therapy in combination with levodopa and other drugs that augment dopaminergic activity. The anticholinergic drugs are more effective in reducing **tremor** than in reducing other manifestations of Parkinson's disease, although they may provide some reduction of bradykinesia and rigidity in patients with mild dysfunction. These drugs also inhibit the neuronal reuptake of dopamine by central dopaminergic neurons and may thereby prolong the action of dopamine.

In addition to being useful in the treatment of **early and advanced Parkinson's disease,** the anticholinergic drugs can also reduce **parkinsonian symptoms caused by dopamine receptor antagonists** (e.g., haloperidol) (see Chapter 22).

Treatment Considerations

Optimal management of Parkinson's disease requires that the disabilities of each patient be carefully assessed before drug treatment is recommended. Early disease of mild intensity can be best managed with exercise, nutrition, and education. Speech, occupational, and physical therapies can also be helpful.

For patients whose clinical manifestations are limited to mild tremor and slowness, anticholinergic drugs or amantadine may be helpful.

For patients with more severe functional disabilities, the dopaminergic drugs are the most effective treatment. Combination therapy with levodopa and carbidopa is usually prescribed for these patients, but monotherapy with a new dopamine receptor agonist (e.g., pramipexole or ropinirole) may provide an effective alternative for patients who have either early or advanced Parkinson's disease. Clinicians should remember that dopaminergic drugs have a delayed onset of action, so improvement in the patient's condition may not be noted until 2 to 3 weeks after therapy is started.

Tolcapone and selegiline inhibit the metabolism of levodopa and dopamine, respectively, and can be used to enhance the effectiveness of levodopa in patients with early or advanced disease. Some clinicians begin selegiline treatment early in the disease in an effort to retard disease progression.

For patients who have more advanced disease and begin to experience the "wearing off" and "on-off" fluctuations of levodopa-carbidopa, it is sometimes helpful to change the drug dosage or formulation. For example, the "wearing off" effect can be minimized by increasing the frequency of doses or using a combination of sustained-release and immediate-release formulations. Alternatively, an additional dopaminergic drug can be added to the treatment regimen. The addition of tolcapone, for example, may reduce motor fluctuations by increasing and stabilizing levodopa concentrations in the striatum. Apomorphine, a nonergoloid dopamine agonist, may provide quick relief from periods of hypomobility.

HUNTINGTON'S DISEASE

Etiology and Pathogenesis

Huntington's disease, or **Huntington's chorea,** is an autosomal dominant hereditary disorder that is characterized by abnormally expansive or choreoathetoid movements (dance-like movements) of the limbs, rhythmic movements of the tongue and face, and mental deterioration that leads to personality disorders, psychosis, and dementia. Patients are usually in their late 30s when the disease begins, and progressive respiratory depression usually causes death in 10 to 15 years.

Huntington's disease is caused by the degeneration of **γ-aminobutyric acid (GABA) neurons** in the **striatum** and elsewhere in the brain. This degeneration can be caused by glutamate-induced neurotoxicity. The loss of GABA neurons that project from the striatum to the lateral globus pallidus leads to disinhibition of thalamic nuclei and to an increase in thalamic input to the motor area of the cortex (see Fig. 24–1).

Treatment

The symptoms of Huntington's disease are consistent with excessive dopaminergic activity in the basal ganglia. Therefore, drugs that block dopamine receptors (e.g., **haloperidol**) and other antipsychotic drugs (see Chapter 22), produce some improvement in motor function and are also helpful in relieving the psychosis that accompanies the disease. **Diazepam** and other benzodiazepine drugs (see Chapter 19) potentiate GABA and can also reduce excess movements in patients with Huntington's disease. The efficacy of benzodiazepines, however, declines significantly with disease progression.

In the future, new treatments may result from identification of the function of *huntingtin*, the abnormal gene product that is synthesized in Huntington's disease. Drugs that inhibit glutamate neurotoxicity might also prove useful in the treatment of this disease.

ALZHEIMER'S DISEASE

Etiology and Pathogenesis

Alzheimer's disease is a type of **progressive dementia** for which no cause is known and no cure has been found. In the United State of America, it accounts for about 60% of all cases of dementia in patients over 65 years of age and is associated with 100,000 deaths each year. The disease has a tremendous negative impact on patients and their families because of its devastating effects on the patient's cognitive, emotional, and physical function.

Alzheimer's disease results from the destruction of **cholinergic and other neurons** in the **cortex** and **limbic structures of the brain,** particularly the amygdala, basal forebrain, and hippocampus. Major changes in these structures include cortical atrophy, neurofibrillary tangles, and neuritic plaques containing β-amyloid protein. The cholinergic neurons destroyed in Alzheimer's disease originate in **Meynert's nucleus** or **nucleus basalis** in the forebrain. These neurons project to the frontal cortex and hippocampus, and they have a critical role in memory and cognition.

Treatment

In patients with Alzheimer's disease, treatment with **donepezil** or **tacrine** has been administered in an effort to improve cholinergic neurotransmission in affected areas of the brain. Although these **centrally acting cholinesterase inhibitors** may slow the deterioration of cognitive function, they do not affect the underlying neurodegenerative process, so the disease is eventually fatal. The adverse effects, contraindications, and drug interactions of donepezil and tacrine are outlined Table 24–1.

Studies in patients with Alzheimer's disease have demonstrated that those treated with donepezil for 24 weeks had significantly better cognitive function than those treated with a placebo. Donepezil is a piperidine-type, reversible cholinesterase inhibitor that selectively inhibits cholinesterase in the CNS and increases acetylcholine levels in the cerebral cortex. The drug is well absorbed after oral administration and crosses the blood–brain barrier. Because it has a long half-life of about 70 hours, it is usually administered once a day. The adverse effects of donepezil include diarrhea, nausea, and vomiting, but these are usually mild and transient. Unlike tacrine, donepezil is not associated with hepatotoxicity.

Tacrine was the first centrally acting cholinesterase inhibitor approved for the treatment of Alzheimer's disease. It has a lower bioavailability and a shorter half-life than does donepezil, and it must be administered several times a day. Tacrine, an acridine compound, is associated with a significant incidence of hepatotoxicity and with peripheral cholinergic side effects such as diarrhea, nausea, and urinary incontinence. Because of these adverse effects, few patients can tolerate the higher doses required to demonstrate cognitive improvement in Alzheimer's disease.

Rivastigmine and **galantamine** are newer centrally acting, reversible acetylcholinestrase inhibitors. Taken in divided doses, they are shown to significantly delay the global cognitive impairment associated with Alzheimer's disease for at least 6 months in clinical trials.

Recently, an agent with a new mechanism of action for the treatment of the dementia of Alzheimer's disease was approved. **Memantine** is a weak, noncompetitive antagonist at the *N*-methyl-D-aspartate (NMDA) receptor. It is hypothesized to work by attenuating the excitotoxic effects of glutamate that may underlie the pathologic process of neuronal loss in Alzheimer's disease.

MULTIPLE SCLEROSIS

Etiology and Pathogenesis

Multiple sclerosis (MS) is a chronic disease characterized by the **demyelination of neurons** in the CNS. Although its etiology is unknown, the disease is postulated to have an autoimmune or viral origin. Demyelination leads to disruption of nerve transmission and is accompanied by an inflammatory response and the formation of plaques in the brain and spinal cord. These plaques typically contain decreased numbers of **oligodendrocytes** (myelin-forming cells). The neurologic symptoms of multiple sclerosis, which depend on the area of the brain that is affected, can include pain, spasticity, weakness, ataxia, fatigue, and problems with speech, vision, gait, and bladder function. Many patients experience relapses and remissions, but some have a more severe and unremitting progression of disease.

Treatment

Interferon beta-1b was the first drug to demonstrate an ability to halt and even reverse the progression of MS. In clinical studies, the drug was found to reduce the frequency of relapses and the number of new lesions detected by magnetic resonance imaging in patients who were ambulatory, had a relapsing-remitting type of multiple sclerosis, and had experienced at least two exacerbations during the last 2 years. Interferon beta-1b is a synthetic analogue of a recombinant interferon-beta produced in *Escherichia coli.* Although the drug's exact mechanism of action is unknown, its effects in patients with MS may be caused by its immunomodulating properties. Interferon beta-1b increases the cytotoxicity of natural killer cells and increases the phagocytic activity of macrophages. In addition, it reduces the amount of interferon-gamma secreted by activated lymphocytes. Because interferon-gamma has been shown to exacerbate the symptoms of MS, a reduction in its secretion may halt the disease. The pharmacologic effects and uses of various interferons are discussed more thoroughly in Chapter 45.

Recently, another interferon product, **interferon beta -1a** was approved to treat the relapsing forms of MS. As with its predecessor, it works as an immunomodulator and is synthesized by recombinant protein pathways.

A monoclonal preparation called **natalizumab** works by blocking the molecular pathway involving cell adhesion and drawing lymphocytes into the CNS. The presence of lymphocytes around neuronal fibers is implicated in the immune processes that contribute to the pathology of MS. **Mitoxantrone** belongs to the class of antineoplastic agents and was recently approved for the treatment of MS. It acts by suppressing the activity of T cells, B cells, and macrophages that are thought to lead the attack on the myelin sheath. **Glatiramer acetate** is a synthetic protein that mimics the structure of **myelin basic protein**, a component of the myelin covering nerve fibers. This drug blocks myelin-damaging T cells by acting as a myelin decoy. In placebo-controlled clinical trials with relapsing-remitting MS, those taking the glatiramer acetate drug had significantly reduced episodes of relapse compared with control subjects.

Spasticity is frequently treated with physical therapy, but **antispastic drugs** (e.g., **baclofen**) (see Table 24–1) may be useful in severe cases. **Tizanidine**, a centrally acting α_2 receptor agonist, is indicated for the management of spasticity. It is thought to reduce spasticity by blocking nerve impulses through presynaptic inhibition of motor neurons, resulting in decreased spasticity without a reduction in muscle strength.

Acute exacerbations are treated with **adrenal corticosteroid drugs** (e.g., **prednisone**). These drugs have anti-inflammatory activity and are discussed in Chapter 33. In patients with multiple sclerosis, corticosteroids shorten the duration of exacerbations and ameliorate symptoms, possibly by decreasing edema. They are administered orally in milder cases and are given parenterally in high doses in more severe cases.

AMYOTROPHIC LATERAL SCLEROSIS

Etiology and Pathogenesis

Amyotrophic lateral sclerosis (ALS), also called **Lou Gehrig's disease,** is a progressive disease of the **motor neurons.** It is characterized by muscle wasting, weakness, and respiratory failure leading to death in 2 to 5 years. The cause of ALS is unknown, but evidence suggests a defect in **superoxide dismutase,** an enzyme that scavenges superoxide radicals.

Treatment

The current treatment for ALS is largely symptomatic. Spasticity can be partly controlled with **baclofen,** a GABA$_B$ agonist whose properties are outlined in Table 24–1. The decline in muscle strength may be slowed by **gabapentin,** an antiepileptic drug discussed in Chapter 20.

Although many drugs have been studied for their potential to reduce the progression of ALS and prolong the length of survival, the first drug that has been specifically approved for use in the treatment of ALS is **riluzole.** This drug has been shown to prolong the time before patients require a tracheostomy and also to prolong life by approximately 3 months. Riluzole is believed to protect motor neurons from the neurotoxic effects of excitatory amino acids (e.g., glutamate) and to prevent the anoxia-related death of cortical neurons. Its exact mechanism of action is unclear, but it may inhibit voltage-gated sodium channels that mediate the release of glutamate from neurons. Clinical studies in patients with ALS indicate that riluzole is more effective in those with bulbar-onset disease than in those with limb-onset disease.

SUMMARY OF IMPORTANT POINTS

■ Parkinson's disease is a chronic disease caused by degeneration of dopaminergic neurons that arise in the substantia nigra. It is characterized by resting tremor, rigidity, and bradykinesia.

■ Parkinson's disease is primarily treated with drugs that increase dopamine levels in the basal ganglia or activate dopamine receptors.

■ Levodopa is converted to dopamine by L-aromatic amino acid decarboxylase (LAAD). It is often coadministered with carbidopa, which inhibits the peripheral decarboxylation of levodopa and increases its brain uptake.

■ Other drugs that increase dopamine levels in the basal ganglia include tolcapone, which inhibits methylation of levodopa, and selegiline, which inhibits the breakdown of dopamine catalyzed by monoamine oxidase type B (MAO-B). Amantadine increases dopamine release and may inhibit its neuronal reuptake.

■ Direct-acting dopamine receptor agonists include bromocriptine, pergolide, pramipexole, and ropinirole. These drugs are often used as adjuncts to levodopa in the treatment of patients whose response to levodopa is inadequate.

■ Levodopa and other dopaminergic drugs can cause significant adverse effects, including nausea, dyskinesias, nightmares, and orthostatic hypotension.

■ Acetylcholine receptor antagonists (anticholinergic drugs) can reduce the tremor seen in Parkinson's disease, but their effectiveness is limited.

■ Huntington's disease is caused by degeneration of γ-aminobutyric (GABA) neurons in the striatum and other parts of the brain. Degeneration of neurons leads to excessive dopamine neurotransmission and choreoathetoid movements. Dopamine receptor antagonists can provide some improvement in affected patients.

■ Alzheimer's disease is a progressive dementia partly caused by loss of cholinergic neurons in the cortex and limbic structures of the brain. Donepezil and tacrine, two centrally acting cholinesterase inhibitors, and memantine, an NMDA antagonist, produce some cognitive improvement in patients with this disease.

■ Multiple sclerosis is a demyelinating disease whose exacerbations may be attenuated with corticosteroid drugs. Treatment with interferon beta-1b, and other immunomodifiers, retards disease progression in some patients.

■ Amyotrophic lateral sclerosis is a progressive disease of the motor neurons. Riluzole, the first drug approved for its treatment, has a limited effect on patient survival.

Review Questions

1. Which of the following is not a mechanism of action for antiparkinsonism agents?
   (A) direct dopamine agonist
   (B) precursor loading
   (C) inhibit dopamine metabolism
   (D) block cholinergic receptors
   (E) selective dopamine reuptake inhibition

2. Cardiac arrhythmias following initial doses of levodopa (L-Dopa) are occasionally observed. Which of the following explanations most likely explain this occurrence?
   (A) direct action on cardiac dopamine receptors
   (B) decreased release of catecholamines
   (C) direct β-adrenergic receptor stimulation
   (D) increased release of dopamine
   (E) interaction with vagal cholinergic receptors

3. Anticholinergic agents are useful in the treatment of Parkinsonism because of which one of the following mechanisms?
   (A) decreased levels of acetylcholine from loss of neurons
   (B) continuing degeneration of dopamine neurons
   (C) neurotransmitter imbalance in the basal ganglia
   (D) increased activity of acetylcholinesterase
   (E) increased release of dopamine in basal ganglia

4. Selegiline, an antidepressant also used for the treatment of Parkinson's disease, has which one of the following mechanisms of action?
   (A) it is a selective MAO-B inhibitor
   (B) it blocks the reuptake of dopamine
   (C) it irreversibly binds to COMT
   (D) increases release of dopamine vesicles
   (E) blocks muscarinic cholinergic receptors

5. Baclofen is used to treat muscle spasticity because of which of the following effects?
   (A) is a receptor agonist at $GABA_B$ receptors
   (B) blocks acetylcholine receptors
   (C) enhances the release of GABA vesicles
   (D) is an antagonist as glutamate receptors
   (E) increases GABA action at Cl^- ion channel

Answers and Explanations

1. The correct answer is E: selective dopamine reuptake inhibition. Although this mechanism of action would be beneficial in the treatment of parkinsonism because it would lead to an increase in synaptic levels of dopamine, no such agents are currently available. Answer (A), direct dopamine agonist, is a mechanism used by dopamine agonists such as bromocriptine. Answer (B), precursor loading, is the mechanism of L-Dopa. Answer (C), inhibit dopamine metabolism, is used by selegiline and tolcapone. Answer (D), block cholinergic receptors, is a mechanism also used for the treatment of parkinsonism by such agents as benztropine.

2. The correct answer is C: direct β-adrenergic receptor stimulation. Metabolism of L-Dopa in the periphery to dopamine can lead to cardiac arrhythmias by direct action of dopamine on cardiac β-adrenergic receptors. Administration of L-Dopa with carbidopa will decrease the formation of dopamine in the periphery and decrease the likelihood of cardiac abnormalities. Answer (A), direct action on cardiac dopamine receptors, may be a possible mechanism if there were significant dopamine receptors in the heart modulating cardiac rhythm, which there are not. Answer (B), decreased release of catecholamines, would decrease cardiac stimulation. Answer (D), increased release of dopamine, is not the best answer because increased peripheral formation is not the same as increased neuronal release. Answer (E), interaction with vagal cholinergic receptors, might affect cardiac function but dopamine or L-Dopa has no interaction with cholinergic receptors.

3. The correct answer is C: neurotransmitter imbalance in the basal ganglia. The decrease of dopamine projections to the striatum results in a relative abundance of acetylcholine activity in the striatum. Acetylcholine (muscarinic) antagonists rebalance this abnormality. Answer (A), decreased levels of acetylcholine from loss of neurons, would not be a reason to give an antagonist to correct this condition. Answer (B), the continuing degeneration of dopamine neurons, is a fact of the progression of the disease state but antimuscarinic agents do not retard the progression of parkinsonism. Answer (D), the increased activity of acetylcholinesterase, is not correct because no evidence of enzyme up-regulation in parkinsonism exists. Answer (E), the increased release of dopamine in basal ganglia, is clearly wrong because the disease is caused by the degeneration of dopamine neurons.

4. The correct answer is A: it is a selective MAO-B inhibitor. Selegiline does retard the progress of parkinsonism by inhibiting the formation of free radicals from the action of MAO-B on dopamine. Answer (B), it blocks the reuptake of dopamine, would be a possible treatment but no drug like this has been tried in the treatment of parkinsonism. Answer (C), it irreversibly binds to COMT, may cause increased dopamine, but this is not the mechanism of selegiline. Answer (D), increases release of dopamine vesicles, is the mechanism of amantadine. Answer (E), blocks muscarinic cholinergic receptors, is the mechanism of anticholinergic agents used for the treatment of parkinsonism.

5. The correct answer is A: is a receptor agonist at $GABA_B$ receptors. Baclofen is presently the only $GABA_B$ receptor agonist approved for the treatment of spasticity. Answers (B) through (E) are incorrect because they are the mechanisms of anticholinergics, amantadine, memantine, and sedative-hypnotic agents, respectively.

SELECTED READINGS

Curran, M. P., and C. M. Perry. Cabergoline: a review of its use in the treatment of Parkinson's disease. Drugs 64(18):2125–2141, 2004.

Fernandez, O. Interferons in relapsing-remitting multiple sclerosis: are there benefits from long-term use? CNS Drugs 18(15):1057–1070, 2004.

Forman, M. S., J. Q. Trojanowski, and V. M. Lee. Neurodegenerative diseases: a decade of discoveries paves the way for therapeutic breakthroughs. Nat Med 10(10):1055–1063, 2004.

Hauser, R. A., and K. E. Lyons. Future therapies for Parkinson's disease. Neurol Clin 22(3 Suppl):S149–S166, 2004.

Schmitt, B., T. Bernhardt, H. J. Moeller, et al. Combination therapy in Alzheimer's disease: a review of current evidence. CNS Drugs 18(13):827–844, 2004.

Standridge, J. B. Pharmacotherapeutic approaches to the prevention of Alzheimer's disease. Am J Geriatr Pharmacother 2(2):119–132, 2004.

Weiner, W. J. Initial treatment of Parkinson disease: levodopa or dopamine agonists. Arch Neurol 61(12):1966–1969, 2004.

Weiss, M. D., P. Weydt, and G. T. Carter. Current pharmacological management of amyotrophic lateral sclerosis and a role for rational polypharmacy. Expert Opin Pharmacother 5(4):735–746, 2004.

CHAPTER 25

Drugs of Abuse

CLASSIFICATION OF DRUGS OF ABUSE

Central Nervous System Depressants

Alcohols and Glycols
- Ethanol
- Methanol
- Ethylene glycol
- Isopropyl alcohol

Barbiturates and Benzodiazepines
- Pentobarbital
- Flunitrazepam
- γ-hydroxybutyrate (GHB)

Opioids
- Heroin
- Oxycodone (OXYCONTIN)

Central Nervous System Stimulants

Amphetamine and Its Derivatives
- Amphetamine
- Methamphetamine
- 3,4-Methylenedioxy-methamphetamine (MDMA)
- Methylphenidate (RITALIN)
- Fenfluramine (and Dexfenfluramine)
- Phentermine

Other Stimulants
- Cocaine
- Caffeine
- Nicotine

Other Psychoactive Drugs

Cannabis and Its Derivatives
- Marijuana
- Dronabinol (MARINOL)

Hallucinogens
- Lysergic acid diethylamide (LSD)
- Mescaline and psilocybin
- Phencyclidine (PCP)

Drugs For Treating Drug-Dependence
- Disulfiram (ANTABUSE)
- Acamprosate calcium (CAMPRAL)
- Naltrexone (TREXAN)
- Methadone
- Buprenorphine (SUBUTEX/SUBOXONE)
- Nicotine (NICORETTE, NICODERM)
- Bupropion (ZYBAN)

OVERVIEW

Drug Abuse

It is human nature that some individuals will experiment with occasional use or become dependent on mind-altering substances. Nearly every society in recorded history sanctioned the use of certain drugs while banning the use of others. In many Western countries, for example, products containing ethanol, nicotine, or caffeine are socially acceptable or at least tolerated by the majority of the population, whereas the use of opioids, cocaine, marijuana, hallucinogens, and other psychoactive drugs are illegal. In other countries, use of alcohol is discouraged and use of other psychoactive drugs, such as marijuana, is socially acceptable. Hence, what constitutes drug abuse from a social or political perspective is highly dependent on cultural attitudes and legal restrictions.

From a medical and psychological perspective, drug abuse can be defined as the use of a drug in a manner that is detrimental to the health or well-being of the drug user, other individuals, or society as a whole. Drug abuse is not restricted to the use of illegal drugs, as the cumulative health and social effects caused by the use of alcoholic beverages and tobacco products in the United States of America (USA) outweighs the negative effects of illicit drug use.

Drug Dependence

Drug dependence is a condition in which an individual feels compelled to repeatedly administer a psychoactive drug. When this is done to avoid physical discomfort or withdrawal, it is known as **physical dependence**; when it has a psychological aspect (the need for stimulation or pleasure, or to escape reality) then it is known as **psychological dependence**. Repeated drug use appears to be a learned behavior that is reinforced, both by the pleasurable effects of the drug and by the negative effects of drug abstinence (withdrawal). These effects are the basis of drug craving in drug-dependent individuals. **Psychological dependence** is caused by the positive reinforcement of drug use that results from the activation of neurons located in the nucleus accumbens. **Physical dependence** is a state in which continued drug use is required to prevent an unpleasant **withdrawal syndrome.** Hence, physical dependence leads to negative reinforcement of drug use. Both psychological and physical dependence appear to result from **neuronal adaptation** to the presence of the drug, albeit in different areas of the brain.

Psychological Dependence

The craving for **alcohol, barbiturates, caffeine, cocaine, opioids,** and **tobacco** is remarkably similar, despite the varied behavioral and physiologic effects that these drugs produce. This similarity supports the hypothesis that psychological dependence is mediated by a common neuronal pathway that leads to **behavioral reinforcement** of drug use. Psychoactive drugs that evoke behavioral reinforcement of their use appear to sensitize dopaminergic neurons that project from the ventral tegmental area to the nucleus accumbens. Other psychoactive drugs that are used for their mind-altering effects, including **lysergic acid diethylamide (LSD),** have a much smaller effect on the dopamine pathway and cause little reinforcement resulting less chronic use of LSD and other agents.

Much evidence indicates that **dopamine** mediates drug reinforcement by binding to dopamine D_1 receptors in the nucleus accumbens. This signal transduction pathway activates adenylyl cyclase, increasing cyclic adenosine monophosphate (cAMP) levels and activating cAMP-dependent kinases. The kinases, in turn, activate other proteins in the signal transduction pathway including **transcription factors**. In the accumbens, the transcription factor, cAMP-response element binding (CREB) protein, increases the synthesis of G proteins, cAMP-dependent protein kinases, and other cell transduction molecules that amplify responses to dopamine. Dopamine release onto accumbens neurons also increases the expression of glutamate receptors, which strengthens synaptic pathways for dopamine neurotransmission much like the molecular mechanisms of learning discovered in the hippocampus. These mechanisms lead to sensitization to dopamine, which underlies the behavioral reinforcement of drug use.

Investigators have observed that the peak of dopamine release in the accumbens occurs at the time of the drug's peak effect on the central nervous system (CNS). The degree of short-term reinforcement of drug use is linked to the rate of increase of dopamine levels in the nucleus accumbens. This relationship appears to account for the propensity of some drugs to produce drug dependence. It also appears to explain the difference in reinforcement effects produced by different routes of administration of a particular drug. For example, the oral administration of an opioid or cocaine causes less reinforcement and psychological dependence than does the intravenous administration or inhalation of an equivalent dose of the same drug. The differences in effect are determined by the rate at which the drug is distributed to the brain and the rate at which dopamine levels in the nucleus accumbens are increased.

Physical Dependence

Physical dependence, also called **neuroadaptation**, results from the adaptations of specific neurons or areas of the brain to the continued presence of a drug. **Physical dependence** is only observed outwardly by the development of a drug-specific withdrawal syndrome if the drug is discontinued or blocked. For this reason, physical dependence contributes to the continued use of a drug to avoid unwanted symptoms. The negative effects of nicotine withdrawal, for example, are responsible for the high relapse rate in persons trying to stop smoking cigarettes. The withdrawal symptoms are often opposite to the drug's acute effect, unmasking the neuroadaptation that acted to balance the effects of chronic drug administration. For example, opioids inhibit neurons regulating the peristaltic tone of the gastrointestinal (GI) tract and cause constipation; diarrhea is a classic sign of opioid withdrawal.

Drug Addiction

Drug addiction usually refers to an extreme pattern of drug abuse in which an individual is continuously preoccupied with drug procurement and use and thus neglects other responsibilities and personal relationships. Addiction is usually associated with a high level of drug dependence. The term 'addict' has a pejorative connotation, however, and the modern treatment of substance abuse as a disease state calls for use of the term 'drug-dependent' individuals or patients.

Classification of Drugs of Abuse

The psychoactive drugs that are used by some individuals for nonmedicinal purposes can be classified as CNS depressants, CNS stimulants, and miscellaneous agents, with the latter group including marijuana, hallucinogens, and phencyclidine. In many cases, drug-dependent individuals are using illegal substances as self-medication for comorbid disorders such as anxiety or depression. After describing the pharmacologic effects of these drugs and any clinical use that they may have, this chapter discusses the treatment of substance abuse. Tables 25–1 through 25–3 provide information about the manifestations and treatment of drug intoxication and withdrawal.

CENTRAL NERVOUS SYSTEM DEPRESSANTS

Alcohols and Glycols

In North America, about 12 million individuals have one or more symptoms of alcoholism, making **alcohol abuse** the number one substance abuse problem. In the USA alone, the

TABLE 25–1. Common Signs and Symptoms of Drug Intoxication

Drug	Motor and Speech Impairment	Emotional and Perceptual Manifestations	Cardiovascular Manifestations	Other Manifestations
Alcohol	Ataxia, incoordination, loquacity, and slurred speech	Euphoria, impaired attention, irritability, mood changes, and sedation	Flushed face	Nystagmus
Amphetamines	Agitation and loquacity	Decreased fatigue, euphoria, grandiosity, hypervigilance, and paranoia	Hypertension or hypotension and tachycardia	Chills, mydriasis, nausea, nystagmus, sweating, and vomiting
Barbiturates	Same as alcohol	Same as alcohol	Hypotension	Nystagmus
Benzodiazepines	Same as alcohol	Same as alcohol	Hypotension	Nystagmus
Cocaine	Same as amphetamines	Altered tactile sensation ("cocaine bugs"), decreased fatigue, euphoria, grandiosity, hypervigilance, and paranoia	Same as amphetamines	Same as amphetamines
Hallucinogens	Dizziness, incoordination, tremor, and weakness	Depersonalization, derealization, hallucinations, illusions, and synesthesia	Tachycardia	Blurred vision, mydriasis, and sweating
Marijuana	Loquacity and rapid speech	Euphoria, hallucinations (with high doses), jocularity, and sensory intensification	Hypertension and tachycardia	Conjunctivitis, dry mouth, increased appetite, and tightness in chest
Opioids	Motor slowness and slurred speech	Apathy, euphoria or dysphoria, impaired attention, and sedation	None	Miosis
Phencyclidine	Agitation, ataxia, muscle rigidity, and slurred speech	Anxiety, delusions, emotional lability, euphoria, and hallucinations	Hypertension and tachycardia	Hostility, miosis, nystagmus, and violent behavior

TABLE 25–2. Emergency Treatment of Drug Intoxication

Drug	Pharmacologic Treatment	Nonpharmacologic Treatment
Alcohol	None	Support vital functions
Amphetamines	Lorazepam for agitation and haloperidol for psychosis	Monitor and support cardiac function
Barbiturates	None	Support vital functions
Benzodiazepines	Flumazenil	Support vital functions
Cocaine	Lorazepam for agitation or seizures	Support vital functions
Hallucinogens	Lorazepam for agitation	Give reassurance and support vital functions
Marijuana	Lorazepam for agitation	Give reassurance and support vital functions
Opioids	Naloxone	Support vital functions
Phencyclidine	Lorazepam for agitation and haloperidol for psychosis	Minimize sensory input

cost of health care, lost work hours, criminal activity, and other problems related to alcohol use is roughly $90 billion each year.

The alcohols and glycols most commonly ingested are ethanol, methanol, and ethylene glycol. Whereas ethanol selectively produces CNS depression, methanol and ethylene glycol affect multiple organ systems and can produce severe or life-threatening toxicity, even when ingested in relatively small doses.

Ethanol

Ethanol, or **ethyl alcohol,** is classified as a CNS depressant and has pharmacologic effects similar to those of the barbiturates and benzodiazepines.

PHARMACOKINETICS. Ethanol has sufficient lipid solubility to enable rapid and almost complete absorption from the gut. It is more rapidly absorbed from the duodenum than from the stomach, and food slows its absorption by slowing the rate of gastric emptying. Ethanol is widely distributed throughout the body and has a volume of distribution that is roughly equivalent to the total body water, or about 38 L/70 kg of body weight.

As shown in Fig. 25–1, ethanol is primarily oxidized by **alcohol dehydrogenase** to form acetaldehyde and is then

TABLE 25–3. **Common Signs and Symptoms of Drug Withdrawal**

Drug	Central Nervous System Manifestations	Musculoskeletal Manifestations	Cardiovascular Manifestations	Other Manifestations
Alcohol	Altered perceptions, insomnia, irritability, and seizures.	Tremor.	Hypertension and tachycardia.	Delirium tremens, nausea, and sweating.
Amphetamines	Depression, drowsiness, dysphoria, fatigue, increased appetite, and sleepiness.	None.	Bradycardia.	None.
Barbiturates	Anxiety, insomnia, irritability, and seizures.	Muscle twitches.	Hypertension and tachycardia.	None.
Benzodiazepines	Agitation, anxiety, dizziness, and insomnia.	Muscle cramps and myoclonic contractions.	Hypertension and tachycardia.	None.
Cocaine	Same as amphetamines.	None.	Bradycardia.	None.
Marijuana	Irritability, mild agitation, and sleep disturbances.	None.	None.	Nausea and stomach cramps.
Nicotine	Anxiety, dysphoria, hostility, impatience, irritability, and restlessness.	None.	Decreased heart rate.	Increased appetite.
Opioids	Anxiety, dysphoria, irritability, restlessness, and sleep disturbances.	Muscle aches.	Hypertension and tachycardia.	Diarrhea, fever, mydriasis, piloerection,* sweating, vomiting, and yawning.

*Because piloerection causes "goose bumps" or "gooseflesh," patients withdrawing from opioids are sometimes described as "going cold turkey."

oxidized by **acetaldehyde dehydrogenase** to form acetate. The acetate derived from ethanol enters the citric acid cycle for further oxidation to carbon dioxide and water. The oxidation of ethanol utilizes significant quantities of nicotinamide adenine dinucleotide (NAD), and the depletion of NAD is responsible for some of the metabolic effects of ethanol that are described below. Ethanol also undergoes oxidation by **cytochrome P450 enzymes.** Unlike alcohol dehydrogenase metabolism, P450 enzyme metabolism is induced by long-term alcohol use. Therefore, P450 induction contributes to alcohol tolerance in heavy drinkers.

About 2% of ethanol is excreted unchanged by the kidneys and lungs. The concentration of ethanol in alveolar air is about 0.05% of that in the blood, and this relationship is used to estimate the **blood alcohol concentration (BAC)** in exhaled air when the **breathalyzer test** is administered. Because ethanol can markedly impair the psychomotor skills required to safely drive a vehicle, all **states** prohibit the operation of motor vehicles while under the influence of alcohol. As of July, 2004, the legal limit of blood alcohol for first-time offenders is a BAC less than 0.08% (80 mg/dL) in all states and federal territories.

The capacity of alcohol dehydrogenase to metabolize ethanol is limited because the enzyme is saturated at relatively low ethanol concentrations. Hence, ethanol metabo-

lism exhibits **zero-order kinetics**, except when serum concentrations of ethanol are very low. For this reason, the BAC is largely determined by the rate of ethanol ingestion. An adult weighing 70 kg usually metabolizes only about 10 mL of absolute ethanol per hour, which is roughly equivalent to the amount of ethanol contained in one alcoholic drink. A BAC of 0.08% to 0.1% in most cases is reached after an adult consumes from two to four drinks (bottles of beer, glasses of wine, or 6 ounces of distilled liquor) within an hour.

CNS EFFECTS, MECHANISMS, AND INTERACTIONS. Ethanol potentiates the actions of γ-aminobutyric acid (GABA) in a manner similar to that of benzodiazepines and barbiturates (see Chapter 19). It thereby produces sedative-hypnotic, anxiolytic, amnesic, and anticonvulsant effects. However, long-term ethanol use or ethanol withdrawal may lower the seizure threshold and thereby cause seizures. Predictably, ethanol potentiates the effects of benzodiazepines and barbiturates, so the combination of any of these drugs with ethanol can produce fatal CNS depression.

Ethanol at low doses produces disinhibition and mild euphoria, which facilitate social interactions by reducing behavioral inhibitions and self-consciousness. These reinforcing effects are related to the rate at which the BAC is rising, which probably determines the rate at which

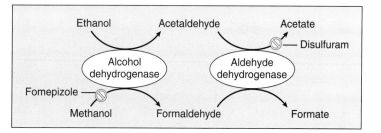

Figure 25-1. Metabolism of ethanol and methanol. Alcohols are oxidized to aldehydes by alcohol dehydrogenase. The aldehydes are oxidized to acetate or formate by aldehyde dehydrogenase. Disulfiram inhibits aldehyde dehydrogenase and leads to the accumulation of acetaldehyde during ethanol ingestion. Fomepizole inhibits alcohol dehydrogenase and is used in methanol or glycol poisoning.

dopamine concentrations increase in the nucleus accumbens. In many individuals, behavioral reinforcement leads to the continued consumption of alcoholic beverages and to ethanol intoxication. This problem is exacerbated by the limited rate at which ethanol can be eliminated from the body.

Ethanol inhibits the release of acetylcholine from CNS neurons, and this action may contribute to the sedation and delirium that occur during alcohol intoxication. Ethanol also inhibits the release of antidiuretic hormone from the pituitary gland and thereby produces a diuretic effect. This diuretic effect is augmented by the consumption of large quantities of alcoholic beverages, such as beer.

Ethanol produces vasodilation and increases heat loss from the body, partly by interfering with temperature regulation by the hypothalamus. Hence, alcohol consumption can contribute to hypothermia during cold weather.

OTHER EFFECTS, MECHANISMS, AND INTERACTIONS. In addition to producing CNS effects, ethanol ingestion produces a variety of short-term and long-term cardiovascular and autonomic effects.

Blood pressure fluctuations are caused by the combination of peripheral vasodilation, depression of regulatory centers in the medulla, and the release of norepinephrine from sympathetic neurons. Consumption of large amounts of ethanol on a long-term basis can eventually lead to alcoholic cardiomyopathy and cardiac arrhythmias.

In alcoholic patients, thiamine deficiency secondary to a poor diet is commonly observed, which leads to nerve demyelination. This, in turn, causes peripheral neuropathies, characterized by paresthesias and reduced sensory acuity. Thiamine deficiency can also cause Wernicke-Korsakoff syndrome, a behavioral disorder characterized by confusion, severe anterograde and retrograde amnesia, ataxia, nystagmus, and ophthalmoplegia. The administration of thiamine substantially reverses all but the amnesic effects seen in patients with this syndrome.

Alcoholic patients can also develop several metabolic disorders. The depletion of NAD (described above) causes several citric acid cycle metabolites and lactate to accumulate and eventually contributes to liver degeneration and impaired glycogenolysis. The resulting hypoglycemia exacerbates the effects of ethanol on the CNS. A dietary deficiency of folate can lead to megaloblastic anemia, whereas a deficiency of other vitamins and antioxidants contributes to the overall tissue damage observed in alcoholism.

The consumption of significant quantities of ethanol during pregnancy is responsible for the occurrence of the **fetal alcohol syndrome,** which is characterized by low birth weight, microcephaly, facial abnormalities (flattening), mental retardation, heart defects, and other abnormalities.

Other Alcohols and Glycols

Methanol, also called **methyl alcohol** or **wood alcohol,** is a highly toxic form of alcohol that can cause profound anion gap metabolic acidosis and severe damage to the eyes. As shown in Fig. 25–1, methanol is converted to formaldehyde and then to formate. Formate is primarily responsible for optic nerve damage, which can result in visual field impairment or permanent blindness. In cases of methanol poisoning, patients are treated with ethanol, which serves to saturate alcohol dehydrogenase and thereby prevent the formation of formaldehyde and formate. Ethanol has a greater affinity for alcohol dehydrogenase than does methanol. Hemodialysis is also used to reduce methanol levels in severe intoxication. Fomepizole, an inhibitor of alcohol dehydrogenase can also be administered, which prevents the formation of toxic metabolites in cases of methanol and ethylene glycol poisoning.

Isopropyl alcohol, which is contained in many formulations of rubbing alcohol, produces more CNS depression than does ethanol or methanol. Isopropyl alcohol is converted to acetone, a substance that can be smelled on the breath. The treatment of intoxication is largely supportive.

Ethylene glycol is contained in antifreeze, and its ingestion can cause anion gap metabolic acidosis and serious toxicity to the kidneys, lungs, and CNS. Ethylene glycol is metabolized to oxalic acid, and calcium oxalate crystals may be found in the urine of patients after ethylene glycol ingestion. Treatment consists of supporting vital functions, giving ethanol or fomepizole, managing acidosis, and performing hemodialysis.

Barbiturates and Benzodiazepines

The pharmacologic properties of barbiturates and benzodiazepines are discussed in Chapter 19. These drugs are sedative-hypnotic agents that are prescribed for the treatment of anxiety disorders, insomnia, and other conditions. They are used recreationally for their euphoric and anxiolytic effects, and some polydrug users use them to reduce the irritability and anxiety associated with cocaine or amphetamine use.

The short-acting barbiturates (e.g., **pentobarbital**) are among the most widely abused sedative-hypnotic drugs. Several benzodiazepines have also been used illicitly, including **flunitrazepam.** Although this drug is not approved for use in the USA, it is used throughout much of the world as an anxiolytic or hypnotic drug. In the USA, it is widely available on the streets and is sometimes referred to as **"roofies,"** derived from its trade name, ROHYPNOL. Flunitrazepam has gained fame as a party drug or 'club drug,' a drug that contributes to date rape. It is an extremely potent benzodiazepine that is tasteless when dissolved in a beverage. Flunitrazepam produces drowsiness, impaired motor skills, and anterograde amnesia. Hence, victims do not recall events that happened the night before. Despite its street reputation, most studies have found that flunitrazepam is no more likely to cause toxicity or dependence than are other benzodiazepines.

Gamma hydroxybutyrate (GHB) usually comes as an odorless liquid, slightly salty to the taste, and sold in small bottles. It has also been found in powder and capsule form. The use of this 'club-drug' has resulted in deaths from CNS depression and mixing with alcohol. It is also listed by the Drug Enforcement Administration (DEA) as a predatory ('date-rape') drug. Its exact mechanism of action is unknown but it is an agonist at $GABA_B$ receptors in the brain.

The long-term use of barbiturate or benzodiazepine drugs can lead to psychological and physical dependence, and their abrupt withdrawal produces symptoms that are similar to those caused by alcohol withdrawal (see Table 25–3).

Opioids

The most commonly abused opioid drug and a popular street drug is **heroin.** This drug is prepared from morphine by the addition of acetyl groups, so it is also called **diacetylmorphine.** Heroin is highly potent and can be easily dissolved in water and injected intravenously. Because it is also highly lipid-soluble and rapidly enters the CNS following injection, heroin can produce an intense euphoric sensation called a "rush." Long-term heroin users develop considerable drug tolerance and physical dependence, and they undergo a wide variety of withdrawal symptoms (see Table 25–3) if they abruptly discontinue their use of the drug.

Other opioids produce effects similar to those of heroin, but usually to a lesser degree. These effects vary with the potency and pharmacokinetic properties of the opioid and with the route of administration. Opioids administered orally tend to produce less euphoria and dependence than do opioids administered by other routes. For this reason, an orally administered drug such as methadone (see Chapter 23) can be used to prevent the craving for heroin as well as the opioid withdrawal reaction without causing significant reinforcement or exacerbating drug dependence. **Oxycodone,** in the slow-release formulation marketed as OXYCONTIN, gained notoriety among street users because a dose meant for long-lasting relief in patients with chronic pain could be crushed and injected intravenously for a powerful rush. This has led to an increase in the number of deaths caused by opioid overdose.

CENTRAL NERVOUS SYSTEM STIMULANTS

The CNS stimulants include amphetamine, amphetamine derivatives, cocaine, caffeine, and nicotine. The amphetamine compounds and cocaine increase the synaptic concentration of norepinephrine and dopamine and exert sympathomimetic effects. They also induce a release of dopamine in the nucleus accumbens because this is the final common pathway for all chronically abused drugs and reinforced behaviors.

Amphetamine and Its Derivatives

Amphetamine and its derivatives (Fig. 25–2A) increase the synaptic concentration of norepinephrine and dopamine by gaining entry into the presynaptic terminal through the reuptake transporter protein and releasing the catecholamines from vesicles. Amphetamine also facilitates the reverse transport of the catecholamines inside the terminal out through the reuptake transporter into the synapse. At high concentrations, amphetamine, but not all derivatives, can also inhibit monoamine oxidase and, by this second mechanism, increase the levels of catecholamines.

The use of amphetamines produces a constellation of central and peripheral effects, including euphoria, insomnia, psychomotor stimulation, anxiety, loss of appetite, increased concentration, decreased fatigue, respiratory stimulation, and hyperthermia. It also produces sympathomimetic effects such as mydriasis, tachycardia, and hypertension. The euphoria and other reinforcing effects are caused by increased dopamine levels in the nucleus accumbens, whereas the jittery and anxious feelings produced by amphetamines primarily result from enhanced release of norepinephrine in the central and peripheral nervous systems.

The amphetamines have a few legitimate medical indications. First, amphetamines or antidepressant drugs can be used to treat **narcolepsy,** a condition characterized by sleep attacks, in which the patient suddenly falls asleep during normal daytime activities. Second, amphetamines can be used to treat **attention deficit disorder (ADD),** a disorder characterized by hyperactivity and the inability to focus attention or concentrate on a task. Amphetamine-type drugs are the most effective treatment for most patients with ADD, and methylphenidate is widely used for this purpose. Third, amphetamine derivatives (e.g., phentermine) can be used as adjuncts in the treatment of **obesity.**

Methamphetamine

Amphetamine and methamphetamine are closely related sympathomimetic amines, and both are drugs of abuse. Of the two, methamphetamine is often preferred by abusers because it causes less norepinephrine to be released and can be more easily pyrolyzed (burned) and smoked. When methamphetamine free base is extracted by ether, pyrolyzed, and smoked, it is called **"ice"** or **"crystal meth."** The euphoria produced by smoking "ice" is much greater than that produced by taking methamphetamine orally, probably because of the faster rate at which dopamine levels are increased by inhaling the drug. The cheap cost and relative ease of making methamphetamine from precursor drugs found in nonprescription cold medicines enabled an illicit cottage industry in small-scale meth labs.

Methylphenidate

Methylphenidate is an amphetamine derivative that usually causes less irritability, anxiety, and anorexia than does amphetamine. When it is used to treat children with ADD, it is administered in the morning and at noontime, with the last dose preferably given no later than 3:00 PM in order to avoid insomnia. Although a causal relationship has not been established, suppression of growth (caused by decreased weight gain) is reported with the long-term use of stimulants in children.

Methylphenidate is not associated with significant dependence when it is used for the treatment of ADD, but it is abused for its CNS stimulant effects.

Phentermine and Fenfluramine

Phentermine and fenfluramine (and its active stereoisomer, dexfenfluramine) are amphetamine derivatives that have been used as appetite suppressants (anorectics) in the treatment of obesity. The drugs act by stimulating the satiety center in the hypothalamus. In comparison with amphetamine, they produce less CNS stimulation and have a lower dependence liability. The combination of phentermine and fenfluramine (Phen-Fen), however, was shown in 1997 to cause valvular heart disease and pulmonary hypertension and both fenfluramine and dexfenfluramine were withdrawn from the market.

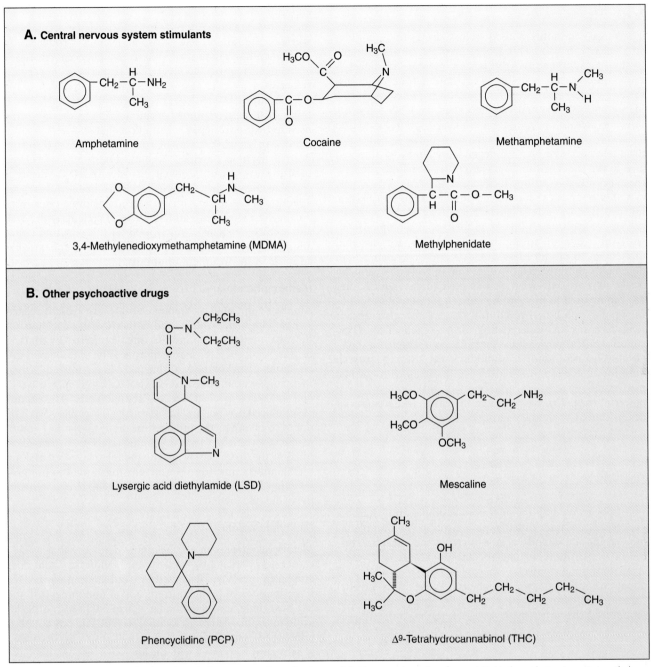

Figure 25-2. Structures of selected central nervous system stimulants and other psychoactive drugs. (A) Methamphetamine, 3,4-methylene-dioxymethamphetamine (MDMA), and methylphenidate are all derivatives of amphetamine. Cocaine is an alkaloid derived from the leaves of *Erythroxylon coca*. (B) Lysergic acid diethylamide (LSD) and mescaline are hallucinogens. Phencyclidine (PCP) was originally developed as a dissociative anesthetic but was withdrawn from the market because it produces hallucinations and delirium, sometimes with hostility and violent behavior. Δ⁹-Tetrahydrocannabinol (THC) is the primary cannabinoid chemical in marijuana.

Phentermine and other anorectics (e.g., **sibutramine**) are still available as an adjunct to dietary restrictions in the treatment of obesity. Tolerance often develops to the anorectic effects of these drugs after a few weeks to a few months of use.

Other Amphetamine Derivatives

Several other amphetamine derivatives have been clandestinely synthesized and sold as **"designer drugs"** on the street.

These include **3,4-methylenedioxymethamphetamine (MDMA)**, a drug called **"ecstasy"** or **"X"**. MDMA produces both psychostimulant and psychotomimetic effects by increasing dopamine and serotonin levels in the brain.

Users of MDMA report that the drug causes euphoria, increases empathy, enhances pleasure, heightens sexuality, and expands consciousness without loss of control. MDMA, however, causes various unpleasant effects (e.g., nausea, anorexia, and anxiety), and its use can be life threatening. In

MDMA users, a number of deaths have resulted from cardiac arrhythmias, hyperthermia, rhabdomyolysis, and disseminated intravascular coagulation. MDMA is neurotoxic to serotonergic neurons, with clear degeneration of serotonergic pathways in animal models. Use of MDMA in humans likely destroys serotonergic brain neurons, which can contribute to some of the associated psychiatric complications, including panic reactions, psychosis, depression, and suicide. These disorders are prevalent in MDMA users today and will probably be observed to a greater extent later in these individuals when neuronal injury is compounded by loss of neurons during aging.

Other Stimulants

Cocaine

Cocaine produces both psychostimulant and local anesthetic activity and has limited clinical use as a local anesthetic (see Chapter 21). The stimulant effects are caused by inhibition of the neuronal reuptake of norepinephrine and dopamine. Cocaine binds to the neurotransmitter transport proteins and causes them to undergo a conformational change that reduces their capacity to transport dopamine or norepinephrine. It is a reuptake blocker in the same manner as an antidepressant. By this mechanism, cocaine increases the synaptic concentration of these neurotransmitters.

Cocaine is an alkaloid derived from the leaves of a plant indigenous to South America, *Erythroxylon coca*. When native South Americans chew the leaves to relieve fatigue, relatively few adverse effects are seen. Use of purified forms of cocaine, however, is associated with significant drug dependence, as well as cardiovascular, pulmonary, and neurotoxicity.

In the past, many cocaine users took powdered cocaine hydrochloride by insufflation (snorting). Cocaine taken in this manner is absorbed across the nasal mucosa and into the circulation. More recently, cocaine free base became available in the form of pellets or rocks, called **"crack,"** because of the cracking sound made during the processing of cocaine powder to the base form. Unlike cocaine hydrochloride, crack cocaine can be smoked. Crack cocaine becomes aerosolized when it is heated, and inhaling the substance into the lungs causes it to be rapidly absorbed into the circulation. Inhalation of crack cocaine produces serum levels that are comparable to those obtained by intravenous administration of the drug. For this reason, crack cocaine produces a euphoric effect that is more intense than that obtained by snorting cocaine. The higher serum levels achieved with crack cocaine use also increase the potential for overdose toxicity, particularly during repeated administration.

The common signs and symptoms of cocaine intoxication are listed in Table 25–1. Unlike other drugs of abuse, cocaine can alter tactile sensation, causing its users to feel as if insects are crawling under their skin (the sensation of "cocaine bugs") and causing them to scratch and produce self-inflicted skin lesions. Cocaine often stimulates respiration at lower doses, and high doses can produce irregular breathing and apnea (Cheyne-Stokes respiration). The local anesthetic actions of cocaine probably contribute to the drug's cardiac toxicity when high doses are administered.

With frank overdoses, the potential for neurotoxicity and cardiac toxicity increases. Cocaine overdose victims often suffer from delirium and can become aggressive and violent. The pulse can become rapid, weak, and irregular. In some cases, cocaine overdose causes tonic–clonic seizures (including status epilepticus), malignant encephalopathy, high-output cardiac failure, or myocardial infarction. When fatalities occur, they typically result from ventricular fibrillation or cardiac arrest. For this reason, the management of cocaine overdose must include cardiovascular and pulmonary support, as well as the administration of a benzodiazepine (e.g., lorazepam) to control agitation or seizures.

Cocaine withdrawal produces fatigue, depression, nightmares or other sleep disturbances, and increased appetite. The management of cocaine withdrawal is largely supportive. **Bromocriptine**, a dopamine receptor agonist, has been used to reduce craving for the drug, but the effectiveness of this treatment for withdrawal has not been firmly established.

Nicotine

Nicotine, the principal alkaloid of plants of the genus *Nicotiana*, is widely available in the form of various tobacco products that can be chewed or smoked.

Nicotine is a lipid-soluble tertiary amine. It is rapidly absorbed into the circulation from the mouth or the respiratory tract and is then quickly distributed to the brain. The drug's CNS effects are rapidly terminated by redistribution from the brain to the peripheral tissues. Although nicotine has a half-life of about 30 minutes, it is metabolized to the active metabolite, cotinine, which has a half-life of about 2 hours. The induction of cytochrome P450 enzymes by tars contained in cigarette smoke accelerates the metabolism of nicotine, and this leads to the development of pharmacokinetic tolerance to the drug. Because the use of cigarettes accelerates the metabolism of β-adrenergic receptor antagonists, benzodiazepines, opioids, and theophylline, cigarette smokers may require higher doses of these drugs to maintain therapeutic serum levels.

Nicotine activates cholinergic nicotinic receptors in the central and peripheral nervous systems and produces a complex constellation of subjective and physiologic effects. The CNS effects of nicotine are similar to those of the psychostimulants and include mild euphoria, increased arousal and concentration, improved memory, and appetite suppression. In addition to activating cholinergic receptors, nicotine inhibits monoamine oxidase. The drug's ability to inhibit this enzyme can partly explain its ability to activate dopaminergic neurotransmission and its dependence liability. The monoamine oxidase inhibitors used in treating depression, however, do not cause significant drug dependence or the intense drug craving associated with nicotine use. More directly, nicotine ultimately increases the release of dopamine in the nucleus accumbens, as with all other addictive drugs and behaviors, and strongly initiates drug dependence.

Caffeine

Caffeine citrate is occasionally administered intravenously to treat **apnea in neonates.** It is also available in nonprescription tablets to prevent **fatigue.**

Caffeine is a methylxanthine that produces mild stimulation by blocking adenosine receptors on neurons throughout the CNS. Because adenosine inhibits dopamine release, caffeine indirectly enhances dopamine neurotransmission. This action is probably responsible for the drug's stimulant effects and dependence liability.

Caffeine is the most widely ingested drug; it is contained in coffee, cola beverages, teas, and other products that are used throughout the world. Caffeine use decreases the desire to sleep, elevates the mood, and causes an increase in alertness, concentration, motivation, and talkativeness. By arousing the sympathetic system, it causes a mild stimulation of heart rate and blood pressure. Caffeine also relaxes most smooth muscles and causes diuresis by increasing renal blood flow.

Because caffeine increases the secretion of gastric acid and pepsin, it can contribute to gastritis and peptic ulcers. High doses of caffeine produce nausea, vomiting, increased muscle tone, and tremors. Although extremely high doses of caffeine can cause delirium, seizures, and even death, these doses are almost impossible to reach by ingesting a caffeinated beverage such as coffee. They can be reached by ingesting caffeine tablets, but abuse of caffeine tablets is limited by the fact that large doses of them produce such unpleasant symptoms.

The manifestations of caffeine withdrawal are relatively mild but include headache, impaired concentration, irritability, depression, anxiety, flulike symptoms, and blurred vision. The withdrawal symptoms can be lessened by reducing caffeine consumption gradually over a period of several weeks.

OTHER PSYCHOACTIVE DRUGS

Cannabis and Its Derivatives

In the USA, a synthetic cannabis derivative called **dronabinol** has been approved for the **treatment of nausea** caused by cancer chemotherapy and for the **stimulation of appetite** in patients who have acquired immunodeficiency syndrome (AIDS) and are suffering from anorexia. The drug is administered orally for these purposes.

The most well-known form of cannabis is **marijuana,** which consists of the dried flowers and leaves of *Cannabis sativa*, and is considered a drug of abuse. The primary cannabinoid in marijuana is Δ^9-**tetrahydrocannabinol (THC)**, a drug whose structure is shown in Fig. 25–2B. When cannabis is inhaled, about 20% of the THC is absorbed into the circulation. In contrast, when cannabis is ingested orally, only about 6% of the THC is absorbed from the gut, owing to the extensive first-pass metabolism. THC has multiple effects on neuronal function. It binds stereospecifically to membrane cannabinoid (CB) receptors in neurons, and this action is linked with inhibition of adenylyl cyclase and cAMP production. The recently discovered endogenous ligand for the CB receptors is called **anandamide**. It also inhibits voltage-gated calcium channels that regulate neurotransmitter release. Through these and other actions, THC appears to modulate the activity of acetylcholine, dopamine, and serotonin.

When marijuana is smoked, pyrolysis releases THC and other substances. The plasma level of THC peaks within several minutes, then it falls rapidly during the first hour, as the drug is redistributed to adipose tissue. Thereafter, it declines slowly, owing to metabolism and excretion in the urine and feces. Because of its high lipophilicity, THC is stored in fat, and the drug and its metabolites can be detected in the body for weeks.

Marijuana use initially causes mild stimulation followed by a depressive phase. The stimulant phase is described as a dreamlike euphoric state characterized by an altered sense of time, increased visual acuity, difficulty in concentrating, and impaired short-term memory. The depressive phase is characterized by drowsiness, lethargy, and increased appetite. The psychoactive effects of marijuana depend somewhat on the environment and the extent of prior use of the drug. For example, first-time users are more likely to experience anxiety than are habitual users.

Marijuana has been implicated as the cause of an 'amotivational syndrome' that is characterized by a lack of desire to work or excel in any part of life. It has also been described as a "gateway drug" whose initial use leads to the subsequent use of other drugs (e.g., cocaine or heroin). Little scientific evidence supports either of these claims. Marijuana, however, causes minor decreases in the levels of testosterone in men, low birth weight in neonates, increased fetal malformations, and decreases ovulation in females. Studies in humans have consistently demonstrated that marijuana reduces aggressive behavior, even though animals injected with THC may show aggression.

Experimental studies have demonstrated that cannabinoids are effective in the treatment of asthma, glaucoma, and vomiting. This is because their use causes bronchodilation, decreased intraocular pressure, and inhibition of nausea. Their use can also cause tachycardia.

The common signs and symptoms of marijuana intoxication and withdrawal are listed in Tables 25–1 and 25–3.

Hallucinogens

Prescription drugs, fever, and disorders such as schizophrenia are all capable of causing hallucinations, which are false perceptions that result from abnormal sensory processing. Unlike prescription drugs, however, drugs such as **lysergic acid diethylamide, mescaline** and **psilocybin** can produce hallucinations without causing delirium. LSD is a synthetic ergot derivative, mescaline is found in the *Peyote* cactus, and psilocybin in mushrooms that grow on cow patties (*Psilocybe coprophilia*). These street drugs are taken orally and usually begin to produce hallucinations within an hour. The effects of LSD can last as long as 12 hours, whereas the effects of mescaline and psilocybin last about 6 hours. The mechanisms responsible for the effects are incompletely understood. Some evidence indicates that LSD selectively activates certain subtypes of serotonin (5-hydroxytryptamine, or 5-HT) receptors in the neocortex, limbic system, and brainstem. According to one hypothesis, the activation of 5-HT$_2$ receptors in the reticular formation leads to the generalization of sensory stimuli to evoke hallucinations.

Although the use of LSD or mescaline usually causes visual hallucinations, it can also cause auditory, tactile, olfactory, gustatory, kinesthetic, and synesthetic hallucinations. Visual hallucinations often follow a temporal pattern in which amorphous bursts of light are followed by geometric forms and then by faces or scenes. Some users also report the occurrence of **synesthesia**, a condition in which one sensory modality assumes the characteristics of another. In a synesthetic hallucination, for example, sounds may be seen or colors may be heard.

The hallucinogens have little effect on cognitive function or arousal. If mood changes occur, they are generally an exaggeration of the predrug mood and are highly context-dependent. They are usually pleasant, but they can be terrifying and cause sufficient anxiety to resemble a panic attack. Mood changes are accompanied by somatic signs of sympathetic activation, including increased heart rate, increased blood pressure, and dilated pupils. Nausea and vomiting can occur, particularly with mescaline use.

Overdoses are rarely serious, but the occasional panic attack ("bad trip") may require intervention that consists of removing the patient to a quiet room and having someone remain with the patient for reassurance.

Phencyclidine

Phencyclidine (PCP) is still a widely used street drug, despite its reputation for causing dangerous side effects and despite efforts to reduce its supply by limiting the sale of chemicals used in its synthesis. PCP was originally developed as a dissociative anesthetic similar to ketamine, but the occurrence of a high incidence of postanesthetic hallucinations and delirium forced its removal from the market.

Sometimes called **"angel dust,"** PCP can be taken via various routes. The drug is incompletely and erratically absorbed from the gut, so it is usually smoked. In some cases, it is sprinkled on tobacco or marijuana and then smoked. In other cases, it is combined with cocaine and heroin before it is used.

Use of PCP produces a unique spectrum of effects that probably result from blockade of glutamate N-methyl-D-aspartate (NMDA) receptors and action at less characterized receptors called **sigma receptors**. As shown in Table 25–1, these effects include euphoria, hallucinations, and psychotomimetic activity, sometimes accompanied by hostility and violent behavior. PCP causes little tolerance, physical dependence, or withdrawal effects.

MANAGEMENT OF DRUG ABUSE

Use of psychoactive drugs can cause several distinct clinical problems, including drug intoxication or overdose, drug withdrawal, and drug dependence. The severity of these problems varies markedly among different classes of drugs

and patterns of drug use. A diagnosis of drug intoxication or dependence in a particular individual is primarily based on the history, psychological assessment, physical examination, and laboratory findings.

Drug Intoxication and Withdrawal

The initial treatment of drug intoxication or overdose consists of supporting cardiovascular and pulmonary functions. **Naloxone** or **flumazenil** can be administered to counteract the acute CNS depression caused by toxic doses of an opioid or a benzodiazepine, respectively (see Table 25–2). **Lorazepam** can be used to control agitation, and an antipsychotic drug (e.g., **haloperidol**) can be administered for psychosis, which can occur with PCP overdose. Haloperidol should not be used in cases of cocaine overdose, however, because it lowers the seizure threshold and can exacerbate or precipitate seizures.

The next stage of treatment is the management of withdrawal reactions that occur as the drug is eliminated from the body. The pharmacologic treatment of withdrawal consists primarily of substitution therapy and symptomatic relief.

A benzodiazepine (e.g., **lorazepam** or **chlordiazepoxide**) can be administered to suppress the acute manifestations of withdrawal from alcohol, including delusions, hallucinations, a coarse tremor, and agitation (**delirium tremens**). The benzodiazepine is then gradually withdrawn over several weeks.

Methadone is usually used to suppress withdrawal reactions in opioid users because it is long-acting and orally effective. Methadone is also given on a long-term basis in the treatment of heroin addiction.

Clonidine, an α_2-adrenergic receptor agonist, is effective in reducing the sympathetic nervous system symptoms of alcohol, opioid, or nicotine withdrawal, and it may facilitate continued abstinence in persons who are dependent on these drugs.

Clinical studies have shown that **bromocriptine,** a dopamine receptor agonist, can lessen the symptoms of cocaine withdrawal, but its role has not been firmly established.

Treatment of Drug Dependence

After treatment of drug intoxication and withdrawal, attention can be directed to the more difficult problem of treating drug dependence. In this endeavor, behavioral therapy and personal motivation are as important as subsequent pharmacologic treatments. Patients are rarely cured, and most clinicians view treatment as a life-long process in which patients are continually recovering. Twelve-step groups, such as Alcoholics Anonymous and Narcotics Anonymous, have been successful in reducing recidivism, partly because they recognize that the individual is always in a state of remission from drug or alcohol dependence and that an ever-present possibility exists of slipping into drug use again.

Pharmacologic agents can be of use in treating drug dependence. Ethanol interacts with drugs that are metabolized by cytochrome P450 enzymes. It also interacts with **disulfiram,** a drug that inhibits acetaldehyde dehydrogenase. When this drug is administered concurrently with ethanol, it leads to the accumulation of acetaldehyde and causes nausea, profuse vomiting, sweating, flushing, palpitations, and dyspnea. Because of its ability to cause these extremely unpleasant symptoms, disulfiram is sometimes prescribed to encourage alcoholic patients to abstain from ethanol use. Other drugs that can cause disulfuram-*like* effects when administered concurrently with ethanol include metronidazole (a drug used in the treatment of protozoal infections) and some of the third-generation cephalosporin antibiotics.

Recently, a new dependence medication for alcohol was approved called **acamprosate calcium**. It is a synthetic compound with a chemical structure similar to that of the endogenous amino acid homotaurine, which is a structural analogue of the amino acid neurotransmitter GABA and the amino acid neuromodulator taurine. The mechanism of action of acamprosate in maintenance of alcohol abstinence is not completely understood. Chronic alcohol exposure is hypothesized to alter the normal balance between neuronal excitation and inhibition. In vitro and in vivo studies in animals have provided evidence to suggest acamprosate can interact with glutamate and GABA neurotransmitter systems centrally, and has led to the hypothesis that acamprosate restores this balance.

Buprenorphine was recently approved for physician out-patient treatment of opioid dependence. It is formulated in a sublingual tablet or oral form in combination with naloxone to prevent intravenous abuse. **Naltrexone** prevents the euphoric and other effects obtained with opioid administration and is used to treat opioid dependence. The patch (transdermal) formulation of naltrexone is ideally suited for this purpose. It is also approved for the treatment of alcohol dependence because opioid receptors play a key role in the reinforcement of the rewarding effects of alcohol and other drugs. **Clonidine,** a centrally acting α_2 agonist, is also used to facilitate abstinence from opioids and nicotine.

Nicotine chewing gum and skin patches have been developed to mitigate nicotine withdrawal reactions in persons who are trying to quit smoking. Another drug used to treat nicotine withdrawal is the antidepressant **bupropion,** which is now available in a long-acting formulation for this purpose. The ability of bupropion to block the reuptake of dopamine can contribute to its effectiveness in treating drug dependence. The combined use of bupropion and nicotine patches is currently being investigated.

Spurred on by both the commercial and medical success of bupropion (ZYBAN) for smoking cessation, government and industry leaders are awakening to the treatment need of drug-dependent individuals. Many anticraving agents and pharmacologic approaches are currently in development. For example, treatment of cocaine dependence by vaccinations to produce anticocaine antibodies is in clinical trials. Other approved agents (e.g., clonidine and bromocriptine) are being tested in drug-dependent populations. Progress on the prevention and management of drug abuse and drug dependence will soon lead to more effective pharmacotherapy for these treatable CNS disorders.

SUMMARY OF IMPORTANT POINTS

■ Drug dependence is a condition in which an individual feels compelled to repeatedly administer a psychoactive drug. The condition is caused by positive reinforcement (psychological dependence) and negative reinforcement (physical dependence) from continued drug use.

■ Reinforcement of drug use results from increased levels of dopamine in the nucleus accumbens and dopamine sensitization of these pathways.

■ Physical dependence, which results from neuronal adaptation to the continued presence of a drug, is usually associated with drug tolerance. Physical dependence results in a characteristic withdrawal syndrome when drug use is discontinued.

■ Alcohol and other central nervous system (CNS) depressants produce motor and cognitive impairment, sedation, euphoria, and behavioral disinhibition.

■ Amphetamines, cocaine, and other CNS stimulants produce euphoria, agitation, hypervigilance, mydriasis, and sympathetic nervous system arousal. Cocaine also produces altered tactile sensation, and cocaine overdose can cause severe cardiovascular and neurotoxicity.

■ Marijuana and cannabis derivatives produce a mild euphoria, talkativeness, conjunctivitis, and increased appetite.

■ Lysergic acid diethylamide (LSD) and other hallucinogens cause hallucinations without producing delirium.

■ The treatment of drug dependence and withdrawal can include some type of substitution therapy: a benzodiazepine substituted for alcohol; methadone substituted for an opioid; and nicotine chewing gum or skin patches substituted for cigarettes.

■ The treatment of alcohol- and opioid-dependent individuals can include naltrexone transdermal patches. Naltrexone is an opioid antagonist that blocks the opioid receptor link in the dopamine reinforcement pathway in the nucleus accumbens.

Review Questions

1. Disulfiram effectively treats alcohol (ethanol) dependence by which of the following mechanisms?
   (A) increasing plasma ethanol concentration
   (B) preventing the conversion of ethanol to methanol in the liver
   (C) increasing circulating acetaldehyde concentrations
   (D) blocking the action of ethanol at its cell membrane receptor
   (E) stabilizing the cell membrane to prevent ethanol disruption

2. The fact that the degree of reinforcement for morphine is less than that of heroin is best explained by which one of the following statements?
(A) morphine is a partial agonist
(B) heroin binds tighter to opioid receptors
(C) morphine is metabolized faster than heroin
(D) morphine is first metabolized to heroin
(E) heroin is distributed quicker to the brain

3. Synesthesia is an acute pharmacologic effect of which drug of abuse?
(A) marijuana
(B) LSD
(C) cocaine
(D) PCP
(E) alcohol

4. Which of the following has NOT been reported as a health hazard of chronic marijuana abuse?
(A) lower birth weight in neonates
(B) decreased testosterone in men
(C) anovulatory cycle in females
(D) increased fetal malformations
(E) increased intraocular pressure

5. Crack cocaine in the 1990s became more problematic than the powder cocaine of the 1980s because of which difference between the two forms of cocaine?
(A) cocaine in crack is more potent than cocaine in powder form
(B) crack cocaine is not metabolized in humans
(C) reinforcement is greater with inhalation vs. insufflation
(D) powder cocaine reaches the brain quicker
(E) coca plants in the 1990s were bred for greater cocaine content

Answers and Explanations

1. The correct answer is C: increasing circulating acetaldehyde concentrations. Disulfiram inhibits the acetaldehyde dehydrogenase, a step in the metabolism of alcohol. Concurrent administration of disulfiram and ethanol causes increased acetaldehyde blood levels, which is associated with flushing, nausea and vomiting, and other ill effects. Answer (A), increasing plasma ethanol concentration, would not be a good ethanol treatment plan because disulfiram is approved for the treatment of alcohol dependence. Answer (B), preventing the conversion of ethanol to methanol in the liver, is simply not true, and answer (D), blocking the action of ethanol at its cell membrane receptor, is also incorrect. Answer (E), stabilizing the cell membrane to prevent ethanol disruption, refers to an older hypothesis of ethanol action in which it was thought that ethanol fluidizes neuronal membranes and thereby disrupts ion channels and neurotransmission. This is clearly not an action of disulfiram.

2. The correct answer is E: heroin is distributed quicker to the brain. Heroin is an illicit opioid made by the addition of two acetyl groups at the 3 and 6 position of the morphine molecule. Because of this diacetylmorphine (heroin) is more lipophilic and crosses the blood–brain barrier quite rapidly to exert its reinforcing effects. Although answers (A), morphine, is a partial agonist and answer (B), heroin, binds tighter to opioid receptors, are wrong, answer (C), morphine, is metabolized faster than heroin, may be generally true because heroin has extra groups to demethylate, the degree of reinforcement is greater with more rapid acting agents. Answer (D), morphine is first metabolized to heroin, is simply wrong.

3. The correct answer is B: LSD. This potent ergot derivative is noted for synesthesia, the phenomenon whereby the perception of sensory modalities cross over such that sounds can be seen and sights can be heard. The drugs of abuse listed as answers (A) and (C) through (E) are not known for such a bizarre CNS effect.

4. The correct answer is E: increased intraocular pressure. This is not an effect of marijuana use and indeed THC, the active ingredient in marijuana, shows promise as a treatment for glaucoma, which is increased intraocular pressure. The other adverse effects listed as answers (A) through (D) are true concerning the chronic use of marijuana.

5. The correct answer is C: reinforcement is greater with inhalation vs. insufflation. The crack epidemic is caused by the switch from insufflation (snorting) to inhalation (smoking) because of the change in cocaine formulation from powder to the free base forms (crack). Answer (A), cocaine in crack is more potent than cocaine in powder form, is not true because the cocaine molecule itself still has the same potency in either form. Answers (B), crack cocaine is not metabolized in humans, and (D), powder cocaine reaches the brain quicker, are simply not true. Answer (E), coca plants in the 1990s were bred for greater cocaine content, may be true but the cocaine molecule itself would not be altered.

SELECTED READINGS

Fudala, P. J., and G. W. Woody. Recent advances in the treatment of opiate addiction. Curr Psychiatry Rep 6(5):339–346, 2004.
Gahlinger, P. M. Club drugs: MDMA, gamma-hydroxybutyrate (GHB), ROHYPNOL, and ketamine. Am Fam Physician 69(11):2619–2626, 2004.
Leweke, F. M., C. W. Gerth, and J. Klosterkotter. Cannabis-associated psychosis: current status of research. CNS Drugs 18(13):895–910, 2004.
Nutt, D., and A. Lingford-Hughes. Infecting the brain to stop addiction? Proc Natl Acad Sci U S A 101(31):11193–11194, 2004.
Piomelli, D. The endogenous cannabinoid system and the treatment of marijuana dependence. Neuropharmacology 47(Suppl 1):359–367, 2004.
Rohsenow, D. J. What place does naltrexone have in the treatment of alcoholism? CNS Drugs 18(9):547–560, 2004.
Rounsaville, B. J. Treatment of cocaine dependence and depression. Biol Psychiatry 56(10):803–809, 2004.

PHARMACOLOGY OF THE RESPIRATORY AND OTHER SYSTEMS

CHAPTER 26

Autacoid Drugs

CLASSIFICATION OF AUTACOID DRUGS

Histamine H₁ Receptor Antagonists

First-generation Antihistamines
- Promethazine (PHENERGAN)
- Diphenhydramine (BENADRYL)
- Chlorpheniramine (CHLOR-TRIMETON)
- Clemastine (TAVIST)
- Dimenhydrinate (DRAMAMINE)
- Hydroxyzine (ATARAX)
- Meclizine (ANTIVERT)

Second-generation Antihistamines
- Fexofenadine (ALLEGRA)
- Loratadine (CLARITIN)
- Desloratadine (CLARINEX)
- Astemizole (HISMANAL)
- Cetirizine (ZYRTEC)

Intranasal Antihistamines
- Azelastine (ASTELIN)

Opthalmic Antihistamines
- Ketotifen (ZADITOR)
- Levocabastine (LIVOSTIN)[a]

Serotonin Agonists
- Buspirone (BUSPAR)

- Sumatriptan (IMITREX)[b]
- Tegaserod (ZELNORM)

Serotonin Antagonists
- Clozapine (CLOZARIL)
- Cyproheptadine (PERIACTIN)
- Methysergide (SANSERT)
- Ondansetron (ZOFRAN)[c]

Prostaglandin Drugs
- Alprostadil (CAVERJECT, MUSE)
- Carboprost tromethamine (HEMABATE)
- Dinoprostone (CERVIDIL)
- Misoprostol (CYTOTEC)
- Epoprostenol (FLOLAN)
- Treprostinil (REMODULIN)
- Latanoprost (XALATAN)[d]

Endothelin-1 Antagonists
- Bosentan (TRACLEER)

[a]also epinastine (ELESTAT), olopatadine (PATANOL)
[b]also zolmitriptan (ZOMIG), rizatriptan (MAXALT), naratriptan (AMERGE), frovatriptan (FROVA), almotriptan (AXERT), eletriptan (RELPAX)
[c]also granisetron (KYTRIL), palonosetron (ALOXI), alosetron (LOTRONEX), dolasetron (ANZEMET)
[d]also bimatoprost (LUMIGAN), travoprost (TRAVATAN)

OVERVIEW

Autacoids (also spelled autocoids), substances produced by neural and non-neural tissues throughout the body, act locally to modulate the activity of smooth muscles, nerves, glands, platelets, and other tissues (Table 26–1). Several autacoids also serve as neurotransmitters in the central nervous system (CNS) or enteric nervous system.

Autacoids regulate certain aspects of **gastrointestinal, uterine, and renal function,** and they are involved in **pain, fever, inflammation, allergic reactions, asthma, thromboembolic disorders,** and **other pathologic conditions.** Drugs that inhibit autacoid synthesis or block autacoid

receptors are helpful in treating these conditions, whereas drugs that activate autacoid receptors are useful for **inducing labor, alleviating migraine headaches, counteracting drug-induced peptic ulcers,** and other purposes.

Autacoids include monoamines (e.g., **histamine** and **serotonin**) as well as fatty acid derivatives (e.g., **prostaglandins** and **leukotrienes**). Autacoids activate specific membrane receptors in target tissues, mostly of the G-protein coupled receptor (GPCR) type. Their effects are usually restricted to the tissue in which they are formed, but under pathologic conditions, extraordinarily large amounts of autacoids can be released into the systemic circulation. These disorders include carcinoid tumor and anaphylactic shock, which cause the release of copious amounts of sero-

TABLE 26-1. Effects of Autocoids

Autacoid	Effects Vascular Smooth Muscle (VSM)	Effects on Nonvascular Smooth Muscle (NVSM)	Other Effects
Histamine	Vasodilation and edema	Contraction of bronchial and other NVSM	Itching; increase in gastric acid secretion
Serotonin	Vasoconstriction in most vascular beds	Contraction of gastrointestinal and other NVSM	Central nervous system neurotransmission; stimulation of platelet aggregation
Eicosanoids			
Leukotrienes	Vasoconstriction or vasodilation	Contraction of bronchial and other NVSM	Inflammatory effects; increase in vascular permeability
Prostaglandin E	Vasodilation	Relaxation of bronchial muscle and contraction of uterine muscle	Inhibition of gastric acid secretion
Prostaglandin F	Vasoconstriction in most vascular beds	Contraction of bronchial and uterine muscle	Increase in aqueous humor outflow
Prostaglandin I	Vasodilation	Contraction	Inhibition of platelet aggregation
Thromboxane A_2	Vasoconstriction	Contraction	Stimulation of platelet aggregation

tonin and histamine, respectively, and exert systemic effects including the CNS. Most autacoids are rapidly metabolized to inactive compounds as seen with prostaglandins, and some autacoids undergo tissue reuptake as evidenced by 5-hydroxytryptamine (5-HT) reuptake transporter proteins in neurons and peripheral cells.

This chapter provides basic information about autacoids and reviews the many types of drugs that influence their effects. Some autacoid drugs are covered completely here, whereas readers are referred to additional chapters for more details on other agents.

HISTAMINE AND RELATED DRUGS

HISTAMINE

Histamine is a biogenic amine produced primarily by mast cells and basophils, which are particularly abundant in the skin, gastrointestinal (GI) tract, and respiratory tract. Histamine is also produced by paracrine cells in the gastric fundus, where it stimulates acid secretion by parietal cells. Histamine also functions as a neurotransmitter in the CNS (see Chapter 18).

Histamine Biosynthesis and Release

Histamine is formed when the amino acid **histidine** is decarboxylated in a reaction catalyzed by the enzyme, L-histidine decarboxylase. Histamine is stored in granules (vesicles) in mast cells and basophils until it is released. It is released from mast cells when membrane-bound **immunoglobulin E (IgE)** interacts with an IgE antigen to cause mast cell degranulation. This process can be blocked by **cromolyn sodium** and related respiratory drugs, as described in Chapter 27. A number of other stimuli can also cause the release of histamine from mast cells (Fig. 26–1). Stimuli that increase cyclic guanosine monophosphate (cGMP) increase histamine release, whereas those that increase cyclic adenosine monophosphate (cAMP) oppose this action.

Mast cell degranulation can also be triggered by bacterial toxins and by drugs such as **morphine** and **tubocurarine.** Some of these stimuli result in the formation of inositol triphosphate (IP_3) and diacylglycerol (DAG). As with neurons, this causes the release of intracellular calcium and the fusion of granule membranes with the plasma membrane, thereby releasing histamine and other compounds. The release of histamine that can occur with morphine administration does not appear to be mediated by opioid receptors because the opioid antagonist, naloxone, does not inhibit morphine-induced histamine release from mast cells.

Histamine is inactivated by methylation and oxidation reactions that are catalyzed by a methyltransferase enzyme and diamine oxidase, respectively.

Histamine Receptors and Effects

Histamine receptors have been classified as H_1, H_2, and H_3. All three types are typical, seven transmembrane GPCR proteins.

H_1 **receptors** are involved in allergic reactions that cause **dermatitis, rhinitis, conjunctivitis,** and **other forms of allergy.** Activation of H_1 receptors in the skin and mucous membranes causes vasodilation, increases vascular permeability, and leads to erythema (heat and redness), congestion, edema, and inflammation. Stimulation of H_1 receptors on mucocutaneous nerve endings can cause pruritus (itching) and in the lungs, initiates the cough reflex. If sufficient histamine is released into the circulation, total peripheral resistance and blood pressure falls and the individual may progress to **anaphylactic shock.** Activation of H_1 receptors also causes bronchoconstriction and contraction of most GI smooth muscles.

H_2 **receptors** are most noted for increasing **gastric acid secretion,** but they are also involved in **allergic reactions.** For this reason, H_2 receptor antagonists are sometimes used in combination with H_1 receptor antagonists in the treatment of allergy. Activation of H_2 receptors in the

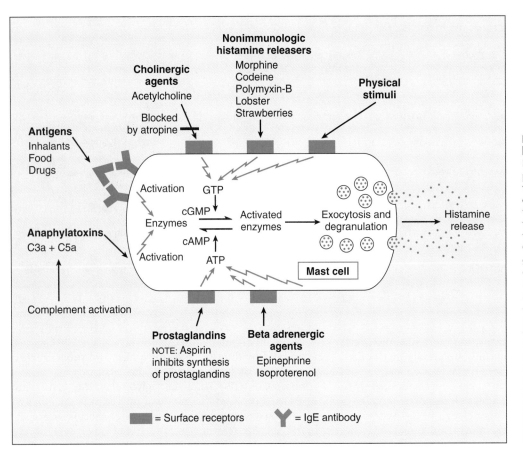

Figure 26–1. Release of histamine from mast cells. Numerous chemical and physical stimuli activate histamine release from mast cells. Complement activation from serum sickness or bacterial endotoxins produces the anaphylactic peptides C3a and C5a, allergic antigens bind to IgE antibodies, and chemicals and other substances increase guanosine triphosphate (GTP) and cyclic guanosine monophosphate (cGMP) to activate enzymes causing increased intracellular calcium and release of histamine granules. β-adrenergic agents and some prostaglandins increase adenosine triphosphate (ATP) and cyclic adenosine monophosphate (cAMP) and reduce activated enzymes.

heart increases the heart rate and contractility, but the cardiac effects of histamine are not prominent under most conditions.

H_3 **receptors** are receptors located in various tissues in the periphery and on nerve terminals. Activation of these presynaptic receptors in the brain inhibits the release of histamine and other neurotransmitters.

ANTIHISTAMINE DRUGS

Antihistamines, or **histamine receptor antagonists,** have been categorized on the basis of their receptor selectivity as H_1 receptor antagonists or H_2 receptor antagonists.

Histamine H_1 Receptor Antagonists

Classification

The following discussion focuses on the properties and uses of four groups of H_1 receptor antagonists. **Chlorpheniramine, clemastine, dimenhydrinate, diphenhydramine, hydroxyzine, meclizine,** and **promethazine** are examples of first-generation drugs. **Astemizole, cetirizine, fexofenadine, loratadine,** and **desloratadine** are examples of second-generation drugs. Drugs in these two groups are administered orally or parenterally. A major difference in the two groups is that the **first-generation antihistamines** are distributed to the CNS and can cause sedation, whereas the **second-generation antihistamines** do not cross the blood–brain barrier significantly. **Azelastine** is an example

of an **intranasal antihistamine,** and **levocabastine, ketotifen, epinastine,** and **olopatadine** are used for **ophthalmic** treatment.

Chemistry, Mechanisms, and Pharmacokinetics

The H_1 antihistamines contain an alkylamine group that resembles the side chain of histamine and permits them to bind to the H_1 receptor and act as competitive receptor antagonists. The drugs can block most of the effects of histamine on vascular smooth muscle and nerves and thereby prevent or counteract allergic reactions.

When antihistamines are administered orally, they are rapidly absorbed and are widely distributed to tissues. Many of them are extensively metabolized in the liver by cytochrome P450 enzymes. Hydroxyzine has an active metabolite that is also available as the drug, cetirizine, and this drug is excreted unchanged in the urine and feces.

Azelastine is a phthalazinone H_1 antihistamine that is marketed as a nasal spray for the treatment of allergic rhinitis. It blocks H_1 receptors and inhibits the release of histamine from mast cells, and it is much more potent than either sodium cromoglycate or theophylline in its inhibiting effect. The systemic bioavailability of azelastine following intranasal administration is about 40%, and the plasma half-life is about 22 hours. Azelastine is metabolized by cytochrome P450 enzymes to desmethylazelastine, a substance whose plasma concentrations are 20% to 30% of azelastine concentrations. Azelastine and its principal

TABLE 26-2. **Pharmacologic Properties of Selected Histamine H1 Receptor Antagonists**

Drug	Duration of Action (Hours)	Sedative Effects	Antiemetic Effects	Anticholinergic Effects
First-generation antihistamines				
Chlorpheniramine	6	Medium	None	Medium
Dimenhydrinate	8	High	Medium	High
Diphenhydramine	8	High	Medium	High
Hydroxyzine	6	High	High	Medium
Meclizine	12	Medium	High	Medium
Promethazine	12	High	High	High
Second-generation antihistamines				
Cetirizine	24	Low	None	Very low
Fexofenadine	12	Very low	None	Very low
Loratadine	24	Very low	None	Very low
Intranasal antihistamines				
Azelastine	12	Low	None	Very low

metabolite both act as antagonists at H_1 receptors. The unchanged drug and its active metabolite are primarily excreted in the feces.

Pharmacologic Effects and Indications

The H_1 antihistamines are all equally effective in treating **allergies,** but they differ markedly in their sedative, antiemetic, and anticholinergic properties (Table 26–2). The second-generation antihistamines cause little or no sedation, so they are often preferred for the treatment of allergies. Antihistamines are usually more effective when administered before exposure to an allergen than afterward. Hence, persons with seasonal allergies, such as allergic rhinitis (see Chapter 27), should take them on a regular basis throughout the period of risk.

First-Generation Antihistamines

Because the first-generation antihistamines have sedative effects, they are occasionally used to produce **sedation.** They are also used to treat **nausea and vomiting,** to prevent **motion sickness** in persons traveling by plane or boat, or to treat **vertigo** (an illusory sense that the environment or one's own body is revolving).

The most sedating drugs are diphenhydramine, hydroxyzine, and promethazine. These drugs have been used to induce sleep or for preoperative sedation. Their sedating properties can also be useful in relieving distress caused by the severe pruritus associated with some allergic reactions. Persons taking these drugs should be cautioned against driving or operating dangerous machinery.

Pheniramine drugs (e.g., chlorpheniramine), which are less sedating than other first-generation drugs, are primarily used in the treatment of allergic reactions to pollen, mold spores, and other environmental allergens.

Meclizine, diphenhydramine, hydroxyzine, and promethazine have higher antiemetic activity than other antihistamines. Meclizine is less sedating than diphenhydramine, hydroxyzine, and promethazine, so it is frequently used to prevent motion sickness or treat vertigo. Dimenhydrinate, which is a mixture of diphenhydramine and 8-chlorotheo-

phylline, is also used for these purposes. Promethazine suppositories are often used to relieve nausea and vomiting associated with various conditions (see Chapter 28).

SECOND-GENERATION ANTIHISTAMINES. The second-generation drugs lack antiemetic activity, so their use is limited to the treatment of **allergies.** None of these drugs causes substantial sedation; however, cetirizine is more likely than astemizole, fexofenadine, or loratadine to cause some sedation. Because fexofenadine has a shorter half-life, it must be taken twice a day, whereas the other second-generation drugs are taken once a day. Fexofenadine and cetirizine are eliminated primarily as the unchanged drug in the feces and urine, respectively. Loratadine and desloratadine are metabolized to active metabolites, which are excreted in the urine and feces.

Intranasal Antihistamines

Azelastine is indicated for the treatment of symptoms of **allergic rhinitis,** including sneezing, nasal itching, and nasal discharge. It is administered as two sprays per nostril twice daily. The drug can cause drowsiness so should be used cautiously when patients are driving or operating dangerous machinery.

Opthalmic Antihistamines

Currently, four antihistamine eyedrop formulations are available. **Levocabastine, epinastine,** and **olopatadine** are selective H_1 antagonists for topical ophthalmic use. They are indicated for the temporary relief of the signs and symptoms of seasonal allergic conjunctivitis. **Ketotifen** is a selective, **noncompetitive** H_1 antagonist and mast cell stabilizer. The action of ketotifen occurs rapidly with an effect seen within minutes after administration and, because of the noncompetitive nature of the receptor antagonism, it has a longer duration of action than the other agents. It is indicated for the temporary prevention of itching of the eye caused by allergic conjunctivitis. All these agents exhibit little to no systemic absorption after administration, so the adverse effects are minor and primarily affect the eyes.

Adverse Effects and Interactions

The H_1 antihistamines produce few serious side effects.

FIRST-GENERATION ANTIHISTAMINES. Sedation is the most common side effect of the first-generation antihistamines. Paradoxically, however, the drugs can produce excitement in infants and children and should be used with caution in these patients.

Diphenhydramine and promethazine have the highest anticholinergic activity (see Table 26–2), but other first-generation drugs also block cholinergic muscarinic receptors. As a result, the drugs can cause dry mouth, blurred vision, tachycardia, urinary retention, and other atropine-like side effects.

Anticholinergic toxicity is the principal manifestation of an overdose of first-generation antihistamines. Administration of physostigmine, a cholinesterase inhibitor that crosses the blood–brain barrier, may be required to counteract the anticholinergic effects of antihistamines in the central nervous system.

SECOND-GENERATION ANTIHISTAMINES. Two of the second-generation drugs, astemizole and terfenadine, may prolong the QT interval on the electrocardiogram and thereby precipitate a cardiac arrhythmia called torsade de pointes. Fexofenadine, is the active metabolite of **terfenadine** (SELEANE). Terfenadine was the first nonsedating H_1 blocker, but was withdrawn from the market by the US Food and Drug Administration (FDA) because it was shown to prolong the QT interval on the electrocardiogram, producing the potential for a type of cardiac arrhythmia called *torsade de pointes*. Fexofenadine does not appear to cause cardiac abnormalities. Cetirizine and loratadine also lack cardiac effects.

INTRANASAL ANTIHISTAMINES. Adverse effects of azelastine are rare and include dizziness, fatigue, headache, nasal irritation, dry mouth, and weight gain.

OPTHALMIC ANTIHISTAMINES. Adverse effects of levocabastine, epinastine, olopatadine and ketotifen are usually limited to the eyes and include transient stinging and burning. These occur in less than 5% of patients.

Histamine H_2 and H_3 Receptor Antagonists

Chapter 28 outlines the properties of H_2 receptor antagonists, which are primarily used to treat **peptic ulcer disease.** There are presently no approved H_3 receptor agents, although clinical trials are underway (see Selected Readings).

SEROTONIN AND RELATED DRUGS

SEROTONIN (5-HT)

Serotonin Biosynthesis and Release

Serotonin, or **5-hydroxytryptamine** (5-HT), is an autacoid and a neurotransmitter that is produced primarily by platelets, enterochromaffin cells in the gut, and neurons. The greatest concentration of serotonin is in the enterochromaf-

fin cells of the GI tract. As illustrated in Fig. 18–3C, serotonin is synthesized from the amino acid **tryptophan** and is converted to **5-hydroxyindoleacetic acid** (5-HIAA) by monoamine oxidase and aldehyde dehydrogenase. 5-HIAA is then excreted in the urine. Serotonin is concentrated in vesicles within the cell and released by calcium-mediated exocytosis.

Serotonin Receptors and Effects

The four main types of **serotonin receptors** are designated as 5-HT_1 through 5-HT_4. The 5-HT_1 and 5-HT_2 receptors have several subtypes that are designated by letters (e.g., 5-HT_{1A} and 5-HT_{1D}). Although most serotonin receptors are G-protein coupled receptors (GPCR), the 5-HT_3 receptor is a ligand-gated cation channel protein. The mechanisms of signal transduction for serotonin receptors are outlined in Table 18–1.

In the peripheral tissues, the physiologic effects of serotonin include platelet aggregation, stimulation of GI motility, and modulation of vascular smooth muscle contraction. Serotonin causes vasoconstriction in most vascular beds and contraction of most smooth muscles. In the CNS, serotonin is involved in the regulation of mood, appetite, sleep, emotional processing, and pain processing (see Chapter 18).

Drugs that affect serotonin activity are classified as serotonin agonists, serotonin antagonists, and serotonin reuptake inhibitors. Examples are mentioned below and discussed in detail in other chapters.

SEROTONIN (5-HT) DRUGS

5-HT Agonists

Serotonin agonists have been developed for use in the management of several specific disorders (Table 26–3). **Buspirone**, a partial agonist that acts at the 5-HT_{1A} receptor, is used to treat **anxiety** and **depression** (see Chapter 19). **Sumatriptan** and related **triptan** compounds, and some

TABLE 26–3.	**Serotonin (5 Hydroxytryptamine, or 5-HT) Receptors and Clinical Uses of Serotonin Agonists and Antagonists**

Drug	5-HT Receptor	Clinical Use
Serotonin agonists		
Buspirone	5-HT_{1A}	Anxiety; depression
Tegaserod	5-HT_4	Irritable bowel syndrome
Sumatriptan	$5\text{-HT}_{1D/1B}$	Migraine headaches
Serotonin antagonists		
Clozapine	5-HT_2	Schizophrenia
Cyproheptadine	5-HT_2	Carcinoid syndrome; pruritus; urticaria
Methysergide	5-HT_2	Carcinoid syndrome; migraine headaches
Ondansetron	5-HT_3	Nausea and vomiting

ergot drugs, are 5-HT$_{1D/1B}$ receptor agonists that are used to treat **migraine headaches** (see Chapter 29).

Cisapride was the first 5-HT$_4$ receptor agonist used for the treatment of **gastroesophageal reflux disease** and **gastrointestinal hypomotility** (see Chapter 28). Activation of 5-HT$_4$ receptors increases the peristaltic action of the GI tract, which is helpful in the above disorders. Cisapride (PROPULSID), however, was pulled from the market in the United States in 2000 after postmarketing surveillance revealed a risk of rare but sometimes fatal prolongation of the QT interval on electrocardiogram records ('long QT syndrome'). A newer 5-HT$_4$ agonist, **tegaserod**, is also a prokinetic agent, but approved for a narrower indication: the short-term treatment of women who have **irritable bowel syndrome (IBS)** with constipation as their main symptom.

5-HT Antagonists

Examples of serotonin antagonists include clozapine, cyproheptadine, methysergide, and ondansetron (see Table 26–3).

Clozapine is an atypical antipsychotic drug that acts partly by blocking 5-HT$_2$ receptors in the CNS. It is used in the treatment of **schizophrenia** (see Chapter 22).

Cyproheptadine is a 5-HT$_2$ receptor antagonist that also has H$_1$ antihistamine activity. This makes it useful in managing **urticaria** (hives) and other allergic reactions in which **pruritus** is a prominent feature. Cyproheptadine is administered orally every 8 to 12 hours and can cause slight to moderate drowsiness.

Methysergide is a 5-HT$_2$ receptor antagonist that is used to prevent **migraine headaches** (see Chapter 29).

Cyproheptadine and **methysergide** are both useful in the care of patients with **carcinoid tumor.** This tumor can produce huge quantities of serotonin, histamine, and other vasoactive substances that cause a constellation of clinical effects called the **carcinoid syndrome.** Affected patients suffer from malabsorption, violent attacks of watery diarrhea and cramping, and paroxysmal vasomotor attacks characterized by sudden red to purple flushing of the face and neck. The malabsorption and diarrhea can be managed by giving cyproheptadine or methysergide in combination with opioid antidiarrheal drugs.

Ondansetron was the first selective 5-HT$_3$ receptor antagonist used as an antiemetic agent in cancer chemotherapy as well as treating nausea and vomiting from other causes. It prevents **nausea and vomiting** by blocking the effects of serotonin in the chemoreceptor trigger zone and in vagal afferent nerves in the GI tract (see Chapter 28). Closely related GI agents sharing the same mechanism of action include **granisetron**, **alosetron**, and **palonosetron**. Granisetron, as with ondansetron, is used to prevent nausea and vomiting caused by cancer chemotherapy and radiation therapy. Alosetron is indicated for treatment of women with IBS whose predominant bowel symptom is diarrhea and who are not constipated. Palonosetron is an injectable-only formulation for the prevention of acute or delayed nausea and vomiting associated with initial and repeat courses of moderately and highly emetogenic cancer chemotherapy.

Serotonin Reuptake Inhibitors

Serotonin reuptake inhibitors are used in the treatment of **depression** and **other central nervous system disorders** (see Chapter 22).

EICOSANOIDS AND RELATED DRUGS

EICOSANOIDS

Eicosanoids are autacoids derived from arachidonic acid (eicosatetraenoic acid) and other 20-carbon fatty acids (*eicos-* is Greek for "twenty").

Eicosanoid Biosynthesis and Release

Eicosanoids are made from arachidonic acid and other 20-carbon, polyunsaturated fatty acids in the cell membrane. They are freed from their esteric attachment to membrane phospholipids by **phospholipase A$_2$**, an enzyme that is activated by numerous chemical stimuli and by physical stimuli such as cell damage. The two main groups of eicosanoids are the **prostaglandins** and the **leukotrienes**, whose formation begins with reactions catalyzed by **cyclooxygenase (COX)** and **5-lipoxygenase**, respectively. As shown in Fig. 26–2, subsequent reactions convert the products of these reactions to specific prostaglandins and leukotrienes.

Each prostaglandin (PG) and each leukotriene is assigned a letter and subscript number (e.g., PGE$_2$). The letter refers to the specific ring structure of the substance, and the subscript number indicates the number of double bonds in the fatty acid chains.

Eicosanoid end products made in individuals consuming a typical Western diet come primarily from arachidonic acid, containing four carbon double bonds. Because the first double bond is located at the sixth carbon, arachidonic acid is known as an **omega-6 fatty acid.** In diets rich in cold-water fish or plants, cell membranes contain an **omega-3 fatty acid**, eicosapentaenoic acid (EPA), with five double bonds starting at the third carbon position. EPA is also a precursor to eicosanoid products and these products have different biological activities than eicosanoids generated from arachidonic acid. For example, prostaglandins derived from omega-6 fatty acids have different vasoactive and platelet-aggregating properties than do prostaglandins derived from omega-3 fatty acids.

After synthesis, eicosanoids are released from the cell to exert local effects on surrounding tissues. Unlike other autacoids, no evidence exists of vesicular storage or calcium-mediated exocytosis for eicosanoid substances within the cell. Because no storage of eicosanoids occurs within the cell, the synthesis of eicosanoids coincides with its release though the cell membrane and into the surrounding tissue.

Eicosanoid Receptors and Effects

All of the naturally released eicosanoids are short-lived and locally acting. Eicosanoid drugs exist as either purified preparations of the same naturally occurring substance or

Figure 26–2. Synthesis of eicosanoids. When phospholipase A_2 is activated by an injury or other stimuli, it catalyzes the hydrolysis of arachidonic acid and other 20-carbon fatty acids from cell membrane phospholipids. Arachidonic acid is converted to prostaglandins and leukotrienes by cyclooxygenase and 5-lipoxygenase, respectively. Other enzymes complete the synthesis of specific eicosanoids. 5-HPETE = 5-hydroperoxyeicosatetraenoic acid.

closely related synthetic analogs. Prostaglandins exert their effects on smooth muscle, platelet aggregation, neurotransmission, glandular secretion, and other biologic activities by activating specific receptors in target tissues. These receptors are GPCR proteins classified by the PG that binds with the highest affinity and selectivity. Accordingly, the prostaglandin receptor for PGD_2 is DP, the receptor for PGE_2 is EP, and so forth for the FP, IP, and TP (thromboxane) receptors. To date, four subtypes of EP receptors have been identified, designated EP_1 through EP_4. **Thromboxanes,** which are substances derived from PG (see Fig. 26–2), also act on smooth muscle and platelet aggregation. Different types of thromboxanes and PG have different physiologic effects, and often are opposite. The particular type of eicosanoid released from a tissue or cell will depend on the particular set of synthetic enzymes contained within the cell.

While **platelet aggregation** is stimulated by thromboxane A_2 (TXA_2), it is inhibited by PGI_2. Prostacyclin is released primarily from vascular endothelial cells and serves to prevent platelet aggregation under normal conditions. In contrast, TXA_2 is produced and released only when a blood vessel is injured, at which time the adherence of platelets to vascular endothelium activates the platelets and leads to the synthesis and release of TXA_2 (see Chapter 16 and Fig. 16–5).

In some cases, the fatty acid precursor of a prostaglandin or thromboxane has a major impact on its biologic activity. For example, thromboxane A_3 (TXA_3), which is synthesized from eicosapentaenoic acid (EPA), an omega-3 fatty acid found in fish oils, produces relatively little platelet aggregation or vasoconstriction in comparison with TXA_2. This difference can largely explain the correlation between increased fish oil consumption and a decreased incidence of thrombotic events (strokes and heart attacks) in certain native populations.

PGE_2 and PGI_2 both cause **vasodilation** in several vascular beds. These PG appear to play a role in maintaining **pulmonary blood flow,** and they also serve to maintain the **patency of the ductus arteriosus** until it is time for its closure. In the kidneys, PGE_2 and PGI_2 produce vasodilation and have important roles in modulating **renal blood flow** and **glomerular filtration.** These actions are particularly important in persons with renal insufficiency and in the elderly. The renal actions of PG also appear to exert an **antihypertensive effect,** partly by increasing water and sodium excretion. Because nonsteroidal anti-inflammatory drugs (NSAID) inhibit PG synthesis, their use can cause or exacerbate renal disorders and may counteract the antihypertensive effect of antihypertensive medications taken concurrently.

Many prostaglandins, including PGE_2 and prostaglandin $F_{2\alpha}$ ($PGF_{2\alpha}$), stimulate **uterine contractions** and increase **gastrointestinal motility.** Their uterine activity is the basis for several therapeutic applications, whereas their gastrointestinal actions can lead to adverse effects (e.g., diarrhea and intestinal cramping). Several PG also produce a **cytoprotective effect on the gastrointestinal mucosa.**

The **leukotrienes** are produced primarily in inflammatory cells, including mast cells, basophils, eosinophils, macrophages, and polymorphonuclear leukocytes. Leukotrienes C_4 and D_4 (LTC_4 and LTD_4) are the main components of the **slow-reacting substance of anaphylaxis (SRS-A).** These two leukotrienes are secreted in the presence

TABLE 26–4. **Effects and Clinical Uses of Selected Prostaglandin (PG) Drugs**

Drug	PG Class	Effect	Clinical Use
Alprostadil	PGE_1	Vasodilation	Erectile dysfunction; patency of the ductus arteriosus
Carboprost tromethamine	$PGF_{2\alpha}$ analogue	Contraction of uterine muscle	Abortifacient; postpartum bleeding
Dinoprostone	PGE_2	Contraction of uterine muscle	Abortifacient; cervical ripening
Epoprostenol	PGI_2	Vasodilation	Pulmonary hypertension
Latanoprost	$PGF_{2\alpha}$ analogue	Increase in aqueous humor outflow	Glaucoma
Misoprostol	PGE_1 analogue	Gastric cytoprotection	Gastric and duodenal ulcers induced by use of nonsteroidal anti-inflammatory drugs (NSAIDs)

of asthma and anaphylaxis and play a major role in bronchospastic disease.

EICOSANOID DRUGS

The effects and clinical uses of prostaglandin drugs are outlined in Table 26–4, and summarized below.

Eicosanoid Synthesis Inhibitors

Among the groups of drugs that inhibit eicosanoid synthesis are **leukotriene inhibitors** (see Chapter 27), **NSAID** (see Chapter 30), and **corticosteroids** (see Chapter 33).

Leukotriene inhibitors act either by inhibiting 5-lipoxygenase or by blocking leukotriene receptors. They are currently used in the management of **asthma,** but other therapeutic applications are being explored.

The NSAID act by inhibiting cyclooxygenase and are primarily used to alleviate **pain** and **inflammation.**

Corticosteroids block the formation of all eicosanoids, partly by inhibiting phospholipase A_2. They have **anti-inflammatory, antiallergic, and antineoplastic effects** and are used in the treatment of a wide variety of adrenal diseases and nonadrenal disorders.

Prostaglandin Drugs

Prostaglandin E₁ and Prostaglandin E₁ Derivatives

Alprostadil is identical to naturally occurring PGE_1 and is available in several formulations for specific clinical uses.

Alprostadil is given by continuous intravenous infusion to maintain the **patency of the ductus arteriosus** in neonates who are awaiting surgery for some types of congenital heart diseases. These include cyanotic heart defects (pulmonary atresia or stenosis, tricuspid atresia, tetralogy of Fallot, and transposition of the great vessels) and acyanotic heart defects (coarctation of the aorta and hypoplastic left ventricle).

Alprostadil is available in injectable, pellet, and cream formulations to treat **erectile dysfunction** in men. For this purpose, the drug is injected into the cavernosa of the penis or slow-release pellets or drops of cream are inserted into the meatus of the urethra. Adverse effects in men treated with

alprostadil include penile pain, penile fibrosis, priapism (persistent erection), flushing, diarrhea, headache, and fever.

Misoprostol is a synthetic PGE_1 analogue available in an orally administered formulation for the prevention of NSAID-induced **gastric ulcers** and **duodenal ulcers** (see Chapter 28). Misoprostol treatment is particularly useful in patients who take NSAID on a long-term basis to alleviate the symptoms of arthritis and other inflammatory conditions. Misoprostol acts locally on the GI mucosa to exert a cytoprotective effect by inhibiting gastric acid secretion and by increasing bicarbonate secretion from mucosal cells. Diarrhea, one of the most common adverse effects of misoprostol use, can be minimized by starting patients on a low dose of the drug and then gradually increasing the dose. In pregnant women, misoprostol is absolutely contraindicated because it can stimulate uterine contractions and cause premature labor.

Misoprostol is also approved for use as an abortifacient in combination with the progesterone receptor antagonist, **mifepristone** (RU86, MIFEREX). When used in combination, mifepristone and misoprostol are 95% to 97% effective within the first 2 weeks of pregnancy.

Prostaglandin E₂ and Prostaglandin F₂α Derivatives

Dinoprostone and **carboprost tromethamine** are prostaglandin drugs that have oxytocic activity and increase the uterine contractions of pregnant women. Dinoprostone is a formulation of naturally occurring PGE_2, whereas carboprost is a synthetic derivative of $PGF_{2\alpha}$.

Dinoprostone is available as a vaginal insert, gel, or suppository. In pregnant women, the vaginal insert or gel is applied to the vagina or cervix to produce **cervical ripening** before labor induction. The insert may provide more accurate dosing than the gel. The suppository is used to **evacuate the uterine contents** in cases of intrauterine fetal death, benign hydatidiform mole, or second-trimester termination of pregnancy.

Carboprost is administered intramuscularly to **control postpartum bleeding** when other measures have failed and to **terminate pregnancy (abortifacient).** It can cause flushing, diarrhea, vomiting, altered blood pressure, blurred vision, respiratory distress, and other adverse reactions.

Latanoprost was the first prostaglandin drug indicated for the treatment of **glaucoma.** It is administered topically as eye drops and is used to treat open-angle glaucoma that is resistant to other pharmacologic treatments. Latanoprost is a $PGF_{2\alpha}$ analogue that acts on FP receptors to increase aqueous humor outflow via the uveoscleral pathway (see Box 6–1). It can alter the color of the iris and cause a permanent eye color change by increasing the amount of melanin in melanocytes. Other synthetic FP receptor agonists developed for the reduction of intraocular pressure in patients with open-angle glaucoma or ocular hypertension are **bimatoprost** and **travoprost.**

Prostaglandin I₂ and Prostaglandin I₂ Derivatives

Epoprostenol is a formulation of naturally occurring PGI_2 (prostacyclin) that is used to treat **pulmonary arterial hypertension (PAH).** Epoprostenol acts on IP receptors to dilate pulmonary blood vessels and increase pulmonary blood flow, thereby counteracting the pathophysiologic consequences of pulmonary hypertension. The drug is administered by continuous intravenous infusion, and the dosage is titrated on the basis of clinical improvement and adverse effects. The most common adverse reactions include flushing, tachycardia, hypotension, diarrhea, nausea, vomiting, and flulike symptoms.

Treprostinil is a stable analogue of prostacyclin which has a half-life of between 2 and 4 hours and can be safely administered by a continuous subcutaneous infusion, via a self-inserted subcutaneous catheter using a micro infusion pump designed specifically for subcutaneous drug delivery. It is approved to diminish the symptoms (e.g., shortness of breath) associated with physical activity in PAH patients.

ENDOTHELIN DRUGS

ENDOTHELIN-1 ANTAGONISTS

Endothelin-1 (ET-1) is a peptide autacoid produced by vascular endothelial cells. It activates ET_A and ET_B receptors in vascular smooth muscle and other tissues. ET-1 may serve physiologically to counteract the vasodilative response to nitric oxide, but elevated levels of ET-1 appear to have a pathophysiologic role in **pulmonary arterial hypertension.** ET-1 also appears to contribute to cardiac dysfunction during coronary reperfusion following thrombolysis in persons with acute myocardial infarction.

Bosentan (TRACLEER) is a dual ET_A and ET_B receptor antagonist that is approved for treating PAH. Clinical trials have shown that bosentan significantly improves 6-minute walking distance in persons with class III or IV PAH, while decreasing pulmonary vascular resistance and dyspnea.

Bosentan is administered orally and is generally well tolerated, but 11% of patients experienced elevated serum aminotransferase levels. For this reason, **liver function tests** should be monitored at baseline and then monthly in persons taking bosentan. Based on animal studies, bosentan is very likely to cause major **birth defects** if used by pregnant women and it is contraindicated in pregnancy and in women of childbearing age who are not using hormonal contraceptives.

SUMMARY OF IMPORTANT POINTS

■ Autacoids include histamine, serotonin, prostaglandins, and leukotrienes. These substances usually act on the same tissue in which they are produced.

■ Histamine is the primary mediator of allergic reactions. Stimulation of H_1 receptors causes vasodilation, edema, congestion, and pruritus. Stimulation of H_2 receptors mediates gastric acid secretion.

■ The first-generation H_1 receptor antagonists (chlorpheniramine, diphenhydramine, meclizine, promethazine, and others) produce varying degrees of sedation and also have anticholinergic side effects. The second-generation drugs (cetirizine, loratadine, fexofenadine, and desloratadine) are largely devoid of central nervous system effects.

■ The H_1 receptor antagonists are primarily used to treat allergies, but meclizine is used to prevent motion sickness and promethazine is used to treat nausea and vomiting.

■ Fexofenadine is the active metabolite of the now-banned terfenadine. Unlike terfenadine, fexofenadine does not prolong the QT interval and cause *torsade de pointes.* Cetirizine, desloratadine, and loratadine also lack cardiac effects.

■ Drugs that affect serotonin (5-hydroxytryptamine, or 5-HT) are classified as serotonin agonists, serotonin antagonists, and serotonin reuptake inhibitors.

■ Some $5\text{-}HT_1$ receptor agonists (e.g., sumatriptan) can be used to treat migraine headaches, whereas some $5\text{-}HT_2$ receptor antagonists (e.g., methysergide) can be used to prevent migraine headaches.

■ Cyproheptadine and methysergide, both of which are $5\text{-}HT_2$ receptor antagonists, are used in the management of carcinoid syndrome, which is caused by excessive production of serotonin and other vasoactive substances in patients with carcinoid tumors from enterochromaffin tissue.

■ Tegaserod is a $5\text{-}HT_4$ receptor agonist used to increase gastrointestinal motility, and ondansetron (among others) is a $5\text{-}HT_3$ receptor antagonist that is used in the treatment of nausea and vomiting.

■ Eicosanoids are derived from arachidonic acid and other precursor 20-carbon fatty acids. The two main groups of eicosanoids are prostaglandins and leukotrienes. The ratio of omega-6 and omega-3 fatty acids in the diet plays an important role in the activity of eicosanoid end products.

■ Alprostadil is PGE_1 and misoprostol is a PGE_1 derivative. Alprostadil is used to maintain patency of the ductus arteriosus in neonates awaiting surgery for heart defects. It is also used to treat erectile dysfunction in men. Misoprostol is used to prevent gastric and duodenal ulcers in persons taking nonsteroidal anti-inflammatory drugs (NSAID).

■ Dinoprostone, the same as PGE_2, is used for cervical ripening before induction of labor and for evacuation of the uterine contents.

■ Carboprost and latanoprost are prostaglandin $F_{2\alpha}$ ($PGF_{2\alpha}$) derivatives. Carboprost is used to control post-partum bleeding and to terminate pregnancy. Latanoprost and other PG antiglaucoma drugs that increase the aqueous humor outflow are used to treat glaucoma.

■ Epoprostenol is PGI_2 (prostacyclin) and treprostinil is a PGI_2 derivative; both are used to treat pulmonary arterial hypertension (PAH). Additionally, bosentan, an endothelin-1 receptor antagonist, is indicated for PAH.

Review Questions

1. Which of the following antihistamines would be best used to treat mild nausea and vomiting due to motion sickness?
   (A) cetirizine
   (B) fexofenadine
   (C) loratadine
   (D) diphenhydramine
   (E) meclizine

2. Which of the following describes the major difference between a first- and second-generation antihistamine?
   (A) selectivity at H_1 receptors
   (B) ability to cross the blood–brain barrier
   (C) effectiveness in treating allergies
   (D) potency at blocking H_1 receptors
   (E) indications for use

3. Of the major serotonin (5-HT) receptors identified and used as targets for therapeutic agents, which one is the only one considered a ligand-gated ion channel?
   (A) 5-HT_{1B}
   (B) 5-HT_{1D}
   (C) 5-HT_2
   (D) 5-HT_3
   (E) 5-HT_4

4. Which of the following drugs is the same as PGI_2 (prostacyclin) and is used for the treatment of pulmonary hypertension?
   (A) misoprostol
   (B) alprostadil
   (C) epoprostenol
   (D) treprostinil
   (E) travoprost

5. Latanoprost is an agonist at the PGF_2 receptors and is effective for the treatment of?
   (A) cornea abrasions
   (B) ocular hypertension and open-angle glaucoma
   (C) ocular albinism
   (D) closed-angle glaucoma
   (E) allergic conjunctivitis

Answers and Explanations

1. The correct answer is E: meclizine. Meclizine is a first-generation antihistamine with higher antiemetic activity than other agents and also less sedating. Answers (A) through (C) are second-generation antihistamines and gain little access to the CNS and thus are nonsedating and ideal for treating allergies, but would be little help for motion sickness. Answer (D), diphenhydramine, does have antiemetic effects but is more sedating than meclizine and thus not the ideal treatment agent. Dimenhydrinate, which is a mixture of diphenhydramine and 8-chlorotheophylline, is used for motion sickness, however.

2. The correct answer is B: ability to cross the blood–brain barrier. The major problem with treatment of allergies with the first-generation antihistamines is the adverse effects of sedation. Answer (A), selectivity at H_1 receptors, may be the case for select first-generation vs. second-generation agents, but is not the major difference between the classes. Answer (C), effectiveness in treating allergies, is not correct because both can effectively treat the symptoms of allergies but second-generation agents can do so without significant sedation. Answer (D), potency at blocking H_1 receptors, is another measure of antagonist affinity and is not correct for the same reasons as (A) above. Answer (E), indications for use, is not correct because both types of agents are used for allergies.

3. The correct answer is D: 5-HT_3 receptors. This type of receptor for serotonin is famous as the only biogenic amine receptor that is ionotropic. The other answers (A) through (C), and (E) are all types of metabotropic receptors, also known as G-protein coupled receptors.

4. The correct answer is C: epoprostenol. Epoprostenol is the same substance as PGI_2 (prostacyclin) and is used for the treatment of pulmonary hypertension. Answer (A) misoprostol, is a synthetic PGE_1 analogue that is available in an orally administered formulation for the prevention of NSAID-induced gastric ulcers and duodenal ulcers. Answer (B), alprostadil, is a naturally occurring prostaglandin but is known as PGE_1. Answer (D), teprostinil, is also used for pulmonary hypertension but is a is a stable analogue of prostacyclin, not the same as prostacyclin itself. Answer (E), travoprost, is a $PGF_{2\alpha}$ analogue and an agonist at FP receptors. It is used for the treatment of open-angle glaucoma.

5. The correct answer is B: ocular hypertensions and open-angle glaucoma. Latanoprost, as well as bimatoprost and travoprost are agonists at the $PGF_{2\alpha}$ receptors and among the most prescribed class of antiglaucoma agents. Answer (A), cornea abrasions, might call for the use of an ocular antihistamine. Answer (C), ocular albinism, might make sense considering the bizarre adverse effect of latanoprost in darkening the color of the iris but is not an FDA-approved indication for latanoprost. Answer (D), closed-angle glaucoma, is usually treated by carbonic anhydrase inhibitors (e.g., acetazolamide) because the pressure rises very high inside the eye and needs to be dropped rapidly. Answer (E), allergic conjunctivitis, is best treated by one of the ocular antihistamines.

SELECTED READINGS

Ahlman, H., O. Nilsson, and M. Olausson. Interventional treatment of the carcinoid syndrome. Neuroendocrinology 80(Suppl 1):67–73, 2004.

Hata, A. N., and R. M. Breyer RM. Pharmacology and signaling of prostaglandin receptors: multiple roles in inflammation and immune modulation. Pharmacol Ther 103(2):147–166, 2004.

Mori, T. A., and L. J. Beilin. Omega-3 fatty acids and inflammation. Curr Atheroscler Rep 6(6):461–467, 2004.

Simmons, D. L., R. M. Botting, and T. Hla. Cyclooxygenase isozymes: the biology of prostaglandin synthesis and inhibition. Pharmacol Rev 56(3): 387–437, 2004.

Simons, F. E. Advances in H_1-antihistamines. N Engl J Med 351(21): 2203–2217, 2004.

Witkin, J. M., and D. L. Nelson. Selective histamine H_3 receptor antagonists for treatment of cognitive deficiencies and other disorders of the central nervous system. Pharmacol Ther 103(1):1–20, 2004.

CHAPTER 27

Drugs for Respiratory Tract Disorders

CLASSIFICATION OF DRUGS FOR RESPIRATORY TRACT DISORDERS

Anti-inflammatory Drugs
Glucocorticoids
- Fluticasone (FLOVENT, FLONASE)[a]
- Prednisone[b]

Mast Cell Stabilizers
- Cromolyn sodium[c]

Leukotriene Inhibitors
- Montelukast (SINGULAIR)[d]

Bronchodilators
Selective β2-Adrenergic Receptor Agonists
- Albuterol (PROVENTIL, VENTOLIN)[e]
- Salmeterol (SEREVENT)
- Formoterol (OXEZE)

Other Bronchodilators
- Ipratropium (ATROVENT)
- Tiotropium (SPIRIVA)
- Theophylline

Immunoglobulin Antagonist
- Omalizumab (XOLAIR)

Antitussives
- Codeine
- Dextromethorphan
- Hydrocodone

Expectorants
- Guaifenesin

Antihistamines
- Fexofenadine (ALLEGRA)[f]
- Diphenhydramine (BENADRYL)

[a]budesonide (PULMICORT, RHINOCORT), beclomethasone, triamcinolone.
[b]also prednisolone, methylprednisolone.
[c]also lodoxamide, nedocromil.
[d]also zafirlukast, zileuton.
[e]also levalbuterol, pirbuterol, terbutaline, fenoterol.
[f]also loratadine (CLARITIN), cetirizine (ZYRTEC).

OVERVIEW

Disorders of the respiratory tract include a wide range of conditions that can be divided into pulmonary disorders and upper respiratory tract disorders. Pulmonary disorders include asthma, chronic obstructive pulmonary disease (COPD), pneumonia, pulmonary fibrosis, and various other conditions. Upper respiratory tract disorders include allergic rhinitis and microbial infections of the nose, sinuses, and throat. This chapter is primarily concerned with the drugs used in the treatment of asthma and rhinitis. The therapy of both of these conditions rests on a foundation of environmental control and preventive anti-inflammatory medication, with other drugs being used chiefly to treat acute exacerbations. Some of the medications used to treat asthma and rhinitis are also used to treat chronic obstructive pul-

monary disease. Drugs used to treat cough and congestion are also discussed in this chapter.

Asthma

Asthma is characterized by airway inflammation and hyperresponsiveness to stimuli that produce bronchoconstriction. These stimuli include **cold air, exercise,** a wide variety of **allergens,** and **emotional stress.**

Exposure to a stimulus triggers the release of various mediators from mast cells, eosinophils, basophils, neutrophils, macrophages, and other cells. Preformed mediators stored in cell granules and include **histamine, adenosine, bradykinin,** and **major basic protein,** whereas lipid mediators are formed from arachidonic acid and include **leukotrienes** and **prostaglandins.** The release of these

299

agents causes inflammation of the airway, edema and desquamation of the bronchial epithelium, and hypertrophy of smooth muscles in the respiratory tract. It also increases the responsiveness of smooth muscles and the permeability of bronchioles to allergens, infectious agents, mediators of inflammation, and other irritants. Increased mucus production then leads to mucus plugging and decreases the ability of the airways to remove these irritants. As a result, patients suffer from airway obstruction and must use accessory muscles to breathe.

Airway obstruction results from a combination of bronchial inflammation, smooth muscle constriction, and obstruction of the lumen with mucus, inflammatory cells, and epithelial debris. Symptoms of obstruction include dyspnea (difficulty in breathing), coughing, wheezing,

headache, tachycardia, syncope, diaphoresis, pallor, and cyanosis. Patients experience a **biphasic reduction in pulmonary function,** with an **early phase** that occurs within 10 to 30 minutes of exposure to an allergen and lasts for 2 to 3 hours and then a **later phase** that occurs 2 to 8 hours after exposure. The late phase is believed to be responsible for inducing and maintaining bronchial hyperreactivity in asthmatic patients. Because of the circadian variation in bronchial responsiveness, some patients have up to an eightfold increase in airway hyperresponsiveness at night, and nearly 70% of asthma-related deaths occur at night.

The drugs used to treat asthma include anti-inflammatory drugs and bronchodilators. The pathophysiology of asthma and sites of anti-inflammatory drug action are shown in Fig. 27–1.

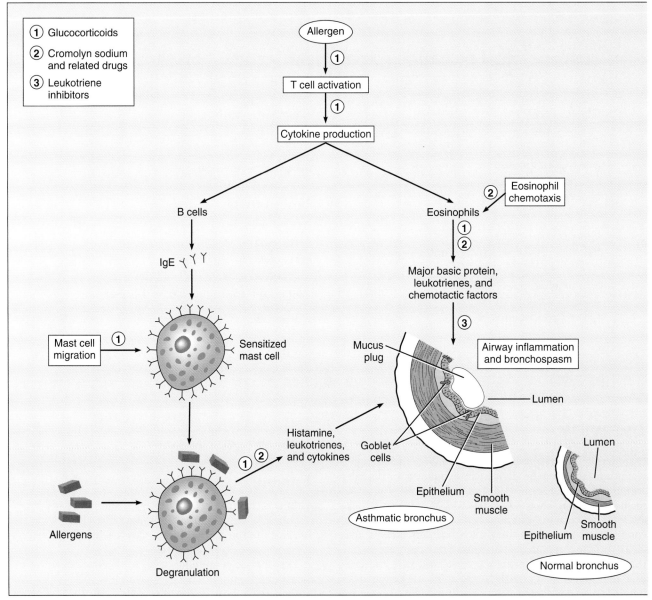

Figure 27-1. Pathophysiology of asthma and sites of anti-inflammatory drug action. When allergens activate T cells, cytokine production is stimulated. The cytokines, in turn, trigger the recruitment, activation, and release of a variety of cells and mediators. Glucocorticoids inhibit numerous steps in this process, including T-cell activation, cytokine production, eosinophil recruitment and activation, and mast cell migration. Glucocorticoids, cromolyn sodium, and other cromolyn-related drugs all inhibit the release of mediators from mast cells and eosinophils. Cromolyn and related drugs also inhibit eosinophil chemotaxis induced by cytokines and other mediators. Leukotriene inhibitors either block leukotriene receptors or inhibit leukotriene synthesis. IgE = immunoglobulin E.

Rhinitis

Rhinitis is most frequently caused by allergic reactions to **pollens, mold spores, dust mites,** and **other environmental allergens** or by infections with **viruses,** such as rhinoviruses and other agents of the common cold.

Allergic rhinitis can be seasonal or nonseasonal (perennial), whereas **viral rhinitis** is an acute, self-limiting condition. Both types of rhinitis are characterized by sneezing, nasal congestion, and rhinorrhea. Nasal pruritus and conjunctivitis are more commonly associated with allergic rhinitis than with viral rhinitis. Malaise, pain, and general discomfort are generally associated with viral rhinitis.

Table 27–1 shows the relative efficacy of various types of respiratory tract drugs, including those used in the treatment of allergic rhinitis and viral rhinitis.

Chronic Obstructive Pulmonary Diseases

Chronic obstructive pulmonary diseases include **chronic bronchitis** and **emphysema.** Chronic bronchitis is characterized by a productive cough associated with inflammation of the bronchioles, whereas emphysema is caused by permanent destruction and enlargement of the airspaces distal to the bronchioles. Both conditions result in airway obstruction, dyspnea (difficult breathing), decreased blood oxygen concentrations, and elevated blood carbon dioxide concentrations. Patients with these conditions have abnormal pulmonary function test values, such as a decreased forced expiratory volume in 1 second (FEV_1). Smoking and advanced age are the primary risk factors for COPD, and smoking cessation can slow disease progression. Although most of the airway obstruction in COPD is irreversible, a portion of the obstruction is caused by smooth muscle spasm and bronchiolar inflammation, and this portion can be reversed by bronchodilator drugs. Patients with COPD often require long-term oxygen therapy, and antibiotics can be used to treat acute exacerbations caused by bacterial infections.

ANTI-INFLAMMATORY DRUGS

Glucocorticoids

Glucocorticoids (corticosteroids), which are effective in the treatment of a wide variety of diseases, are available for oral, parenteral, topical, and inhalational administration. The discussion here focuses on the use of glucocorticoids for **asthma** and **allergic rhinitis.** Chapter 33 provides a detailed description of drug properties and discusses other indications for glucocorticoid use.

The recognition that asthma is primarily an inflammatory disease has increased the role of glucocorticoids in asthma therapy. For persons with moderate to severe asthma, glucocorticoids have become the cornerstone of therapy, and some patients with mild asthma may derive significant benefit from their use as well. Although glucocorticoids are the most efficacious anti-inflammatory drugs available for the treatment of both asthma and allergic rhinitis (see Table 27–1), they have the potential to cause the greatest number of adverse effects. The incidence of adverse effects is markedly reduced when these drugs are given by inhalation, so this route of administration is used under most circumstances. Other routes are reserved for the treatment of chronic severe asthma or acute exacerbations of asthma.

Among the glucocorticoids available as metered-dose inhalers are **beclomethasone, budesonide, fluticasone,** and **triamcinolone.** Beclomethasone and triamcinolone are usually administered three or four times a day, whereas fluticasone and budesonide need to be administered only twice a day. The proper use of metered-dose inhalers requires considerable skill and the utilization of a spacer device between the mouth and the inhaler. The spacer decreases the amount of drug that is deposited in the mouth and upper airway and facilitates the delivery of the drug to the bronchioles.

As with other anti-inflammatory drugs, glucocorticoids are primarily used on a long-term basis to prevent asthmatic attacks, rather than to treat acute bronchospasm. The maximal response to glucocorticoids usually requires up to 8 weeks to develop. Glucocorticoids can reduce the number

TABLE 27–1. **Relative Efficacy of Anti-inflammatory Drugs, Bronchodilators, and Miscellaneous Agents in the Management of Respiratory Tract Disorders***

Drug	Asthma	COPD	Allergic Rhinitis	Viral Rhinitis
Anti-inflammatory drugs				
Glucocorticoids	++++	0 to ++	++++	0
Mast cell stabilizers	+++	0 to ++	+++	0
Leukotriene inhibitors	+++	0 to+	Unknown	0
Bronchodilators				
Selective β_2-adrenergic receptor agonists	++++	++	0	0
Other bronchodilators				
– Ipratropium	+	+++	++	++
– Theophylline	++ to +++	++ to +++	0	0
Miscellaneous agents				
Analgesics	0	0	0	+++
Antihistamines	0 to ++	0	++++	+
Decongestants	0 to ++	0 to ++	+++	+++

*COPD = chronic obstructive pulmonary disease (e.g. emphysema). Ratings range from 0 (not efficacious) to ++++ (highly efficacious).

and severity of symptoms and decrease the need for β_2-adrenergic receptor agonists and other bronchodilators.

Adverse effects associated with inhaled glucocorticoids are usually mild. Excessive deposition of the drugs in the mouth and upper airway can lead to oral candidiasis (thrush). Also, concern exists about the potential for glucocorticoids to suppress growth in children. This problem is difficult to evaluate because asthmatic children may have growth disturbances related to their disease. A meta-analysis of 21 studies, however, concluded that inhaled beclomethasone does not cause growth impairment. Another study showed that 95% of children who received inhaled budesonide for an average of 9 years reached their target adult height despite initial growth retardation (Agertoft and Pedersen, 2000).

Mast Cell Stabilizers

Cromolyn Sodium

CHEMISTRY AND MECHANISMS. Cromolyn sodium and related drugs are nonsteroidal compounds that stabilize the plasma membranes of mast cells and eosinophils and thereby prevent degranulation and release of histamine, leukotrienes, and other mediators of allergic reactions that lead to airway inflammation (see Fig. 27–1). For this reason, these drugs are often called mast cell stabilizers. Inhibition of mediator release by cromolyn compounds is thought to result from blockade of calcium influx into mast cells. Cromolyn and related drugs do not interfere with the binding of immunoglobulin E (IgE) to mast cells or with the binding of antigen to IgE. The drug is not a bronchodilator, and its beneficial effects in asthma and other conditions are largely prophylactic.

PHARMACOKINETICS. Cromolyn and other mast cell stabilizers are rather insoluble in body fluids, and minimal systemic absorption occurs following their oral administration or inhalation. The oral bioavailability of cromolyn is about 1%. When the drug is administered by inhalation, its major effect is exerted on the respiratory tract and very little is absorbed into the circulation. Most of the drug is swallowed following inhalation, and about 98% of it is excreted in the feces.

INDICATIONS. Cromolyn is administered by inhalation to treat **asthma** or **allergic rhinitis** and is available in an ophthalmic solution to treat **vernal (seasonal) conjunctivitis.** Cromolyn and related compounds are primarily used for the long-term prophylaxis of asthmatic bronchoconstriction and allergic reactions, and they have no role in the treatment of acute bronchospasm. For perennial asthma, the drug is usually given several times a day at regular intervals until symptoms resolve. Improvement can require several weeks, and then the dosage can be reduced to the lowest effective level. For exercise-induced asthma, cromolyn is inhaled not more than 1 hour before the anticipated exercise or other precipitating factor. For allergic rhinitis or vernal conjunctivitis, cromolyn is administered several times a day at regular intervals.

Cromolyn is administered orally before meals and at bedtime to treat **systemic mastocytosis,** a rare condition characterized by infiltration of the liver, spleen, lymph nodes, and gastrointestinal tract with mast cells. A similar dosage schedule has been used to treat **ulcerative colitis** and **food allergy.**

ADVERSE EFFECTS AND INTERACTIONS. Cromolyn and other mast cell stabilizers are remarkably nontoxic, partly because of their low solubility and systemic absorption. In some patients, however, cromolyn inhalation can irritate the throat and cause cough and bronchospasm. Administration of a β_2-adrenergic receptor agonist can prevent or relieve this reaction. Nasal and ocular preparations can cause localized pain and irritation, but these effects are usually mild and transient. Cromolyn does not interact significantly with other drugs.

Lodoxamide and Nedocromil

Lodoxamide is formulated as an ophthalmic solution to treat ocular allergies, including **vernal keratitis** and **vernal conjunctivitis.** As with other mast cell stabilizers, lodoxamide appears to prevent calcium influx into mast cells and mast cell degranulation. It can cause ocular discomfort but is generally well tolerated.

Nedocromil has properties that are similar to those of cromolyn. Nedocromil, however, is only available as an aerosol for the prevention of bronchoconstriction in patients with **asthma.** It is initially administered as two inhalations four times a day at regular intervals, but the frequency of doses can be reduced to two or three times a day in persons whose asthma is well controlled.

Leukotriene Inhibitors

Leukotrienes are a group of arachidonic acid metabolites formed via the **5-lipoxygenase pathway** (see Chapter 26). These substances serve as mediators in the inflammatory events that contribute to bronchospasm in patients with asthma.

Two leukotriene receptor antagonists, zafirlukast (ACCOLATE) and montelukast (SINGULAIR), are now available. Zileuton is a **leukotriene synthesis inhibitor**.

Zafirlukast and Montelukast

CHEMISTRY AND MECHANISMS. Zafirlukast and montelukast each have a complex structure that contains a sulfur moiety and resembles the structure of the **cysteinyl leukotrienes,** which are called **sulfidopeptide leukotrienes** or **leukotrienes C_4, D_4, and E_4** (LTC$_4$, LTD$_4$, and LTE$_4$). Because of their structural resemblance, the drugs can compete with the leukotrienes for their receptor, the **CysLT$_1$ receptor.** This receptor mediates airway inflammation, edema, bronchoconstriction, and the secretion of thick, viscous mucus. The leukotriene antagonists have been shown to inhibit both the early and the late phases of bronchoconstriction induced by antigen challenge.

PHARMACOKINETICS. Zafirlukast and montelukast are administered orally and are well absorbed from the gut. They are both highly bound to plasma proteins (>99%) and are extensively metabolized by hepatic cytochrome P450 enzymes. The half-life of zafirlukast is about 10 hours, whereas that of montelukast is only about 4 hours. Nevertheless, montelukast is administered as a single daily dose in the evening, whereas zafirlukast is usually given twice a day. It would appear that the biologic activity of montelukast persists longer than the serum levels of the drug.

PHARMACOLOGIC EFFECTS AND INDICATIONS. The leukotriene receptor antagonists are considered alternatives to other anti-inflammatory drugs for the long-term control of mild to moderate **asthma.** The receptor antagonists improve pulmonary function, control symptoms, and can significantly reduce the incidence of asthmatic attacks. Their beneficial effects appear to be cumulative, and maximal effectiveness may require several weeks to months of therapy. Their main benefit seems to be a reduction in airway inflammation, but they also produce significant bronchodilation within 1 hour of administration. Although they are not indicated for the treatment of acute bronchospasm, they do enhance the bronchodilating effect of β_2-adrenergic receptor agonists, and they reduce the need for acute treatment of bronchospasm.

Leukotriene receptor antagonists offer the advantages of convenient oral administration and minimal side effects, but they are not as efficacious as glucocorticoids in the management of moderate to severe asthma. Furthermore, they are not recommended as monotherapy for the management of exercise-induced asthma.

ADVERSE EFFECTS AND INTERACTIONS. The leukotriene receptor antagonists are relatively free of serious adverse effects. Allergic granulomatous angiitis (Churg-Strauss syndrome), however, has developed in some patients who were being withdrawn from glucocorticoid therapy while receiving zafirlukast, so careful monitoring is necessary under these circumstances.

Zafirlukast inhibits the CYP2C9 and CYP3A4 isozymes of cytochrome P450 and may thereby interfere with the metabolism of phenytoin and warfarin (drugs metabolized by CYP2C9) and of felodipine, lovastatin, and triazolam (drugs metabolized by CYP3A4). Montelukast does not inhibit these isozymes or exhibit significant drug interactions. Hence, its use may be preferred in patients receiving concomitant drug therapy.

Zileuton

MECHANISMS. Zileuton (ZYELO) inhibits 5-lipoxygenase, the enzyme responsible for catalyzing the formation of leukotrienes from arachidonic acid. By blocking leukotriene synthesis, the drug protects the airways from the inflammatory and bronchoconstricting effects of leukotrienes.

PHARMACOKINETICS. Zileuton is administered orally four times a day (with meals and at bedtime). It is rapidly absorbed from the gut but undergoes some first-pass hepatic inactivation. Once in the systemic circulation, it is almost entirely metabolized by glucuronidation, with an elimination half-life of about 2 hours.

PHARMACOLOGIC EFFECTS AND INDICATIONS. Studies have shown that leukotriene synthesis increases during an asthmatic attack and that this increase can be prevented by the long-term use of zileuton in patients with mild to moderate **asthma.**

ADVERSE EFFECTS AND INTERACTIONS. Because zileuton must be taken four times a day, patient noncompliance is some-times a problem. Mild and transient adverse reactions to zileuton use include a flulike syndrome, headache, drowsiness, and dyspepsia. Zileuton elevates hepatic enzyme levels, so patients taking the drug should be closely monitored for signs of hepatitis. Patients with transaminase levels greater than three times the upper limit of normal should not take the drug. Zileuton should also be used cautiously in patients who consume substantial quantities of alcohol.

Zileuton inhibits isozymes CYP1A2 and CYP3A4, and it may elevate plasma concentrations of theophylline and warfarin. Patients who take these drugs concurrently with zileuton should be closely monitored, and doses of these drugs may need to be reduced.

BRONCHODILATORS

The bronchodilators include selective β_2-adrenergic receptor agonists, muscarinic receptor antagonists, and theophylline. All of these drugs relax bronchial smooth muscle and prevent or relieve bronchospasm. The β_2 receptor agonists are the only type of bronchodilator used to counteract an acute asthmatic attack. Muscarinic antagonists, which are less useful in asthma, are primarily used to treat patients with COPD. Theophylline can be administered on a long-term basis to prevent bronchoconstriction in patients with either asthma or emphysema.

Selective β_2-Adrenergic Receptor Agonists

The selective β_2-adrenergic receptor agonists are the primary bronchodilators used in the treatment of **asthma.** By activating β_2 receptors, these drugs increase cyclic adenosine monophosphate (cAMP) concentrations in smooth muscle and thereby cause the muscle to relax (Fig. 27–2). The selective β_2 receptor agonists relax bronchial smooth muscle without producing as much cardiac stimulation as do their nonselective counterparts, which also activate β_1 receptors in the heart (Fig. 27–3). The selectivity of β_2 receptor agonists is limited, however, and higher doses can activate cardiac β_1 receptors and thereby increase heart rate and contractility.

Chapter 8 describes the pharmacologic and other properties of various types of adrenergic receptor agonists, and Table 27–2 compares the properties of selective β_2-adrenergic receptor agonists that are administered by inhalation.

Rapid-acting β_2 receptor agonists (e.g., **albuterol, levalbuterol, fenoterol, pirbuterol,** and **terbutaline**) are usually given by the inhalational route to prevent or treat **acute bronchospasm.** Although oral formulations of albuterol and terbutaline are available for children or adults who are unable to use a metered-dose inhaler, the oral formulations have a slower onset of action and can cause more systemic side effects. Pirbuterol is available only as an aerosol inhaler for adults.

Levalbuterol (XOPENEX), the (R)-enantiomer of racemic albuterol, is claimed to cause less tachycardia, palpitations, and tremors than albuterol. A clinical study comparing albuterol and levalbuterol therapy in children with asthma,

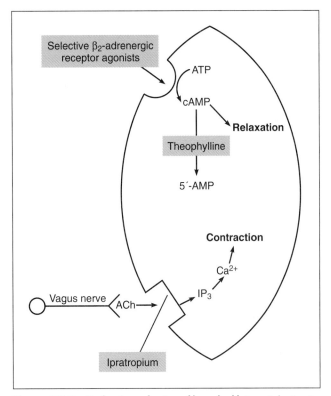

Figure 27–2. Mechanisms of action of bronchodilators. Selective β₂-adrenergic receptor agonists activate β₂ receptors. This increases cyclic adenosine monophosphate (cAMP) concentrations in smooth muscle and causes the muscle to relax. Theophylline inhibits phosphodiesterase isozymes and blocks the degradation of cAMP to 5'-AMP. Ipratropium and tiotropium block the stimulation of muscarinic receptors by acetylcholine (ACh) released from vagus nerves and thereby attenuate reflex bronchoconstriction. The effect of ACh is mediated by IP₃-induced calcium release and leads to smooth muscle contraction. ATP = adenosine triphosphate; and IP₃ = inositol triphosphate.

however, found no significant difference in heart rates or number of emergency department visits (Carl et al., 2003).

Salmeterol (SEREVENT) and **formoterol** (OXEZE) are slower- and longer-acting β₂ receptor agonists that are given twice daily by inhalation for the long-term treatment of asthma. They are particularly useful in preventing **nocturnal asthmatic attacks,** which are sometimes life-threatening, and preventing **exercise-induced asthma.** Salmeterol and formoterol also inhibit the late phase of **allergen-induced bronchoconstriction,** which usually occurs after the bronchodilating effects of shorter-acting drugs have dissipated. These drugs are not indicated for the treatment of acute bronchospasm, for which a rapid-acting β₂ agonist should be used. Salmeterol is available in a combination product that also contains fluticasone (ADVAIR).

Other Bronchodilators

Ipratropium and Tiotropium

Ipratropium (ATROVENT) and tiotropium (SPIRIVA) are muscarinic receptor antagonists. Ipratropium is the isopropyl derivative of atropine, whose properties are described in Chapter 7. The addition of the isopropyl group results in a quaternary ammonium compound that is not well absorbed into the circulation. Tiotropium is a synthetic quaternary ammonium compound. Both drugs are administered by oral inhalation for pulmonary disease, and produce very few systemic side effects. Ipratropium is also available as a nasal spray for rhinitis. These drugs produce their bronchodilating effects by blocking the bronchoconstricting effect of vagus (parasympathetic) nerve stimulation (see Fig. 27–2).

In patients with a **chronic obstructive pulmonary disease** (e.g., **chronic bronchitis** and **emphysema**), the bronchodilating effect of ipratropium is slower to develop than that of albuterol (a β₂ receptor agonist described above), but it lasts longer. In one study, for example, investigators found that the effect of ipratropium was sustained after 12 weeks of treatment, whereas the effect of albuterol on FEV₁ appeared to diminish over a 12-week period. Other studies have demonstrated that ipratropium improves the quality of life in patients with moderate to severe COPD, reduces rhinorrhea in patients with **allergic or viral rhinitis,** and benefits infants with **acute bronchitis.**

Ipratropium is less effective than a β₂ receptor agonist in the treatment of most patients with **asthma.** Some studies indicate, however, that combined therapy with ipratropium and a β₂ receptor agonist has a greater bronchodilating effect than either drug alone in patients who have acute asthma. Ipratropium is useful as a "rescue" therapy, in combination with other drugs, for children with acute severe asthma.

Tiotropium is the first once-daily inhaled treatment for patients with COPD. It improves lung function for a full 24 hours and may become a preferred treatment for patients with mild to severe COPD. Clinical studies found that the mean peak improvement in FEV₁ was 0.28 to 0.31 L (28% to 31%) after 1 week of therapy, and this improvement was maintained throughout the 6-month study period. As with ipratropium, the most common adverse effect of tiotropium is dry mouth.

Theophylline

CHEMISTRY, MECHANISMS, AND PHARMACOLOGIC EFFECTS. As with caffeine, theophylline is a **methylxanthine drug.** These drugs produce various degrees of central nervous system (CNS) stimulation, bronchodilation, diuresis, and other pharmacologic effects. In comparison with caffeine, for example, theophylline produces less CNS stimulation and more bronchodilation.

Theophylline has several actions at the cellular level, including inhibition of phosphodiesterase (PDE) isozymes, antagonism of adenosine receptors, inhibition of calcium influx, and enhancement of catecholamine secretion. All of these effects are purported to contribute to the drug's beneficial bronchodilating effects in patients with asthma, yet each has also been subject to criticism. Recently, theophylline has also been found to elicit several anti-inflammatory and immunosuppressant effects that may contribute to its efficacy in asthma. It seems likely that theophylline exerts its beneficial effects through multiple actions and interactions involving numerous types of cells and receptors.

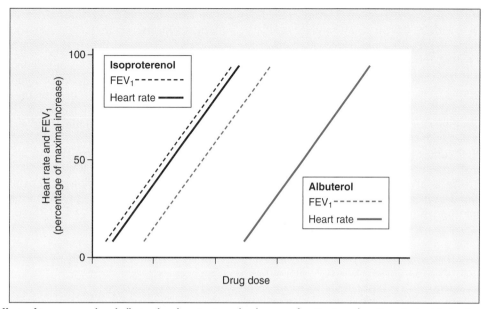

Figure 27–3. Effects of isoproterenol and albuterol on heart rate and pulmonary function in asthmatic patients. Albuterol, a selective β_2-adrenergic receptor agonist, increases the forced expiratory volume in 1 second (FEV$_1$) at doses that produce relatively little cardiac stimulation. Isoproterenol, a nonselective β_1 and β_2-adrenergic receptor agonist, has equipotent effects on heart rate and FEV$_1$.

Theophylline is a nonspecific inhibitor of several PDE isozymes found in bronchial smooth muscle and inflammatory cells. As discussed above and shown in Fig. 27–2, cAMP mediates the bronchodilating effect of β_2 receptor agonists, and the traditional understanding has been that theophylline produces its bronchodilating effect by inhibiting PDE isozymes that catalyze the degradation of cAMP. Some studies have suggested that therapeutic levels of theophylline do not produce significant PDE inhibition. When asthmatic patients are compared with healthy individuals, however, it now appears that the asthmatic patients have higher PDE levels in their airways and that theophylline has a greater effect on their airways. Furthermore, studies show that investigational drugs that selectively inhibit type III and IV PDE can also relax human bronchial smooth muscle. Therefore,

most authorities believe that inhibition of PDE remains a viable mechanism for the bronchodilating effect of theophylline and related drugs.

Evidence also indicates that theophylline exerts anti-inflammatory and immunomodulating effects that may be relevant to the treatment of asthma. Some of these actions are mediated by PDE inhibition, whereas others are caused by inhibition of T lymphocyte proliferation and cytokine production. In patients with asthma, theophylline reduces the number of eosinophils, lymphocytes, and monocytes that infiltrate the airway epithelium. It also impairs the release of cationic basic protein and eosinophil-derived neurotoxin, which are substances that contribute to the pathogenesis of asthma by damaging the epithelial lining of bronchioles.

PHARMACOKINETICS. After oral administration, theophylline is well absorbed from the gut and has relatively little first-pass inactivation. The drug is widely distributed and crosses the blood–brain barrier to enter the CNS. Via the actions of a cytochrome P450 isozyme called CYP1A2, theophylline is extensively metabolized to inactive agents. These metabolites are primarily excreted in the urine, along with 10% of the parent drug. The half-life of theophylline is about 8 hours in adults who do not smoke. In contrast, it is about 4.5 hours in adults who smoke and in children from 1 to 9 years of age, because these populations metabolize the drug more rapidly. Cigarette smoke contains compounds that induce CYP1A2 enzyme synthesis. Hence, children and persons who smoke cigarettes may require larger theophylline doses per kg than do non-smoking adults.

Because of theophylline's narrow margin of safety, theophylline serum levels should be monitored, especially when therapy is initiated. Therapeutic serum levels are considered to be in the range of 5 to 15 mg/L. Higher levels are associ-

TABLE 27–2.	Pharmacologic Properties of Selective β_2-Adrenergic Agonists Administered by Inhalation		
Drug	**Onset of Action (Minutes)**	**Duration of Action (Hours)**	**Dosage**
Albuterol	5	3–8	2 puffs every 4–6 hours
Pirbuterol	5	5	2 puffs every 4–6 hours
Salmeterol	20	12	2 puffs every 12 hours
Terbutaline	5–15	3–6	2 puffs every 4–6 hours

ated with a greater risk of adverse reactions. The use of theophylline has declined with the advent of safer and more efficacious bronchodilators and with the increased emphasis on anti-inflammatory drug therapy for asthma. Today, theophylline is primarily used to treat patients not controlled by other drugs alone.

INDICATIONS. Theophylline is primarily used to treat chronic obstructive lung disorders and asthma, but it is also used to treat apnea.

In patients with **chronic obstructive pulmonary disease**, theophylline is an effective bronchodilator whose long-term use is associated with a 20% increase in FEV_1 and with improvement in minute ventilation and gas exchange. Treatment with theophylline is reported to reduce dyspnea, increase diaphragmatic contractility, improve the exercise performance and sense of well-being of patients, and reduce fatigue. Theophylline can also increase the central respiratory drive and has favorable cardiovascular effects, including a reduction in pulmonary artery pressure and vascular resistance and an increase in right and left ventricular ejection fractions. The drug's other beneficial effects include increased mucociliary clearance and reduced airway inflammation. Hence, a good rationale exists for using theophylline to treat COPD in patients whose symptoms are not controlled with optimal doses of β_2 receptor agonists and ipratropium or tiotropium. Theophylline is most beneficial in patients with moderate to severe COPD.

Although the use of theophylline in the management of **asthma** is declining, recent studies support a continuing role for this drug in specific situations. It is useful in controlling nocturnal asthma, and it can improve pulmonary function in patients who require large doses of glucocorticoids. Patients who have moderate to severe asthma and are already being treated with glucocorticoids and β_2 receptor agonists may benefit from the addition of theophylline to their regimen, and the drug may be particularly useful in controlling refractory symptoms in patients with severe asthma.

Theophylline is an important drug for the treatment of **recurrent apnea in premature infants.** The drug appears to act via adenosine antagonism to increase both the sensitivity of respiratory centers to carbon dioxide and the contractility of respiratory muscles. Theophylline has also been used to treat **obstructive sleep apnea** and periodic breathing. The drug, however, can reduce sleep quality via CNS stimulation.

ADVERSE EFFECTS. Major adverse effects of theophylline include gastrointestinal distress, CNS stimulation, and cardiac stimulation.

Adverse gastrointestinal effects (e.g., abdominal pain, nausea, and vomiting) may be minimized by taking the drug with food or antacids or with a full glass of water or milk.

Central nervous system effects include headache, anxiety, restlessness, insomnia, dizziness, and seizures. A reduction in dosage will often eliminate these problems.

Theophylline can affect the cardiovascular system, causing hypotension, bradycardia, extra systoles, premature ventricular contractions, and tachycardia. These events are usually mild and transient, but serious reactions occasionally develop. Seizures and serious arrhythmias can occur at concentrations over 25 mg/L.

INTERACTIONS. Cimetidine inhibits CYP1A2 and thereby prevents the metabolism of theophylline in the liver. Erythromycin and other macrolide antibiotics can reduce theophylline clearance and increase theophylline plasma concentrations, but the interaction only seems significant when theophylline concentrations are already in the high therapeutic range. Other drugs that can reduce the clearance and increase the plasma concentrations of theophylline include fluoroquinolone antimicrobial drugs, isoniazid, and verapamil. Careful monitoring of patients is important, because it is difficult to predict which patients will require dosage adjustments when these drugs are given concomitantly.

MANAGEMENT OF ASTHMA

The management of asthma is based on the severity and frequency of asthmatic episodes, as determined by the number of days and nights with symptoms per week, and by the FEV_1 expressed as a percent of the predicted normal FEV_1. Based on these criteria, asthma can be classified as mild intermittent or as mild, moderate, or severe persistent asthma. The pharmacologic therapy for asthma falls into two categories. Some medications are administered daily to suppress airway inflammation and prevent bronchospasm, whereas other treatments are used as rescue therapy to counteract bronchospasm when acute exacerbations occur.

For mild, intermittent asthma, no daily medications are required and acute asthma episodes are treated with a short-acting β_2 agonist. For mild, persistent asthma, a low-dose of an inhaled corticosteroid administered with a nebulizer or a metered dose inhaler is the preferred therapy for preventing asthma exacerbations. Alternatives include cromolyn compounds, a leukotriene antagonist, or a sustained-release theophylline preparation.

The preferred treatment to prevent acute exacerbations in persons with moderate, persistent asthma is a low-dose inhaled corticosteroid plus a long-acting β_2 agonist, or a medium dose inhaled corticosteroid alone. Alternatively, a leukotriene antagonist or theophylline can be added to low to medium doses of an inhaled corticosteroid. Long-term preventive therapy for severe, persistent asthma is usually a medium dose of an inhaled corticosteroid plus a long-acting β_2 agonist.

Persons 12 years of age and older with moderate to severe allergic asthma may benefit from injections of an immunoglobulin E (IgE) antagonist known as omalizumab (XOLAIR), which is given subcutaneously every 2 to 4 weeks in combination with inhaled corticosteroid therapy. Omalizumab, however, can cause various allergic reactions itself, including anaphylaxis.

Mild acute exacerbations of asthma are usually managed with one or two treatments of an inhaled β_2 agonist (e.g., albuterol or levalbuterol), given 4 to 6 hours apart. Medical attention is required if the patient does not respond to these treatments, and may consist of multiple treatments of albuterol alone or in combination with ipratropium, oxygen, and possibly fluid replacement. In addition, short-course "burst" treatments of systemic corticosteroids (e.g., prednisone, prednisolone, or intravenous methylprednisolone) may be initiated for these episodes. Antibiotics should also be prescribed for documented bacterial infections. Severe attacks that do not respond to normal therapy, termed *status asthmaticus*, are more aggressively treated with oxygen, systemic steroids, and back-to-back or continuous β_2 agonist treatments.

ANTITUSSIVES

Coughing usually serves a beneficial purpose by expelling irritating substances such as dust, pollen, and accumulated fluids and inflammatory cells from the upper airways. An incessant nonproductive cough, however, can lead to loss of sleep, rib fractures, pneumothorax, rupture of surgical wounds, or even syncope. Antitussive drugs are frequently used to **suppress coughing,** but the first-line therapy consists of determining and controlling the infection, allergy, or other condition responsible for the cough.

The **cough reflex** is initiated by stimulation of sensory receptors on afferent nerve endings located between mucosal cells of the pharynx, larynx, and larger airways. The impulses ascend via the vagus nerve to the dorsal medulla. The efferent limb of the reflex consists of somatic nerves innervating the larynx and thoracoabdominal muscles. Some antitussives act locally to anesthetize the afferent nerves that initiate the cough reflex, whereas others act by inhibiting the cough center in the medulla.

The locally acting antitussives include **menthol and related drugs** that are administered as throat sprays or lozenges. The centrally acting antitussives consist of **opioids,** and these are usually administered orally. Almost all of the opioid agonist drugs will exert an antitussive effect, but opioids that have a higher ratio of antitussive effects to analgesic and euphoric effects are usually used for this purpose. These include **dextromethorphan, codeine,** and **hydrocodone.**

Dextromethorphan is the D-isomer of a potent opioid agonist. Although dextromethorphan has potent antitussive activity, it will not cause drowsiness, euphoria, analgesia, or other CNS effects, except at extremely high doses. For these reasons, it is available in many nonprescription products for cough and other respiratory tract conditions, and it is the most widely used opioid antitussive drug.

Codeine and hydrocodone are moderate opioid agonists whose analgesic effects are described in Chapter 23. These drugs exhibit excellent antitussive activity at doses that produce relatively little CNS depression or euphoria. They are available in a number of liquid cough preparations that may also include guaifenesin, antihistamines, and decongestants.

EXPECTORANTS

An expectorant is a drug that facilitates the coughing up of mucus and other material from the lungs. **Guaifenesin** is an oral nonprescription drug that has been used for this purpose for many years. It is purported to reduce the adhesiveness and surface tension of respiratory tract secre-

tions and thereby facilitate their expectoration, but the exact mechanism by which the drug produces this effect is unknown. Through its expectorant effect, guaifenesin can also reduce the frequency of coughing. The drug may be useful in patients with **thick, tenacious respiratory tract secretions;** in patients with **dry, nonproductive coughing;** and in patients with **sinusitis** to increase airway hydration.

MANAGEMENT OF RHINITIS

Allergic Rhinitis

The effective management of allergic rhinitis includes environmental control of exposure to allergens, prophylactic use of anti-inflammatory medications, and control of symptoms with antihistamine drugs and decongestants. Although some patients with mild symptoms can be adequately treated with an antihistamine drug used alone or in combination with a decongestant, patients with moderate to severe rhinitis usually benefit from anti-inflammatory therapy.

Glucocorticoids are the most efficacious anti-inflammatory drugs for allergic rhinitis (see Table 27–1), and inhalational formulations of **budesonide** (RHINOCORT), **fluticasone** (FLONASE), and other glucocorticoids are available for this purpose. These products are convenient and effective, and they cause very few adverse reactions. **Cromolyn sodium** is slightly less effective but can be used in patients who do not tolerate glucocorticoids.

Whereas anti-inflammatory drugs can significantly reduce symptoms in most cases, some patients will continue to experience symptoms during peak seasonal exposure to mold spores or pollens (e.g., ragweed pollen). At that time, antihistamines can be added to the treatment regimen. A long-acting, nonsedating antihistamine such as **loratadine** (CLARITIN) or **fexofenadine** (ALLEGRA) (see Chapter 26) is suitable for most patients. Diphenhydramine (BENADRYL) is a sedating antihistamine that can be used for relief of nocturnal symptoms.

If anti-inflammatory drugs and antihistamines do not control nasal congestion, a decongestant drug such as **pseudoephedrine** (see Chapter 8) can also be added to the regimen. Decongestants, however, are often not needed if patients begin taking anti-inflammatory drugs before the onset of seasonal allergies and if they add an antihistamine drug at the first sign of allergic symptoms.

Ipratropium is used occasionally for the treatment of rhinorrhea associated with rhinitis. A nasal spray formulation is available for this purpose, but it does not relieve nasal itching or congestion.

Ocular inflammation, discomfort, and pruritus can be a particularly troublesome aspect of seasonal allergies. **Cromolyn** and **lodoxamide** are available in topical ocular formulations that are effective in preventing symptoms of allergic conjunctivitis. Mild ocular symptoms can be treated with topical decongestants and oral or topical antihistamines, such as azelastine (OPTIVAR) and olopatadine (PATANOL). More severe ocular symptoms may be controlled with a topical nonsteroidal anti-inflammatory drug such as **ketorolac** (ACULAR) (see Chapter 30).

Topical corticosteroids are not usually used for allergic conjunctivitis, because their long-term use is associated with adverse effects such as increased intraocular pressure and cataracts.

Viral Rhinitis

Viral rhinitis (the common cold) is a self-limiting condition that is best treated conservatively. Analgesics such as **acetaminophen** or **ibuprofen** (see Chapter 30) can be used to relieve the aches and discomfort associated with viral rhinitis. An increased intake of **zinc** has been advocated, and some data support its antiviral activity. Decongestants such as **pseudoephedrine** (see Chapter 8) can be used to relieve nasal congestion, and **ipratropium** is approved for the treatment of rhinorrhea in persons with viral or allergic rhinitis. Some clinicians advocate the short-term use (≥10 days) of herbal products containing *Echinacea purpurea*, which stimulates the immune system and may thereby shorten the duration and severity of viral rhinitis. Long-term use of *Echinacea* may suppress the immune system, however.

SUMMARY OF IMPORTANT POINTS

- Drugs used in the management of asthma are classified as anti-inflammatory agents or bronchodilators, but some drugs exhibit both anti-inflammatory and bronchodilating action.

- Glucocorticoids, the most efficacious anti-inflammatory drugs, are usually given by inhalation on a long-term basis to prevent asthmatic attacks. Orally or parenterally administered glucocorticoids are used for the management of chronic severe asthma or acute exacerbations of asthma.

- Cromolyn sodium and related drugs are used prophylactically in the management of mild to moderate asthma, allergic rhinitis, and related disorders. They have few adverse effects.

- Leukotriene inhibitors have anti-inflammatory and bronchodilating activity and offer convenient oral therapy for the prevention of asthmatic attacks. Montelukast and zafirlukast are leukotriene receptor antagonists, and zileuton is a leukotriene synthesis inhibitor.

- Short-acting β₂-adrenergic receptor agonists are the most efficacious bronchodilators for the treatment of acute bronchospasm. Examples are albuterol, pirbuterol, and terbutaline. Long-acting β₂ agonists, salmeterol and formoterol, are used to prevent bronchospasm.

- Ipratropium and tiotropium are muscarinic receptor antagonists that are used to treat chronic obstructive pulmonary disease (COPD) but have less efficacy in the treatment of asthma.

- Theophylline has anti-inflammatory and bronchodilating activity and is useful for the treatment of asthma

and COPD. The metabolism of theophylline is affected by smoking and by the concurrent administration of drugs that inhibit cytochrome P450. Children metabolize theophylline more rapidly than do adults.

- Theophylline levels should be monitored to ensure efficacy and prevent toxicity. Adverse effects include gastrointestinal, central nervous system, and cardiac toxicity.

- Antitussives are used to suppress dry, nonproductive coughing. Dextromethorphan is available without a prescription, whereas codeine and hydrocodone are contained in many prescription cough preparations.

- Guaifenesin is an expectorant that appears to facilitate removal of mucus and other material from the airways. It is also used in the treatment of sinusitis.

- Allergic rhinitis is managed with anti-inflammatory drugs (glucocorticoids and cromolyn compounds), antihistamines, and decongestants.

Review Questions

For each numbered drug description, select the corresponding drug from the lettered choices.

1. This orally administered drug blocks leukotriene receptors.
2. This drug inhibits the degradation of cyclic adenosine monophosphate.
3. This drug prevents the release of leukotrienes and histamine from mast cells.
4. This drug prevents bronchoconstriction elicited by vagus nerve stimulation.
5. This long-acting inhaled glucocorticoid is used to prevent bronchospasm.

   (A) nedocromil
   (B) zileuton
   (C) fexofenadine
   (D) formoterol
   (E) budesonide
   (F) montelukast
   (G) prednisone
   (H) theophylline
   (I) tiotropium

Answers and Explanations

1. The correct answer is F: montelukast. Montelukast is a competitive leukotriene receptor antagonist, whereas zileuton inhibits leukotriene synthesis. Both act as anti-inflammatory agents to suppress airway inflammation and prevent bronchospasm in asthmatic patients.

2. The correct answer is H: theophylline. Theophylline inhibits phosphodiesterase enzymes that degrade cyclic adenosine monophosphate (cAMP), thereby elevating concentrations of cAMP in bronchial smooth muscle and causing muscle relaxation.

3. The correct answer is A: nedocromil. Nedocromil, cromolyn, and lodoxamide are mast cell stabilizers that prevent the release of histamine, leukotrienes, and other mediators of inflammation from mast cells and eosinophils. By this and other mechanisms, these drugs reduce bronchial inflammation and prevent bronchospasm in asthmatic patients.

4. The correct answer is I: tiotropium. Tiotropium and ipratropium are muscarinic receptor antagonists that block vagus nerve-induced bronchoconstriction and thereby produce bronchodilation in persons with chronic bronchitis or emphysema.

5. The correct answer is E: budesonide. Budesonide is a potent glucocorticoid (corticosteroid) drug administered twice daily by inhalation to prevent acute exacerbations of asthma. Prednisone and related drugs are given orally or parenterally to treat severe asthmatic exacerbations and for chronic severe asthma.

SELECTED READINGS

Agertoft, L., and S. Pedersen. Effect of long-term treatment with inhaled budesonide on adult height in children with asthma. N Engl J Med 343:1064–1069, 2000.

Carl, J. C., T. R. Myers, and H. L. Kirchner, et al. Comparison of racemic albuterol and levalbuterol for treatment of acute asthma. J Pediatr 143:731–736, 2003.

Redding, G. J, and S. W. Stoloff. Changes in recommended treatments for mild and moderate asthma. J Fam Pract 53:692–700, 2004.

Schoening, S. K. Management and treatment of reversible airway disease. Am J Manag Care 10(5 Suppl):S127–S128, 2004.

CHAPTER 28

Drugs for Gastrointestinal Tract Disorders

CLASSIFICATION OF DRUGS FOR GASTROINTESTINAL TRACT DISORDERS*

Drugs That Reduce Gastric Acidity
Histamine H$_2$ Receptor Antagonists
- Famotidine (PEPCID)[a]

Proton Pump Inhibitors
- Omeprazole (PRILOSEC)[b]

Gastric Antacids
- Aluminum and magnesium hydroxides
- Calcium carbonate

Cytoprotective Drugs
- Misoprostol (CYTOTEC)
- Sucralfate

Drugs for Inflammatory Bowel Diseases
- Mesalamine (ASACOL)
- Infliximab (REMICADE)
- Hydrocortisone

Prokinetic Drugs
- Metoclopramide (REGLAN)
- Tegaserod (ZELNORM)

Drugs for Constipation
- Bisacodyl (DULCOLAX)
- Magnesium oxide and sodium phosphate

- Psyllium (METAMUCIL)
- Docusate (COLACE, SURFAK)

Antidiarrheal Agents
- Loperamide (IMODIUM)
- Diphenoxylate (LOMOTIL)
- Polycarbophil

Antiemetics
Serotonin 5-HT$_3$ Receptor Antagonists
- Ondansetron (ZOFRAN)[c]

Neurokinin-1 (NK$_1$) Receptor Antagonists
- Aprepitant (EMEND)

Other Agents
- Meclizine (ANTIVERT)[d]
- Dronabinol (MARINOL)
- Dexamethasone (DECADRON)
- Prochlorperazine (COMPAZINE)

[a]also cimetidine (TAGAMET), ranitidine (ZANTAC), nizatidine (AXID).
[b]also rabeprazole (ACIPHEX), pantoprazole (PROTONIX), esomeprazole (NEXIUM).
[c]also granisetron (KYTRIL), dolasetron (ANZEMET), palonosetron (ALOXI), alosetron (LOTRONEX).
[d]also promethazine (PHENERGAN), dimenhydrinate (DRAMAMINE).

OVERVIEW

Gastrointestinal tract disorders are among the most common reasons that people seek assistance from health care providers. Many drugs are available to treat the causes and relieve the various symptoms of gastrointestinal diseases. This chapter focuses on drugs used in the management of peptic ulcer disease, inflammatory bowel diseases, gastrointestinal motility disorders, dyspepsia, constipation, diarrhea, nausea, and vomiting.

Peptic Ulcer Disease

Peptic ulcer disease is characterized by inflamed lesions or excavations (ulcers) of the mucosa and underlying tissue of the upper gastrointestinal tract. The ulcers are the result of damage to the mucous membrane that normally protects the esophagus, stomach, and duodenum from gastric acid and pepsin. This damage can be caused by several factors, including excessive acid and pepsin production, bile acid reflux, advancing age, ischemia, inhibition of prostaglandin synthesis, and infection with *Helicobacter pylori.*

In Western countries, the number of persons who harbor *H. pylori* increases from under 5% at birth to about 20% at the age of 45 years. Only a small proportion of persons harboring this bacterial organism, however, will develop peptic ulcer disease. Those at greatest risk include individuals who smoke, ingest excessive amounts of alcohol or nonsteroidal anti-inflammatory drugs (NSAID), are elderly, or have gastrointestinal ischemia. Prolonged use of glucocorticoids can also be a risk factor for peptic ulcer disease.

H. pylori-induced gastritis is believed to precede the development of peptic ulcers in most persons. *H. pylori* is found in the gastrointestinal tract of almost all patients with **duodenal ulcers** and about 80% of patients with **gastric ulcers.** Evidence indicates that the organism can penetrate the mucosa, attach to mucosal epithelial cells, release enzymes that damage the mucous membrane and mucosal cells, and cause inflammation and tissue destruction. Evidence also suggests that the eradication of *H. pylori* heals peptic ulcers and significantly reduces the recurrence rate for gastric and duodenal ulcers.

The agents used to treat peptic ulcer disease include drugs that reduce gastric acidity (primarily histamine H_2 receptor antagonists and proton pump inhibitors), drugs that eliminate *H. pylori*, and drugs that exert a cytoprotective effect on the gastrointestinal mucosa.

Inflammatory Bowel Diseases

The two most common inflammatory bowel diseases are **ulcerative colitis** and **Crohn's disease.** In ulcerative colitis, inflammation of the gastrointestinal mucosa is limited to the colon and rectum. In Crohn's disease, inflammation is transmural and can occur in any part of the gastrointestinal tract. Crohn's disease is sometimes incorrectly described as regional enteritis.

Abdominal cramping and diarrhea are among the most common complaints of patients with an inflammatory bowel disease. The clinical presentation of the disease can vary widely. Many patients experience acute exacerbations separated by periods of remission, but prolonged illness can occur in persons with severe disease. Because the symptoms and clinical course of ulcerative colitis and Crohn's disease are similar, a definitive diagnosis is often difficult and may require extensive laboratory, endoscopic, and radiologic testing.

Ulcerative colitis and Crohn's disease are generally treated with glucocorticoids, mesalamine, and infliximab.

Gastrointestinal Motility Disorders

A number of gastrointestinal tract disorders are characterized by inadequate gastrointestinal motility. These include gastroesophageal reflux disease (GERD), gastroparesis, and irritable bowel syndrome (IBS).

Gastroesophageal reflux disease, which is characterized by esophagitis, is caused by the reflux of gastric acid into the esophagus. The disease is often associated with excessive secretion of gastric acid and decreased pressure in the lower esophageal sphincter. Pharmacologic agents used in the treatment of GERD include drugs that reduce gastric acidity (e.g., H_2 receptor antagonists and proton pump inhibitors) and drugs that increase esophageal sphincter pressure (e.g., cisapride). Also useful are nonpharmacologic measures that include avoidance of certain foods (e.g., chocolate), avoidance of bedtime snacks, and elevation of the upper body during sleep. Because obesity contributes to GERD, weight reduction can help alleviate symptoms.

Acute gastroparesis is a delay in gastric emptying that is typically seen in patients recovering from surgery, trauma, or abdominal infections. **Chronic gastroparesis** is seen in patients with neuropathies that affect the stomach, such as patients with diabetes mellitus. As with other forms of gastroparesis, **diabetic gastroparesis** can be treated with prokinetic drugs (e.g., metoclopramide).

Irritable bowel syndrome is a common, noninflammatory disorder characterized by abnormal bowel movements, which can consist of diarrhea, constipation, or both. The bowel is anatomically normal. Prokinetic drugs can be helpful in patients with IBS.

Dyspepsia

Dyspepsia, or **heartburn,** is characterized by epigastric discomfort following meals. It is often associated with impaired digestion and excessive stomach acidity, but it is also caused by other factors. Several low-dose formulations of H_2 receptor antagonists are available as nonprescription drugs for the prevention and treatment of dyspepsia.

Constipation

Constipation can be an acute or chronic condition and it is characterized by the difficult passage of hard, dry feces. The treatment of constipation rests on a foundation of increased dietary fiber ingestion, adequate fluid intake, and regular exercise. Patients should be encouraged to eat fruits, vegetables, and whole grain foods that add bulk to the diet. If dietary modifications are not sufficient to alleviate constipation, a laxative can be used to facilitate peristalsis. Bulk-forming laxatives can be used on a long-term basis without noticeable side effects, but the other types of laxatives described below should be used only to relieve acute constipation.

Diarrhea

The frequency of elimination and consistency of stools vary from person to person. Diarrhea is a condition characterized by an increase in the number and liquidity of a person's stools. Diarrhea has many causes, and it ranges in severity from mild to life-threatening. Most cases of diarrhea are self-limiting and subside within 1 or 2 days without treatment. Severe diarrhea caused by bacterial infections and other causes can lead to significant loss of fluids and electrolytes and should be treated promptly.

If fever and systemic symptoms (e.g., anorexia and volume depletion) are absent, patients with acute diarrhea can usually be managed with dietary restrictions and with fluid and electrolyte replacement. An antidiarrheal agent can be given as adjunct treatment. Dietary guidelines usually consist of avoiding solid food and milk products for 24 hours. As bowel movements decrease, a bland diet can be started. Several preparations that contain the correct proportions of glucose and electrolytes are available for fluid and electrolyte replacement.

If fever or systemic symptoms are present, patients with diarrhea should be examined for microbial or parasitic infections. If cultures are positive, an appropriate antimicrobial or antiparasitic drug should be given. Chronic diarrhea is defined as diarrhea lasting for 14 days or longer. This condition requires a more thorough diagnostic work-up to determine the underlying cause and enable the selection of appropriate therapy.

A number of drugs can cause diarrhea, including antibiotics that eradicate the normal intestinal flora and predispose patients to superinfections. Limited evidence suggests that administration of *Lactobacillus* preparations can help restore the normal bowel flora and reduce diarrhea in these patients.

Nausea and Vomiting

Emesis, or vomiting, is a physiologic response to the presence of irritating and potentially harmful substances in the gut or blood stream. It sometimes occurs as a result of excessive vestibular stimulation (motion sickness) or psychological stimuli such as fear, dread, or obnoxious sights and odors. Vomiting is frequently preceded by nausea. Many antiemetic drugs are available to prevent vomiting.

DRUGS THAT REDUCE GASTRIC ACIDITY

The physiology of gastric acid secretion and sites of drug action are illustrated in Fig. 28–1.

The principal physiologic stimulants of gastric acid secretion are **gastrin, acetylcholine,** and **histamine.** Gastrin is a hormone secreted by G cells in the gastric antrum, whereas acetylcholine is released from vagus nerve terminals. Gastrin and acetylcholine directly stimulate acid secretion by parietal cells, and they also stimulate the release of histamine from paracrine (enterochromaffin-like) cells. Histamine stimulates H_2 receptors located on parietal cells and provokes acid secretion via cyclic adenosine monophosphate (cAMP) stimulation of the proton pump (H^+, K^+-ATPase).

The vagus nerve mediates the cephalic phase of gastric acid secretion evoked by the smell, taste, and thought of food. Gastrin mediates the gastric phase of acid secretion evoked by the presence of food in the stomach. Histamine contributes to the cephalic and gastric phases of acid secretion, and it also mediates basal acid secretion in the fasting state.

The level of gastric acidity can be reduced either by neutralizing gastric acid (as occurs with antacids) or by inhibiting gastric acid secretion (as occurs with histamine H_2 receptor antagonists, proton pump inhibitors, or muscarinic receptor antagonists). Today, the most widely used drugs to

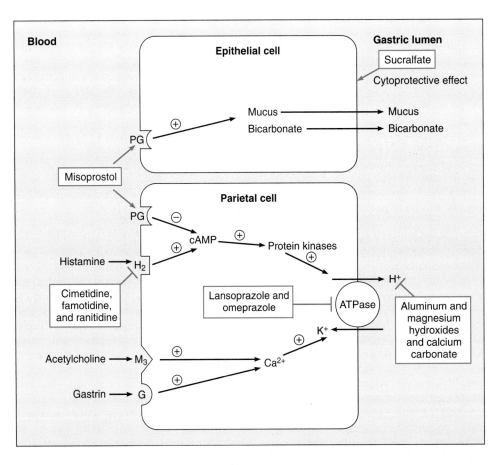

Figure 28–1. Physiology of gastric acid secretion and sites of drug action. Gastric acid is secreted by the proton pump (H^+, K^+-ATPase) located in the luminal membrane of parietal cells. H^+, K^+-ATPase is stimulated by histamine, acetylcholine, and gastrin, and it is irreversibly blocked by the proton pump inhibitors (lansoprazole and omeprazole). The effect of histamine is blocked by H_2 receptor antagonists (cimetidine, famotidine, and ranitidine). Prostaglandins (e.g., misoprostol) inhibit gastric acid secretion and stimulate secretion of mucus and bicarbonate by epithelial cells. Sucralfate binds to proteins of the ulcer crater and exerts a cytoprotective effect, whereas antacids (aluminum and magnesium hydroxides and calcium carbonate) neutralize acid in the gastric lumen. PG = prostaglandin receptor; H_2 = histamine H_2 receptor; M_3 = muscarinic M_3 receptor; G = gastrin receptor; and cAMP = cyclic adenosine monophosphate.

Figure 28-2. Structures of histamine and serotonin and their antagonists. Cimetidine is a histamine H_2 receptor antagonist whose structure is similar to that of histamine. Ondansetron is a serotonin 5-HT_3 receptor antagonist whose structure is similar to that of serotonin. The parts of the structures that are similar are unshaded.

inhibit gastric acid secretion are the H_2 receptor antagonists and the proton pump inhibitors.

Histamine H_2 Receptor Antagonists

The H_2 receptor antagonists, or **H_2-blockers,** include **cimetidine, famotidine,** and **ranitidine.**

CHEMISTRY, MECHANISMS, AND PHARMACOLOGIC EFFECTS. The H_2-blockers each contain a five-membered imidazole, thiazole, or furan ring with an attached side chain. The structure of H_2-blockers is similar to that of histamine (Fig. 28–2), and this enables the drugs to compete with histamine for binding to H_2 receptors on gastric parietal cells (see Fig. 28–1). The H_2-blockers have been shown to be potent inhibitors of both meal-stimulated secretion and basal secretion of **gastric acid.** When they reduce the volume and concentration of gastric acid, they produce a proportionate decrease in the production of **pepsin** because gastric acid catalyzes the conversion of inactive pepsinogen to pepsin. The H_2-blockers also reduce the secretion of **intrinsic factor,** but not enough to significantly reduce vitamin B_{12} absorption. They have no effect on gastric emptying time, esophageal sphincter pressure, or pancreatic enzyme secretion.

PHARMACOKINETICS. The H_2-blockers are well absorbed from the gut and undergo varying degrees of hepatic inactivation before being excreted in the urine. Although the half-life of most H_2-blockers is only 2 to 3 hours, their duration of action is considerably longer (Table 28–1). Therefore, these drugs can be administered only once or twice daily.

INDICATIONS. The H_2-blockers are used to treat several conditions associated with excessive acid production. These include **dyspepsia, peptic ulcer disease,** and **gastroesophageal reflux disease.** An H_2-blocker is also occasionally used in combination with an H_1-blocker for the treatment of **allergic reactions** that do not respond when an H_1-blocker is used alone.

For the prevention or treatment of dyspepsia, several low-dose formulations of H_2-blockers are available as nonprescription drugs. These formulations are most effective when taken 30 minutes before ingestion of a dyspepsia-provoking meal.

For the treatment of peptic ulcer disease, H_2-blockers are administered once or twice daily at doses that raise the gastric pH above 4 for about 13 hours a day. Most authorities currently recommend giving a single daily dose at bedtime on an empty stomach and continuing the treatment for 6 to 8 weeks. The bedtime dose ensures that acid secretion is suppressed all night.

When cimetidine was introduced as the first H_2-blocker, it quickly revolutionized the treatment of peptic ulcers and became the most profitable drug marketed at the time. Studies have shown that cimetidine and other H_2-blockers rapidly suppress acid secretion and relieve pain in persons with peptic ulcers, and they heal about 70% of ulcers in 4 weeks and about 85% in 8 weeks. According to controlled trials, all of the available H_2-blockers produce comparable healing rates. Unfortunately, 80% to 90% of patients who undergo monotherapy with an H_2-blocker have an ulcer recurrence within 1 year after discontinuing this therapy. In

TABLE 28-1.	**Properties of Selected Drugs for Peptic Ulcer Disease**		
Drug Class	**Duration of Action (Hours)**	**Duration of Therapy (Weeks)**	**Recurrence Rate* (%)**
Antimicrobial agents	Varies	2	<5
Cytoprotective drugs (sucralfate)	6–12	6–8	80–90
Gastric antacids	3–4	6–8	80–90
Histamine H_2 receptor antagonists	12	6–8	80–90
Proton pump inhibitors	24–48	6–8	80–90

*Recurrence rates are high when patients with peptic ulcer disease are not treated for *Helicobacter pylori* infection. To reduce the recurrence rate, patients should be treated concomitantly with two or three appropriate antimicrobial agents (e.g. amoxicillin, bismuth, clarithromycin, metronidazole, and tetracycline) for 2 weeks plus an inhibitor of gastric acid secretion (either a histamine H_2 receptor antagonist or a proton pump inhibitor) for 6 to 8 weeks.

contrast, fewer than 5% of patients who undergo therapy with both an H_2-blocker and clarithromycin, an agent to eliminate *H. pylori* infection, have an ulcer recurrence. For this reason, combination therapy is recommended.

ADVERSE EFFECTS. Cimetidine has weak antiandrogenic activity and can cause gynecomastia in elderly men, but this reaction is less common with other H_2-blockers. The fact that the H_2-blockers have proved remarkably nontoxic has led to their approval as nonprescription drugs.

INTERACTIONS. Cimetidine is a well-known inhibitor of cytochrome P450 isozymes CYP2C9, CYP2D6, and CYP3A4. These isozymes are involved in the metabolism of numerous drugs, including alprazolam, carbamazepine, cisapride, disopyramide, felodipine, lovastatin, phenytoin, saquinavir, triazolam, and warfarin. The dosage of these drugs may need to be reduced in patients taking cimetidine concurrently, and patients should be monitored closely for signs of toxicity. Another H_2-blocker, such as ranitidine or famotidine, is often used instead of cimetidine in patients receiving concomitant drug therapy, because these H_2-blockers are much less likely to cause drug interactions.

Proton Pump Inhibitors

The proton pump inhibitors include **lansoprazole** and **omeprazole.**

CHEMISTRY AND PHARMACOKINETICS. The proton pump inhibitors are benzimidazole compounds.

The proton pump inhibitors are acid-labile prodrugs that are administered orally as sustained-release, enteric-coated preparations. After they are absorbed from the gut, the prodrugs are distributed to the secretory canaliculi in the gastric mucosa and converted to active metabolites that bind to the proton pump. These drugs are eventually metabolized to inactive compounds in the liver, primarily by cytochrome P450 2C19, and these compounds are excreted in the urine and feces. Persons with the 2C19 extensive metabolizer phenotype may require higher doses of proton pump inhibitors to cure peptic ulcer.

MECHANISMS AND PHARMACOLOGIC EFFECTS. The active metabolites of proton pump inhibitors form a covalent disulfide link with a cysteinyl residue in the proton pump (H^+,K^+-ATPase) located in the luminal membrane of gastric parietal cells (see Fig. 28–1). This enables the drugs to irreversibly inhibit the proton pump and to prevent the secretion of gastric acid for an extended period of time. The drugs can produce a dose-dependent inhibition of up to 95% of gastric acid secretion, and a single dose can inhibit acid secretion for 1 to 2 days. This makes the proton pump inhibitors more efficacious and longer-acting than the H_2-blockers (see Table 28–1).

INDICATIONS. Proton pump inhibitors are useful in the treatment of **peptic ulcer disease.** They typically heal 75% to 80% of peptic ulcers in 4 weeks, whereas H_2-blockers heal about 70% in 4 weeks. Patients who have been treated with proton pump inhibitors appear to relapse at the same rate as those who have been treated with H_2-blockers. Because the recurrence of ulcers is usually caused by persistent *H. pylori*

infection, experts recommend that proton pump inhibitors be given in combination with drugs that eliminate *H. pylori* infection.

Proton pump inhibitors are the drugs of choice for patients with **Zollinger-Ellison syndrome,** a condition characterized by severe ulcers resulting from **gastrin-secreting tumors (gastrinomas).** Higher doses are required for treating patients with this condition than for treating patients with typical peptic ulcer disease.

Proton pump inhibitors are also the most effective drugs for treating **gastroesophageal reflux disease.** Omeprazole is available in a nonprescription product for the treatment of dyspepsia and heartburn.

ADVERSE EFFECTS. Proton pump inhibitors are usually well tolerated. Minor gastrointestinal and central nervous system (CNS) side effects have occurred in some patients, and skin rash and elevated hepatic enzyme levels have also been reported. Patients with GERD, however, have been treated for several years without significant side effects.

Muscarinic Receptor Antagonists

Atropine and related drugs such as dicyclomine (see Chapter 7), are often used to relieve irritable bowel symptoms such as intestinal cramping and pain. Before H_2-blockers and proton pump inhibitors were developed, muscarinic receptor antagonists (see Chapter 7) were used to treat peptic ulcer disease. Although administering high doses of atropine can effectively reduce gastric acid secretion, it often causes blurred vision, urinary retention, and other intolerable side effects, and these drugs are rarely used for this purpose today. **Pirenzepine** is a selective muscarinic M_1 antagonist that reduces gastric acid secretion at doses that produce fewer adverse effects than atropine produces. The M_1 receptor appears to mediate the release of histamine from gastric paracrine cells. Pirenzepine is available in Canada but not in the United States. As with nonselective muscarinic antagonists, pirenzepine can cause blurred vision.

Gastric Antacids

MECHANISMS AND PHARMACOLOGIC EFFECTS. Gastric antacids chemically neutralize stomach acid. This raises the gastrointestinal pH sufficiently to relieve the pain of dyspepsia and acid indigestion and to enable peptic ulcers to heal.

PHARMACOKINETICS AND ADVERSE EFFECTS. The most commonly used antacids are **aluminum and magnesium hydroxides** and **calcium carbonate.** These substances are available in chewable tablets and in liquid suspensions. When used alone, aluminum hydroxide can cause constipation, whereas magnesium hydroxide often causes diarrhea. For this reason, the combination of aluminum and magnesium hydroxides usually has a relatively neutral effect on gastrointestinal motility. Calcium carbonate can also cause constipation, and large doses of calcium carbonate can lead to a rebound in acid secretion.

INDICATIONS. Antacids are available without a prescription and are commonly used to treat **acid indigestion** and **dyspepsia.** Nonprescription products containing a low dose of a histamine H_2 antagonist and an antacid are also available for this purpose.

Although some studies have shown that antacids can be as effective as acid secretion inhibitors for treating **peptic ulcer disease,** antacids are more difficult for patients to use correctly. For antacids to be effective, they must be taken in large quantities at frequent intervals. For example, 30 mL (1 ounce) of the aluminum and magnesium hydroxide suspension must be taken several times a day (1 to 3 hours after each meal and at bedtime) for 6 to 8 weeks. Nocturnal acid secretion is particularly difficult to control with antacids and may require multiple nighttime doses. For these reasons, antacids are not widely used as the primary treatment for peptic ulcer disease today.

In addition to its utility as a gastric antacid, calcium carbonate is also used as a **calcium supplement.**

CYTOPROTECTIVE DRUGS

Sucralfate and misoprostol (CYTOTEC) both protect the gastrointestinal mucosa, but they do so by different means (see Fig. 28–1).

Sucralfate

CHEMISTRY, MECHANISMS, AND PHARMACOLOGIC EFFECTS. Sucralfate is a viscous polymer of sucrose octasulfate and aluminum hydroxide. This sulfated polysaccharide adheres to ulcer craters and epithelial cells, and it inhibits pepsin-catalyzed hydrolysis of mucosal proteins. Sucralfate also stimulates prostaglandin synthesis in mucosal cells. These actions contribute to the formation of a protective barrier to acid and pepsin and thereby facilitate the healing of ulcers.

PHARMACOKINETICS. Sucralfate is administered orally as a tablet or suspension. The drug is not absorbed significantly from the gut, and it is primarily excreted in the feces. Patients absorb a small amount of aluminum from the drug, so sucralfate should be used cautiously in patients with renal impairment.

INDICATIONS. In the management of **peptic ulcer disease,** sucralfate can be used to treat active ulcers or to suppress the recurrence of ulcers. Because it is somewhat less effective than drugs that inhibit gastric acid secretion, it is primarily used in patients who cannot tolerate H_2-blockers or proton pump inhibitors.

ADVERSE EFFECTS AND INTERACTIONS. Although sucralfate causes very few systemic adverse effects, constipation, other gastrointestinal disturbances, and laryngospasm have been reported occasionally. The use of sucralfate can impair the absorption of other drugs (e.g., digoxin, fluoroquinolones, ketoconazole, and phenytoin). To prevent this problem, sucralfate should be ingested 2 hours before or after these other drugs are taken.

Misoprostol

As discussed in Chapter 26, misoprostol is a prostaglandin E_1 analogue. The drug exerts a cytoprotective effect by inhibiting gastric acid secretion and promoting the secretion of mucus and bicarbonate. It is primarily indicated for the prevention of **gastric and duodenal ulcers** in patients who are taking NSAID on a long-term basis for the treatment of arthritis and other conditions. Because misoprostol is expensive, it is usually reserved for patients at high risk of NSAID-induced ulcers, including the elderly and those with a history of peptic ulcer disease.

Misoprostol is administered orally four times daily with food for the duration of NSAID therapy. Diarrhea and intestinal cramping are the most common adverse effects, but other gastrointestinal reactions can also occur.

Misoprostol can stimulate uterine contractions and induce labor in pregnant women, so its use is contraindicated during pregnancy.

DRUGS FOR *HELICOBACTER PYLORI* INFECTION

The discovery that *H. pylori* infection plays a role in peptic ulcer disease has led to the development of effective methods to treat infections caused by this bacterium. Single-drug therapy is rarely effective in eradicating *H. pylori* organisms. Therefore, multiple-drug therapy must be used, despite that it is complicated and costly and is sometimes associated with compliance problems and significant side effects.

For the treatment of **peptic ulcer disease,** most regimens include a gastric acid secretion inhibitor (either a proton pump inhibitor or H_2-blocker, as described above) and two or more of the following agents: **amoxicillin, bismuth, clarithromycin, metronidazole,** and **tetracycline.** Currently, experts recommend that gastric acid secretion inhibitors be given for 6 to 8 weeks and that antimicrobial agents be given for 2 weeks. Studies indicate that three-drug regimens consisting of one proton pump inhibitor and two antimicrobial agents achieve eradication rates of about 90%. Based on some reports, regimens that include clarithromycin may provide higher eradication rates in a shorter period of time (7 to 10 days) than do regimens that include antimicrobial agents other than clarithromycin.

The properties of antimicrobial agents are discussed in the chapters of Section VII.

DRUGS FOR INFLAMMATORY BOWEL DISEASES

Glucocorticoids

Hydrocortisone and other glucocorticoids (see Chapter 33) have been extensively used for the treatment of both **ulcerative colitis** and **Crohn's disease.** In cases of mild ulcerative colitis, they may be effectively administered as rectal enemas. In cases of Crohn's disease or more severe ulcerative colitis, they are usually administered orally or parenterally.

Glucocorticoids are often able to induce the remission of ulcerative colitis or Crohn's disease, but they have proved less valuable in maintaining remission, particularly without causing significant toxicity. The long-term maintenance of remission usually requires treatment with an aminosalicylate.

Aminosalicylates

Sulfasalazine and its active metabolite, **mesalamine (ASACOL),** are used to induce and maintain the remission of inflammatory bowel diseases.

Sulfasalazine has been used to treat **ulcerative colitis** for many years, and it is also helpful in the treatment of **Crohn's disease.** The drug is a modified sulfonamide compound (see Chapter 40) and is not well absorbed from the gut. In the gastrointestinal tract, bacteria convert sulfasalazine to 5-aminosalicylic acid (5-ASA, or **mesalamine**) and sulfapyridine. Although 5-ASA is believed to mediate the inflammatory effects of sulfasalazine, the exact mechanism is uncertain. Some investigators hypothesize that 5-ASA acts by inhibiting prostaglandin synthesis or by inhibiting the migration of inflammatory cells into the bowel wall. Others hypothesize that 5-ASA is a superoxide-free radical scavenger.

Mesalamine can be administered as a rectal suppository, rectal suspension, or delayed-release oral tablet. It acts primarily in the gut, but about 15% of the drug is absorbed into the circulation.

Other Agents

Although the primary therapy for inflammatory bowel disease consists of glucocorticoids and aminosalicylates, a few other agents have also been used. Immunosuppressive agents (see Chapter 45) are reserved for the treatment of patients who fail to respond to glucocorticoid therapy. **Metronidazole** is an antimicrobial agent that has demonstrated value in some cases of Crohn's disease and may work by eradicating bacteria that contribute to mucosal inflammation in this disease. **Infliximab (REMICADE)** is a monoclonal antibody to tumor necrosis factor-α (TNF-α), a substance believed to play a role in the pathogenesis of Crohn's disease. According to one study, a single 2-hour intravenous infusion of infliximab resulted in improvement in 82% of patients with moderate to severe Crohn's disease.

PROKINETIC DRUGS

Prokinetic drugs are used in the management of a number of disorders characterized by gastrointestinal hypomotility. Prokinetic drugs and laxatives both increase gastrointestinal motility, but they do so by different means. Prokinetic drugs increase the activity of gastrointestinal smooth muscle throughout the gastrointestinal tract, whereas laxatives stimulate intestinal peristalsis primarily by increasing the amount of water and bulk in the intestinal lumen.

The prokinetic drugs include metoclopramide, which acts by blocking **dopamine D$_2$ receptors**, and tegaserod, which activates **serotonin 5-HT$_4$ receptors.**

Metoclopramide

MECHANISMS AND PHARMACOLOGIC EFFECTS. Metoclopramide is believed to increase gastrointestinal motility primarily by blocking dopamine D$_2$ receptors, which prevents relaxation of gastrointestinal smooth muscle produced by dopamine. For example, dopamine infusions reduced gastric muscle tone in human volunteers and delayed gastric emp-

tying. In addition to blocking the direct effects of dopamine on gastrointestinal smooth muscle, metoclopramide also blocks presynaptic dopamine receptors that inhibit the release of acetylcholine from cholinergic motor neurons in the enteric nervous system. It thereby promotes the release of acetylcholine and increases stimulation of muscarinic receptors in gastrointestinal smooth muscle. By facilitating cholinergic neurotransmission, metoclopramide enhances propulsive activity in a coordinated manner, leading to increased tone and motility in the esophagus and stomach.

Metoclopramide accelerates gastric emptying by preventing relaxation of the gastric body and increasing phasic contractions of the antrum. At the same time, it relaxes the proximal duodenum so that it can accept gastric material as antral contractions arrive at the pyloric sphincter. Metoclopramide also increases the resting pressure of the lower esophageal sphincter and thereby reduces reflux of acid from the stomach into the esophagus.

PHARMACOKINETICS. Metoclopramide can be administered orally or parenterally. It is rapidly absorbed from the gut and has an average bioavailability of 85%. The drug is conjugated with sulfate and glucuronate, and these metabolites are excreted in the urine, along with 20% of the parent compound. The terminal half-life is about 4 hours.

INDICATIONS. Metoclopramide is used to treat **gastroesophageal reflux disease**, **diabetic gastroparesis,** and **intractable hiccup.** It is sometimes used to facilitate **intubation of the small bowel** during radiologic examination. In addition, metoclopramide exerts **antiemetic effects** by blocking dopamine D$_2$ and serotonin 5-HT$_3$ receptors in the chemoreceptor trigger zone (see the discussion of antiemetics, below).

ADVERSE EFFECTS. The major adverse effects of metoclopramide are CNS reactions (e.g., drowsiness, extrapyramidal effects, and seizures). Hyperprolactinemia, diarrhea, and hematologic toxicity have also been reported. Metoclopramide is contraindicated in persons with seizure disorders, mechanical obstruction of the gastrointestinal tract, gastrointestinal hemorrhage, or pheochromocytoma.

Tegaserod

Irritable bowel syndrome is a complex biopsychosocial disorder characterized by chronic abdominal pain or discomfort that is relieved by defecation and is associated with altered bowel habits. Some patients complain primarily of diarrhea, whereas constipation predominates in others. Many patients with IBS also experience nausea, bloating, and flatulence.

Tegaserod (ZELNORM) is a **prokinetic (promotility) agent** that is approved for treating women with IBS whose predominant symptom is constipation. Tegaserod relieves constipation and other symptoms of IBS by augmenting the peristaltic reflex throughout the gastrointestinal tract, possibly by increasing the number of circular muscle contractions during peristalsis. Its effectiveness in men has not been established, partly because IBS occurs primarily in women.

Tegaserod is a partial agonist at **serotonin 5-HT$_4$ receptors.** It is believed to produce its promotility effect by activating 5-HT$_4$ receptors on sensory neurons in the enteric nervous system whose stimulation leads to the release of neurotransmitters (e.g., **calcitonin gene-related peptide**).

Tegaserod is given orally twice a day before meals. The drug is rapidly absorbed but undergoes extensive presystemic metabolism resulting in an absolute bioavailability of only 10% when taken on an empty stomach. Taking the drug with food reduces bioavailability by an additional 50%. Tegaserod is converted to inactive glucuronide metabolites before undergoing renal excretion.

The most common adverse effect associated with tegaserod use is diarrhea, which is usually mild and transient. Rare cases of more severe diarrhea and **ischemic colitis** have also occurred in persons taking tegaserod.

LAXATIVES

Laxatives are drugs that stimulate intestinal peristalsis and increase the movement of material through the bowel. By these actions, laxatives decrease the intestinal transit time and facilitate defecation. Laxatives are used to **treat constipation** and to **evacuate the bowel before surgery or diagnostic examination.** They are also used to **eliminate drugs or poisons from the intestinal tract** in cases of drug overdose or poisoning.

Laxatives are classified according to their mechanism of action as bulk-forming, surfactant, osmotic, or stimulant. Lubricant laxatives, such as mineral oil, are essentially obsolete.

Of the various types of laxatives, only the bulk-forming ones can be used on a long-term basis without noticeable side effects. Long-term use of osmotic or stimulant laxatives can lead to electrolyte depletion, serum electrolyte abnormalities, and dependence on laxative use. Patients with renal impairment are particularly susceptible to these adverse effects, because they may not be able to properly excrete osmotic substances that are absorbed into the circulation.

Bulk-Forming Laxatives

Bulk-forming laxatives are undigestible hydrophilic substances, such as **psyllium hydrophilic mucilloid** (METAMUCIL) and **calcium polycarbophil** (FIBERCON) that resemble natural dietary fiber. They absorb and retain water in the intestinal lumen and thereby increase the mass of intestinal material. These actions cause mechanical distention of the intestinal wall and stimulate peristalsis. Bulk-forming laxatives are available in several preparations, including fiber tablets and packets of psyllium granules. They must be taken with a full glass of water to ensure adequate hydration of the preparation and avoid intestinal obstruction. Bulk-forming laxatives are the safest and most physiologic type of laxative, and they rarely cause adverse effects. For this reason, they are the preferred drugs for the management of chronic constipation. Because of their ability to absorb water and irritant substances such as bile salts, these drugs are also used in the treatment of diarrhea (see below).

Surfactant Laxatives

The surfactant laxatives include **docusate sodium** (COLACE) and docusate calcium (SURFAK). These laxatives are also called **stool softeners** because they facilitate the incorporation of water into fatty intestinal material and thereby soften the feces. Stool softeners are primarily beneficial when fecal materials are hard or dry and when their passage is irritating and painful (e.g., as occurs with anorectal conditions such as hemorrhoids). They are also useful when patients must avoid straining during defecation (e.g., after having abdominal or other surgery). Surfactants produce few adverse effects.

Osmotic (Saline) Laxatives

Osmotic laxatives consist of poorly absorbed inorganic salts, such as **magnesium oxide** (milk of magnesia) and **sodium phosphate.** These substances attract and retain water in the intestinal lumen and increase intraluminal pressure, thereby stimulating peristalsis. They can be taken orally as a liquid or chewable tablet, or they can be administered as an enema. Sufficient doses of osmotic laxatives act rapidly to stimulate defecation. Sodium phosphate is often used to evacuate the bowel in patients scheduled for surgery or diagnostic examination or in patients suffering from drug overdose or poisoning. Lower doses of magnesium oxide can be used to prevent constipation in some patients, such as those receiving opioid analgesics. Use of osmotic laxatives, however, can lead to excessive loss of fluids and electrolytes, so these laxatives are generally not well suited for the treatment of chronic constipation.

Stimulant (Secretory) Laxatives

The stimulant laxatives include a large group of natural and synthetic compounds that act directly on the intestinal mucosa to alter fluid secretion and stimulate peristalsis. These compounds include natural products (e.g., castor oil, plant extracts of senna, or cascara), and synthetic compounds such as **bisacodyl** (DULCOLAX). Bisacodyl is available in oral and rectal suppository formulations that are used in evacuating the bowel before surgery or examination. The stimulant laxatives can cause a number of adverse effects, including abdominal cramping and significant electrolyte and fluid depletion. For this reason, the use of these drugs should be limited to the short-term treatment of acute constipation.

ANTIDIARRHEAL AGENTS

Diarrhea can be acute or chronic; it can range in severity from mild to life-threatening and has many causes and pathophysiologic mechanisms. For example, **secretory diarrhea** can be caused by microbial toxins, laxatives, vasoactive intestinal polypeptide (VIP) secreted by a pancreatic tumor, excessive bile acids, or unabsorbed fat in malabsorption syndromes (steatorrhea). Most of the mediators of secretory diarrhea act by stimulating cAMP formation or inhibiting membrane Na$^+$-K$^+$-ATPase, and this leads to an increase in the secretion of water and electrolytes by the intestinal mucosa. Cholera toxin, for instance, stimulates adenylyl cyclase activity and increases cAMP levels in intestinal cells which, in turn, causes active secretion of electrolytes and water into the intestinal lumen. Some mediators of diarrhea also inhibit ion absorption by intestinal cells.

General guidelines for the treatment of diarrhea are outlined at the beginning of this chapter. In cases of severe or chronic diarrhea, efforts should focus on eliminating or controlling the underlying cause and giving appropriate fluid and electrolyte replacement. Antidiarrheal agents can be used as adjuncts to provide symptomatic relief. These agents include systemically acting opioid drugs and locally acting drugs.

Opioid Drugs

The opioids are the most efficacious antidiarrheal drugs. They exert a nonspecific effect that can control diarrhea from almost any cause. Opioids act by inducing a sustained segmental contraction of intestinal smooth muscle, which prevents the rhythmic waves of contraction and relaxation of smooth muscle that occur with normal peristalsis.

The effects of opioids are mediated by activation of **opioid receptors** in smooth muscle. All of the more potent opioid receptor agonists are effective antidiarrheal compounds. In most cases, the opioid chosen for treatment of diarrhea is one that selectively activates intestinal opioid receptors while having relatively little effect on the CNS. **Diphenoxylate** (LOMOTIL) and **loperamide** (IMODIUM) are the opioid agonists with the greatest ratio of intestinal smooth muscle activity to CNS activity, so they are the most widely used opioids for treating diarrhea. Loperamide is available without a prescription and can effectively control mild diarrhea.

Locally Acting Drugs

Psyllium hydrophilic mucilloid and **calcium polycarbophil** (MITROLAN, EQUALACTIN) control diarrhea by acting locally within the intestinal tract to adsorb water and irritant substances such as bile acids. These substances are suitable for the treatment of mild diarrhea.

Bismuth subsalicylate appears to produce its antidiarrheal effect by inhibiting intestinal secretions. It is most effective in treating infectious diarrhea, which often has a strong secretory component. In patients with traveler's diarrhea and other forms of infectious diarrhea, clinical studies demonstrated that bismuth subsalicylate caused a greater reduction in the number of diarrheal episodes than did a placebo. Bismuth subsalicylate suspension, however, must be given frequently and repeatedly for maximal efficacy (30 mL every 30 minutes for up to eight doses per day). This preparation causes few side effects, but excessively large doses can expose the patient to bismuth or salicylate toxicity.

ANTIEMETICS

Emesis, or **vomiting,** is initiated by a nucleus of cells located in the medulla and called the **vomiting center** (emesis center). This center coordinates a complex series of events involving pharyngeal, gastrointestinal, and abdominal wall contractions that lead to expulsion of the gastric contents. These include orally migrating intestinal contractions (reverse peristalsis), gastric contractions, contractions of the diaphragm and abdominal wall, and relaxation of the esophageal sphincter and wall. The reverse intestinal contractions are associated with **nausea,** which is an intensely unpleasant feeling of the imminent need to vomit. Nausea can also occur in the absence of vomiting.

The neural pathways involved in emesis and the sites of antiemetic drug action are shown in Fig. 28–3. The vomiting center can be activated by afferent fibers arising from the gut, **chemoreceptor trigger zone** (CTZ), cerebral cortex, or vestibular apparatus. The CTZ is located in the area postrema and responds to blood-borne substances, including cytotoxic cancer chemotherapy drugs. These substances activate the CTZ via stimulation of **serotonin 5-HT$_3$, dopamine D$_2$, or muscarinic M$_1$ receptors.** The vestibular apparatus activates the vomiting center via fibers that project to the cerebellum and release acetylcholine or histamine. Noxious substances in the gut can activate vagal afferent pathways to the solitary tract nucleus, which projects to the vomiting center, as well as pathways to the nerve tracts that stimulate the CTZ. The D$_2$, 5-HT$_3$, and neurokinin 1 (NK$_1$) receptors also have a major role in these pathways.

Most antiemetic drugs act by blocking **dopamine, serotonin, muscarinic, or histamine receptors.** Some drugs appear to inhibit several pathways that lead to vomiting center activation. The D$_2$ and 5-HT$_3$ receptor antagonists inhibit activation of both the CTZ and the solitary tract nucleus. Muscarinic receptor antagonists can block the CTZ, solitary tract, and vestibular pathways involved in emesis.

Serotonin 5-HT$_3$ Receptor Antagonists

Ondansetron (ZOFRAN) was the first selective 5-HT$_3$ receptor antagonist to be developed for the treatment of cancer chemotherapy-induced nausea and vomiting. It was found to significantly reduce the number of episodes of emesis in patients treated with cisplatin, which is one of the most highly emetogenic chemotherapy agents. Other first-generation 5-HT$_3$ antagonists were subsequently developed and include **granisetron** (KYTRIL) and **dolasetron** (ANZEMET). All of the first-generation 5-HT$_3$ antagonists have similar pharmacologic properties and clinical efficacies. **Palonosetron** (ALOXI) is a newer drug that has been called a second-generation 5-HT$_3$ antagonist because of its greater affinity for 5-HT$_3$ receptors and its much longer half-life and duration of action.

CHEMISTRY, MECHANISMS, AND PHARMACOLOGIC EFFECTS. The 5-HT$_3$ antagonists (e.g., ondansetron) have structures that resemble the structure of serotonin (see Fig. 28–2). Cancer chemotherapy is associated with nausea and vomiting when serotonin released from enterochromaffin cells of the small intestine activates 5-HT$_3$ receptors located on vagal afferents and activates the vomiting reflex (see Fig. 28–3). Anticancer drugs also stimulate the CTZ that activates the vomiting center in the medulla. Ondansetron and related drugs competitively block 5-HT$_3$ receptors located on visceral afferent

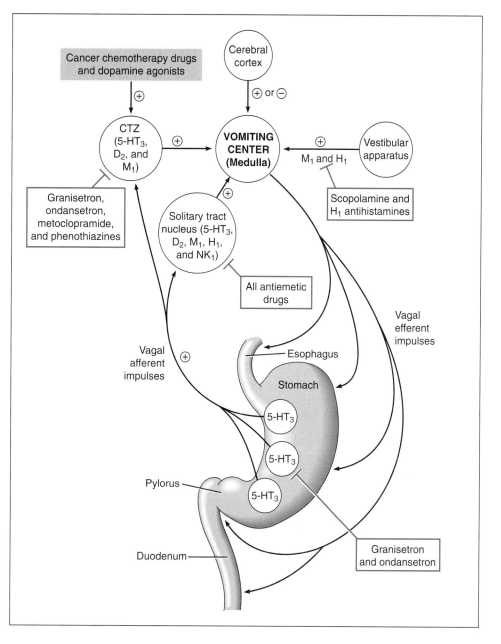

Figure 28-3. Physiology of emesis and sites of drug action. Emetic stimuli travel from the gastrointestinal tract via the solitary tract nucleus to arrive at the vomiting center in the medulla. Emetic stimuli also reach the vomiting center via afferent fibers from the chemoreceptor trigger zone (CTZ), cerebral cortex, and vestibular apparatus. Granisetron and ondansetron prevent emesis by blocking serotonin 5-HT$_3$ receptors in the gastrointestinal tract, solitary tract nucleus, and CTZ. Metoclopramide and phenothiazines prevent emesis by blocking dopamine D$_2$ receptors in the solitary tract nucleus and CTZ. Aprepitant blocks neurokinin 1 (NK$_1$) receptors in the solitary tract. Scopolamine and the H$_1$ antihistamines prevent emesis by blocking muscarinic M$_1$ receptors, histamine H$_1$ receptors, or both types of receptors in the vestibular tracts that project to the vomiting center and in the solitary tract nucleus and CTZ. Note that cancer chemotherapy drugs and dopamine agonists cause emesis, in part, by stimulating the CTZ.

nerves in the gastrointestinal tract, in the solitary tract nucleus, and in the CTZ. This enables these drugs to prevent both peripheral and central stimulation of the vomiting center.

PHARMACOKINETICS AND INDICATIONS. Some of the 5-HT$_3$ receptor antagonists (e.g., ondansetron) can be administered orally or intravenously, whereas others (e.g., palonosetron) are only given intravenously. These drugs are metabolized by cytochrome P450, and the metabolites are primarily eliminated in the urine. The half-lives of granisetron, ondansetron, and dolasetron are 4, 6, and 7 hours, respectively. Palonosetron has a half-life of about 40 hours, which confers a much longer duration of action than other 5-HT$_3$ antagonists.

All of the 5-HT$_3$ antagonists are primarily used for the prevention of **cancer chemotherapy-induced emesis.**

Ondansetron and dolasetron are also approved for the prevention and treatment of **postoperative emesis**, whereas ondansetron and granisetron are used to prevent **nausea and vomiting caused by radiation therapy**.

First-generation 5-HT$_3$ antagonists are usually administered just before chemotherapy and continued for 3 to 5 days after the course of chemotherapy is completed. Because of its longer duration of action, a single dose of palonosetron may prevent nausea and vomiting for up to 7 days following chemotherapy. One study found that a single intravenous dose of 0.25 mg palonosetron was significantly superior to 32 mg of intravenous ondansetron in the prevention of acute and delayed chemotherapy-induced nausea and vomiting (Gralla et al., 2003).

Other antiemetic drugs appear to exert an additive or synergistic effect in combination with 5-HT$_3$ antagonists. Studies have shown that a combination of ondansetron and dexamethasone, for example, could control emesis in persons who had failed to respond to ondansetron alone. Studies have also confirmed the usefulness of ondansetron in controlling postoperative nausea and vomiting. In patients who underwent laparoscopic cholecystectomy, for example, ondansetron was found to be more effective than metoclopramide or a placebo in controlling emesis.

ADVERSE EFFECTS AND INTERACTIONS. The serotonin 5-HT$_3$ antagonists are well tolerated and usually produce few adverse effects. The most common side effects are headache, constipation, and diarrhea. Less common reactions include hypertension and elevated hepatic enzyme levels. In several cases, use of ondansetron resulted in an anaphylactoid reaction consisting of bronchospasm, angioedema, hypotension, and urticaria. Clinically significant drug interactions with 5-HT$_3$ receptor antagonists have not been identified, although ketoconazole appears to inhibit the metabolism of granisetron.

Dopamine D$_2$ Receptor Antagonists

The D$_2$ receptor antagonists include **metoclopramide** and a large number of **phenothiazine drugs** such as **prochlorperazine.** All of the D$_2$ receptor antagonists appear to act primarily on the CTZ to inhibit stimulation of the vomiting center, but they may also inhibit afferent impulses from the gut by antagonizing receptors in the solitary tract nucleus. In addition to blocking D$_2$ receptors, high doses of metoclopramide appear to inhibit vomiting by blocking 5-HT$_3$ receptors in the gut and CNS.

The phenothiazines, as a class, have antiemetic, antipsychotic, anticholinergic, antihistamine, and sedative properties (see Chapter 22). Prochlorperazine has been one of the most widely used phenothiazines for the management of **nausea and vomiting in a wide range of clinical applications.** It can be administered parenterally or as a rectal suppository in patients who are unable to take oral medication. In patients with **cancer chemotherapy-induced emesis,** the efficacy of prochlorperazine and other phenothiazines appears to be less than that of ondansetron, dexamethasone, or metoclopramide. Higher doses of phenothiazines are more effective than lower doses but often cause considerable hypotension and extrapyramidal side effects.

Metoclopramide is a D$_2$ receptor antagonist that also has prokinetic activity (see above). Metoclopramide has been found to be somewhat less effective than ondansetron and other 5-HT$_3$ antagonists for the prevention of **cisplatin-induced emesis.**

With the advent of selective 5-HT$_3$ receptor antagonists such as ondansetron, the use of D$_2$ receptor antagonists for cancer chemotherapy-induced emesis appears to be declining. Phenothiazine compounds and metoclopramide, however, remain viable options for treating nausea and vomiting from other causes.

Aprepitant

Substance P is a peptide of the **tachykinin** family that acts as a neurotransmitter in the gut and brain. Substance P is released from vagal afferent fibers in the solitary tract where it activates **neurokinin 1** receptors and thereby produces emesis (see Fig. 28–3). **Aprepitant** (EMEND) is a nonpeptide

NK$_1$ receptor antagonist that has been found to prevent emesis induced by various stimuli in animal models. The drug is intended to be used in combination with a 5-HT$_3$ antagonist (e.g., ondansetron) and dexamethasone to prevent acute and delayed nausea and vomiting occurring with highly emetogenic cancer chemotherapy, including cisplatin (see chapter 45).

Aprepitant is administered orally and is metabolized primarily by cytochrome P450 3A4 with a terminal half-life of 9 to 13 hours. Drugs that inhibit CYP 3A4 can elevate plasma concentrations of aprepitant. In phase III clinical trials, the incidence of adverse effects in patients receiving aprepitant was similar to that of the control group.

Other Antiemetics

Dronabinol, an oral formulation of **Δ^9-tetrahydrocannabinol** (THC), is approved for the treatment of **cancer chemotherapy-induced emesis** when conventional antiemetic drugs have failed. Dronabinol is usually administered several hours before chemotherapy and is then administered every 4 to 6 hours during a 12-hour period after chemotherapy. The drug probably acts on the vomiting center in the medulla, but its exact site and mechanism of action are uncertain. It has about the same antiemetic efficacy as the phenothiazines, but it is usually less effective than ondansetron or metoclopramide. Dronabinol is also approved as an **appetite stimulant** for anorexic patients with acquired immunodeficiency syndrome (AIDS).

Several histamine H$_1$ receptor antagonists (H$_1$ antihistamines) have antiemetic actions and are discussed in Chapter 26. Two of these agents, **dimenhydrinate** (DRAMAMINE) and **meclizine** (ANTIVERT), are used in the management of **motion sickness.** Another of these agents, **promethazine** (PHENERGAN), is an H$_1$ antihistamine that also has significant antimuscarinic activity and is used to prevent and treat **nausea and vomiting** induced by medications, anesthetics, and a wide variety of neurologic, psychogenic, and gastrointestinal stimuli. Promethazine is usually administered as a rectal suppository or by injection.

Scopolamine is a muscarinic receptor antagonist that is similar to atropine and is primarily used to prevent **motion sickness.** In addition to being used by persons traveling in cars, planes, or boats for extended times, it has been used by astronauts in space. Scopolamine is available as a skin patch that slowly releases the drug over 72 hours.

SUMMARY OF IMPORTANT POINTS

■ Drugs used to treat peptic ulcers include inhibitors of gastric acid secretion, cytoprotective agents, and drugs for *H. pylori* infection. The histamine H$_2$ receptor antagonists (cimetidine, famotidine, ranitidine, and others) and the proton pump inhibitors (omeprazole and others) are the primary gastric acid inhibitors. Gastric antacids (aluminum and magnesium hydroxides and calcium carbonate) are also used.

■ The H$_2$ receptor antagonists inhibit basal and meal-stimulated acid secretion and can be used to treat gastroesophageal reflux disease (GERD) and dyspepsia as well as peptic ulcer disease. Cimetidine inhibits cytochrome P450 isozymes and may increase the plasma concentrations of many other drugs, leading to potential toxicity.

■ Omeprazole and related drugs irreversibly inhibit the proton pump (H^+,K^+-ATPase) and acid secretion. They are the most efficacious drugs for treating GERD, and they are the drugs of choice for use in patients with gastrin-secreting tumors (gastrinomas) and Zollinger-Ellison syndrome.

■ Sucralfate is a cytoprotective drug that binds to the ulcer crater and forms a barrier to acid and pepsin. Misoprostol is a prostaglandin E_1 analogue that increases the production of mucus and bicarbonate while reducing the secretion of gastric acid. Misoprostol is used to prevent ulcers caused by long-term therapy with nonsteroidal anti-inflammatory drugs (NSAID).

■ Inflammatory bowel diseases (ulcerative colitis and Crohn's disease) are primarily treated with glucocorticoids, aminosalicylates (sulfasalazine and mesalamine), and infliximab (an antibody to tumor necrosis factor-α).

■ Prokinetic drugs increase gastrointestinal motility and are used to treat GERD, diabetic gastroparesis, and other disorders. Metoclopramide inhibits dopamine D_2 receptors and blocks dopamine-induced smooth muscle relaxation while increasing acetylcholine release in the gut.

■ Tegaserod is a serotonin 5-HT_4 partial agonist that increases gastrointestinal motility and relieves constipation and other symptoms of irritable bowel disease.

■ Laxatives are drugs used to facilitate defecation and evacuate the bowels. They include bulk-forming laxatives (psyllium), surfactant laxatives (docusate sodium), osmotic laxatives (magnesium oxide and sodium phosphate), and stimulant laxatives (bisacodyl and others). Bulk-forming laxatives are preferred for the treatment of chronic constipation. Osmotic and stimulant laxatives are used to clear the bowels of patients preparing for intestinal surgery or diagnostic examination and patients being treated for a drug overdose or poisoning.

■ Opioids are the most efficacious antidiarrheal drugs. Loperamide and diphenoxylate cause little or no central nervous system effects at doses that control diarrhea.

■ Serotonin 5-HT_3 receptor antagonists (ondansetron and others) are the most efficacious antiemetics for the management of cancer chemotherapy-induced nausea and vomiting. Aprepitant, a neurokinin 1 receptor antagonist, also prevents chemotherapy-induced emesis. Metoclopramide and other D_2 receptor antagonists (e.g., prochlorperazine) are also effective antiemetics.

■ Promethazine is used for mild nausea and vomiting caused by drugs, infections, and other stimuli. Motion sickness can be prevented by meclizine and dimenhydrinate (H_1 receptor antagonists), or by scopolamine, a muscarinic receptor antagonist.

Review Questions

For each patient described, select the lettered drug class that would be the most appropriate treatment for that patient.

1. A woman with a history of motion sickness is planning airline travel.

2. A woman with irritable bowel syndrome has recurrent episodes of constipation.

3. A diabetic patient experiences chronic gastric retention and bloating.

4. Medical tests show that a man has chronic heartburn caused by reflux of gastric acid.

5. A man undergoing cancer chemotherapy requires medication to prevent nausea and vomiting.

    (A) serotonin 5-HT_3 receptor antagonist
    (B) serotonin 5-HT_4 agonist
    (C) H^+/K^+-ATPase inhibitor
    (D) opioid receptor agonist
    (E) histamine H_1 receptor antagonist
    (F) dopamine D_2 receptor antagonist

Answers and Explanations

1. The correct answer is E: a histamine H_1 receptor antagonist. Antihistamines such as meclizine and diphenhydrinate are often used to prevent motion sickness. Antimuscarinic drugs such as scopolamine are also used for this purpose. These drugs act by blocking neurotransmission from the vestibular apparatus in the inner ear to the vomiting center in the brainstem.

2. The correct answer is B: a serotonin 5-HT_4 agonist. Tegaserod is a partial agonist at 5-HT_4 receptors and acts to increase the number of circular muscle contractions during peristalsis and thereby relieve constipation.

3. The correct answer is F: a dopamine D_2 receptor antagonist. Metoclopramide is a D_2 receptor antagonist that inhibits gastrointestinal smooth muscle relaxation produced by dopamine and thereby increases motility throughout the gastrointestinal tract. It is used to treat delayed gastric emptying (gastroparesis) in diabetic patients and for other purposes.

4. The correct answer is C: a H^+/K^+-ATPase inhibitor. Omeprazole and related drugs inhibit the proton pump (H^+/K^+-ATPase) and reduce acid secretion by gastric parietal cells. By this action, these drugs reduce acid reflux in persons with symptoms of gastroesophageal reflux disease.

5. The correct answer is A: serotonin 5-HT_3 receptor antagonist. Ondansetron and other 5-HT_3 antagonists prevent emesis caused by stimulation of the chemoreceptor trigger zone (CTZ) by antineoplastic drugs. Dopamine D_2 receptor antagonists such as metoclopramide are also used to prevent emesis caused by these drugs, but they are not as effective as 5-HT_3 antagonists when used alone.

SELECTED READINGS

Camilleri, M. Treating irritable bowel syndrome: overview, perspective and future therapies. Br J Pharmacol 141:1237–1248, 2004.

Ford, A. C., B. C. Delaney, D. Forman, et al. Eradication therapy in Helicobacter pylori positive peptic ulcer disease: a systematic review and economic analysis. Am J Gastroenterol 99:1833–1855, 2004.

Gralla, R., M. Lichinitser, and S. Van Der Vegt, et al. Palonosetron improves prevention of chemotherapy-induced nausea and vomiting following moderately emetogenic chemotherapy: results of a double-blind randomized phase III trial comparing single doses of palonosetron and ondansetron. Ann Oncol 14:1570–1577, 2003.

Hesketh, P. J. New treatment options for chemotherapy-induced nausea and vomiting. Support Care Cancer 12:550–554, 2004.

Metz, D. C. Managing gastroesophageal reflux disease for the lifetime of the patient: evaluating the long-term options. Am J Med 117(Suppl 5A): 49S–55S, 2004.

Welage, L. S. Pharmacologic properties of proton pump inhibitors. Pharmacother 23:74S–80S, 2003.

CHAPTER 29

Drugs for Headache Disorders

CLASSIFICATION OF DRUGS FOR HEADACHE DISORDERS*

Drugs for Migraine Headaches
Drugs for Preventing Migraine Headaches
Anticonvulsants and antidepressants
- Divalproex sodium (DEPAKOTE)
- Amitriptyline (ELAVIL)
- Fluoxetine (PROZAC)
- Phenelzine (NARDIL)

Nonsteroidal Anti-inflammatory Drugs
- Aspirin
- Naproxen (NAPROSYN, ALLEVE)
- Fenoprofen (NALFON)[a]

β-Adrenergic Receptor Antagonists
- Propranolol (INDERAL)
- Timolol (TIMOLIDE)

Calcium Channel Blockers
- Verapamil (CALAN)
- Nimodipine (NIMOTOP)

Serotonin 5-HT$_2$ Receptor Antagonists
- Methysergide (SANSERT)

Other Drugs or Agents for Preventing Migraine
- Gabapentin (NEURONTIN)
- Feverfew/ginger (GELSTAT MIGRAINE)
- Vitamin B$_2$ (RIBOFLAVIN)

Drugs for Aborting Migraine Headaches
Serotonin 5-HT$_{1D/1B}$ receptor agonists
- Dihydroergotamine (DHE 45, MIGRANAL)
- Ergotamine (ERGONAL)
- Sumatriptan (IMITREX)
- Zolmitriptan (ZOMIG)
- Rizatriptan (MAXALT)
- Naratriptan (AMERGE)[b]

Other drugs for aborting migraine
- Isometheptene (MIDRID)
- Tramadol (ULTRAM)
- Butorphanol (STADOL NS)
- Acetaminophen/codeine (TYLENOL WITH CODEINE #3)
- Acetaminophen/caffeine/butalbital (FIORICET)
- Naproxen (NAPROSYN, ALLEVE)
- Prochlorperazine (COMPAZINE)

Drugs for other Headaches
See Table 29–1

Note that some drugs are listed more than once.
[a]also flurbiprofen (ANSAID), ketoprofen (ORUDIS), mefenamic acid (PONSTEL)
[b]also frovatriptan (FROVA), almotriptan (AXERT), eletriptan (RELPAX)

OVERVIEW

The International Headache Society divides headache disorders into two large groups. The first, **primary headache disorders,** includes **cluster, migraine, and tension headaches.** The characteristics and management of these three types of headaches, which together account for 97% to 98% of all headaches, are compared in Table 29–1. The second group includes **secondary headache disorders,** which arise from organic disorders (e.g., hemorrhage, infection, neuropathy, stroke, and tumor), are responsible for the remaining 2% to 3% of headaches. In patients with secondary headaches, management focuses on treating the underlying disorder.

Because migraine is the most common headache disorder, it is the focus of this chapter.

TABLE 29–1. **Classification and Pharmacologic Management of Headache Disorders***

Classification	Characteristics	Drugs for Preventing Headaches	Drugs for Aborting Headaches
Primary headaches			
Cluster headaches	Severe, unilateral, retro-orbital; clustered over time.	Lithium, methysergide, and verapamil	DHE, ergotamine, glucocorticoids, lidocaine, oxygen, and sumatriptan
Migraine headaches	Moderate or severe, often unilateral, usually pulsatile; occur with or without aura.	β-Adrenergic receptor antagonists, anticonvulsants, antidepressants, calcium channel blockers, NSAIDs, and serotonin 5-HT$_2$ receptor antagonists	DHE, ergotamine, isometheptene, NSAIDs, tramadol, and triptans[†]
Tension headaches	Mild or moderate, bilateral, nonpulsatile; exert bandlike pressure.	Amitriptyline	Muscle relaxants and NSAIDs
Secondary headaches	Characteristics vary, depending on the underlying cause.[‡]	None	None (treat underlying disorder)

*DHE = dihydroergotamine; and NSAIDs = nonsteroidal anti-inflammatory drugs.
[†]Triptans include naratriptan, rizatriptan, sumatriptan, and zolmitriptan.
[‡]Examples of causes are hemorrhage, infection, neuropathy, stroke, and tumor.

CHARACTERISTICS AND PATHOGENESIS OF MIGRAINE HEADACHES

In the United States of America, approximately 24 million people suffer from migraine headache disorder. The pathophysiologic mechanisms of the disorder are not completely understood, but the headaches appear to result from neurovascular dysfunction caused by an imbalance between excitatory and inhibitory neuronal activity at various levels in the central nervous system (CNS). This imbalance can be triggered by hormones, stress, fatigue, hunger, and circulating food- or drug-derived substances.

About 15% of patients who have migraine headache disorder report that they experience an **aura** that precedes each headache attack and lasts for about 15 to 20 minutes. A **visual aura** can take the form of brightly flashing lights or rippling images that spread from the corner of the visual field (teichopsia). A **sensory aura** can take the form of a paresthesia that involves the arm and face and tends to "march" sequentially from the fingers to the hand and then to the body. Auras are believed to result from the cerebral vasoconstriction and ischemia that precipitate migraine attacks. A migraine without an aura (previously known as a common migraine) is often accompanied by an attack of photophobia, phonophobia, nausea, or vomiting.

Each migraine attack has two phases. The **first phase** is characterized by **cerebral vasoconstriction** and **ischemia.** The release of **serotonin,** or **5-hydroxytryptamine** (5-HT), from CNS neurons and circulating platelets contributes to this phase. Hence, antiplatelet drugs and serotonin receptor antagonists have demonstrated efficacy in the prevention of migraine headaches. The **second phase,** which is longer than the first one, is characterized by **cerebral vasodilation** and **pain.** The trigeminal neurovascular system appears to play a central role in the second phase. Neurons in the trigeminal complex release various peptides, including **substance P** and **calcitonin gene-related peptide** (CGRP). The peptides trigger vasodilation and inflammation of pial and dural vessels which, in turn, stimulates nociceptive fibers of the trigeminal nerve and causes pain. Fig. 29–1 depicts these events and the mechanisms of drugs that are used to terminate migraine headaches.

DRUGS FOR MIGRAINE HEADACHES

The drugs used to manage patients with migraine headaches can be classified as **prophylactic drugs** and **abortive (symptomatic) drugs.** Many prophylactic drugs act by preventing the vasoconstrictive phase of the disorder, whereas abortive drugs reverse the vasodilative phase of migraine or relieve pain and inflammation.

Several drugs for migraine are antagonists or agonists at specific types of **serotonin receptors.** These receptors have been classified into four main types, 5-HT$_1$ through 5-HT$_4$.

The **5-HT$_2$ receptors** are widely distributed in the CNS, smooth muscle, and platelets, where they mediate vasoconstriction and platelet aggregation. Drugs that block 5-HT$_2$ receptors (e.g., methysergide) can prevent the vasoconstrictive phase of migraine and are used as migraine prophylactics.

The **5-HT$_1$ receptors** are the predominant serotonin receptors in the CNS, and many of them function as presynaptic autoreceptors whose activation inhibits the release of serotonin and other neurotransmitters. The 5-HT$_1$ receptors also mediate cerebral vasoconstriction. Drugs that activate these receptors (e.g., sumatriptan) are used to terminate a migraine attack.

DRUGS FOR MIGRAINE PREVENTION

Numerous classes of drugs are used to prevent migraine headaches in persons who experience frequent attacks. These

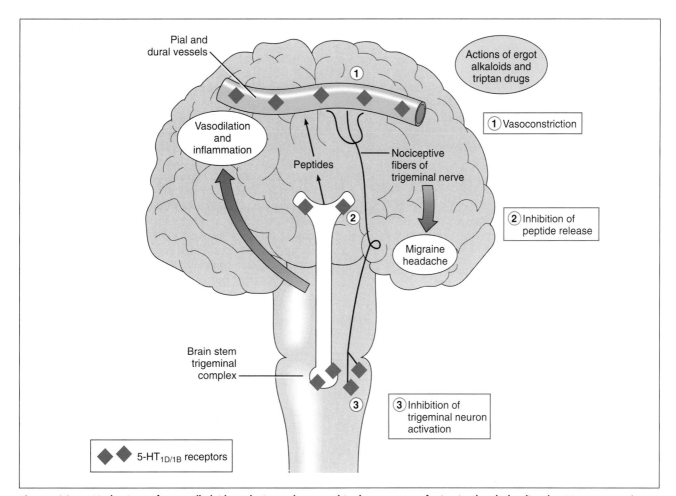

Figure 29–1. Mechanisms of ergot alkaloids and triptan drugs used in the treatment of migraine headache disorder. Migraine attacks are thought to result from trigeminal neurovascular dysfunction. When neurons in the trigeminal complex release peptides such as substance P and calcitonin gene-related peptide (CGRP), this causes vasodilation and inflammation of pial and dural vessels. These events activate nociceptive trigeminal fibers and cause the moderate to severe pain that is characteristic of migraine headaches. Ergot alkaloids and triptan drugs terminate the pain by activating serotonin 5-HT$_{1B/1D}$ receptors at several sites: (1) They activate receptors on pial and dural vessels and thereby cause vasoconstriction. (2) They activate presynaptic receptors to inhibit the release of peptides and other mediators from trigeminal neurons. (3) They activate receptors in the brainstem, which is believed to inhibit activation of trigeminal neurons responsible for migraine attacks.

include anticonvulsants, antidepressants, anti-inflammatory drugs, β-adrenergic receptor antagonists, calcium channel blockers, and serotonin receptor antagonists. A trial of several different types of drugs may be useful to determine the most effective drug for a particular patient. Each drug requires several weeks of therapy before its effectiveness can be observed.

Anticonvulsants and Antidepressants

The properties of anticonvulsants and antidepressants are described in Chapters 20 and 22, respectively. Studies have shown that these two classes of drugs can prevent migraine in some persons, but the mechanisms underlying their effect are poorly understood.

Valproate (divalproex) is the most widely used anticonvulsant for migraine prophylaxis. Its onset of efficacy (2 to 3 weeks) is somewhat shorter than that of other prophylactic drugs. Its common adverse effects include sedation, tremor, and weight gain.

Three types of antidepressants can be used to prevent migraine. The first consists of selective serotonin reuptake inhibitors (SSRI), such as **fluoxetine.** The second consists of tricyclic antidepressants. In this second group, tertiary amines such as **amitriptyline** are more potent inhibitors of serotonin reuptake and may be more effective in preventing migraine than are secondary amines such as desipramine. The third group consists of monoamine oxidase (MAO) inhibitors, such as **phenelzine.** MAO inhibitors can block serotonin degradation and are occasionally used in persons who fail to respond to other antidepressants.

Patients must take antidepressants for 3 to 4 weeks before the drugs become effective in preventing headaches or in alleviating the symptoms of depression. The inhibition of serotonin reuptake by the antidepressants leads to down-regulation of postsynaptic serotonin receptors and a compensatory increase in the firing rate of serotonin neurons. The relationship between these actions and migraine prophylaxis, however, has not been clearly established.

Serotonin reuptake inhibitors sometimes cause anxiety, insomnia, tremor, anorexia, and sexual dysfunction. Tricyclic antidepressants can cause drowsiness, tremor, and anticholinergic effects such as dry mouth, blurred vision, and urinary retention. MAO inhibitors can cause a hypertensive crisis if they are taken with tyramine-containing foods or with sympathomimetic amine drugs.

Nonsteroidal Anti-inflammatory Drugs

Nonsteroidal anti-inflammatory drugs (NSAID), including **naproxen,** can be used for the prevention and treatment of migraine. As discussed in Chapter 30, these drugs act by blocking thromboxane synthesis and platelet aggregation and thereby reducing the release of serotonin. NSAID can be used continuously or on an intermittent basis to prevent predictable headaches. For example, administration beginning 1 week before menses and continuing through menstruation may prevent associated migraine headaches.

β-Adrenergic Receptor Antagonists

Of the various types of β-adrenergic receptor antagonists that are available (see Chapter 9), only the β-blockers that lack intrinsic sympathomimetic activity are effective for the prevention of migraine headaches. One example of these β-blockers is **timolol.** Another example, **propranolol,** has been widely used for migraine prophylaxis but can cause more CNS side effects than timolol.

The mechanism of action of β-blockers in migraine prophylaxis is uncertain. The drugs may attenuate the vasodilative phase of migraine by blocking β_2-adrenergic receptor-mediated vasodilation. They may also reduce platelet aggregation and thereby decrease the release of serotonin from platelets.

Calcium Channel Blockers

Although **verapamil** and other calcium channel blockers have been used for migraine prophylaxis, some authorities believe that the calcium channel blockers are less effective in preventing migraine attacks than are other classes of drugs.

Calcium channel blockers probably act by preventing the vasoconstrictive phase of migraine headaches. The properties of these drugs are described in Chapter 10.

5-HT$_2$ Receptor Antagonists

Methysergide is a drug that blocks 5-HT$_2$ receptors and thereby prevents the vasoconstrictive phase of migraine from occurring. Because of the drug's potential toxicity, however, other prophylactic drugs are usually chosen initially for migraine prophylaxis.

The drug is associated with a number of relatively mild adverse effects, including abdominal pain, weight gain, and hallucinations. It is also associated with a risk of life-threatening retroperitoneal, pleural, and cardiac valve fibrosis. For this reason, it should not be used longer than 6 months without a 1-month, drug-free period initiated by a 2-week taper of the drug dosage. Serum creatinine measurements

should be monitored and chest x-rays studies should be done to detect early signs of fibrosis in patients treated with methysergide.

Other Drugs or Agents for Migraine Prevention

Gabapentin is an agent approved for the treatment of seizure disorders (see Chapter 20) and postherpetic neuralgia. It is moderately effective with little adverse effects in preventing occurrence of migraines. Although gabapentin is known to enhance γ-aminobutyric acid (GABA) action in the treatment of seizure disorder, its actions in migraine treatment are unclear.

The result of a 3-month double-blind, placebo-controlled study of patients with migraines showed that **riboflavin (vitamin B$_2$)** can significantly reduce the frequency and duration of migraine attacks. This study found that a daily dose of 400 mg produced a significant decrease in the number of migraine attacks as well as the total days with headache pain. The effect was not evident until after 2 months of administration, however, and the mechanism of action is unknown.

Feverfew is an herbal remedy that has low to moderate efficacy in preventing migraines, with little side effects. It is available without a prescription as a combination of the extracts of *Pyrethrum parthenium* (feverfew) and *Zingiber officinale* (ginger) in a rapidly dissolving formulation. The active ingredient in feverfew is parthenolide, which has anti-inflammatory activity. As with NSAID, parthenolide can prevent inflammation associated with migraine headaches.

DRUGS FOR MIGRAINE TERMINATION

Numerous drugs can be used to terminate a migraine headache after it has begun. Most of these drugs are serotonin 5-HT$_{1D/1B}$ receptor agonists, and their sites of action are shown in Fig. 29–1. The structures of serotonin and two of the receptor agonists are illustrated in Fig. 29–2A and 29–2B.

5-HT$_{1D/1B}$ Receptor Agonists

Ergot Agents

Ergotamine and **dihydroergotamine (DHE), ergot alkaloids,** are effective in the treatment of migraine headaches and cluster headaches. A number of other ergot alkaloids are available and are used in the treatment of Parkinson's disease, hyperprolactinemia, and other disorders. The potent hallucinogen, lysergic acid diethylamide (LSD) is also an ergot derivative.

CHEMISTRY AND MECHANISMS. As with other ergot alkaloids, ergotamine and DHE are isolated from *Claviceps purpurea*, a fungus that grows primarily on rye. Ergotamine and DHE relieve migraine primarily by activating serotonin 5-HT$_{1D/1B}$ receptors at several levels in the trigeminal neurovascular system. Activation of 5-HT$_{1D/1B}$ receptors in cerebral blood vessels produces vasoconstriction, thereby reversing the

A. Serotonin

B. Drugs for migraine headaches

Ergotamine

Sumatriptan

Figure 29-2. Structures of serotonin (A) and selected drugs for migraine headaches (B). Serotonin is also called 5-hydroxytryptamine (5-HT). Ergotamine is an ergot alkaloid, and sumatriptan is a structural analogue of serotonin. Both drugs are serotonin 5-HT$_{1B/1D}$ receptor agonists.

vasodilation that contributes to the throbbing migraine headache. Stimulation of presynaptic 5-HT$_{1D/1B}$ receptors on trigeminal nerve endings inhibits the release of peptides that cause vasodilation, neurogenic inflammation, and pain. Finally, stimulation of 5-HT$_{1D/1B}$ receptors in the brainstem prevents activation of trigeminal nerves involved in migraine headache.

PHARMACOKINETIC AND PHARMACOLOGIC EFFECTS. The ergot alkaloids are most effective when they are given early in a migraine attack.

Ergotamine is marketed in parenteral, oral, and rectal formulations. When it is given orally, it has a relatively slow onset of action because of its poor oral bioavailability. Although it is available as a rectal suppository for use by persons with nausea and vomiting, it can actually worsen these symptoms by stimulating the vomiting center. Some oral and rectal ergotamine preparations contain caffeine, which appears to increase the absorption of ergotamine and may exert a mild vasoconstrictive effect that helps relieve migraine.

Dihydroergotamine is available in intranasal and injectable preparations. The intranasal preparation, which was recently approved by the FDA, offers patients a convenient method of administering DHE and has a moderately rapid onset of action. The injectable DHE preparation, which is usually more rapid acting and reliable than the

various ergotamine preparations, can be administered subcutaneously, intramuscularly, or intravenously. When administered parenterally, DHE is often given with an antiemetic drug (e.g., metoclopramide) to prevent drug-induced nausea and vomiting.

ADVERSE EFFECTS. The relatively mild adverse effects of ergot alkaloids include nausea and vomiting, diarrhea, muscle cramps, cold skin, panesthesia, and vertigo.

Ergotamine and DHE can cause peripheral vasoconstriction by stimulating α-adrenergic receptors and by directly stimulating vascular smooth muscle. These drugs, therefore, are contraindicated in persons with coronary artery disease or peripheral vascular disease. Excessive doses of ergotamine or DHE can cause severe cerebral vasoconstriction, ischemia, and rebound vasodilation and headache. A rebound headache can last several days, and hospitalization may be required to wean the patient from ergotamine and alleviate the pain. Strict dosage guidelines must be followed to prevent rebound headache and other forms of toxicity. To prevent cumulative toxicity, daily use of ergotamine should be avoided.

INTERACTIONS. Concomitant use of ergot alkaloids and β-adrenergic receptor antagonists can cause severe peripheral ischemia resulting from α-adrenergic receptor-mediated vasoconstriction that is unopposed by β$_2$-adrenergic receptor-mediated vasodilation. Hence, this drug combination should be avoided.

Triptan Agents

Sumatriptan was the first of a new group of selective serotonin 5-HT$_{1D/1B}$ agonists to be developed. These so-called **triptan drugs** include **naratriptan, rizatriptan,** and **zolmitriptan.** Although these four triptans have amassed the most data on their effectiveness in aborting a migraine attack, newer agents such as **frovatriptan, almotriptan,** and **eletriptan,** are also available. The newer triptans are similar to sumatriptan, but their improved pharmacokinetic properties may be advantageous in some cases.

CHEMISTRY AND MECHANISMS. Sumatriptan and other 5-HT$_{1D/1B}$ agonists are structural analogues of serotonin (see Fig. 29–2). Their mechanisms for terminating migraine headaches appear to be similar to those of ergotamine and DHE (see previous text).

PHARMACOKINETIC AND PHARMACOLOGIC EFFECTS. A sumatriptan preparation for subcutaneous administration was introduced in 1992, and oral and intranasal preparations were introduced several years later. Peak plasma levels of sumatriptan are achieved most rapidly with subcutaneous administration and least rapidly with oral administration. Relief of migraine usually takes an hour when the drug is given subcutaneously but can take up to 2 hours when it is given orally.

Naratriptan, rizatriptan, and zolmitriptan are currently limited to oral administration. In comparison with sumatriptan, these newer triptan drugs are more lipophilic, have higher oral bioavailabilities, and achieve higher concentrations in the CNS. The fact that they penetrate the CNS more readily may enable them to inhibit the brainstem mechanisms involved in migraine more effectively than does sumatriptan.

In a clinical trial comparing the effects of sumatriptan treatment with those of DHE treatment in patients who suffer from migraine headache disorder, subcutaneously administered sumatriptan was found to relieve 85% of migraine attacks and to be slightly superior to DHE in this regard. Nevertheless, studies show that sumatriptan is not efficacious in 10% to 20% of patients who have migraine headache disorder, and about 40% of patients who initially obtain relief with sumatriptan have a recurrence of their headache on the same day. Recurrences are more prevalent in patients who have more severe and longer attacks. If a headache recurs, treatment can be repeated at specified intervals until a maximal daily dose has been administered. Because sumatriptan and other triptan drugs cost more than ergotamine alkaloids, the need to repeat doses may be a factor in drug selection.

According to some clinical trials, the newer triptans have a 10% to 20% greater efficacy than sumatriptan, and their rates of headache recurrence are lower (30% for newer triptans vs. 40% for sumatriptan). Naratriptan has a longer half-life than sumatriptan, and this may explain its lower rate of headache recurrence. Further clinical studies are needed to confirm these differences.

ADVERSE EFFECTS AND INTERACTIONS. In clinical trials, the incidence of chest tightness, weakness, somnolence, and dizziness in subjects treated with a triptan agent was nearly 50%, whereas the incidence in subjects treated with a placebo was about 30%. The incidence of adverse effects appears to be similar for all triptan drugs.

The triptans have been reported to cause abnormal tingling or burning sensations in the skin on various parts of the body. These sensations are benign, but they can be mistaken for a serious adverse effect by the patient.

Triptan drugs can cause coronary vasospasm and should not be used in patients with a history of angina pectoris, myocardial infarction, or other coronary artery disease. As with ergots, triptan agents can increase blood pressure so they should not be given to patients with uncontrolled hypertension. The triptans should not be used concurrently with MAO inhibitors, nor should they be used within 24 hours of administering an ergot alkaloid or methysergide.

Other Drugs for Migraine Termination

An NSAID, such as **naproxen,** can be used either to prevent or to abort a migraine attack. Combination formulations of acetaminophen, butalbital (a barbiturate), and caffeine are also effective in aborting migraine headaches.

Isometheptene, an agent that acts as a sympathomimetic, can terminate migraine headaches. It is available in a preparation that also contains acetaminophen and a mild sedative drug.

Opioid analgesics can relieve the pain of migraine headaches, but their use should be reserved for patients in whom other agents are contraindicated or ineffective. **Tramadol** has been particularly useful in chronic pain syndromes (see Chapter 23) and is one of the most widely used

opioid drugs for the treatment of migraine. Tramadol acts as an agonist at μ opioid receptors, and it also inhibits norepinephrine and serotonin reuptake in the CNS. The latter action may contribute to the drug's analgesic effect. **Butorphanol** acts as an agonist at κ opioid receptors and a mixed agonist-antagonist at μ opioid receptors. It is available in a nasal spray formulation. **Acetaminophen with codeine,** or other NSAID–opioid combinations, is also effective in patients resistant to other drug treatments.

The antipsychotic agent, **prochlorperazine,** is effective in aborting unremitting migraine headache when given intravenously.

GUIDELINES FOR MANAGING MIGRAINE HEADACHES
Prophylactic Treatment of Migraines

Nonpharmacologic measures can play a significant role in the prevention of migraine attacks. These measures include appropriate patient education; the identification and avoidance of factors that contribute to migraine attacks, including particular foods, beverages, and environmental factors; biofeedback and relaxation therapy; and psychotherapy. Acupuncture and physiotherapy may be beneficial, but their efficacy has not been established in controlled trials.

Many pharmacologic agents are known to prevent migraine attacks. The efficacy of these agents varies from patient to patient, however, so finding a drug that works well is largely a matter of trial and error. The characteristics of individual patients should help guide drug selection. For example, β-blockers have negative effects on cardiac output, so they are usually less suitable than other drugs for competitive athletes. The goal of prophylactic drug use is to reduce the frequency of migraine attacks by at least 50%, and the criteria for evaluating the efficacy of particular drugs should be clearly established and understood by the physician and patient. It usually takes 3 to 4 weeks of therapy before the benefit of a given drug is observed, so authorities recommend a trial of 4 to 6 weeks before switching to another drug.

Acute Treatment of Migraines

The ideal drug to terminate migraine headaches would act rapidly, be highly efficacious, and have a low potential to cause serious adverse effects. No available drug meets all of these criteria. The newer serotonin agonists (triptans) appear to be less toxic and slightly more effective than the ergot preparations. DHE, however, has the advantage of a longer duration of action than the triptan drugs. Intranasal preparations of sumatriptan and DHE offer a more rapid onset of action than do oral preparations, and they are more convenient than parenteral therapy.

The optimal use of abortive treatment requires prudent drug selection and reasonable restrictions on drug use to avoid toxicity or habituation. The effectiveness of a given drug varies widely from patient to patient, so a judicious trial of several drugs is usually required to determine the most effective drug for a particular patient. Some authorities recommend starting abortive therapy with an NSAID (e.g., naproxen). If use of an NSAID consistently fails to relieve pain within an hour, then the patient should be encouraged to switch to a different agent, such as a triptan drug or DHE. Although this approach may work well for some patients, others may derive more benefit from the initial use of a triptan or DHE. To evaluate the effects of drug therapy, the patient should be instructed to keep an accurate log of drug dosage and symptom severity, especially during a trial period.

The overuse of abortive drugs can lead to serious toxicity, so patients must be properly instructed about limiting their use of these drugs. According to the guidelines of the National Headache Foundation, patients should limit their use of ergotamine to eight treatment days per month, with an ample interval between treatment days. They should limit their use of sumatriptan and other triptan drugs to six treatment days per month and two treatment days per week, and they should limit their use of opioid drugs to two treatment days per week.

CHARACTERISTICS AND TREATMENT OF CLUSTER HEADACHES

Cluster headaches are severe, unilateral, retro-orbital headaches that tend to group or cluster over time. Patients often describe a searing or burning pain that arises behind one eye, occurs without warning, and can be excruciating. Pain often lasts from 15 minutes to 3 hours and usually occurs at the same time each day. Unlike patients with migraine headaches, who are highly sensitive to movement and external stimuli, those with cluster headaches often pace in an agitated fashion, apply pressure to the orbit, or even strike the face to provide distraction from the pain. The incidence of cluster headache disorder is low, however, affecting less than 0.5% of the population.

Drugs to prevent cluster headaches include lithium (see Chapter 22), methysergide, and verapamil. As with migraine headaches, cluster headaches can be aborted by administering DHE, ergotamine, or sumatriptan. Other agents that are effective in aborting cluster headaches include inhaled oxygen, intranasal lidocaine, and glucocorticoids. Guidelines for selecting drugs to manage cluster headaches are similar to those outlined above for migraine headaches.

CHARACTERISTICS AND TREATMENT OF TENSION HEADACHES

Tension headaches are characterized by bilateral, nonpulsatile, bandlike pressure that is mild or moderate in intensity. This common type of headache often responds to physiologic approaches that correct cervical or dental alignment or visual refractive error. Nonpharmacologic therapies (e.g., biofeedback, acupuncture, and physiotherapy) are also useful in controlling both episodic and chronic tension headaches. Pharmacologic therapy usually consists of NSAID and muscle relaxants, but patients with chronic tension headaches may also respond to prophylactic use of

amitriptyline. This drug is usually tolerated better when therapy is initiated with a low dose at bedtime and the dosage is gradually increased over a period of several weeks.

SUMMARY OF IMPORTANT POINTS

■ Migraine, the most common headache disorder, is believed to result from neurovascular dysfunction at several levels in the central nervous system. Cerebral vasoconstriction and ischemia are followed by vasodilation, inflammation, and a unilateral, pulsatile headache.

■ Drugs for migraine prophylaxis should aim to reduce the frequency of migraine attacks by 50%. These include anticonvulsants (valproate), antidepressants (amitriptyline and fluoxetine), nonsteroidal anti-inflammatory drugs (NSAID, such as naproxen), β-adrenergic receptor antagonists (propranolol, timolol), calcium channel blockers (verapamil, nimodipine), and serotonin 5-HT$_2$ receptor antagonists (methysergide).

■ Prophylactic drugs often must be taken for 3 to 4 weeks before benefits are observed.

■ Drugs for aborting migraine headaches include ergot alkaloids (ergotamine and dihydroergotamine) and so-called triptan drugs (sumatriptan and others). These drugs act primarily by stimulating serotonin 5-HT$_{1D/1B}$ receptors. This stimulation causes cerebral vasoconstriction, inhibits the release of peptides and other mediators of inflammation and vasodilation from trigeminal neurons, and inhibits activation of the trigeminal nucleus in the brainstem.

■ Ergot alkaloids and triptan drugs can cause marked vasoconstriction, so their dosage and frequency of use must be restricted to avoid rebound headache and adverse effects. Common adverse effects of ergots include nausea, vomiting, and muscle cramps; those of triptans include chest tightness and drowsiness. Use of ergots or triptans is contraindicated in patients with coronary artery disease.

■ Other agents for aborting migraine headaches include NSAID (e.g., naproxen), opioid analgesics (e.g., tramadol), and a sympathomimetic drug called isometheptene.

■ Cluster headaches can be prevented with lithium, methysergide, or verapamil. They can be terminated with ergot alkaloids, sumatriptan, inhaled oxygen, intranasal lidocaine, or glucocorticoids.

■ Tension headaches often respond to NSAID and muscle relaxants. Nonpharmacologic therapies (e.g., biofeedback and physiotherapy) are also useful.

Review Questions

1. Which of the following agents has not shown effectiveness in the prophylactic treatment of migraine headache?
   (A) zolmitriptan
   (B) methysergide

(C) verapamil
(D) naproxen
(E) amitriptyline

2. Use of sumatriptan is contraindicated in which one of the following conditions?
    (A) postpartum women
    (B) uncontrolled hypertension
    (C) moderate to unresponsive severe migraines
    (D) hepatic insufficiency
    (E) renal dysfunction

3. The therapeutic effect of the triptan class of drugs is caused by which mechanism of action?
    (A) antagonism at serotonin 5-HT$_2$ receptors
    (B) stimulation of serotonin 5-HT$_{1D}$ receptors
    (C) antagonism at dopamine receptors
    (D) antagonism at α-adrenergic receptors
    (E) direct inhibition of substance P receptors in the vasculature

4. Methysergide is indicated for the treatment of migraine because it has which one the following effects?
    (A) it prevents the release of serotonin
    (B) it is a 5-HT$_{1B/D}$ agonist
    (C) it inhibits the COX-2 enzyme
    (D) it is an antagonist at 5-HT$_2$ receptors
    (E) it blocks calcium channels

5. A 35-year-old women with a history of migraine reports to her physician that the last time she used her medicine to stop an acute attack, she felt numbness and tingling in her extremities and blanching and cyanosis of her fingers. Which one of the following medications did she take?
    (A) methysergide
    (B) sumatriptan
    (C) dihydroergotamine
    (D) tramadol
    (E) naproxen

Answers and Explanations

1. The correct answer is A: zolmitriptan. The triptan agents are only effective in the acute treatment of a migraine headache. They are agonists at 5-HT$_{1B/1D}$ receptors in cerebral blood vessels that produces vasoconstriction, on trigeminal nerve endings inhibiting the release of inflammatory substances, and in the brainstem to prevent activation of trigeminal nerves. Answers (B) through (E) have shown various degrees of effectiveness in preventing migraines in controlled studies.

2. The correct choice is B: uncontrolled hypertension. Triptans can increase blood pressure by constriction of peripheral smooth muscle. This is also a contraindication for using ergot agents such as DHE and ergotamine. Answers (A), (C), (D), and (E) are not conditions warranting contraindications for triptan use.

3. The correct answer is B: stimulation of serotonin 5-HT$_{1D}$ receptors. These agents are agonists at 5-HT$_{1B/1D}$ receptors. Answers (A) and (C) though (E) are mechanisms of other agents unrelated to the clinically used triptan drugs.

4. The correct answer is D: it is an antagonist at 5-HT$_2$ receptors. Methysergide is indicated for the treatment of migraine or, better stated, the prophylactic treatment to prevent migraine attacks because of its antagonist activity at serotonin receptors. Other answer choices are not the primary mechanism of action of methysergide.

5. The correct choice is C: dihydroergotamine. DHE is an ergot alkaloid and these agents are known to cause vasoconstriction and paresthesia in the extremities, especially at high doses. Answer (A), methysergide, is also an ergot but not used for acute treatment of migraine attacks. Answer (B), sumatriptan, is a triptan also used for acute attacks and can cause vasoconstriction but not as common as observed with DHE. Answer (D), tramadol, is a dual-action opioid-antidepressant agent, helpful in the acute treatment of migraine but not producing the patient's constellation of adverse effects. Answer (E), naproxen, is a NSAID agent that can cause increased release of norepinephrine and possible vasoconstriction, but is not as common as DHE is producing these effects.

SELECTED READINGS

Ashkenazi, A., and S. D. Silberstein. Headache management for the pain specialist. Reg Anesth Pain Med 29(5):462–475, 2004.

Beck, E., W. J. Sieber, and R. Trejo. Management of cluster headache. Am Fam Physician 71(4):717–724, 2005.

Colombo, B., P. O. Annovazzi, and G. Comi. Therapy of primary headaches: the role of antidepressants. Neurol Sci 25(Suppl 3):S171–S175, 2004.

Gladstone, J. P., and D. W. Dodick. Revised 2004 International Classification of Headache Disorders: new headache types. Can J Neurol Sci 31(3):304–314, 2004.

Grazzi, L. Primary headaches in children and adolescents. Neurol Sci 25(Suppl 3):S232–S233, 2004.

Lipton, R. B., and M. E. Bigal. Headache: triumphs in translational research. Lancet Neurol 4(1):11–12, 2005.

Narbone, M. C., M. Abbate, and S. Gangemi. Acute drug treatment of migraine attack. Neurol Sci 25(Suppl 3):S113–S118, 2004.

Smith, T. R., and J. Stoneman. Medication overuse headache from antimigraine therapy: clinical features, pathogenesis and management. Drugs 64(22):2503–2514, 2004.

CHAPTER 30

Drugs for Pain, Inflammation, and Arthritic Disorders

CLASSIFICATION OF DRUGS FOR PAIN, INFLAMMATION, AND ARTHRITIC DISORDERS*

Nonsteroidal Anti-inflammatory Drugs
Nonselective Cyclooxygenase Inhibitors
- Aspirin and other salicylates
- Acetaminophen (TYLENOL)
- Ibuprofen (MOTRIN, ADVIL)
- Ketoprofen (ORUDIS)
- Naproxen (NAPROSYN, ALLEVE)
- Indomethacin (INDOCIN)
- Sulindac (CLINORIL)
- Ketorolac (TORADOL)
- Piroxicam (FELDENE)
- Nabumetone (RELAFEN)
- Etodolac (LODINE)
- Meloxicam (MOBIC)

Selective Cyclooxygenase-2 Inhibitors
- Celecoxib (CELEBREX)
- Rofecoxib (VIOXX)
- Valdecoxib (BEXTRA)

Disease-Modifying Antirheumatic Drugs
Gold Salts
- Auranofin (RIDAURA)
- Gold sodium thiomalate (MYOCHRYSINE, AUROLATE)
- Aurothioglucose (SOLGANAL)

Glucocorticoids
- Prednisone (DELTASONE)

Other Disease-modifying Antirheumatic Drugs
- Methotrexate (RHEUMATREX)
- Leflunomide (ARAVA)
- Hydroxychloroquine (PLAQUENIL)
- Etanercept (ENBREL)
- Infliximab (REMICADE)
- Adalimumab (HUMIRA)
- Anakinra (KINERET)
- Penicillamine (CUPRIMINE)
- Sulfasalazine (AZULFIDINE)

Drugs for Gout
Drugs to Prevent Gout Attacks
- Probenecid (BENEMID)
- Sulfinpyrazone (ANTURANE)
- Allopurinol (ZYLOPRIM)

Drugs to Treat Gout Attacks
- Colchicine
- Indomethacin and other NSAID

*Note that some drugs are listed more than once.

OVERVIEW

A variety of medical disorders and injuries are characterized by pain and inflammation. This chapter describes the pharmacologic properties of **nonsteroidal anti-inflammatory drugs (NSAID)**, which are widely used to alleviate the symptoms of rheumatoid arthritis, osteoarthritis, and gout, as well as to relieve the pain and fever that accompany many nonarthritic disorders. The chapter also discusses **disease-modifying antirheumatic drugs (DMARD)** and drugs for the **prevention and treatment of gout.**

RHEUMATOID ARTHRITIS

Rheumatoid arthritis (RA) is an autoimmune disorder of unknown etiology. RA is characterized by symmetric joint inflammation and most patients with RA experience a chronic, fluctuating course of disease that, despite therapeutic measures, can result in progressive joint destruction, deformity, disability, and premature death. Rheumatoid arthritis affects 2% to 3% of the US population, making it the most common systemic inflammatory disease. It is three times more common in women than in men. RA is characterized by symmetric joint inflammation. Those most frequently affected are the small joints of the hands, wrists, and feet, but the joints of the ankles, elbows, hips, knees, and shoulders can also be involved. Cardiopulmonary, neurologic, and ocular inflammation are commonly found in patients with RA, and many patients develop rheumatoid nodules on the extensor surfaces of the elbows, forearms, and hands. In addition, many patients have extra-articular manifestations, such as vasculitis, lymphadenopathy, and splenomegaly.

As shown in Fig. 30–1, rheumatoid arthritis is triggered by autoimmune mechanisms that lead to the destruction of synovial tissue and other connective tissue. Both humoral and cellular immune mechanisms are involved in the pathogenesis of the disease. These mechanisms include the cytokine-mediated activation of T and B lymphocytes and the recruitment and activation of macrophages. The inflammatory leukocytes then release a variety of prostaglandins, cytotoxic compounds, and free radicals that cause joint inflammation and destruction. Patients with RA show elevated levels of IgRF complexes and extracorporeal filtering of these complexes using immunoabsorption apheresis has helped some patients.

In patients with rheumatoid arthritis, NSAID are used to relieve pain and inflammation, and DMARD are used to suppress the underlying disease process and slow the progression of joint destruction. The sites of action of selected antirheumatic drugs are depicted in Fig. 30–1 and discussed below.

OSTEOARTHRITIS

Osteoarthritis, also called **degenerative joint disease,** is the most common joint disease in the world. It affects about 10% of persons over 60 years of age, and radiographic evidence of osteoarthritis can be found in most persons over 65. The disease is not simply associated with aging, however. Other factors that increase the risk for osteoarthritis include obesity, osteoporosis, smoking, heredity, repetitive use of joints through work or leisure activities, and joint trauma.

Osteoarthritis primarily affects weight-bearing joints and causes deformity, limitation of motion, and progressive disability. The cartilage undergoes thickening, inflammation, splitting, and thinning. Eventually, the cartilaginous layer is completely destroyed, leading to erosion and microfractures

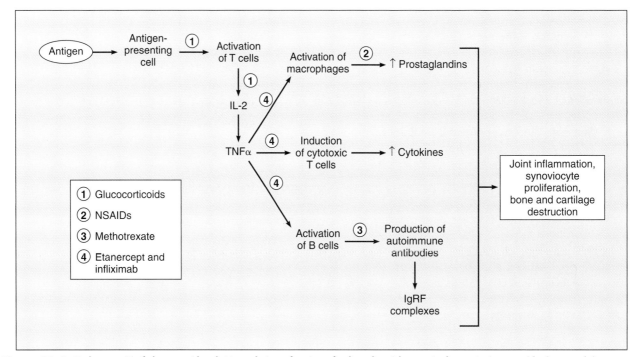

Figure 30–1. Pathogenesis of rheumatoid arthritis and sites of action of selected antirheumatic drugs. In this simplified view of the immune system, antigen-presenting cells phagocytose antigens and present them to T cells, thereby activating the T cells. Activated T cells produce cytokines (IL-2, IL-1, TNFα and others) that stimulate the production of B and T cells. B cells produce plasma cells that form antibodies. T helper cells activate macrophages and cytotoxic T cells. Together, T cells, macrophages, and cytotoxic T cells produce cytotoxic cytokines and prostaglandins that cause joint inflammation, synovial proliferation, and bone and cartilage destruction. Glucocorticoids inhibit T-cell activation and interleukin-2 (IL-2) production by regulation of gene transcription. Glucocorticoids and nonsteroidal anti-inflammatory drugs (NSAID) inhibit the formation of prostaglandins. Methotrexate inhibits the proliferation and activity of T cells and B cells. Etanercept and infliximab inactivate a cytokine called tumor necrosis factor-α (TNFα). Immunoglobin G-rheumatoid factor (IgRF) complexes are detected in the blood of patients with rheumatoid arthritis.

in the underlying bone. The major symptoms of osteoarthritis are pain, stiffness, and muscle weakness around affected joints.

Nonpharmacologic measures for treating osteoarthritis include joint protection and splinting, physiotherapy, orthotic prostheses to support the feet, and joint replacement surgery. Pharmacologic measures include NSAID, local glucocorticoid injections, and experimental chondroprotective drugs (e.g., chondroitin sulfate and glucosamine). Recently, sodium hyaluronate (SUPARTZ) was approved for intra-articular injection as a type of joint fluid replacement in the treatment of osteoarthritis. It is a sterile, viscoelastic solution prepared from chicken combs.

GOUT

Gout is an arthritic syndrome caused by an inflammatory response to crystals of **monosodium urate monohydrate** in joints, renal tubules, and other tissues. The deposition of these crystals occurs as a consequence of **hyperuricemia,** which can result from overproduction or underexcretion of uric acid. Other risk factors for gout include obesity, alcohol consumption, and hypertension.

Acute gout is treated with an NSAID or colchicine to relieve joint inflammation. Subsequent attacks of gout can be prevented by long-term therapy with a drug that either increases uric acid excretion or inhibits uric acid formation and thereby reduces the serum level of uric acid.

NONSTEROIDAL ANTI-INFLAMMATORY DRUGS (NSAID)

MECHANISM OF ACTION

The nonsteroidal anti-inflammatory drugs comprise a large family of weakly acidic drugs whose pharmacologic effects result primarily from the inhibition of **cyclooxygenase (COX)**, an enzyme that catalyzes the first step in the synthesis of **prostaglandins** from arachidonic acid and other precursor fatty acids (see Chapter 26). COX is a microsomal enzyme, existing as a dimer (two molecules linked to form a functional unit) in the lumen and membrane of the endoplasmic reticulum. NSAID decrease COX activity primarily by competitive inhibition; however, aspirin forms a covalent, irreversible inhibition of COX (Fig. 30–2). The net effect of NSAID administration is a decrease in the production of prostaglandins.

Prostaglandin Effects

Prostaglandins play an important role in the development of pain, inflammation, and fever.

Prostaglandins are released from cells in response to chemical stimuli or physical trauma. They sensitize sensory nerves to nociceptive stimuli and thereby amplify the formation of pain impulses. They also promote tissue inflammation by stimulating inflammatory cell chemotaxis, causing vasodilation and increasing capillary permeability and edema.

Fever, defined as the elevation of body temperature to a level above 37°C (98.6°F), often results from an alteration of hypothalamic thermoregulatory mechanisms. Bacterial toxins and other pyrogens stimulate the production of cytokines by leukocytes, and these cytokines increase prostaglandin synthesis in the preoptic area of the hypothalamus. The prostaglandins then act to reset the body's thermostat to a new point above 37°C. This, in turn, activates temperature-raising mechanisms, such as a reduction in heat loss via cutaneous vasodilation, and causes the temperature to rise. All NSAID relieve fever by inhibiting prostaglandin synthesis in the hypothalamus, but these drugs are not capable of reducing body temperature below normal.

Cyclooxygenase Isozymes

Cyclooxygenase is now known to occur in two major isoforms: **cyclooxygenase-1 (COX-1)** and **cyclooxygenase-2 (COX-2).** COX-1 is a constitutive or "housekeeping" enzyme that is found in relatively constant levels in various tissues. COX-1 participates in the synthesis of prostaglandins that have a cytoprotective effect on the gastrointestinal (GI) tract. It also catalyzes the formation of thromboxane A_2 in platelets, leading to platelet aggregation and hemostasis. In contrast, COX-2 is an inducible enzyme. Its levels are normally very low in most tissues but are rapidly upregulated during the inflammatory process by proinflammatory substances (e.g., cytokines, endotoxins, and tumor promoters). Both COX-1 and COX-2 appear to participate in renal homeostasis.

Most of the NSAID available today are nonselective inhibitors of COX-1 and COX-2. The discovery of COX isozymes led to the development of selective COX-2 inhibitors, the first one being **celecoxib.** These selective inhibitors are effective anti-inflammatory drugs, and they produce less GI bleeding and ulcers than do the nonselective COX inhibitors.

A third COX isozyme (**COX-3**), which was recently discovered, appears to be a splice variant of COX-1. Acetaminophen shows the greatest inhibition of this enzyme form and this finding likely explains the reason that acetaminophen has little anti-inflammatory action.

SPECIFIC AGENTS

Nonselective Cyclooxygenase Inhibitors

Among the nonselective COX inhibitors are many well-known NSAID that are available without a prescription, including aspirin, ibuprofen, ketoprofen, and naproxen. Acetaminophen is only a weak anti-inflammatory agent, but it is also included in this class of drugs because it exerts analgesic and antipyretic effects via inhibition of COX. As shown in Table 30–1, the NSAID vary greatly in potency and half-life, but most of them are administered from two to four times a day with food.

Lower doses of NSAID are usually sufficient to treat mild to moderate pain and counteract fever, whereas higher doses are generally needed to relieve inflammation associated with

Figure 30–2. Mechanism of action for aspirin. (A) The COX enzyme exists as a homodimer with two interlocking identical molecules each providing an active channel for its substrates. Aspirin is chemically known as acetylsalicylate acid. (B) Aspirin molecules enter the active channel of COX and add an acetyl group to an amino acid R-group in the active site of COX. The acetyl group is attached to serine at the 530 position in COX-1 and to serine at the 516 position in COX-2. This produces irreversible or noncompetitive inhibition. (C) The aspirin molecule without the acetyl group is called salicylic acid or salicylate, which is a competitive inhibitor of COX.

TABLE 30–1. **Properties of Nonsteroidal Anti-inflammatory Drugs**

Drug	Relative Potency	Half-Life (Hours)	Daily Doses
Nonselective cyclooxygenase inhibitors			
Acetaminophen	1	3	4
Aspirin	1	2*	4
Ibuprofen	4	2	2–4
Indomethacin	40	4	1–3
Ketoprofen	20	2	2–4
Ketorolac	100	7	4
Naproxen	4	14	2
Selective cyclooxygenase-2 inhibitors			
Celecoxib	20	11	2

*For aspirin, the value shown is the half-life of the active metabolite, salicylic acid.

arthritic disorders and injuries. NSAID are particularly effective in relieving pain caused by tissue inflammation or by bone or joint trauma, and they can be combined with opioid analgesics to obtain a greater analgesic effect and reduce the need for higher doses of opioids. For example, NSAID are widely used in the treatment of postoperative pain, either alone or in combination with an opioid.

Recent studies have shown that NSAID can delay or slow the progress of Alzheimer's disease. The neurodegeneration that occurs in this disease is accompanied by inflammatory mechanisms that involve COX and the activation of the complement cascade.

Increased expression of COX-2 is seen in some cancer cells and the angiogenesis essential to tumor growth requires COX-2. Overexpression of COX-2 leads to increased expression of vascular endothelial growth factor (VEGF). Regular use of NSAID has been shown to decrease the risk of developing colorectal cancer. This can be especially so with the COX-2 selective NSAID.

Although NSAID are effective in relieving the pain of chronic disorders, their long-term use is associated with a number of adverse effects, including GI bleeding, peptic ulcers, and renal and hepatic dysfunction. Acetaminophen produces fewer GI problems than do other nonselective COX inhibitors, but it also lacks significant antiplatelet and anti-inflammatory activity. Although acetaminophen can be used concurrently with another NSAID for supplemental analgesia, alternative combinations of two NSAID should generally be avoided, not only because they increase the risk of GI and other side effects but also because they sometimes have adverse interactions. For example, aspirin and other salicylates displace some NSAID (e.g., ketorolac) from plasma proteins and thereby increase their serum levels significantly.

The NSAID can interact with a large number of other drugs through pharmacokinetic and pharmacodynamic mechanisms. Most NSAID inhibit the renal excretion of lithium and can increase lithium serum levels and toxicity. NSAID can reduce the clearance of methotrexate and aminoglycoside drugs. NSAID can also interfere to varying degrees with the antihypertensive effect of diuretics, β-adrenergic receptor antagonists, angiotensin inhibitors, and other antihypertensive drugs. When given with potassium-sparing diuretics, NSAID can cause potassium retention and lead to hyperkalemia. Some drug interactions are only associated with particular NSAID. For example, high doses of salicylates exert a hypoglycemic effect that can alter the effects of antidiabetic drugs. Indomethacin reduces the natriuretic effect of diuretics and can cause nephrotoxicity when given with triamterene.

Low doses of acetaminophen can be safely used for analgesia and antipyresis during pregnancy. The use of other NSAID during the second half of pregnancy is generally not recommended, however, because of potential adverse effects to the fetus. These effects result from prostaglandin inhibition and include GI bleeding, platelet inhibition, renal dysfunction, and premature closure of the ductus arteriosus.

Aspirin and Other Salicylates

The therapeutic value of salicylates was originally recognized when they were identified as the active ingredients of willow bark and other plant materials used in folk medicine to relieve pain and fever. Aspirin was synthesized in 1899 during a search for a salicylate derivative that would be less irritating to the stomach than salicylic acid. Aspirin soon became widely used around the world as an analgesic, antipyretic, and anti-inflammatory drug.

CHEMISTRY. Salicylic acid derivatives include aspirin (acetylsalicylic acid, ASA) and several nonacetylated drugs, such as salsalate, choline magnesium salicylate, and methyl salicylate (oil of wintergreen).

PHARMACOLOGIC EFFECTS AND INDICATIONS. In adults, the salicylates can be used in the management of **pain, fever,** and **inflammation,** as well as in the prophylaxis of **myocardial infarction, stroke, and other thromboembolic disorders.** In children, the use of salicylates should be avoided, because the risk of Reye's syndrome appears to be increased in virus-infected children who are treated with these drugs.

The analgesic, antipyretic, and anti-inflammatory effects of aspirin and other salicylates result from nonspecific inhibition of COX in peripheral tissues and the central nervous system. Aspirin irreversibly acetylates platelet COX and has a longer-lasting effect on thromboxane synthesis than do other salicylates. The antiplatelet effect of aspirin persists for about 14 days, whereas that of most other NSAID is much shorter. The effect is long-lived, because platelets lack a nucleus and do not make new COX enzyme.

The salicylates are usually administered orally, but formulations are also available for topical and rectal administration. The oral dosage of aspirin that is needed to inhibit platelet aggregation is somewhat lower than the oral dosage needed to obtain analgesic and antipyretic effects, and it is much lower than the oral dosage needed to relieve inflammation caused by arthritic and other inflammatory disorders. Fig. 30–3 shows the relationship between the dosage of aspirin and the pharmacologic and toxic effects of the drug.

PHARMACOKINETICS. Aspirin is well absorbed from the gut. Although its concurrent administration with antacids may slow its absorption rate, it will not significantly reduce its bioavailability. Aspirin is rapidly hydrolyzed to salicylic acid by plasma esterase, and this accounts for its short plasma half-life (about 15 minutes). Most of the pharmacologic effects of aspirin are attributed to its salicylic acid metabolite, which has a half-life of about 2 hours. Aspirin itself, however, is responsible for irreversible inhibition of platelet COX and platelet aggregation.

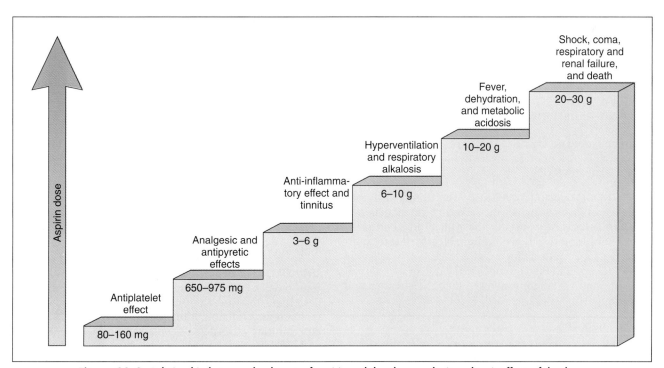

Figure 30–3. Relationship between the dosage of aspirin and the pharmacologic and toxic effects of the drug.

Most of the salicylic acid formed from aspirin and other salicylate drugs is conjugated with glycine to form salicyluric acid. This substance is then excreted in the urine, along with about 10% of free salicylate and a similar amount of glucuronide conjugates. The rate of excretion of salicylate is affected by urine pH. For this reason, alkalinization of the urine by administration of sodium bicarbonate has been used to increase the ionization and elimination of salicylic acid in cases of drug overdose (see Chapter 2).

When a therapeutic dose of aspirin or other salicylate is ingested, the rate of metabolism and the rate of excretion of salicylic acid are proportional to the drug's plasma concentration (first-order elimination). When an excessive dose is taken, the elimination pathways become saturated, giving rise to zero-order elimination. For this reason, larger doses can rapidly elevate plasma salicylate concentrations to toxic levels, especially in the elderly, who are at greatest risk of aspirin toxicity.

ADVERSE EFFECTS. The use of aspirin in children with chickenpox and other viral infections has been associated with Reye's syndrome. As mentioned, treatment with salicylates, therefore, should be avoided in children.

Therapeutic doses of aspirin can cause gastric irritation and contribute to GI bleeding and peptic ulcers. Moderately high therapeutic doses can cause tinnitus, which is described as an abnormal auditory sensation or noise.

Excessive doses of aspirin produce the toxic effects shown in Fig. 30–3. Hyperventilation is caused by direct and indirect stimulation of the respiratory center in the medulla, and it often leads to increased exhalation of carbon dioxide and respiratory alkalosis. Higher plasma salicylate concentrations can cause fever, dehydration, and severe metabolic acidosis. If not treated promptly, these events can culminate in shock, coma, organ system failure, and death. Excessive doses of aspirin can also cause a hypoprothrombinemic effect that impairs hemostasis and causes bleeding.

Aspirin hypersensitivity is an uncommon but serious condition that can result in severe and potentially fatal anaphylactic reactions. Symptoms of aspirin intolerance include vasomotor rhinitis, angioedema, and urticaria (hives). Aspirin sensitivity occurs most frequently in persons with asthma, nasal polyps, or chronic urticaria. Persons who have had a severe hypersensitivity reaction to aspirin or another salicylate should not be treated with another type of NSAID, because a 5% risk of cross-sensitivity exists between salicylates and other NSAID.

TREATMENT OF SALICYLATE OVERDOSE. The treatment of salicylate poisoning may include the following: (1) induction of vomiting and gastric lavage to remove unabsorbed drug; (2) intravenous administration of **sodium bicarbonate** to counteract metabolic acidosis, increase the ionization of salicylate in the kidneys, and thereby enhance the rate of excretion of salicylate; and (3) administration of fluids, electrolytes, and other supportive care, as needed.

Acetaminophen

CHEMISTRY, PHARMACOLOGIC EFFECTS, AND INDICATIONS. For more than 100 years, acetaminophen has been available for the treatment of **mild pain and fever.** The drug is a *p*-aminophenol derivative that exerts analgesic and antipyretic effects at doses that are well tolerated and produce remarkably few adverse effects during short-term administration. Unlike aspirin use, acetaminophen use has not been associated with Reye's syndrome, so acetaminophen can be safely given to patients with fever caused by viral illnesses.

Acetaminophen has only weak anti-inflammatory activity, partly because it is inactivated by peroxides produced in the cells of inflamed tissue. Recent evidence suggests the existence of a third COX isoform, designated COX-3, with roles in mediating pain and fever, and subject to inhibition by acetaminophen. Acetaminophen has little effect on COX-1 or COX-2 and, thus, lacks anti-inflammatory activity. Although acetaminophen is not considered a first-line drug for patients with arthritic disorders, it is sometimes used as an analgesic in those with **mild arthritis.** Because acetaminophen lacks the ability to inhibit thromboxane synthesis and platelet aggregation, it is not used for the prophylaxis of myocardial infarction, stroke, or other thromboembolic disorders.

PHARMACOKINETICS. Acetaminophen is rapidly absorbed from the gut, exhibits minimal binding to plasma proteins, and is widely distributed to peripheral tissues and the central nervous system.

As shown in Fig. 30–4, acetaminophen is extensively metabolized by several pathways in the liver. Most of the drug is conjugated with sulfate and glucuronide, and these metabolites are excreted in the urine. A small amount of acetaminophen is converted by cytochrome P450 to a potentially hepatotoxic quinone intermediate. When a therapeutic dose of acetaminophen is taken, the quinone intermediate is rapidly inactivated by conjugation with glutathione. Toxic doses of acetaminophen, however, deplete hepatic glutathione, cause accumulation of the quinone intermediate, and lead to hepatic necrosis. To prevent liver damage, patients who ingest an overdose and are determined to be at risk for hepatotoxicity can be given acetylcysteine, a sulfhydryl compound that conjugates the quinone intermediate and renders it harmless.

ADVERSE EFFECTS. Some epidemiologic evidence indicates that long-term use of acetaminophen is associated with an increased risk of renal dysfunction.

Although therapeutic doses of acetaminophen are remarkably nontoxic, the ingestion of 20 to 30 tablets is sufficient to cause life-threatening hepatotoxicity.

TREATMENT OF ACETAMINOPHEN OVERDOSE. Because hepatotoxicity gradually progresses over several days following an acetaminophen overdose, prompt treatment with **acetylcysteine** can prevent or significantly reduce hepatotoxicity.

Ibuprofen, Ketoprofen, and Naproxen

CHEMISTRY, PHARMACOLOGIC EFFECTS, AND INDICATIONS. Ibuprofen, ketoprofen, and naproxen are propionic acid derivatives that are among the most widely used NSAID for **pain and inflammation caused by trauma, infection, autoimmune disorders, neoplasms, joint degeneration, and other factors.** By reversibly and nonselectively inhibiting COX isozymes, these drugs can exert their analgesic, antipyretic, and anti-inflammatory effects. Low-dose for-

Figure 30–4. Acetaminophen metabolism and hepatotoxicity. Acetaminophen is primarily metabolized by conjugation with sulfate and glucuronide. A minor pathway involves oxidation of acetaminophen by cytochrome P450 enzymes to form a potentially toxic intermediate, N-acetyl-benzoquinoneimine. When a therapeutic dose of acetaminophen is taken, this quinone intermediate is conjugated with glutathione and excreted in the urine. When a toxic dose of acetaminophen is taken, glutathione stores are depleted, and the quinone intermediate attacks hepatic cell macromolecules. This process results in hepatic necrosis. Acetylcysteine (MUCOMYST) given to treat acetaminophen overdose protects the liver by maintaining or restoring the glutathione levels, or by acting as an alternate substrate for conjugation with, and thus, detoxification of the reactive metabolite.

mulations of the drugs are now available without prescription for the treatment of mild pain and inflammation. The higher-dose formulations used to treat most arthritic disorders still require a prescription.

PHARMACOKINETICS. Ibuprofen, ketoprofen, and naproxen are administered orally, are widely distributed, and are extensively metabolized to inactive metabolites in the liver before undergoing renal excretion. Naproxen has a longer half-life (14 hours) than does ibuprofen or ketoprofen (2 hours each). For this reason, naproxen is given twice daily, whereas ibuprofen or ketoprofen is usually administered from two to four times a day.

ADVERSE EFFECTS. Ibuprofen and related drugs produce dose-dependent gastric irritation, nausea, dyspepsia, and bleeding. Long-term administration of high doses has been associated with peptic ulcer disease, but short-term use of low doses causes very few serious adverse effects. Among the serious effects that have been reported are hepatic toxicity and renal toxicity. In some cases, acute renal failure occurred following short-term use of therapeutic doses by patients who failed to ingest adequate fluids and became dehydrated.

Indomethacin, Sulindac, and Ketorolac

Indomethacin, an indoleacetic acid derivative, is often regarded as one of the most potent inhibitors of COX isozymes. Because of its greater tendency to cause adverse effects, this drug is usually reserved for the management of **moderate to severe acute inflammatory conditions.** It is also used to treat infants with a **patent ductus arteriosus.** In these infants, indomethacin inhibits the synthesis of prostaglandins and thereby causes closure of the ductus.

The incidence of GI and central nervous system side effects is higher with the use of indomethacin than with the use of many other NSAID. Indomethacin therapy is also associated with a risk of serious hematologic toxicity. Hence, therapy should be limited to short-term use whenever possible, and patients should be closely monitored.

Sulindac, which is structurally related to indomethacin, is actually a prodrug converted to an active sulfide metabolite. The parent compound, sulindac sulfoxide, is inactive in COX inhibition assays done in vitro as biotransformation in the liver produces the active metabolite. It is noted for having a 'renal-sparing' effect such that at moderate doses alters the renal prostaglandin production less than other NSAID. Besides sulindac use in the treatment of RA, it is also administered to treat adenomas in polyp disease.

Ketorolac is an arylacetic acid derivative. It has potent analgesic activity and is one of the few NSAID that is available for parenteral use for either intravenous or intramuscular administration.

In studies of mild to moderate postoperative pain, ketorolac produced a level of analgesia comparable to that produced by morphine but caused less nausea, vomiting, and drowsiness. Ketorolac, therefore, has been widely used for the short-term management of **moderate pain,** such as **postoperative pain associated with dental surgery.** Although the drug has also been used to treat **migraine headaches,** it does not appear to be superior to ibuprofen for treatment of musculoskeletal pain. The ophthalmic solution for ketorolac is used to treat **allergic conjunctivitis** and **postoperative ocular inflammation.**

Ketorolac causes fewer adverse GI and central nervous system effects than do opioid analgesics, but it poses a significant risk of hematologic toxicity and other adverse effects. For this reason, oral or parenteral therapy with the drug must be limited to 5 or fewer days. In patients with renal or hepatic disease, ketorolac should be used with caution because it is associated with an increased risk of severe renal or hepatic impairment. A similar drug, **bromfenac** (DURACT), was withdrawn from the market in 1998, following postmarketing reports of hepatic failure and death.

Piroxicam and Nabumetone

Piroxicam is an effective anti-inflammatory agent with a potency equal to aspirin or naproxen for the chronic treatment of RA. The main advantage of piroxicam is its 50 hour plasma half-life. This allows a single daily dose in most patients, although it can take up to 2 weeks to achieve maximal therapeutic effect.

One of the few nonacid NSAID, **nabumetone,** is a ketone prodrug with weak COX inhibitory activity in vitro. It is converted to one or more active metabolites in vivo and a potent inhibition of COX activity occurs with these metabolites. It also has the advantage that a half-life of 20 hours allows once daily dosing in most patients.

Etodolac and Meloxicam

Other NSAID, including **meloxicam** and **etodolac,** which have been marketed in Europe or the United States as safer NSAID, were found after the discovery of COX-2 to be preferential inhibitors of this enzyme. They are more selective for COX-2 than typical NSAID but not as selective as the COX-2 inhibitors.

Selective Cyclooxygenase-2 Inhibitors

Celecoxib, Rofecoxib, and Valdecoxib

The selective cyclooxygenase-2 inhibitors are a new group of drugs that appear to provide potent anti-inflammatory activity without causing significant GI toxicity. **Celecoxib** (CELEBREX), the first selective COX-2 inhibitor to be marketed, was soon followed by the release of **rofecoxib** (VIOXX) and **valdecoxib** (BEXTRA). Together, these agents are known as 'coxibs.' In late 2004, the makers of rofecoxib voluntarily withdrew the drug from the market after data were analyzed from a clinical trial testing rofecoxib's effectiveness in preventing recurrence of colorectal polyps. This study found an increased relative risk for confirmed cardiovascular events (e.g., heart attack and stroke) beginning after 18 months of treatment in the patients taking rofecoxib compared with those taking placebo. Valdecoxib has also shown an increased risk for cardiovascular events in patients after heart surgery. Serious skin reactions (e.g., toxic epidermal necrolysis, Stevens-Johnson syndrome, and erythema multiforme) have been reported in patients receiving valdecoxib. Some of these reactions have resulted in fatalities. For these reasons, the US Food and Drug Administration (FDA) removed valdecoxib from the market in 2005.

With regard to celecoxib, patients in a colon cancer clinical trial taking 400 mg of celecoxib twice daily had a 3.4 times greater risk of cardiovascular events compared with those taking placebo. For patients in the trial taking 200 mg of celecoxib twice daily, the risk was 2.5 times greater. The FDA strengthened the warnings for use of the remaining COX-2 inhibitor, celecoxib. At the time of this writing, it is not clear if all COX-2 inhibitors share the same cardiovascular risk or if newer agents, still in development, will show less cardiovascular risk and make it to the market.

CHEMISTRY, PHARMACOLOGIC EFFECTS, AND INDICATIONS. Celecoxib is a potent analgesic, antipyretic, and anti-inflammatory agent. This drug does not inhibit platelet aggregation, because platelets contain only the COX-1 isozyme.

In clinical studies of **osteoarthritis** and **rheumatoid arthritis,** celecoxib was shown to be as efficacious as naproxen without causing significant side effects. In a study of postoperative pain management, however, celecoxib was reported to provide insufficient analgesia to control pain after general surgery. In laboratory studies, investigators found that celecoxib was more effective than nonselective COX inhibitors in protecting against **colon carcinogenesis.** This finding suggested a role for prophylactic coxib use in persons with a high risk of colon cancer; however, clinical trials were halted because of cardiovascular events (see above).

PHARMACOKINETICS. Celecoxib is available for oral administration and is usually taken twice daily. The drug is rapidly absorbed from the gut, is metabolized by cytochrome P450 isozyme CYP2C9, and is excreted in the feces and urine. The half-life is about 11 hours.

ADVERSE EFFECTS AND INTERACTIONS. Besides the risk of cardiovascular events, celecoxib appears to cause a low incidence of adverse reactions, the most common of which are diarrhea, dyspepsia, and abdominal pain. This drug is associated with a much lower incidence of gastroduodenal ulcers than the nonselective NSAID (e.g., ibuprofen and naproxen).

Because celecoxib is metabolized by CYP2C9, drugs such as fluconazole, fluvastatin, and zafirlukast may inhibit its metabolism and increase its serum concentration. Lower doses of celecoxib should be used in patients treated concurrently with these interacting drugs.

DISEASE-MODIFYING ANTIRHEUMATIC DRUGS

The disease-modifying antirheumatic drugs (DMARD) are agents capable of slowing the progression of joint erosions in patients with RA. Examples of DMARD are gold salts, glucocorticoids, hydroxychloroquine, methotrexate (MTX), and a number of newer immunologic agents, including leflunomide, etanercept, and infliximab. These drugs have a delayed onset of action and require several weeks to months before their antirheumatic benefits are observed. Several studies suggest that using a combination of DMARD is more effective than using a single DMARD in many patients with RA.

Disease-modifying antirheumatic drugs act by various mechanisms to suppress the proliferation and activity of lymphocytes and polymorphonuclear leukocytes and thereby counteract their ability to cause joint inflammation and destruction. Because joint erosion is usually found within the first 2 years of RA, many rheumatologists prescribe DMARD at the time of diagnosis. The utility of DMARD, however, is often limited by their toxicity or by their loss of efficacy over time, and many patients must cease taking them within 5 years of commencing therapy.

GOLD SALTS

Gold salts were first used to treat RA in the late 1920s, from the finding of Robert Koch in 1890 that elemental gold inhibited the growth of *Mycobacterium tuberculosis* and the mistaken belief that the swollen joints characteristic of RA were caused by these infectious agents. They were once used extensively in the management of this disease, but their popularity has declined with the introduction of newer DMARD, which tend to be more efficacious and less toxic. Both oral and parenteral gold preparations are available. The oral compound, **auranofin,** is poorly absorbed from the gut, however, and may be less efficacious than parenteral preparations, such as **gold sodium thiomalate** (also called **sodium aurothiomalate**). A second preparation of gold for intravenous administration is available as **aurothioglucose.** The antirheumatic effects of gold salts are usually not observed until 3 to 6 months after starting therapy.

Gold salts can cause a variety of adverse hematologic, dermatologic, GI, and renal effects. Flushing, hypotension, and tachycardia are sometimes observed. Skin rash and stomatitis are commonly observed and require discontinuation of treatment until they resolve.

GLUCOCORTICOIDS

For many years, **prednisone** and other glucocorticoids have played an important role in the treatment of RA. These drugs induce the formation of lipocortin, a protein that inhibits phospholipase A_2 activity. By this mechanism, they inhibit the release of arachidonic acid from cell membranes and the formation of prostaglandins. Glucocorticoids also inhibit the production of numerous cytokines, including interleukins and tumor necrosis factor (TNF), by regulation of their gene transcription.

Glucocorticoids act more rapidly than other DMARD, but their long-term use is limited by the development of serious adverse effects. In light of these facts, glucocorticoids have been used in various ways to manage patients with RA or other inflammatory joint diseases. For example, they have been used to induce a remission in the disease at the time that therapy with another (slower-acting) DMARD is started; to provide short courses of therapy during disease flare-ups; and to provide continuous low-dose background therapy in patients being treated with other DMARD and NSAID.

OTHER DISEASE-MODIFYING ANTIRHEUMATIC DRUGS

Methotrexate

Methotrexate is an antineoplastic and immunomodulating drug whose properties are discussed in detail in Chapter 45. The drug was first used to treat RA in the 1980s, and it remains the single most effective DMARD available today.

Methotrexate has several mechanisms of action. It inhibits human folate reductase and thereby reduces the availability of active forms of folate that are required for thymidylate and DNA synthesis. It also inhibits lymphocyte proliferation and the production of cytokines and rheumatoid factor. In addition, it interferes with polymorphonuclear leukocyte chemotaxis and reduces the production of cytotoxins and free radicals that damage the synovial membrane and bone.

Methotrexate is considered the DMARD of choice for most patients with RA. The drug can be given orally or intramuscularly and has a fairly rapid onset of action, with benefits observed as early as 2 to 3 weeks after therapy is started. From 45% to 55% of patients continue therapy for at least 5 to 7 years, and sustained efficacy for up to 15 years has been demonstrated in some patients. The combined use of MTX and other DMARD is often more effective than single-drug therapy.

Treatment with MTX is generally well tolerated by patients with RA, but it can cause adverse GI, hematologic, hepatic, and pulmonary reactions. Elevated liver enzyme levels are found in up to 15% of patients treated with MTX, but serious hepatotoxicity is rare. The administration of folic acid supplements does not reduce the drug efficacy and may prevent some of these adverse effects.

The use of MTX is contraindicated in pregnancy.

Leflunomide

Leflunomide is a newer immunosuppressive drug that acts as a powerful inhibitor of mononuclear and T-cell proliferation. The active metabolite of leflunomide inhibits a key enzyme in pyrimidine synthesis, dihydroorotate dehydrogenase, and thereby prevents replication of DNA and synthesis of RNA and protein in immune cells. Leflunomide is converted to its active metabolite in the intestinal wall and liver. The active metabolite is further metabolized and excreted in the urine and feces, with an elimination half-life of about 2 weeks.

Leflunomide is marketed as an alternative to MTX for the first-line management of RA. In a controlled trial, 41% of patients treated with leflunomide showed significant improvement in tender and swollen joints, compared with 35% of those treated with MTX and 19% given a placebo.

The adverse effects of leflunomide include diarrhea and reversible alopecia. The drug can increase serum levels of hepatic enzymes and increase the risk of hepatotoxicity when it is used in combination with MTX. The active metabolite of leflunomide inhibits CYP2C9 and may thereby increase the serum level of many drugs, including ibuprofen and some of the other NSAID.

Leflunomide is teratogenic, so its use is contraindicated in pregnancy.

Hydroxychloroquine

Hydroxychloroquine, an antimalarial drug related to chloroquine, has been extensively used as a DMARD. It inhibits the function of lymphocytes, reduces the chemotaxis and phagocytosis of polymorphonuclear leukocytes, and decreases the production of superoxide radicals by these cells. The drug has a slow onset of action and can require 6 months of therapy before benefits are observed. It does not produce the myelosuppressive, hepatic, and renal toxicities that many other DMARD produce. Hydroxychloroquine occasionally causes GI disturbances, and patients undergoing hydroxychloroquine treatment must be monitored for adverse ocular effects, including blurred vision, scotomas, and night blindness.

Immunomodulators

Etanercept, Infliximab, and Adalimumab

Etanercept, infliximab, and adalimumab are immunologic agents that exert their antirheumatic effects by binding to and inactivating **tumor necrosis factor.** TNF is one of the proinflammatory cytokines produced by macrophages and activated T cells. Elevated levels of TNF are found in the synovial fluid of joints and play an important role in both the pathologic inflammation and the joint destruction that are hallmarks of RA (see Fig. 30–1).

Etanercept is a protein formed by recombining human p75 (75-kd) TNF receptors with Fc fragments of human immunoglobulin G1 (IgG1). In comparison with the original protein, the recombined protein can antagonize TNF to a greater extent and has a longer half-life. Experimental studies in several animal models of RA have found etanercept treatment to be effective, as have subsequent clinical trials in patients with this disease. According to a 3-month clinical study, 75% of patients with RA had a significant improvement in the signs and symptoms of their disease. The drug was generally well tolerated, although injection site reactions were common.

Etanercept must be administered subcutaneously twice a week and is expensive (a 6-month supply costs about $6300). The drug is currently intended for use in patients whose RA is refractory to treatment with MTX or other DMARD. Etanercept can be used alone or in combination with MTX in these patients.

Infliximab is a chimeric human-murine monoclonal antibody that inactivates TNF. It has been used in the treatment of Crohn's disease and RA. In one clinical trial, infliximab treatment resulted in an improvement of RA manifestations in 80% of patients whose disease was refractory to other drugs. In another study, infliximab was found to be more effective when combined with MTX than when used alone. Infliximab is administered intravenously at 4- to 12-week intervals.

Adalimumab is a human IgG1 monoclonal antibody specific for human TNF. It is made by recombinant DNA technology in a mammalian cell expression system and purified to exclude viral particles. For adult patients, adalimumab (40 mg) is administered every other week as a subcutaneous injection. During adalimumab treatment, administration of MTX, glucocorticoids, salicylates, NSAID, analgesics or other DMARD can continue safely. Some patients not taking concomitant MTX may see additional benefits by increasing the frequency of adalimumab to 40 mg every week.

All TNF blocking agents, including adalimumab, produced serious infections and sepsis, some fatal, during clinical trials. Many of the serious infections were seen in patients on concomitant immunosuppressive therapy that, in addition to their RA, could predispose them to infections. Tuberculosis and invasive opportunistic fungal infections have also been noted during treatment with TNF blockers.

Lymphomas have also been reported in patients treated with TNF blocking agents. In clinical trials, patients with RA, particularly those with highly active disease, were at increased risk (up to several fold) for the development of lymphoma. The role of TNF blockers in the development of malignancy is not known.

Anakinra

Anakinra is a recombinant form of the human interleukin-1 receptor antagonist (IL-1Ra), differing only by the addition of a single methionine residue at its amino terminus. It blocks the biologic activity of IL-1 by competitively inhibiting IL-1 binding to the interleukin-1 type I receptor (IL-1RI). IL-1 production is induced in response to inflammatory stimuli and mediates inflammatory and immunologic responses. IL-1 has a broad range of activities, including cartilage degradation by its induction of the rapid loss of proteoglycans, as well as stimulation of bone resorption. The levels of the naturally occurring IL-1Ra in synovial fluid of patients with RA are not sufficient to compete with the increased production of IL-1.

The recommended dose of anakinra is 100 mg/day administered daily by subcutaneous injection. The adverse effects are the same as for the TNF blockers, with serious infections and lymphoma of most concern.

Sulfasalazine and Penicillamine

Sulfasalazine was originally used in the treatment of RA in 1930s, but only recently was it approved for this indication by the FDA. In the 1920s and 1930s, scientists theorized that RA was an inflammatory disease caused by an infection in the GI tract. Consistent with that hypothesis, sulfasalazine was developed and is a formulation combining an anti-inflammatory drug, 5-amino salicylic acid, with an antibacterial drug, sulfapyridine. Recent experiments suggest that it is sulfapyridine that is active against RA, but the exact mechanism is not known. Because sulfasalazine is a 'sulfa' drug, people who are allergic to sulfa drugs should not take it.

D-penicillamine is a penicillin-derived compound used frequently in the past, but its use today has declined with the increasing use of other disease modifying anti-rheumatic drugs (e.g., methotrexate). It is not understood exactly how penicillamine provides a benefit in RA but it is known to reduce the blood levels of inflammatory cytokines. Penicillamine effects can take up to 3 months to manifest; however, if no effect is seen in a year, it should be stopped.

DRUGS FOR THE TREATMENT OF GOUT

The effective management of gout often requires the use of various agents to prevent and treat acute attacks.

DRUGS FOR PREVENTING GOUT ATTACKS

Gout attacks can be prevented by lowering the serum concentration of uric acid. Probenecid and sulfinpyrazone accomplish this goal by increasing the excretion of uric acid, whereas allopurinol does so by inhibiting the synthesis of uric acid. Uric acid metabolism and sites of drug action are depicted in Fig. 30–5.

Probenecid

A **uricosuric drug,** such as probenecid, is used to prevent gout attacks in persons who under-excrete uric acid, as indicated by a 24-hour uric acid excretion that is less than 800 mg.

Probenecid is a weak acid that competitively inhibits the reabsorption of uric acid by renal tubules and thereby increases the excretion of uric acid. The drug is taken orally and should be swallowed with a full glass of water to ensure adequate fluid intake. Treatment should begin with a low dose, and the dosage should be gradually increased until an adequate uricosuric effect is obtained or the maximal dosage is reached. Probenecid treatment is usually well tolerated.

The use of aspirin and other salicylates can alter or interfere with the uricosuric effect of probenecid, so patients should avoid concurrent use of these agents. High doses of salicylates inhibit uric acid reabsorption and exert a uricosuric effect. Low doses of salicylates, however, inhibit uric acid secretion by renal tubules and thereby increase serum concentrations of uric acid.

Sulfinpyrazone

Sulfinpyrazone is another uricosuric agent that competitively inhibits the active reabsorption of urate at the proximal renal tubule. As with probenecid, it increases the urinary

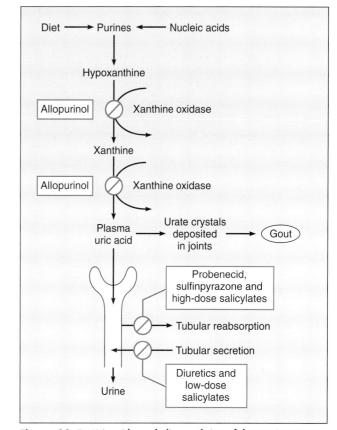

Figure 30–5. Uric acid metabolism and sites of drug action. Purines obtained from the diet or from catabolism of nucleic acids are converted to hypoxanthine. Under normal conditions, xanthine oxidase converts hypoxanthine to xanthine and then to uric acid. Allopurinol acts by inhibiting xanthine oxidase. Probenecid, sulfinpyrazone, and high-dose salicylates inhibit the renal tubular reabsorption of uric acid, whereas diuretics and low-dose salicylates inhibit the renal tubular secretion of uric acid.

excretion of uric acid and lowers serum urate concentrations. Although sulfinpyrazone lacks clinically useful anti-inflammatory or analgesic activity, it inhibits prostaglandin synthesis and shares some of the risks associated with NSAID, including the potential for causing GI, renal, or hematologic adverse effects.

Allopurinol

Allopurinol is used to prevent gout attacks in persons who overproduce uric acid, as indicated by a 24-hour uric acid excretion that is greater than 800 mg. It is also sometimes used to prevent hyperuricemia and gout in persons who are having cancer chemotherapy and whose rate of purine catabolism is high because of the death of neoplastic cells.

Allopurinol and its active metabolite, **oxipurinol** (also called alloxanthine), decrease the production of uric acid by inhibiting xanthine oxidase, the enzyme that converts hypoxanthine to xanthine and xanthine to uric acid. Allopurinol is a competitive inhibitor of **xanthine oxidase.** In contrast to uricosuric drugs, allopurinol causes a decrease in uric acid excretion and a corresponding increase in the urinary excretion of hypoxanthine. In addition, allopurinol increases reutilization of hypoxanthine and xanthine for nucleotide and nucleic acid synthesis via an action on enzyme hypoxanthine-guanine phosphoribosyltransferase (HGPRTase). The resultant increase in nucleotide concentration leads to increased feedback inhibition of *de novo* purine synthesis. By lowering both serum and urine concentrations of uric acid below its solubility limits, allopurinol prevents or decreases urate deposition, thereby preventing the occurrence or progression of both gouty arthritis and urate nephropathy.

Allopurinol is administered orally. Most of the drug is rapidly converted to its active metabolite, oxypurinol, in the liver. Oxypurinol has a half-life of about 20 hours, and most of this metabolite is excreted unchanged in the urine.

About 25% of patients are unable to tolerate allopurinol because of its adverse effects, which include nausea, vomiting, hepatitis, skin rashes, and other forms of hypersensitivity. Because allopurinol inhibits the catabolism of azathioprine and mercaptopurine, doses of these drugs may need to be reduced if allopurinol is given concurrently with either of them.

DRUGS FOR TREATING GOUT ATTACKS

Indomethacin

In patients with acute gout, a potent anti-inflammatory drug is given for the rapid relief of pain. Although **indomethacin** (see previous text) is widely used for this purpose, other NSAID are often effective when used in an adequate dosage. If these drugs do not provide relief or cannot be tolerated by the patient, **colchicine** can be given orally or parenterally.

Colchicine

Colchicine was traditionally used to treat acute gout, but it is less frequently used today because of its unpleasant side effects, which include nausea, vomiting, diarrhea, and abdominal cramps. The drug is believed to act by inhibiting the motility of inflammatory leukocytes and thereby blocking their ability to cause crystal-induced joint inflammation. Colchicine is rapidly absorbed after oral administration. It is partly metabolized in the liver, and the drug and its metabolites are excreted by the biliary and fecal route. If colchicine treatment causes the adverse effects noted above, treatment should be stopped to avoid more serious toxicity.

SUMMARY OF IMPORTANT POINTS

■ Nonsteroidal anti-inflammatory drugs (NSAID) act primarily by inhibiting cyclooxygenase (COX) and the synthesis of prostaglandins. The drugs exhibit varying degrees of analgesic, anti-inflammatory, and antipyretic activity. Most of them also inhibit platelet aggregation. Long-term use of NSAID can lead to renal or hepatic toxicity.

■ Nonselective COX inhibitors include acetaminophen, aspirin, ibuprofen, indomethacin, ketoprofen, ketorolac, and naproxen. Except for acetaminophen, the agents in

this group can cause gastric irritation and bleeding, and their long-term use can lead to peptic ulcers.

■ Acetaminophen is an effective analgesic and antipyretic agent, but it lacks significant anti-inflammatory and antiplatelet activity. A minor metabolite of acetaminophen is a potentially hepatotoxic quinone. This quinone metabolite is normally inactivated by conjugation with glutathione, but toxic doses of acetaminophen can deplete glutathione and cause fatal liver failure.

■ Acetylcysteine, a sulfhydryl compound that conjugates and inactivates the quinone metabolite of acetaminophen, is used as an antidote for acetaminophen hepatotoxicity.

■ Low doses of aspirin have potent antiplatelet effects because they acetylate and irreversibly inhibit platelet COX. Low doses of aspirin also produce analgesic and antipyretic effects, but higher doses are needed to counteract inflammation.

■ High therapeutic doses of aspirin can cause tinnitus. Toxic doses cause hyperventilation and respiratory alkalosis, followed by metabolic acidosis. In cases of severe aspirin toxicity, sodium bicarbonate can be given to counteract acidosis and increase urinary excretion of salicylic acid.

■ Ibuprofen, ketoprofen, and naproxen are potent NSAID that are widely used as analgesic, antipyretic, and anti-inflammatory agents. Ketorolac is a potent analgesic that can be given orally or parenterally. To avoid hematologic toxicity, ketorolac use should be limited to a few days.

■ Indomethacin is a potent COX inhibitor that can be used to treat moderate to severe acute inflammatory conditions. It is also used to cause closure of the ductus arteriosus in infants.

■ Celecoxib, the first selective COX-2 inhibitor, is a potent analgesic, antipyretic, and anti-inflammatory drug. Its associated incidence of gastrointestinal bleeding and peptic ulcers is lower than that of nonselective COX inhibitors. Rofecoxib and valdecoxib are also selective COX-2 inhibitors, or coxibs, but increased risk of cardiovascular events for all three coxibs has resulted in rofecoxib and valdecoxib withdrawal from the market and uncertain status of coxib therapy.

■ Disease-modifying antirheumatic drugs (DMARD) are agents capable of slowing the progression of joint erosions in patients with rheumatoid arthritis. These drugs have a slow onset of action and can cause considerable toxicity. DMARD act by inhibiting the proliferation and activity of lymphocytes and polymorphonuclear leukocytes.

■ Methotrexate (MTX), the most widely used and effective DMARD, can be combined with other drugs in this class for enhanced activity. It is generally well tolerated and can be used effectively for many years.

■ Etanercept, infliximab, and adalimumab and infliximab are DMARD that bind to and inactivate tumor necrosis factor (TNF). Anakinra, a recombinant form of the human interleukin-1 receptor antagonist (IL-1Ra), blocks the biologic activity of IL-1 by competitively inhibiting IL-1 binding to the interleukin-1 type I receptor (IL-1RI). These drugs are administered intermittently by injection and appear to benefit many patients with rheumatoid arthritis, but all carry the risk of increased infections.

■ Other DMARD include gold salts, glucocorticoids, leflunomide, hydroxychloroquine, sulfasalazine, and penicillamine.

■ Gout is caused by hyperuricemia and the deposition of urate crystals in joints. Uricosuric drugs (e.g., probenecid and sulfinpyrazone) increase uric acid excretion, whereas allopurinol inhibits uric acid formation. These drugs are used to prevent gout attacks.

■ Acute gout is treated with an anti-inflammatory drug (e.g., indomethacin) another NSAID, or colchicine. Colchicine inhibits the motility of leukocytes and thereby prevents their migration into joints and their ability to cause urate crystal-induced joint inflammation.

Review Questions

1. Aspirin is often used in low doses to prevent platelet aggregation by inhibiting the synthesis of which substance?
(A) leukotriene
(B) prostacyclin (PGI_2)
(C) thromboxane A_2
(D) arachidonic acid
(E) phospholipase A_2

2. Acetaminophen is a potent analgesic and antipyretic NSAID, but differs from other agents in that it has no anti-inflammatory action. Which of the following reasons explains this unique aspect of acetaminophen?
(A) the distribution of acetaminophen does not reach peripheral sites of inflammation
(B) acetaminophen it is not an inhibitor of the cyclooxygenase (COX) enzyme
(C) anti-inflammatory doses of acetaminophen are too high and toxic
(D) it is selective for a newly discovered isozyme of cyclooxygenase
(E) acetaminophen undergoes significant first-pass metabolism

3. Which of the following agents augments the physiologic concentration of interleukin-1 receptor antagonist proteins in the treatment of rheumatoid arthritis?
(A) adalimumab
(B) leflunomide
(C) etanercept
(D) infliximab
(E) anakinra

4. With respect to antigout therapy, inhibition of tubulin polymerization into microtubules is important given the role of which process in which aspect of the disease?

(A) leukotriene synthesis
(B) uric acid production
(C) kidney reabsorption of uric acid
(D) leukocyte migration
(E) plasma binding of uric acid

5. A 45-year old obese male with a history of alcohol abuse and hypertension presents with complaints of joint swelling and pain. His urate excretion rate is 950 mg/day. Which of the following agents is the best treatment for his condition?
(A) probenicid
(B) allopurinol
(C) piroxicam
(D) sulfinpyrazone
(E) colchicine

Answers and Explanations

1. The correct answer is C: thromboxane A_2. Aspirin binds irreversibly to COX enzyme in platelets and because the platelets do not have a nucleus and cannot synthesize new COX protein, the effect of aspirin persists until the platelet is taken out of circulation. Thromboxane A_2 (TXA_2) produces vasoconstriction and promotes the formation of clots, therefore aspirin can prevent clot formation and coronary thrombosis. Answer (B), prostacyclin (PGI_2), is also inhibited by aspirin because it is a COX product but the particular enzyme to synthesize PGI_2 is not found in platelets. The other agents are not affected by aspirin administration.

2. The best answer is D: it is selective for a newly discovered isozyme of cyclooxygenase. This isozyme, called COX-3, appears to be a splice variant of COX-1 (from the same gene, but different posttranscriptional processing of the RNA). It is also sometimes mentioned that the peroxide formation at sites of inflammation inhibits the activity of acetaminophen, but this may be less of a factor now that COX-3 is recognized. Answers (A) through (C) are not correct and answer (E) is not true to a greater degree than other NSAID that do have anti-inflammatory action.

3. The correct answer is E: anakinra. Anakinra, a recombinant form of the human interleukin-1 receptor antagonist protein (IL-1Ra), blocks the biologic activity of IL-1 by competitively inhibiting IL-1 binding to the interleukin-1 type I receptor (IL-1RI). Answer (A), adalimumab, is a human IgG1 monoclonal antibody specific for human tumor necrosis factor (TNF). Answer (B), leflunomide, is an immunosuppressive drug that inhibits mononuclear and T-cell proliferation. Answer (C), etanercept, is a protein formed by recombining human p75 TNF receptors with Fc fragments of human immunoglobulin G1 (IgG1). Answer (D), infliximab, is a chimeric human-murine (mouse) monoclonal antibody that inactivates TNF and is approved for the treatment of Crohn's disease and rheumatoid arthritis.

4. The correct answer is D: leukocyte migration. The invasion of leukocytes (macrophages, and so on) into the joint capsule and subsequent release of inflammatory

cytokines is a key process in the progression of rheumatoid arthritis. The agent that disrupts tubulin formation is colchicine. Other processes given as answers are not important with regard to colchicine action.

5. The correct answer is (B) allopurinol. The two main strategies for treating gout are to increase the excretion of uric acid with a uricosuric agent (probenecid or sulfinpyrazone) or decrease the production of uric acid by inhibiting xanthine oxidase with allopurinol. The 24-hour rate of uric acid excretion provides a guideline for which therapy to use. Less than 800 mg, use a uricosuric because there is too little excretion of uric acid; and more than 800 mg, use allopurinol because there is too much uric acid being made.

SELECTED READINGS

Bieber, J. D., and R. A. Terkeltaub. Gout: on the brink of novel therapeutic options for an ancient disease. Arthritis Rheum 50(8):2400–2414, 2004.

Hinz, B., and K. Brune. Pain and osteoarthritis: new drugs and mechanisms. Curr Opin Rheumatol 16(5):628–633, 2004.

Minghetti, L. Cyclooxygenase-2 (COX-2) in inflammatory and degenerative brain diseases. J Neuropathol Exp Neurol 63(9):901–910, 2004

Roberts, L., and G. J. McColl. Tumour necrosis factor inhibitors: risks and benefits in patients with rheumatoid arthritis. Intern Med J 34(12):687–693, 2004.

Schlesinger, N. Management of acute and chronic gouty arthritis: present state-of-the-art. Drugs 64(21):2399–2416, 2004.

Subramanian, S., and R. Handa. Biological agents in rheumatoid arthritis. J Postgrad Med 50(4):293–299, 2004.

Zha, S., V. Yegnasubramanian, W. G. Nelson, et al. Cyclooxygenases in cancer: progress and perspective. Cancer Lett 215(1):1–20, 2004.

ENDOCRINE PHARMACOLOGY

CHAPTER 31

Hypothalamic and Pituitary Drugs

CLASSIFICATION OF HYPOTHALAMIC AND PITUITARY DRUGS

Anterior Pituitary Hormones and Releasing Hormones

Corticotropin and Related Drugs
- Cosyntropin
- Corticorelin ovine triflutate (ACTHREL)

Growth Hormone and Related Drugs
- Somatropin[a]
- Octreotide (SANDOSTATIN)
- Pegvisomant (SOMAVERT)

Gonadotropins and Related Drugs
- Chorionic gonadotropin and menotropins
- Leuprolide (LUPRON)[b]
- Abarelix (PLENAXIS)

Other Drugs
- Cabergoline (COSTINEX)[c]

Posterior Pituitary Hormones and Related Drugs
- Desmopressin and vasopressin
- Oxytocin
- Atosiban

[a] also somatrem and sermorelin
[b] also gonadorelin, goserelin, nafarelin
[c] also bromocriptine (PARLODEL)

OVERVIEW

The hypothalamus and pituitary gland constitute an important neuroendocrine system that regulates growth, reproduction, metabolic rates, and other important body functions. The pituitary gland is divided into two major lobes: the adenohypophysis (anterior lobe) and the neurohypophysis (posterior lobe). Various hormones are secreted by each of these lobes and by the hypothalamus.

Adenohypophysis and Hypothalamus

The adenohypophysis secretes six hormones: (1) **corticotropin** (adrenocorticotropic hormone, ACTH); (2) **somatotropin** (growth hormone, GH); (3) **follicle-stimulating hormone** (FSH); (4) **luteinizing hormone** (LH); (5) **thyrotropin** (thyroid-stimulating hormone, TSH); and (6) **prolactin**. The actions of these **anterior pituitary hormones** are summarized in Fig. 31–1.

The secretion of anterior pituitary hormones is controlled by several hormone-releasing and hormone-inhibiting factors that are formed in the hypothalamus. These **hypothalamic hormones** include the following: (1) **corticotropin-releasing hormone** (CRH); (2) **growth hormone-releasing hormone** (GHRH); (3) **somatostatin** (growth hormone-inhibiting hormone, GIH); (4) **gonadotropin-releasing hormone** (GnRH); (5) **thyrotropin-releasing hormone** (TRH); and (6) **prolactin-inhibiting hormone** (PIH). Evidence also suggests the presence of one or more prolactin-releasing factors. The various hypothalamic hormones are secreted by the arcuate and other hypothalamic nuclei, and they are transported to the anterior pituitary via the hypophysioportal circulation.

The anterior pituitary hormones are transported to their target organs via the systemic circulation. In the target organs, they stimulate growth, development, and the secretion of other hormones, which both activate specific functions in various organs and exert negative feedback inhibition of the corresponding hypothalamic and pituitary hormones.

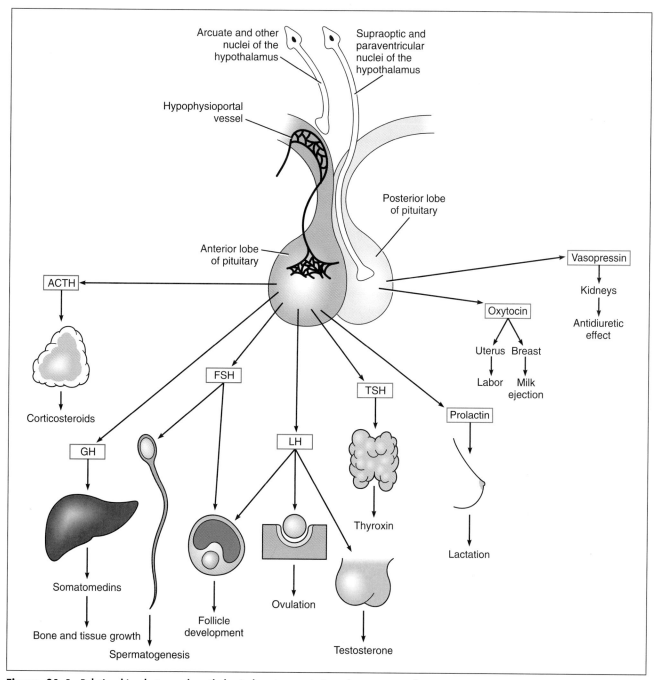

Figure 31-1. Relationships between hypothalamic hormones, pituitary hormones, and target organs. Numerous hormone-releasing and hormone-inhibiting factors formed in the arcuate and other hypothalamic nuclei are transported to the anterior pituitary by hypophysioportal vessels. In response to hypothalamic hormones, the anterior pituitary secretes the following: corticotropin, which evokes corticosteroid secretion by the adrenal cortex; growth hormone (GH), which elicits production of insulin-like growth factors (IGF) by the liver; follicle-stimulating hormone (FSH), which stimulates spermatogenesis and facilitates ovarian follicle development; luteinizing hormone (LH), which elicits testosterone secretion by the testes, facilitates ovarian follicle development, and induces ovulation; thyroid-stimulating hormone (TSH), which stimulates thyroxin secretion by the thyroid gland; and prolactin, which induces breast tissue growth and lactation. The posterior pituitary hormones, which are formed in the supraoptic and paraventricular nuclei, are transported by nerve axons to the posterior lobe, where they are released by physiologic stimuli. Oxytocin induces milk ejection by the breast and stimulates uterine contractions during labor. Vasopressin increases water and sodium reabsorption by the kidneys.

Neurohypophysis

The neurohypophysis secretes **oxytocin** and **vasopressin.** These **posterior pituitary hormones** are synthesized in the cell bodies of neurons in the supraoptic and paraventricular nuclei of the hypothalamus. The hormones are transported down the nerve axons to their endings in the posterior pituitary, where they are released in response to electrical activity in the nerve terminals.

Uses of Hypothalamic and Pituitary Hormones

Hypothalamic and pituitary hormones are used for both diagnostic and therapeutic purposes. Hypothalamic hormone-releasing factors are helpful in assessing the functional capacity of the anterior pituitary to secrete particular pituitary hormones. Anterior pituitary hormones are used to evaluate the functional capacity of their target organs, to stimulate hypofunctional target organs, and to provide replacement therapy in hormone deficiency states. Posterior pituitary hormones are used therapeutically to activate specific physiologic functions.

All of the hypothalamic and pituitary hormones are peptides or small proteins that are extensively degraded in the gut following oral administration. For this reason, most of these hormones are administered parenterally. A few of them are available as a spray for intranasal administration.

ANTERIOR PITUITARY HORMONES

Corticotropin and Related Drugs

Corticotropin is a 39-amino-acid peptide that is released from the anterior pituitary in response to CRH stimulation. Corticotropin then stimulates the adrenal cortex to produce cortisol, aldosterone, and adrenal androgens by increasing the activity of the enzyme that converts cholesterol to pregnenolone and is the rate-limiting enzyme in corticosteroid production.

Corticotropin Preparations

Two corticotropin preparations are available for clinical use: porcine **corticotropin** and a synthetic form of human corticotropin called **cosyntropin.** Cosyntropin contains the first 24 amino acids of human corticotropin, which are the ones necessary for its biologic activity. Cosyntropin is preferable for clinical use because it produces fewer allergic reactions.

Cosyntropin is used in two diagnostic tests. First, it is used to distinguish **congenital adrenal hyperplasia** from **ovarian hyperandrogenism.** Second, and more commonly, it is used to diagnose **adrenal insufficiency** in a test that measures plasma cortisol levels before and after a cosyntropin injection. Cosyntropin increases cortisol levels in healthy individuals but fails to increase cortisol levels in persons with adrenal insufficiency. Then to distinguish primary adrenal insufficiency from secondary adrenal insufficiency, endogenous plasma corticotropin concentrations are measured. In patients with primary adrenal insufficiency, corticotropin concentrations are high because of the lack of negative feedback inhibition of the hypothalamus and pituitary gland by the adrenal corticosteroids. In patients with secondary adrenal insufficiency, corticotropin concentrations are low because of inadequate production of corticotropin by the pituitary gland.

Corticotropin-Releasing Hormone

Corticorelin ovine triflutate (ACTHREL) is a preparation containing recombinant ovine corticotropin-releasing hormone. Intravenous administration of this preparation stimulates secretion of corticotropin and cortisol in normal subjects. Corticorelin is used as a diagnostic test to determine whether the excessive levels of cortisol that occur in persons with Cushing's syndrome are caused by excessive corticotropin secretion from a pituitary adenoma or by excessive secretion of cortisol by an adrenal tumor.

Growth Hormone and Related Drugs

Growth hormone (somatotropin), a large peptide that contains 191 amino acids, is produced by the anterior pituitary, and has both direct and indirect actions on target organs. GH acts directly to stimulate lipolysis and antagonize insulin to elevate blood glucose levels. Most of the effects of GH, however, are mediated by **insulin-like growth factors** (IGF), which are peptides produced in the liver and cartilage. The IGF stimulate skeletal growth, amino acid transport, protein synthesis, nucleic acid synthesis, and cell proliferation.

The secretion of GH is stimulated by GHRH and is inhibited by GIH (somatostatin). Several preparations of GH, GHRH, and somatostatin are available for use in the diagnosis and treatment of **growth disorders** associated with excessive or inadequate secretion of GH.

Growth Hormone Preparations

Growth hormone preparations obtained from animal sources are not active in humans. In the past, GH obtained from human cadavers was used to treat patients with **growth hormone deficiency and short stature,** but some of the patients subsequently developed Creutzfeldt-Jakob disease. This fatal disease, as with mad cow disease and kuru, is characterized by spongiform encephalopathy and is thought to be transmitted by unconventional neurotoxic agents called prions.

Today, two biosynthetic GH preparations are available for treatment of GH deficiency. One that is identical to human GH is called **somatropin, recombinant.** The other, a human GH analogue that contains one additional amino acid, is called **somatrem.** These preparations have been used to treat children with a variety of growth disorders including GH deficiency, Turner syndrome, chronic renal failure, Prader-Willi syndrome, and cystic fibrosis. GH preparations have been clearly shown to improve height velocity and final height in these conditions. Children who received craniospinal irradiation for treatment of a childhood malignancy are less responsive to GH replacement than children with idiopathic growth hormone deficiency and they have a tendency to enter puberty at an earlier age. These children may respond to supraphysiologic doses of GH preparations and suppression of early puberty using a gonadotropin releasing hormone analogue (see below). Somatropin and somatrem are usually administered subcutaneously once daily to persons with growth hormone deficiency. GH deficiency is often accompanied by other pituitary hormone deficiencies, which should also be treated with appropriate hormones.

Growth Hormone-Releasing Hormone Preparations

Sermorelin, a synthetic analogue of GHRH, is available for use in a test to determine whether **growth hormone deficiency** is secondary to **hypothalamic insufficiency** or to **pituitary insufficiency.** In this test, plasma levels of GH are measured before and after a single injection of sermorelin. A normal response indicates that the pituitary is capable of secreting GH and that the patient's GH deficiency is caused by hypothalamic insufficiency.

Sermorelin has orphan drug status for the treatment of GH deficiency and the treatment of weight loss associated with acquired immunodeficiency syndrome (AIDS).

Growth Hormone-Inhibiting Hormone Preparations

Somatostatin (growth hormone-inhibiting hormone) inhibits GH secretion, but it also exerts effects on several endocrine glands, including the pancreas, and this limits its therapeutic usefulness. Scientists searching for GIH preparations that were more selective for GH inhibition discovered **octreotide** (SANDOSTATIN), a somatostatin analogue that consists of 8 amino acids. In comparison with somatostatin, octreotide is 45 times more potent in inhibiting GH secretion but only 2 times as potent in inhibiting insulin secretion by the pancreas.

Octreotide is used to treat patients with **acromegaly.** This endocrine disorder, which is caused by excessive GH secretion, is characterized by acral enlargement and soft tissue overgrowth of the hands and feet, coarsening of facial features, thickening and oiliness of the skin, and increased sweating. It is often accompanied by numerous other metabolic and endocrine abnormalities. Octreotide also has been used successfully in the treatment of several **neoplastic diseases,** including **carcinoid syndrome, pituitary adenomas that secrete thyrotropin,** and **tumors that produce vasoactive intestinal polypeptide** (VIP).

Octreotide is usually administered subcutaneously every 8 hours. A sustained-release preparation for intramuscular administration has also been developed. Adverse effects of octreotide treatment include nausea, vomiting, abdominal cramps, steatorrhea (excessive fat in the feces), and gallstones.

In patients with acromegaly, the use of **cabergoline** (see below) and other dopamine agonists can reduce circulating levels of GH, IGF, and prolactin. These drugs are particularly useful in the treatment of persons with elevated GH and prolactin secretion.

Growth Hormone Receptor Antagonist

Pegvisomant (SOMAVERT) is a pegylated analogue of GH that acts as a GH receptor antagonist in target organs and thereby normalizes serum IGF-I concentrations in 97% of persons with acromegaly. **Pegylation** (addition of polyethylene glycol to the molecule) significantly increases the half-life of peptide drugs. Pegvisomant significantly improves

signs and symptoms of GH excess in these persons, including patients who were wholly or partially resistant to somatostatin analogues such as octreotide. In one study of persons with acromegaly, pegvisomant reduced serum IGF levels and finger ring size in a dose-dependent manner while improving symptoms of tissue swelling, arthralgia, headache, perspiration, and fatigue. The drug appears to have a good safety profile, but liver function tests should be regularly monitored.

Gonadotropins and Related Drugs

The pituitary secretes two gonadotropins, namely, FSH and LH, in response to pulsatile stimulation by GnRH. The frequency and amplitude of the GnRH pulses at a particular time determine which gonadotropin is secreted. In females, FSH stimulates ovarian follicle maturation, whereas LH assists FSH in follicle development, induces ovulation, and stimulates the corpus luteum to produce progesterone and androgens. In males, FSH stimulates spermatogenesis, whereas LH stimulates Leydig's cells in the testes to produce testosterone.

Gonadotropin Preparations

Several gonadotropin preparations are available for the treatment of infertility and hypogonadism. One of them contains both FSH and LH, is called **menotropins** (human menopausal gonadotropin, or hMG), and is obtained from the urine of menopausal women. Another primarily contains LH, is called **chorionic gonadotropin** (human chorionic gonadotropin, or hCG), and is produced by the placenta and isolated from the urine of pregnant women.

In women with **infertility** caused by failure to ovulate, menotropins and chorionic gonadotropin are used sequentially. A dose of menotropins is administered each day for 9 to 12 days to stimulate maturation of the ovarian follicle. On the day after the last dose is given, a single dose of chorionic gonadotropin is administered to induce ovulation. In men with **hypogonadotropic hypogonadism,** menotropins therapy is used to stimulate spermatogenesis. In prepubertal boys with **cryptorchidism** (undescended testes) and hypogonadism, chorionic gonadotropin is administered to stimulate testosterone production and descent of the testes.

Gonadotropin-Releasing Hormone Preparations

Two classes of drugs target pituitary receptors for gonadotropin-releasing hormone: the GnRH agonists and the GnRH antagonist called abarelix (PLENAXIS).

The GnRH agonists include **gonadorelin, goserelin, leuprolide,** and **nafarelin.** Gonadorelin is a synthetic version of natural GnRH, and the other preparations are synthetic GnRH analogues. As with natural GnRH, these synthetic drugs affect the release of gonadotropins. The way in which they are administered determines their effects on the body. **Pulsatile administration** mimics the natural secretion of GnRH and is used therapeutically to stimulate the release of FSH and LH from the anterior pituitary. In contrast, continuous administration of GnRH agonists leads to down-regulation of GnRH receptors and decreased secretion of FSH and LH. GnRH agonists are used in this manner to suppress gonadotropin stimulation of target organs.

Gonadorelin has a half-life of about 5 minutes. Unlike the other GnRH preparations, gonadorelin can be administered in a pulsatile manner via a portable infusion pump that injects a small bolus of the drug subcutaneously every 60 to 120 minutes. In women with infertility caused by **hypothalamic amenorrhea,** pulsatile treatment for 10 to 20 days is given to induce ovulation. Ovulation rates exceeding 90% are achieved by this method, and most women become pregnant within 6 months of therapy. Gonadorelin is also used diagnostically to evaluate the functional capacity of the gonadotropin-secreting cells of the pituitary. For this purpose, plasma gonadotropin concentrations are measured before and after a single dose of gonadorelin is injected.

Goserelin, leuprolide, and nafarelin are administered continuously and act to down-regulate pituitary GnRH receptors and thereby reduce gonadotropin secretion. By suppressing gonadotropin secretion, these GnRH analogues reduce testosterone levels in males and estrogen levels in females. This, in turn, decreases testosterone stimulation of the prostate gland and estrogen stimulation of the breast and uterus. For this reason, the GnRH analogues are effective in the treatment of **precocious puberty** in boys or girls and in the treatment of **prostate cancer, breast cancer,** and **endometriosis** in adults.

Nafarelin (SYNAREL) is used to manage endometriosis in women and central precocious puberty in children. It is administered as a nasal spray. Leuprolide (LUPRON) and goserelin (ZOLADEX) are administered as pellets that slowly release the drug following subcutaneous implantation. They are used to treat advanced prostate cancer, breast cancer, and endometriosis. Because these drugs cause a transient increase in testosterone levels when treatment of prostate cancer is begun, they should be given in combination with a testosterone antagonist (e.g., flutamide or bicalutamide) until testosterone levels fall. These drugs can cause a number of adverse effects because of decreased sex steroid levels, including hot flashes. Nafarelin, leuprolide, and goserelin have half-lives of about 3 hours.

Gonadotropin-Releasing Hormone Antagonist

Abarelix (PLENAXIS) is the newest development in the treatment of advanced prostate cancer. It is a synthetic decapeptide that blocks GnRH receptors and thereby reduces pituitary secretion of LH and FSH, leading to reduced secretion of testosterone. More than 90% of men achieved medical castration, defined as a serum testosterone level less than 50 ng/dL, 4 weeks after a single intramuscular injection of abarelix. Although testosterone levels can increase in some patients over time, about 75% of men maintained testosterone levels below 50 ng/dL for 1 year. Unlike GnRH agonists, abarelix does not cause a transient increase in testosterone levels and concurrent treatment with testosterone antagonists is not necessary. A small percentage of men experienced an immediate hypersensitivity reaction following abarelix administration. The drug appears to be suitable for treating advanced symptomatic prostate cancer in men who are not good candidates for GnRH agonists and who refuse surgical castration.

Thyrotropin and Related Drugs

Thyrotropin is secreted in response to stimulation of the anterior pituitary by thyrotropin-releasing hormone. Both **thyrotropin** and a TRH preparation called **protirelin** have been used as diagnostic agents, but their use has been largely supplanted by other methods.

Prolactin and Related Drugs

Prolactin contains 198 amino acids and acts on the mammary gland to stimulate tissue growth and promote lactation (milk production) in the presence of adequate levels of estrogens, progestins, and other hormones. Prolactin does not have any current clinical use.

The secretion of prolactin is inhibited by prolactin-inhibiting hormone (dopamine) and is stimulated by hypothalamic prolactin-releasing factors. Excessive prolactin secretion causes **hyperprolactinemia** and often leads to **galactorrhea** (excessive milk production), **hypogonadism,** and **infertility.** In some cases, hyperprolactinemia occurs secondary to **prolactin-secreting pituitary adenomas.**

Both the idiopathic and secondary forms of hyperprolactinemia can be treated with a dopamine agonist such as **cabergoline** (DOSTINEX) or bromocriptine. Each drug mimics the action of PIH and thereby reduces prolactin secretion. In patients with prolactin-secreting adenomas, treatment with either drug also produces a significant reduction in tumor size.

Bromocriptine and cabergoline are both ergot alkaloid derivatives. The pharmacologic properties of bromocriptine, a drug that is also used to treat Parkinson's disease, are described in Chapter 24. In comparison with bromocriptine, cabergoline appears to be more effective and better tolerated in patients with hyperprolactinemia. Cabergoline selectively activates dopamine D_2 receptors in the pituitary gland and thereby suppresses the secretion of prolactin. It is also useful in persons with a mixed **growth hormone and prolactin-secreting pituitary adenoma.** The drug has an elimination half-life of about 65 hours, which provides a long duration of action. The most common adverse effects of cabergoline are nausea, headache, and dizziness.

POSTERIOR PITUITARY HORMONES

Oxytocin and vasopressin are nonapeptides that are released from the posterior pituitary in response to specific physiologic stimuli (see Fig. 31–1).

Oxytocin and Related Drugs

Oxytocin is a hormone that increases the strength of uterine contractions and causes milk ejection (milk let-down) by contracting myoepithelial cells that line the ducts of the breast. The hormone is released via a reflex that is triggered by dilation of the uterine cervix, uterine contractions, or breast suckling. During late pregnancy, the uterus becomes highly sensitive to the actions of oxytocin owing to an increased number of oxytocin receptors. The sensitivity of the uterus is enhanced by estrogen and is inhibited by progesterone.

Synthetic oxytocin has several uses in obstetrics. The drug is given intravenously to **induce or enhance uterine contractions during labor,** and it is injected intramuscularly to **prevent postpartum uterine hemorrhage** by causing the uterine muscle to contract. In addition, a nasal spray preparation of oxytocin is available to **stimulate milk letdown in nursing mothers.** The spray is inhaled 2 to 3 minutes before breast-feeding. Adverse reactions to oxytocin are uncommon. They include cardiac arrhythmias, central nervous system stimulation, excessive uterine contraction, and hyponatremia.

Use of synthetic oxytocin is contraindicated in instances of fetal distress, abnormal fetal presentation, prematurity, or cephalopelvic disproportion.

Atosiban, a peptide of 9 amino acids, acts as a competitive antagonist of oxytocin and has been approved in European countries for the treatment of **premature labor.** Although the benefit of drugs that inhibit labor (**tocolytic drugs**) in women with premature labor remains controversial, a role appears to exist for short-term tocolysis to gain time so that corticosteroids can be administered to enhance fetal lung maturation before birth. Atosiban appears to be well tolerated, and unlike the adrenergic β_2 agonists, atosiban does not increase fetal heart rate. Additional clinical trials are needed to establish the safety and efficacy of tocolysis in premature labor and to identify the most effective drugs for this purpose.

Vasopressin and Related Drugs

Vasopressin (arginine vasopressin) is secreted by the posterior pituitary in response to a decrease in extracellular fluid volume or an increase in plasma osmotic pressure. The hormone interacts with two types of **vasopressin receptors** to exert its antidiuretic and vasoconstrictive effects.

To increase water reabsorption by the kidney, vasopressin stimulates the insertion of water channels (aquaporins) in the luminal membranes of renal tubule cells in the collecting ducts. This action concentrates the urine and reduces the urine volume. For this reason, vasopressin is also called **antidiuretic hormone** (ADH). The renal actions of vasopressin are mediated by V_2 **receptors** via production of cyclic adenosine monophosphate (cAMP).

Vasopressin causes vasoconstriction in several vascular beds by stimulating V_1 **receptors** in vascular smooth muscle.

A deficiency of pituitary vasopressin secretion leads to **diabetes insipidus,** a condition characterized by excessive water excretion (polyuria) and subsequent increased water intake (polydipsia). Diabetes insipidus is usually treated with **desmopressin,** a long-acting synthetic analogue of vasopressin. This agent has potent antidiuretic activity but causes much less vasoconstriction than does natural vasopressin. Desmopressin solutions are available for subcutaneous, intramuscular, or intravenous administration. Desmopressin nasal spray is also available and it is used to prevent nocturnal urine production and enuresis in patients with diabetes insipidus. Desmopressin overdosage can result in dilutional hyponatremia.

Synthetic vasopressin is available as an injectable preparation for the treatment of **bleeding caused by esophageal varices or colonic diverticula.** In these conditions, the drug acts by producing vasoconstriction. Vasopressin should be used cautiously in persons with coronary artery disease.

SUMMARY OF IMPORTANT POINTS

- Cosyntropin is a synthetic corticotropin analogue used to diagnose adrenal insufficiency, whereas corticorelin ovine triflutate is a corticotropin-releasing hormone used as a diagnostic test to distinguish adrenal and pituitary origins of Cushing's syndrome.

- Recombinant somatropin and somatrem are growth hormone preparations used to treat growth hormone deficiency in children with a low growth rate.

- Octreotide is a synthetic growth hormone-inhibiting hormone (somatostatin) analogue used in the treatment of acromegaly, carcinoid syndrome, pituitary adenomas that secrete thyrotropin, and tumors that secrete vasoactive intestinal polypeptide.

- Pegvisomant is a growth hormone analogue and growth hormone receptor antagonist used to treat acromegaly.

- Menotropins and chorionic gonadotropin are human gonadotropin preparations used to induce ovulation in infertile women. Chorionic gonadotropin is also used to stimulate spermatogenesis in men with hypogonadotropic hypogonadism and to treat cryptorchidism in prepubertal boys.

- Gonadorelin is a gonadotropin-releasing hormone (GnRH) preparation administered in pulsatile fashion to induce ovulation in women with hypothalamic amenorrhea.

- Goserelin and leuprolide are synthetic GnRH preparations administered continuously to suppress gonadotropin secretion in children with precocious puberty and in adults with prostate cancer, breast cancer, and endometriosis.

- Nafarelin is a GnRH preparation administered as a nasal spray to treat precocious puberty in children and endometriosis in women.

- Abarelix is a GnRH antagonist that reduces gonadotropin and gonadal steroid secretion, and is used to treat advanced prostate cancer.

- Dopamine agonists, cabergoline and bromocriptine, are used to suppress prolactin secretion in women with hyperprolactinemia. This condition is often associated with galactorrhea, hypogonadism, and infertility. Cabergoline may also reduce excessive growth hormone secretion in some persons with acromegaly and hyperprolactinemia.

- Oxytocin, which stimulates uterine contractions at term, is used to induce or augment labor, to prevent postpartum uterine hemorrhage, and to stimulate milk let-down in nursing women. Atosiban is an oxytocin antagonist being studied for treatment of premature labor.

■ Desmopressin is a synthetic vasopressin analogue that retains the antidiuretic activity of the natural hormone but lacks the vasoconstrictive effect. It is administered parenterally and intranasally to treat diabetes insipidus resulting from deficient pituitary vasopressin secretion. Synthetic vasopressin is used to control gastrointestinal bleeding by causing vasoconstriction.

Review Questions

1. Which drug is used to reduce secretion of gonadotropins and gonadal steroids in children with precocious puberty?
   (A) cabergoline
   (B) menotropins
   (C) leuprolide
   (D) gonadorelin
   (E) octreotide

2. Which drug for treating acromegaly acts by blocking receptors for growth hormone?
   (A) pegvisomant
   (B) somatropin
   (C) octreotide
   (D) sermorelin
   (E) cabergoline

3. By which mechanism does cabergoline relieve symptoms of hyperprolactinemia in persons with a prolactin-secreting pituitary adenoma?
   (A) blocking prolactin receptors
   (B) blocking receptors for prolactin releasing hormone
   (C) a cytotoxic effect on pituitary adenoma cells
   (D) activating receptors for prolactin-inhibiting hormone
   (E) stimulating the breakdown of prolactin

4. Which drug acts to block receptors for gonadotropin-releasing hormone in persons with advanced prostate cancer?
   (A) goserelin
   (B) abarelix
   (C) leuprolide
   (D) octreotide
   (E) pegvisomant

5. Octreotide is correctly described by which of the following statements?
   (A) It is identical to naturally occurring somatostatin.
   (B) It is used to treat growth hormone deficiency.
   (C) It is administered orally.
   (D) It is a more potent inhibitor of growth hormone secretion than is somatostatin.
   (E) It contains more than 100 amino acids.

Answers and Explanations

1. The answer is C: leuprolide. Leuprolide is an agonist at pituitary receptors for gonadotropin-releasing hormone (GnRH). When administered continuously, rather than in a physiologically pulsatile manner, leuprolide and other GnRH agonists cause down-regulation of GnRH receptors, leading to decreased secretion of gonadotropins (luteinizing hormone [LH] and follicle-stimulating hormone [FSH]). This action reduces secretion of gonadal steroids and thereby slows the onset of puberty in children with precocious puberty.

2. The answer is A: pegvisomant. Pegvisomant represents a new approach to treating acromegaly. It acts by blocking receptors for growth hormone and thereby reduces the formation of insulin-like growth factors (IGF) that mediate the growth-stimulating and other effects of growth hormone. Other drugs used to treat acromegaly act by reducing growth hormone secretion (octreotide and cabergoline).

3. The answer is D: activating receptors for prolactin-inhibiting hormone. Prolactin secretion is ordinarily restrained by tonic secretion of prolactin-inhibiting hormone (PIH or dopamine). Cabergoline and bromocriptine are dopamine receptor agonists that act to mimic the effect of endogenous prolactin-inhibiting hormone and thereby reduce excessive prolactin secretion in persons with prolactin-secreting pituitary adenomas.

4. The answer is B: abarelix. Abarelix is a gonadotropin-releasing hormone (GnRH) antagonist that blocks pituitary receptors for GnRH and thereby inhibits gonadotropin secretion in men with advanced prostate cancer. Unlike the GnRH agonists (e.g., leuprolide and goserelin), abarelix does not cause a transient increase in gonadotropin secretion when the drug is first given.

5. The answer is D: It is a more potent inhibitor of growth hormone secretion than is somatostatin. Octreotide only contains 8 amino acids is not identical to somatostatin (answers A and E). It is not administered orally (answer C) and it is not used to treat growth hormone deficiency (answer B). In fact, octreotide is used to treat acromegaly caused by excessive growth hormone secretion.

SELECTED READINGS

Antoniazzi, F., and G. Zamboni. Central precocious puberty: current treatment options. Paediatr Drugs 6:211–231, 2004.

Muller, A. F., and A. J. van der Lely. Pharmacological therapy for acromegaly: a critical review. Drugs 64:1817–1838, 2004.

Paisley, A. N., P. Trainer, and W. Drake. Pegvisomant: a novel pharmacotherapy for the treatment of acromegaly. Expert Opin Biol Ther 4:421–425, 2004.

Tsatsaris, V., B. Carbonne, and D. Cabrol. Atosiban for preterm labour. Drugs 64:375–382, 2004.

Van der Lely, A. J. Justified and unjustified use of growth hormone. Postgrad Med J 80:577–580, 2004.

CHAPTER 32

Thyroid Drugs

CLASSIFICATION OF THYROID DRUGS

Thyroid Hormone Preparations
- Levothyroxine (LEVOXYL, SYNTHROID)
- Liothyronine (CYTOMEL)

Antithyroid Agents

Thiourea Drugs
- Methimazole (TAPAZOLE)
- Propylthiouracil

β-Adrenergic Receptor Antagonists
- Propranolol

Other Antithyroid Agents
- Potassium iodide solution
- Sodium iodide I 131 (^{131}I)

OVERVIEW

The thyroid gland synthesizes and secretes **triiodothyronine** (T_3) and **tetraiodothyronine** (T_4, thyroxine). These **thyroid hormones** are necessary for normal growth and development, and they play a role in a number of metabolic processes, including those involved in the synthesis and degradation of essentially all other hormones. Thyroid hormones also augment sympathetic nervous system function, primarily by increasing the number of adrenergic receptors in target tissues.

Synthesis of Thyroid Hormones

Thyroid hormones are synthesized in a process that involves the uptake and organification of **iodide** and the subsequent coupling of iodotyrosine residues of **thyroglobulin**. These steps are illustrated in Fig. 32–1.

Iodide is actively transported into thyroid follicle cells. It diffuses across the cells to the apical membrane, where it is oxidized and attached to tyrosine residues of thyroglobulin. This process is called iodide organification. The iodinated tyrosine residues, monoiodotyrosine (MIT) and diiodotyrosine (DIT), are then coupled to form T_3 and T_4. Iodide organification and the coupling reactions are catalyzed by peroxidase.

T_4 accounts for about 80% of the hormones secreted by the thyroid, and T_3 accounts for the remainder. These hormones are transported to target organs by thyroid-binding globulin, thyroid-binding prealbumin, and albumin. In peripheral tissues, some of the T_4 is converted to T_3 and reverse T_3 (rT_3) by 5′-deiodinase and 5-deiodinase, respectively. T_3 is about five times more active than T_4, whereas rT_3 in completely inactive. For this reason, the deiodinase enzymes have an important role in controlling the level of thyroid activity. T_3 and rT_3 are eventually metabolized by deiodinase and sulfotransferase reactions to diiodothyronine sulfate.

When T_3 enters the cell nucleus, it binds to specific receptors that activate gene transcription, leading to increased synthesis of proteins necessary for growth, development, and calorigenesis (heat production).

Release of Thyroid Hormones

As discussed in Chapter 31, the secretion of thyroid hormones is modulated by an anterior pituitary hormone called **thyroid-stimulating hormone** (TSH, or thyrotropin) and by a hypothalamic hormone called **thyrotropin-releasing hormone** (TRH).

Thyroglobulin is stored as colloid in the follicular lumen. It reenters the follicular cell by endocytosis, and it undergoes proteolysis during release of the thyroid hormones. This release is stimulated by TSH via the formation of cyclic adenosine monophosphate (cAMP) in thyroid follicular cells.

The production of thyroid hormones is controlled in two ways. First, it is controlled by T_3, which inhibits TRH and TSH secretion by the hypothalamus and pituitary. Second, it is controlled by the rate of conversion of T_4 to T_3 and rT_3 in peripheral tissues. This rate, in turn, is affected by a variety of hormones, nutrients, and disease states.

353

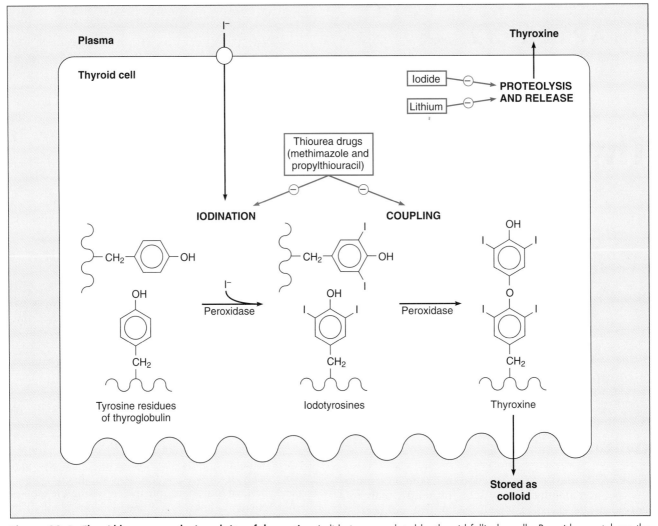

Figure 32–1. Thyroid hormone synthesis and sites of drug action. Iodide is accumulated by thyroid follicular cells. Peroxidase catalyzes the iodination of tyrosine residues of thyroglobulin and the coupling of iodotyrosines to form triiodothyronine (T_3) and tetraiodothyronine (T_4, thyroxine). Thyroglobulin is stored as colloid in thyroid follicles and undergoes proteolysis to release T_4 when stimulated by thyroid-stimulating hormone (TSH, or thyrotropin). Thiourea drugs inhibit the synthesis of thyroid hormones by inhibiting iodination and coupling of tyrosine residues. Elevated iodide concentrations and lithium inhibit the release of thyroid hormones.

Normal and Abnormal Thyroid Function

Normal thyroid function, or **euthyroidism,** is maintained via feedback inhibition of TSH secretion. This inhibition keeps the plasma concentration of free (circulating or unbound) T_4 within a narrow range.

Thyroid disorders are diagnosed primarily on the basis of clinical manifestations and plasma T_4 and TSH levels. **Hypothyroidism** is characterized by low T_4 and high TSH levels, which impair growth and development and cause a decrease in metabolic activity. In contrast, **hyperthyroidism** is associated with high T_4 and low TSH levels, which cause hyperactivity of organ systems (particularly the nervous and cardiovascular systems) and speed up the metabolism.

THYROID DISORDERS

Thyroid disorders are relatively common. In many cases, patients seek medical attention because they notice a diffuse or nodular thyroid gland enlargement (**goiter**) or suffer from other manifestations of abnormal thyroid function.

Hypothyroidism

In infants and children, hypothyroidism causes irreversible mental retardation and impairs growth and development. In adults, hypothyroidism is associated with impairment of physical and mental activity and with slowing of cardiovascular, gastrointestinal, and neuromuscular function. Hypothyroid patients may complain of lethargy, cold intolerance, weight gain, and constipation. The skin may become coarse, dry, and cold. Eventually, hypothyroidism causes **myxedema,** which is described as a dry, waxy swelling of the skin with nonpitting edema. **Myxedema coma** is characterized by hypothermia, hypoglycemia, weakness, stupor, and shock and is the end stage of long-standing, untreated hypothyroidism.

Many patients with mild hypothyroidism have a T_4 level within the normal range. As the disease progresses, however, the T_4 level usually falls below normal.

The most common cause of hypothyroidism in adults is **autoimmune thyroiditis (Hashimoto's disease).** Other causes include thyroid surgery or radioactive iodine (RAI) treatment for hyperthyroidism; dietary iodine deficiency; and thyroid hypoplasia or enzymatic defects. Pituitary or hypothalamic dysfunction can cause secondary hypothyroidism.

Several types of drugs can induce thyroid disorders. Lithium inhibits the release of thyroid hormones by the thyroid gland (see Fig. 32–1) and can cause hypothyroidism by this mechanism. Amiodarone is an iodine-containing antiarrhythmic drug that can cause either hypothyroidism or hyperthyroidism through a variety of mechanisms that alter multiple thyroid functions.

The treatment for all forms of hypothyroidism is replacement therapy with a thyroid hormone preparation.

Hyperthyroidism

Manifestations of hyperthyroidism, or **thyrotoxicosis,** can include nervousness, emotional lability, weight loss despite an increased appetite, heat intolerance, palpitations, proximal muscle weakness, increased frequency of bowel movements, and irregular menses.

Most cases of hyperthyroidism are associated with overproduction of thyroid hormones by the thyroid gland, as indicated by the finding of increased RAI uptake. Excessive thyroid hormone production can result from excessive TSH, as occurs in patients with **TSH-secreting pituitary adenomas,** or it can result from gland stimulation by thyroid antibodies, as occurs in patients with **Graves' disease.**

Graves' disease results from the formation of antibodies directed against the TSH receptor on the surface of thyroid cells. The antibodies stimulate the receptor in the same manner as TSH, resulting in overproduction of thyroid hormones. Graves' disease is characterized by hyperthyroidism, thyroid enlargement, and exophthalmus (abnormal protrusion of the eyeball). Exophthalmus results from stimulation of orbital muscles by thyroid antibodies.

Excessive thyroid hormone production also occurs in persons with thyroid nodules that are independent of pituitary gland control. **Inflammatory thyroid disease (subacute thyroiditis)** can cause a transient form of hyperthyroidism that is caused by the release of preformed thyroid hormone from thyroid follicles.

Three treatment modalities are used in hyperthyroidism: antithyroid agents, surgery, and RAI treatment. The goals of therapy are to eliminate excessive thyroid hormone production and to control the symptoms of hyperthyroidism. The choice of treatment depends on the type and severity of hyperthyroidism and on the individual characteristics of the patient. Antithyroid agents are primarily used for the short-term treatment of hyperthyroidism, either to induce remission of Graves' disease or to control the symptoms of hyperthyroidism before thyroid surgery or RAI treatment. Surgery or RAI treatment can permanently cure hyperthyroidism. Either of these treatment modalities, however, often results in chronic hypothyroidism, which necessitates life-long thyroid hormone replacement therapy.

THYROID HORMONE PREPARATIONS

Natural Hormone Preparations

The natural thyroid hormone preparations include **thyroid [USP]** and **thyroglobulin [USP].** Thyroid [USP] is desiccated hog, beef, or sheep thyroid gland that contains a standardized quantity of T_4 and T_3 in each tablet. Thyroglobulin [USP] is a purified hog gland extract that contains a standardized amount of T_4 and T_3 in a ratio of 25:1.

Because the stability of natural thyroid hormone preparations is unpredictable and because some persons are allergic to the animal proteins contained in them, these preparations have been largely replaced by synthetic hormone preparations for the treatment of hypothyroidism.

Synthetic Hormone Preparations

The synthetic thyroid hormone preparations include **levothyroxine** (T_4), **liothyronine** (T_3), and **liotrix** (a mixture containing T_4 and T_3 in a ratio of 4:1). Little justification exists for using liotrix to treat hypothyroidism, so it is not discussed further. The pharmacologic and pharmacokinetic properties of levothyroxine and liothyronine are discussed below and compared in Table 32–1.

Levothyroxine

PHARMACOKINETICS. The oral bioavailability of levothyroxine (LEVOTHROID, LEVOXYL, SYNTHROID) is about 80%. Different brands and generic formulations of levothyroxine vary in hormone content and bioavailability, however, so the substitution of one formulation for another should be undertaken with caution. Because the half-life of levothyroxine is about 7 days, once-daily administration of the drug produces little fluctuation in plasma hormone levels. About 35% of T_4 is converted to T_3 in peripheral tissues. Therefore, exogenous administration of levothyroxine produces physiologic levels of both T_4 and T_3. For this reason, levothyroxine may be considered a prodrug. The exogenously administered hormones are degraded in the same manner as their natural counterparts.

INDICATIONS. Levothyroxine is the drug of choice for **thyroid hormone replacement** in patients with **hypothyroidism,** because it is chemically stable, nonallergic, and can be given orally once a day. Levothyroxine administration produces a stable pool of T_4 that is converted to T_3 at a steady and consistent rate. Levothyroxine tablets are available in a

Property	Levothyroxine	Liothyronine
Relative potency	1	4
Oral bioavailability	80% (variable)	95%
Elimination half-life	7 days	1 day
Daily doses	1	1–3

TABLE 32–1. **Pharmacologic and Pharmacokinetic Properties of Levothyroxine (T_4) and Liothyronine (T_3)**

wide range of doses to accommodate individualized therapy based on clinical and laboratory data. Therapy is usually begun with a lower dose, particularly in elderly patients and those with long-standing hypothyroidism. The dose is then increased at monthly intervals until a full replacement dose is achieved. A gradual increase in the dose prevents excessive stress on the cardiovascular and other organ systems and thereby causes fewer adverse reactions. Children usually require higher doses per kilogram of body weight than do adults.

The steady-state maintenance dose of levothyroxine is determined on the basis of the patient's clinical response, TSH levels, and T_4 levels. Many clinicians consider the TSH level to be the most sensitive test for determining thyroid replacement dosage. An elevated TSH level indicates that the levothyroxine dose is not sufficient. The expected range of T_4 levels in patients receiving thyroid replacement therapy is higher than that in healthy individuals, because a higher level of T_4 is required in patients to maintain adequate T_3 levels in the absence of endogenous T_3 production by the thyroid gland.

Levothyroxine is also the drug of choice for **suppressive therapy** in patients with **thyroid nodules, diffuse goiters,** or **thyroid cancer.** In these conditions, levothyroxine acts to suppress TSH production and reduce stimulation of abnormal thyroid tissue. Suppressive therapy thereby reduces goiter size and thyroid gland volume.

Myxedema coma is a medical emergency that requires intravenous administration of a loading dose of levothyroxine and then requires smaller daily maintenance doses.

ADVERSE EFFECTS. Thyroid hormone preparations rarely cause adverse reactions if dosing is appropriate and is carefully monitored during the initial treatment of hypothyroidism and periodically thereafter. The effects of excessive doses are similar to the manifestations of hyperthyroidism.

INTERACTIONS. Aluminum hydroxide, cholestyramine, ferrous sulfate, and sucralfate are among the drugs that interfere with the absorption of levothyroxine. These drugs should be administered 2 hours before or after levothyroxine is administered. Estrogens, androgens, and glucocorticoids can alter thyroid-binding globulin and total T_4 and T_3 levels, but free T_4 and TSH levels usually remain normal in patients taking these steroid hormones. For this reason, the dosage of levothyroxine usually does not need to be adjusted in persons who are taking steroid hormones.

Liothyronine

As shown in Table 32–1, liothyronine (T_3, CYTOMEL) is more potent than levothyroxine (T_4) and has a higher oral bioavailability. It is seldom used in the treatment of hypothyroidism, however, because it has several disadvantages. Liothyronine has a much shorter half-life than levothyroxine, so multiple daily doses may be needed to obtain a smooth response during hormone replacement therapy. Liothyronine does not increase plasma T_4 levels, so it is difficult to monitor the response to treatment. Liothyronine also causes more adverse cardiac effects and is more expensive than levothyroxine.

ANTITHYROID AGENTS

Antithyroid agents used in the treatment of hyperthyroidism include thiourea drugs, β-adrenergic receptor antagonists (β-blockers), iodide salts, and radioactive iodine.

The thiourea drugs inhibit the synthesis of thyroid hormones, whereas sufficient doses of iodide salts inhibit the release of these hormones. The β-blockers are used to control the cardiovascular symptoms of hyperthyroidism until definitive treatment becomes effective. The β-blockers, the corticosteroids, some thiourea derivatives (see below), and some iodinated contrast agents (e.g., **ipodate**) also inhibit the peripheral conversion of T_4 to T_3. Because of this action, ipodate is being investigated for the treatment of acute thyrotoxicosis.

Thiourea Drugs

The thiourea (thioureylene and thioamide) drugs include **methimazole** (TAPAZOLE) and **propylthiouracil** (PTU). Their structures are shown in Fig. 32–2.

Drug Properties

MECHANISMS. As discussed earlier in this chapter, the synthesis of thyroid hormones requires oxidation of trapped iodide, formation of iodotyrosines, and the coupling of iodotyrosines to form T_3 and T_4. Methimazole and PTU both inhibit peroxidase-catalyzed steps in this process (see Fig. 32–1). In addition, PTU (but not methimazole) inhibits the conversion of T_4 to T_3 in peripheral tissues. The contribution of this action to the therapeutic efficacy of PTU is uncertain, however, because PTU and methimazole appear to be therapeutically equivalent.

PHARMACOKINETICS. The thiourea drugs are well absorbed from the gut following oral administration. They are actively concentrated in the thyroid gland, which may account for their relatively long duration of action despite having relatively short half-lives. The thiourea drugs are extensively metabolized before undergoing renal excretion.

Methimazole   Propylthiouracil   Thiourea

Figure 32–2. Structures of methimazole and propylthiouracil, two antithyroid agents that contain a thiourea moiety.

INDICATIONS. In patients with **Graves' disease,** a thiourea drug can be used in an attempt to induce remission or as a means to control symptoms before surgery or RAI treatment. The effects of thiourea drugs are delayed because it takes about 4 to 8 weeks of therapy before the glandular hormone stores are depleted and circulating hormone levels start to return to the normal range. At this time, doses can be gradually tapered at monthly intervals to achieve the desired steady-state thyroid hormone level. If the objective is long-term remission of Graves' disease, patients usually remain on the drug for 12 to 24 months. About 45% of patients will eventually obtain a permanent remission. The mechanisms responsible for remission are uncertain but may involve a reduction in the thyroid-stimulating activity of thyroid antibodies or an alteration of the immunologic defect that stimulated antibody production. Persons with persistent thyroid-stimulating antibodies have a higher incidence of relapse than do persons without persistent antibodies.

ADVERSE EFFECTS. Pruritic maculopapular **rash,** arthralgia, and fever occur in up to 5% of persons treated with a thiourea drug. Less frequently, a lupus erythematosuslike syndrome, hepatitis, or gastrointestinal distress is reported.

Many patients experience benign and transient **leukopenia,** with a white blood cell count of less than $4000/\mu L$. This condition does not appear to be associated with the more severe **agranulocytosis** that sometimes occurs and is characterized by a granulocyte count of less than $250/\mu L$. Severe agranulocytosis usually develops during the first 3 months of therapy and can be prevented by advising patients to stop treatment and immediately contact their physician if they experience fever, malaise, sore throat, or other flulike symptoms.

Methimazole and PTU exhibit cross-sensitivity in about 50% of patients. For this reason, patients who have experienced a major adverse reaction should not be switched to the other drug.

Specific Drugs

Although methimazole and PTU appear to be clinically equivalent, they have minor differences. The plasma half-lives of methimazole and PTU are about 7 and 2 hours, respectively. Either drug, however, can be administered once or twice a day. Unlike methimazole, PTU inhibits the peripheral conversion of T_4 to T_3. Nevertheless, the clinical effects of the drugs are primarily related to inhibition of hormone synthesis and depletion of glandular stores.

About 70% of PTU is bound to plasma proteins. Methimazole is not bound to plasma proteins, and it readily crosses the placenta and appears in breast milk. Contrary to older studies, which indicated that PTU crosses the placenta less readily, newer evidence indicates that fetal blood concentrations of PTU are greater than maternal blood concentrations. Hence, both drugs must be used cautiously during pregnancy.

β-Adrenergic Receptor Antagonists

Thyroid hormones and the sympathetic nervous system act synergistically on cardiovascular function. This explains why increased levels of thyroid hormones can cause tachycardia, palpitations, and arrhythmias. β-Adrenergic receptor antagonists (e.g., **propranolol**) are used to reduce cardiovascular stimulation associated with hyperthyroidism. They act immediately and are particularly useful during **severe acute thyrotoxicosis (thyroid storm).** They are also used to control symptoms of hyperthyroidism in patients awaiting surgery or a response to RAI treatment.

Other Antithyroid Agents

Iodide Salts

Iodide salts are contained in **potassium iodide solutions,** such as **saturated solution of potassium iodide** (SSKI) and **Lugol's solution.** They are used on a short-term basis to treat patients with acute thyrotoxicosis, to prepare patients for thyroid surgery, and to inhibit the release of thyroid hormones following RAI treatment. Iodide salts can also be used to competitively block RAI uptake by the thyroid gland in the event of a nuclear reactor accident or other accidental exposure to toxic levels of RAI.

When administered in sufficient doses, iodide salts act immediately to inhibit the release of thyroid hormones from the thyroid gland. Plasma hormone levels then gradually decline as the circulating hormones are degraded. Patients with hyperthyroidism usually obtain symptomatic improvement within 2 to 7 days after starting iodide therapy. This effect is limited to several weeks, however, because the thyroid gland eventually escapes from the inhibitory effects of iodide salts. A thiourea drug can be used concurrently with iodide salts to further inhibit thyroid function and to provide a longer-lasting antithyroid effect.

In patients scheduled for thyroid surgery, a potassium iodide solution is usually administered preoperatively for 7 to 14 days to reduce the size and vascularity of the thyroid gland. As an adjunct to RAI treatment, potassium iodide is given 3 to 7 days following the administration of RAI.

The adverse effects of iodide salts are usually mild and can include skin rashes and other hypersensitivity reactions, salivary gland swelling, metallic taste, sore gums, and gastrointestinal discomfort.

Radioactive Iodine

Radioactive iodine is usually administered as a colorless and tasteless solution of **sodium iodide I 131** (^{131}I). The isotope is rapidly absorbed from the gut and concentrated by the thyroid gland. In the gland, it emits beta particles that destroy thyroid tissue. The particles have a tissue penetration of 2 mm, and the isotope has a half-life of 8 days. As thyroid tissue is destroyed, the circulating thyroid hormone levels gradually return to normal over several weeks.

β-Adrenergic receptor antagonists usually are used to control symptoms of hyperthyroidism while the patient is awaiting the response to RAI treatment. Methimazole or PTU can be used if β-blockers alone are not adequate to control these symptoms. Pretreatment with thiourea drugs before RAI treatment, however, appears to reduce the cure rate and cause a higher incidence of post-treatment recurrence or persistence of hyperthyroidism. For this reason, thiourea drugs should be withdrawn several days before RAI treatment and reinstituted several days after it.

Iodide salts are used after RAI treatment to inhibit thyroid hormone release. They should not be used before RAI treatment, however, because nonradioactive iodide would compete with ^{131}I for uptake by the thyroid gland.

Treatment with RAI is absolutely contraindicated in pregnant women, because it destroys fetal thyroid tissue.

■ RAI (^{131}I) is concentrated by the thyroid gland and emits beta particles that destroy thyroid tissue. It is used in the treatment of Graves' disease and other forms of hyperthyroidism. RAI treatment is absolutely contraindicated in pregnant women.

SUMMARY OF IMPORTANT POINTS

■ The thyroid gland synthesizes and secretes triiodothyronine (T_3) and tetraiodothyronine (T_4, thyroxine).

■ The steps in thyroid hormone synthesis include active iodide uptake by the thyroid gland, incorporation of iodide into tyrosine residues of thyroglobulin, and coupling of iodotyrosines to form T_3 and T_4. The secretion of T_3 and T_4 is modulated by thyroid-stimulating hormone (TSH, or thyrotropin) and by thyrotropin-releasing hormone (TRH).

■ The thyroid hormones, which activate cytoplasmic receptors, are translocated to the cell nucleus. In the nucleus, they activate gene transcription and thereby increase the metabolic rate and accelerate a wide range of cellular activities required for normal growth and development and for the maintenance of normal metabolism.

■ Levothyroxine (synthetic T_4) is the drug of choice for all forms of hypothyroidism. It has a long half-life (7 days) and can be administered orally once a day.

■ Liothyronine (synthetic T_3) is more potent than levothyroxine and has a higher oral bioavailability. It has a shorter half-life, however, and may need to be given several times a day.

■ Methimazole and propylthiouracil (PTU) are thiourea drugs that inhibit peroxidase-catalyzed steps in the synthesis of thyroid hormone. PTU also inhibits the peripheral conversion of T_4 to T_3. The onset of action of these drugs is delayed because of the time required to deplete glandular stores of thyroid hormone.

■ In patients with Graves' disease, methimazole or PTU is used in an attempt to induce remission or as a means to control symptoms before surgery or radioactive iodine (RAI) treatment.

■ β-Adrenergic receptor antagonists are used to control the cardiovascular symptoms of hyperthyroidism in patients who are suffering from acute thyrotoxicosis, are awaiting surgery, or are awaiting a response to RAI treatment.

■ The iodide salts in potassium iodide solutions act rapidly to inhibit the release of thyroid hormones from the thyroid gland. They produce symptomatic improvement in 2 to 7 days as circulating levels of thyroid hormones decline. Potassium iodide solutions are used to control symptoms of acute thyrotoxicosis, to reduce the vascularity and size of the thyroid gland before surgery, and to inhibit thyroid hormone release following RAI treatment.

Review Questions

For each drug described, select the corresponding drug from the lettered choices.

1. This drug is used to reduce the size and vascularity of the thyroid gland before surgery for hyperthyroidism.

2. This drug inhibits thyroid hormone synthesis and is used to induce remission in persons who present with a goiter, exophthalmos, and an elevated serum tetraiodothyronine (T_4) level.

3. This drug is used to control tachycardia and palpitations in persons with acute symptoms of hyperthyroidism.

4. This drug would be administered once daily to achieve euthyroidism in persons who had undergone total thyroidectomy.

5. This drug may cure hyperthyroidism while permanently causing hypothyroidism.

  (A) liothyronine
  (B) methimazole
  (C) propranolol
  (D) potassium iodide solution
  (E) levothyroxine
  (F) radioactive sodium iodide (^{131}I)

Answers and Explanations

1. The answer is D: potassium iodide solution. Potassium iodide solution can be administered for 2 weeks before surgery for hyperthyroidism to reduce the size and vascularity of the gland, thereby facilitating surgical excision of the gland.

2. The answer is B: methimazole. Methimazole and propylthiouracil are thiourea drugs that block catalase, the enzyme that catalyses the iodination of tyrosine residues of thyroglobulin, and couples iodothyronines to form thyroid hormones. These drugs are used for chronic suppression of hyperthyroidism in persons with Graves' disease.

3. The answer is C: propranolol. Propranolol and other adrenergic β-blockers can be used for short-term management of the excessive cardiovascular stimulation that often occurs in persons with severe acute hyperthyroidism. The β-blockers are used to control tachycardia and palpitations until antithyroid drugs reduce excessive thyroid hormone levels.

4. The answer is E: levothyroxine. Levothyroxine is the drug of choice for chronic thyroid hormone replacement therapy in persons with hypothyroidism. A single daily

dose of levothyroxine provides relatively stable physiologic levels of both T_4 and T_3 because a portion of the drug is converted to T_3 in peripheral tissues. Liothyronine, or synthetic T_3, is usually less desirable for this purpose because its shorter half-life leads to greater fluctuations in hormone levels and effects between doses.

5. The answer is F: radioactive sodium iodide (^{131}I). By destroying thyroid tissue, ^{131}I may permanently cure hyperthyroidism and cause hypothyroidism.

SELECTED READINGS

Bonnema, S. J., F. N. Bennedbaek, A. Veje, et al. Propylthiouracil before ^{131}I therapy of hyperthyroid diseases: effect on cure rate evaluated by a randomized clinical trial. J Clin Endocrinol Metab 89:4439–4444, 2004.

Iskandar, S. B., R. M. Jordan, and A. N. Peiris. Treating amiodarone-induced thyrotoxicosis with radioactive iodine. Tenn Med 97:408–410, 2004.

Siegmund, W., K. Spieker, A. I. Weike, et al. Replacement therapy with levothyroxine plus triiodothyronine is not superior to thyroxine alone to improve well-being and cognitive performance in hypothyroidism. Clin Endocrinol (Oxf) 60:750–757, 2004.

Topliss, D. J., and C. J. Eastman. Diagnosis and management of hyperthyroidism and hypothyroidism. Med J Aust 180:186–193, 2004.

CHAPTER 33

Adrenal Steroids and Related Drugs

CLASSIFICATION OF ADRENAL STEROIDS AND RELATED DRUGS

Adrenal Steroid Preparations
Mineralocorticoids
- Fludrocortisone (FLORINEF)

Glucocorticoids
- Cortisone and hydrocortisone
- Dexamethasone (DECADRON)[a]
- Prednisone[b]
- Desoximetasone (TOPICORT)[c]

Adrenal Androgens
- Dehydroepiandrosterone

Adrenal Steroid Inhibitors
Corticosteroid Synthesis Inhibitors
- Aminoglutethimide
- Ketoconazole
- Metyrapone

Corticosteroid Receptor Antagonists
- Mifepristone
- Spironolactone

[a]also betamethasone, budesonide, triamcinolone
[b]also prednisolone, methylprednisolone
[c]also desonide, fluticasone, fluocinonide, betamethasone, clobetasol

OVERVIEW

SYNTHESIS OF ADRENAL STEROIDS

The adrenal cortex occupies about 90% of the adrenal gland, consists of three layers, and produces three types of steroid hormones, or **corticosteroids.** These hormones can be classified as **mineralocorticoids, glucocorticoids,** and **adrenal androgens.** The mineralocorticoids are primarily produced in the outer layer (zona glomerulosa), whereas the glucocorticoids and adrenal androgens are produced in the middle layer (zona fasciculata) and inner layer (zona reticularis).

The major pathways for mineralocorticoid, glucocorticoid, and androgen biosynthesis are shown in Fig. 33–1. In humans, **aldosterone** is the major mineralocorticoid, **cortisol** is the major glucocorticoid, and **dehydroepiandrosterone** (DHEA) is the major adrenal androgen.

SECRETION OF ADRENAL STEROIDS

The secretion of adrenal steroids is affected by **physical and mental stress** and by the actions of two hormones: **corticotropin** (adrenocorticotropic hormone, ACTH), which is secreted by the anterior pituitary, and **corticotropin-releasing hormone** (CRH), which is secreted by the hypothalamus.

The secretion of aldosterone is partly stimulated by corticotropin but is chiefly regulated by the **renin-angiotensin system.** In contrast, the secretion of cortisol and adrenal androgens is controlled by corticotropin.

Various types of physical and mental stress are powerful activators of CRH secretion, and increased CRH secretion leads to increased corticotropin and cortisol production. As shown in Fig. 33–2, however, cortisol and other glucocorticoids act as feedback inhibitors of both CRH and corticotropin. This is why exogenously administered glucocorticoids can suppress the hypothalamic-pituitary-adrenal axis and inhibit endogenous cortisol production, leading to adrenal insufficiency when the exogenous glucocorticoid is withdrawn.

Although exogenously administered glucocorticoids have several actions that increase the body's resistance to stress, people who become dependent on these drugs often require larger doses of them during periods of stress, including stress caused by surgery, infection, and other trauma or disease states.

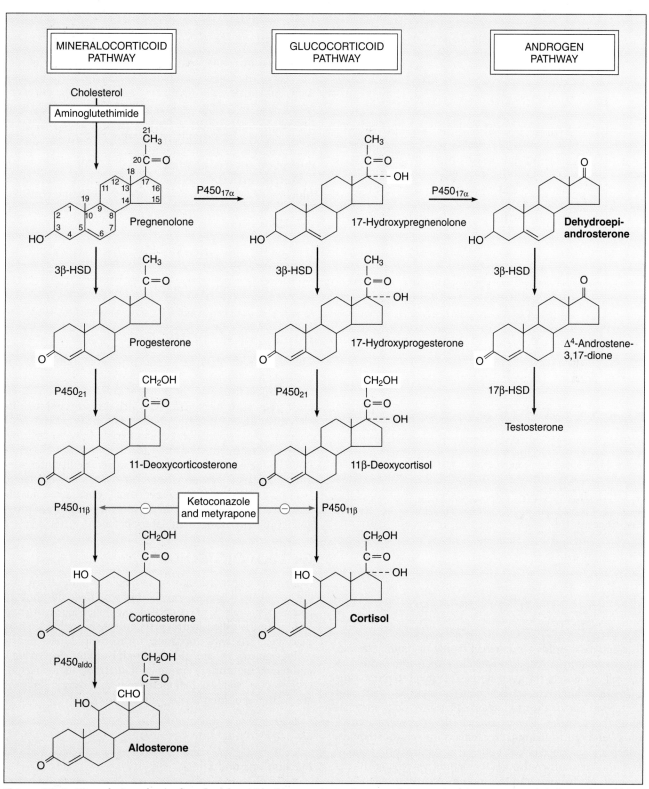

Figure 33–1. Biosynthetic pathways for adrenal steroids. Major pathways for mineralocorticoid, glucocorticoid, and androgen biosynthesis are shown. Important enzymes include 3β-hydroxysteroid dehydrogenase (3β-HSD), steroid 21-hydroxylase (P450$_{21}$), steroid 11β-hydroxylase (P450$_{11\beta}$), aldosterone synthase (P450$_{aldo}$), steroid 17α-hydroxylase (P450$_{17\alpha}$), and 17β-hydroxysteroid dehydrogenase (17β-HSD). The structural changes produced by each reaction are unshaded. Aminoglutethimide blocks the synthesis of all adrenal steroids by inhibiting the conversion of cholesterol to pregnenolone. Ketoconazole and metyrapone inhibit P450$_{11\beta}$. The most common defect causing congenital adrenal hyperplasia is P450$_{21}$ deficiency.

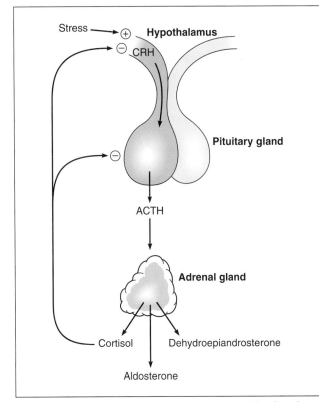

Figure 33–2. Regulation of the secretion of cortisol by the adrenal cortex. Stress and other stimuli increase the release of corticotropin-releasing hormone (CRH) from hypothalamic paraventricular nuclei. CRH is carried by hypophysioportal vessels to the anterior pituitary, where it stimulates the release of corticotropin (ACTH). Corticotropin acts on the adrenal cortex to increase the release of adrenal steroids, although the release of aldosterone is primarily regulated by the renin-angiotensin system. Cortisol exerts feedback inhibition on the hypothalamus and pituitary to inhibit the release of CRH and Corticotropin.

BINDING OF ADRENAL STEROIDS TO RECEPTORS

The adrenal steroids act on target tissues by binding to specific cytoplasmic receptors, which are then translocated to the cell nucleus. In the nucleus, the activated receptors stimulate or inhibit the transcription of specific genes and thereby modulate the production of key metabolic enzymes and other proteins. These actions lead to the various metabolic and anti-inflammatory effects of glucocorticoids, which are described below. In the renal tubules, activation of the mineralocorticoid receptor stimulates the synthesis of sodium channels and the sodium-potassium adenosine triphosphatase (ATPase) that are involved in sodium reabsorption. This mechanism is responsible for the salt-retaining effects of mineralocorticoids.

The **glucocorticoid receptor** has a high affinity for cortisol but a much lower affinity for aldosterone, whereas the **mineralocorticoid receptor** has a high affinity for both aldosterone and cortisol. This enables cortisol to exert both glucocorticoid and mineralocorticoid actions.

USES OF ADRENAL STEROIDS AND RELATED DRUGS

The glucocorticoids are most frequently used clinically because of the anti-inflammatory effects produced by supraphysiologic doses of them. Less commonly, the glucocorticoids and the mineralocorticoids are used as replacement therapy in the treatment of **adrenal insufficiency** and in the treatment of **adrenogenital syndromes** that produce excessive quantities of adrenal androgens and insufficient quantities of other corticosteroids.

Adrenocortical hyperfunction (Cushing's syndrome), which is caused by excessive levels of circulating corticosteroids, is treated with surgery, irradiation, and adrenal steroid inhibitors.

ADRENAL STEROID PREPARATIONS

The properties and structures of selected adrenal steroids are shown in Table 33–1 and Fig. 33–3.

MINERALOCORTICOIDS

Aldosterone, the major mineralocorticoid in humans, is not available for clinical use.

Fludrocortisone is the mineralocorticoid that is used most frequently. In patients with **primary adrenal insufficiency (Addison's disease),** fludrocortisone is given to supplement the mineralocorticoid effects of hydrocortisone (cortisol) treatment. The need for fludrocortisone is indicated by the continued presence of hyperkalemia after adequate doses of hydrocortisone have been administered. Fludrocortisone is administered orally once a day in the morning. The drug's salt-retaining potency is about 20 times greater than its anti-inflammatory potency.

GLUCOCORTICOIDS

Numerous glucocorticoids are available for clinical use and are frequently classified on the basis of their duration of action (see Table 33–1). **Cortisol,** the major glucocorticoid in humans, is called **hydrocortisone** when used as a pharmaceutical. As with **cortisone,** hydrocortisone is a short-acting glucocorticoid. **Methylprednisolone, prednisone,** and **triamcinolone** are examples of intermediate-acting glucocorticoids, whereas **betamethasone** and **dexamethasone** are examples of long-acting glucocorticoids.

Drug Properties

Mechanisms and Effects

Although the glucocorticoids were named for their role in the regulation of glucose metabolism, they have a number of other important physiologic actions.

EFFECTS ON CARBOHYDRATE, LIPID, AND PROTEIN METABOLISM. Glucocorticoids induce enzymes involved in gluconeogenesis (the formation of glucose from amino acids), promote glucose formation, and have an anti-insulin effect. This is why glucocorticoid insufficiency can lead to hypoglycemia

TABLE 33-1. Pharmacologic Properties of Adrenal Steroids

Drug*	Route of Administration	Duration of Action (Hours)	Mineralocorticoid (Salt-Retaining) Potency	Glucocorticoid (Anti-inflammatory) Potency
Short-acting drugs				
Hydrocortisone (cortisol)	Oral, parenteral, or topical	8–12	1	1
Cortisone	Oral, parenteral, or topical	8–12	0.8	0.8
Fludrocortisone	Oral	8–12	200	10
Intermediate-acting drugs				
Methylprednisolone	Oral, parenteral, or topical	12–36	0.5	5
Prednisone	Oral	12–36	0.7	3.5
Triamcinolone	Oral, parenteral, or topical	12–36	0	5
Long-acting drugs				
Betamethasone	Oral, parenteral, or topical	24–72	0	30
Dexamethasone	Oral, parenteral, or topical	24–72	0	30

*Fludrocortisone is classified as a mineralocorticoid, while the other drugs are classified as glucocorticoids.

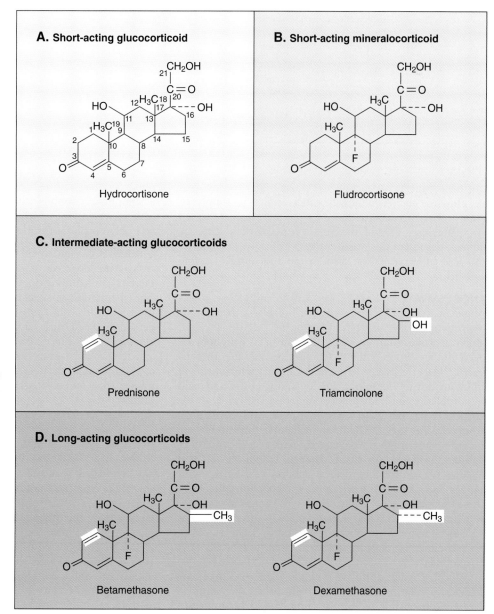

Figure 33–3. Structures of selected adrenal steroids. Hydrocortisone (cortisol) is a natural steroid. In the synthetic steroids, glucocorticoid potency is enhanced by the introduction of a double bond at the 1,2 position or the introduction of a hydroxyl or methyl group at the 16 position. These structural modifications are unshaded. Betamethasone and dexamethasone differ only in the configuration of the methyl group at the 16 position: in betamethasone (solid line) and in dexamethasone (dashed line). Both glucocorticoid and mineralocorticoid activities are increased by a fluorine substitution at the 9 position.

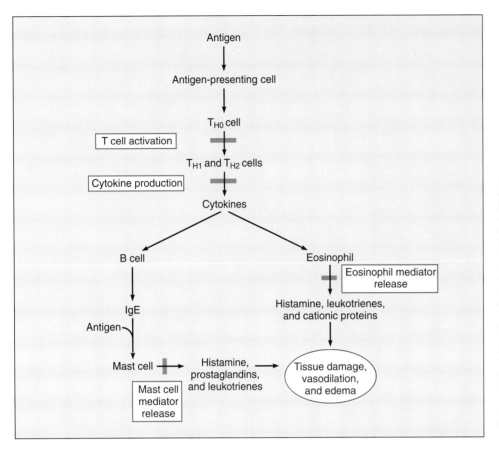

Figure 33–4. Anti-inflammatory actions of glucocorticoids. During the inflammatory process, undifferentiated T helper cells (T$_{H0}$) become activated T cells (T$_{H1}$ and T$_{H2}$) and produce cytokines. In addition to stimulating antibody production by B cells, cytokines recruit and activate eosinophils. Glucocorticoids act by suppressing T-cell activation, suppressing cytokine production, and preventing mast cells and eosinophils from releasing various chemical mediators of inflammation, including histamine, prostaglandins, leukotrienes, and other substances that cause tissue damage, vasodilatation, and edema. Glucocorticoids have additional anti-inflammatory effects that are described in the text. IgE = immunoglobulin E.

during stress. Glucocorticoids also activate enzymes involved in protein catabolism, thereby increasing the supply of amino acids needed for gluconeogenesis. Glucocorticoids stimulate lipolysis and inhibit the uptake of glucose by adipose tissue. For this reason, excessive glucocorticoid levels can lead to abnormal fat distribution and muscle wasting (see below).

ANTI-INFLAMMATORY EFFECTS. The anti-inflammatory effects of glucocorticoids are primarily attributable to their multiple actions on several types of leukocytes (Fig. 33–4). First, glucocorticoids suppress the activation of T lymphocytes. Second, they suppress the production of cytokines by activated T helper cells. Cytokines normally play a major role in inflammation by recruiting and activating eosinophils and by stimulating antibody production by B cells. Third, glucocorticoids prevent mast cells, basophils, and eosinophils from releasing various chemical mediators of inflammation, including histamine, prostaglandins, leukotrienes, and other substances that cause tissue damage, vasodilatation, and edema. Fourth, glucocorticoids stabilize lysosomal membranes and prevent the release of catabolic enzymes from these organelles. Finally, glucocorticoids cause vasoconstriction and decrease capillary permeability by direct actions as well as by inhibiting the actions of kinins, bacterial toxins, and chemical mediators released from mast cells and eosinophils.

Glucocorticoids also have multiple effects on circulating leukocytes. Pharmacologic doses of glucocorticoids suppress lymphoid tissue and reduce the number of circulating lymphocytes. They also reduce the concentration of circulating eosinophils, basophils, and monocytes while at the same time increasing the concentration of erythrocytes, platelets, and polymorphonuclear leukocytes.

OTHER EFFECTS. Glucocorticoids increase bone catabolism and antagonize the effect of vitamin D on calcium absorption, thereby contributing to the development of osteoporosis (see Chapter 36). Glucocorticoids also have several effects on the central nervous system. They alter the mood in some persons and can cause euphoria or psychosis. Large doses of glucocorticoids stimulate gastric acid and pepsin production and may thereby exacerbate peptic ulcers. Glucocorticoids can also reduce the secretion of thyroid-stimulating hormone (TSH) and follicle-stimulating hormone (FSH) by the pituitary gland.

Chemistry

In addition to showing the chemical structure of hydrocortisone, Fig. 33–3 shows the structures of several synthetic glucocorticoids that were developed to provide greater glucocorticoid (anti-inflammatory) potency than hydrocortisone. In the synthetic steroids, glucocorticoid potency is enhanced by the introduction of a double bond at the 1,2 position or the introduction of a hydroxyl or methyl group at the 16 position. Both glucocorticoid and mineralocorticoid activities are increased by a fluorine substitution at the 9 position. Table 33–1 shows the ratio of glucocorticoid potency to mineralocorticoid potency in numerous adrenal steroids.

Indications

Glucocorticoids are used for the diagnosis and treatment of adrenal diseases and for the treatment of a diverse group of nonadrenal disorders.

ADRENAL INSUFFICIENCY. In **primary adrenal insufficiency (Addison's disease)**, all regions of the adrenal cortex are destroyed. This gives rise to deficiencies in cortisol and aldosterone and to a reduction in androgen secretion. **Secondary adrenal insufficiency** has several causes, but it most commonly results when steroid drugs are used for a prolonged time, thereby suppressing the hypothalamic-pituitary-adrenal axis. Secondary disease is characterized by low levels of cortisol and androgens but normal levels of aldosterone.

Acute adrenal insufficiency (**adrenal crisis, addisonian crisis**) is a medical emergency that must be treated promptly with intravenously administered hydrocortisone for up to 48 hours. Once the patient's condition is stabilized, long-term oral hydrocortisone treatment can be instituted.

In the treatment of **chronic adrenal insufficiency,** hydrocortisone is administered orally in a manner that mimics the circadian secretion of cortisol by the normal adrenal gland, with two thirds of the daily dose given in the morning and one third given in the evening. If hyperkalemia is still present after the oral hydrocortisone dose is stabilized, the addition of a mineralocorticoid to the treatment regimen is usually required. A single daily dose of fludrocortisone is often used for this purpose.

Congenital adrenal hyperplasia (CAH) refers to a group of disorders caused by specific enzyme deficiencies that impair the synthesis of cortisol and aldosterone. Impaired synthesis leads to a compensatory increase in corticotropin secretion by the pituitary and results in adrenal hyperplasia. Because of the enzyme deficiencies, the steroid biosynthetic pathway shifts to the production of adrenal androgens, thereby resulting in virilism (masculinization) and hirsutism (excessive hair growth). The most common defect is **21-hydroxylase deficiency,** which accounts for 90% of cases of CAH. The second most common defect is **11β-hydroxylase deficiency,** which accounts for 9% of cases. CAH is treated by giving hydrocortisone to suppress the secretion of corticotropin. Fludrocortisone can be given to provide additional mineralocorticoid activity for salt-losing patients with CAH.

CUSHING'S SYNDROME. Cushing's syndrome is caused most often by a pituitary adenoma that produces excessive quantities of corticotropin, leading to adrenal hyperplasia and excessive cortisol production. Other causes of Cushing's syndrome include adrenal adenomas, adrenal carcinomas, and ectopic corticotropin-secreting tumors.

The diagnosis of Cushing's syndrome is often based on the free cortisol level in urine samples and on the results of testing with dexamethasone. In the **low-dose dexamethasone suppression test,** a single dose of dexamethasone is given orally at 11:00 pm, and cortisol levels in plasma are measured at 8:00 am the following morning. In healthy individuals, dexamethasone will suppress corticotropin secretion by the pituitary and cause plasma cortisol levels to be under 5 μg/dL. In persons with Cushing's syndrome, dexamethasone will not suppress corticotropin secretion, so the

cortisol level will usually exceed 10 μg/dL. The **high-dose dexamethasone suppression test** can be used to differentiate adrenal hyperplasia from other causes of hyperadrenocorticism.

Cushing's syndrome is usually treated by surgical excision of the pituitary adenoma or the hyperplastic adrenal glands. Patients must receive hydrocortisone parenterally in large doses during the surgical procedure. The dose is then gradually tapered to normal replacement levels.

INFLAMMATION, ALLERGY, AND AUTOIMMUNE DISORDERS. The glucocorticoids are most frequently used to suppress inflammation and immune dysfunction associated with diseases affecting almost every organ in the body. Glucocorticoids counteract inflammation evoked by physical trauma, extreme temperatures, noxious chemicals, radiation damage, and microbial pathogens. They also suppress inflammation caused by allergic and autoimmune reactions and other disease states.

CANCER. Because of their lymphotoxic effects, glucocorticoids are used in the treatment of **lymphocytic leukemias and lymphomas** (see Chapter 45). Dexamethasone is a long-acting glucocorticoid used in combination with other drugs to prevent emesis during cancer chemotherapy.

RESPIRATORY DISTRESS SYNDROME. Betamethasone is used to prevent respiratory distress syndrome in premature infants. It acts by promoting fetal lung maturation in the same manner as endogenous cortisol does. Betamethasone is used because it is not highly protein bound and will readily enter the placental circulation.

DERMATOLOGIC CONDITIONS. Corticosteroids are often used to treat a wide range of dermatologic conditions, including atopic (contact) dermatitis, pruritis (itching) from various causes, psoriasis, sarcoidosis, seborrheic dermatitis, sunburn, and a number of other conditions. Topical corticosteroids are grouped according to their relative anti-inflammatory potency (high, medium, and low). Low-potency drugs are preferred for treating areas with thinner skin (e.g., the face, eye) and intertriginous areas where skin is folded or overlapped. Low- to medium-potency steroids can be used on the ears, trunk, arms, legs, and scalp. Medium- to very high-potency drugs may be needed to treat disorders in areas of thicker skin (e.g., the palms and soles).

The type of lesion influences the choice of vehicle for drug administration. Ointments are preferred to treat disorders involving dry, cracked, scaly, or hardened skin. Lotions and creams are best for treating moist, weeping lesions or conditions with intense inflammation. Lotions and gels are usually more convenient for applying steroids to hairy areas.

Low-potency topical corticosteroids include hydrocortisone, which is available without prescription for treating minor allergic reactions (e.g., insect bites). Other low-potency topical steroids include desonide (DESOWEN) and dexamethasone. Medium-potency topical steroids include triamcinolone (KENALOG) and fluticasone (CUTIVATE). Desoximetasone (TOPICORT) and fluocinonide (LIDEX) are high-potency topical corticosteroids, whereas betamethasone dipropionate (DIPROLENE) and clobetasol (TEMOVATE) are very high-potency steroids.

OTHER DISORDERS. Glucocorticoids are used to treat **hypercalcemia,** and they are the drugs of choice for managing **sarcoidosis.** Glucocorticoids are also used as immunosuppressant drugs to prevent **organ graft rejection** (see Chapter 45).

Pharmacokinetics

Many glucocorticoids are available for oral, parenteral, and topical use. Some are available for inhalational administration.

ORAL PREPARATIONS. When administered orally, glucocorticoids are extremely lipid soluble and are well absorbed from the gut. In the circulation, the glucocorticoids are highly bound to corticosteroid-binding globulin and albumin. Glucocorticoids are oxidized by cytochrome P450 enzymes and conjugated with sulfate or glucuronide in the liver before undergoing renal excretion. The biologic half-life and duration of action of glucocorticoids are primarily determined by their potency at the glucocorticoid receptor. The highly potent glucocorticoids evoke a longer-lasting stimulation of gene transcription than do the less potent drugs.

Glucocorticoids are administered orally to treat serious allergic reactions, autoimmune disorders, neoplastic diseases, and many other conditions. Prednisone or another intermediate-acting drug is often used for these purposes. For acute allergic reactions and other acute disorders, glucocorticoids are often more effective when they are given initially in large doses. The dose is then gradually tapered over several days until treatment is discontinued. For severe autoimmune and inflammatory disorders (e.g., **systemic lupus erythematous** and polymyositis with dermatomyositis), large doses of prednisone must be given daily for several months until a remission is achieved, and then the dose is slowly tapered and continued for 1 to 2 years or longer. In some conditions, it may be possible to convert the patient to alternate-day therapy, in which all or most of the dose is given on alternate days. This dosage schedule appears to reduce the severity of adverse effects and produces less suppression of the hypothalamic-pituitary-adrenal axis by allowing more time for recovery between doses.

PARENTERAL PREPARATIONS. Glucocorticoids are administered parenterally to treat acute adrenal crises, acute allergic reactions, and similar emergencies. In some cases, the drugs are given intravenously. In other cases, they are given intramuscularly, either as a rapidly absorbed solution or as a slowly absorbed drug suspension (depot preparation). Depot preparations are useful in providing a sustained level of the drug for several weeks, as is sometimes necessary in the treatment of a severe allergic reaction.

TOPICAL AND INHALATIONAL PREPARATIONS. Whenever possible, topical or inhalational administration is preferred because it is usually well tolerated and avoids most systemic adverse effects. Topical administration is widely used in the treatment of allergic or inflammatory conditions affecting the skin (see previous text), mucous membranes, or eyes. For example, glucocorticoids are administered topically in the eye to treat allergic conjunctivitis and acute uveitis (inflammation of the iris, ciliary body, or choroid). Glucocorticoids are given by inhalation to treat allergic rhinitis, aspiration pneumonia, asthma, and other respiratory conditions (see Chapter 27).

Adverse Effects

The administration of supraphysiologic doses of glucocorticoids for more than 2 weeks produces a series of tissue and metabolic changes that resemble Cushing's syndrome. The face becomes rounded and puffy (moon facies) as fat is redistributed to the face and trunk from the extremities. Fat accumulation in the supraclavicular and dorsocervical areas contributes to the development of a "buffalo hump." Increased hair growth (hirsutism), weight gain, and muscle wasting and weakness are often observed. Dermatologic changes can include acne (steroid acne), bruising, and thinning of the skin.

Other metabolic and physiologic changes caused by glucocorticoid administration include hyperglycemia, glucose intolerance, osteoporosis, and hypertension. Some changes, such as sodium retention, potassium loss, and hypertension, are more common when cortisone or hydrocortisone is used because these drugs have greater mineralocorticoid activity than do other glucocorticoids.

Long-term use of glucocorticoids can cause posterior subcapsular **cataracts** and **glaucoma,** can exacerbate the manifestations of peptic ulcer disease, and can mask the symptoms and signs of mycotic and other infections. In children, long-term use can cause growth retardation.

Glucocorticoids are contraindicated or should be used with caution in patients with psychoses, peptic ulcers, heart diseases, hypertension, diabetes, osteoporosis, and certain infections.

Specific Drugs

Short-Acting Glucocorticoids

Hydrocortisone and cortisone have a duration of action of 8 to 12 hours, have equal glucocorticoid and mineralocorticoid effects, and are the preferred glucocorticoids when replacement therapy is needed for patients with adrenal insufficiency. These drugs are also used as anti-inflammatory agents, but more potent glucocorticoids are often preferred for patients with severe inflammatory, allergic, and autoimmune disorders.

Intermediate-Acting Glucocorticoids

Prednisone, prednisolone, methylprednisolone, and triamcinolone are the glucocorticoids used most often for systemic treatment. In the body, prednisone is rapidly converted to prednisolone, a substance that is itself available as a drug. The intermediate-acting glucocorticoids have a duration of action of 12 to 36 hours and are often used to treat cancer, inflammation, allergy, and autoimmune disorders.

Long-Acting Glucocorticoids

Betamethasone (CELESTONE) and dexamethasone (DECADRON) are stereoisomers that differ in the configuration of the methyl group at the 16 position. Betamethasone is available for systemic use, and it is also used in the topical treatment of a number of skin disorders, including psoriasis, seborrheic or atopic dermatitis, and neurodermatitis.

Dexamethasone is used in dexamethasone suppression tests (see above) and in the treatment of a variety of neoplastic, infectious, and other inflammatory conditions that require the use of a potent and long-acting drug. Budesonide (ENTOCORT EC) is another long-acting corticosteroid drug.

Inhalational Glucocorticoids

Several glucocorticoids, including **beclomethasone** (BECLOVENT, VANCERIL), are available for nasal inhalation or oral inhalation to treat allergic rhinitis or asthma, respectively. Inhaled glucocorticoids are often first-line therapy for these disorders, and their administration and use are described in Chapter 27.

ADRENAL ANDROGENS

Dehydroepiandrosterone is the major androgen secreted by the adrenal cortex. Smaller quantities of androstenedione and testosterone are also secreted by the adrenal gland.

Dehydroepiandrosterone is an extremely weak androgen, but it is partly converted to testosterone in the body. In humans, studies show that the production of DHEA by the adrenal gland declines in a linear fashion after the age of 20 years. In animals, studies indicate that DHEA protects against the development of diabetes mellitus, immune disorders, and cancer. DHEA also appears to prevent weight gain and prolong life in some species. For these reasons, the use of DHEA supplements has been adopted uncritically by the health food culture. Although some evidence suggests beneficial effects of DHEA in the elderly and other people, much remains to be learned about the clinical utility of this steroid.

Because DHEA is a weak androgen, it should not be used by men with prostate cancer.

ADRENAL STEROID INHIBITORS

CORTICOSTEROID SYNTHESIS INHIBITORS

Fig. 33–l shows the sites of action of three inhibitors of corticosteroid synthesis: aminoglutethimide, metyrapone, and ketoconazole.

Aminoglutethimide

Aminoglutethimide inhibits the conversion of cholesterol to pregnenolone, an early and rate-limiting step in adrenal steroid biosynthesis. Because the synthesis of all steroids is reduced by aminoglutethimide, it has been used in the treatment of **breast cancer** and **malignant adrenocortical tumors.** It also has been used in combination with metyrapone to treat **Cushing's syndrome.**

Metyrapone

Metyrapone inhibits the synthesis of glucocorticoids by inhibiting the 11 ß-hydroxylase enzyme that catalyzes the final step in the glucocorticoid pathway. As a result of this action, the steroid biosynthetic pathway is shifted to the production of adrenal androgens. Metyrapone is occasionally used to treat **Cushing's syndrome** in patients who are refractory to other treatments and are not candidates for surgery. Metyrapone is also sometimes used in tests of adrenal function.

Ketoconazole

Ketoconazole is an antifungal drug that inhibits several cytochrome P450 enzymes involved in steroid biosynthesis, including 11 β-hydroxylase. When used in the treatment of **Cushing's syndrome,** the drug can lower the amount of cortisol to the normal range for most patients. It also inhibits androgen synthesis, however, and may cause gynecomastia in male patients.

CORTICOSTEROID RECEPTOR ANTAGONISTS

Spironolactone

Spironolactone is a synthetic steroid that competes with aldosterone for the mineralocorticoid (aldosterone) receptor in the renal tubules. It is used as a **potassium-sparing diuretic** (see Chapter 13) and as an agent for the treatment of hyperaldosteronism. Spironolactone is the drug of choice for **primary hyperaldosteronism** caused by bilateral adrenal hyperplasia, whereas surgery is the treatment of choice for hyperaldosteronism caused by an aldosterone-producing adenoma. **Secondary hyperaldosteronism** associated with heart failure, Bartter's syndrome, and other causes may also be improved by the administration of spironolactone.

Mifepristone

Mifepristone is an antagonist at both progesterone and glucocorticoid receptors (see Chapter 34). It is undergoing investigation for the treatment of **Cushing's syndrome** and appears to be highly effective in reversing the effects of **hyperadrenocorticism.**

SUMMARY OF IMPORTANT POINTS

■ The adrenal gland secretes mineralocorticoids (primarily aldosterone), glucocorticoids (primarily cortisol), and adrenal androgens (primarily dehydroepiandrosterone).

■ Mineralocorticoids have salt-retaining activity. They include fludrocortisone, a short-acting drug that is used to supplement hydrocortisone (cortisol) treatment in patients with adrenal insufficiency.

■ Glucocorticoids increase gluconeogenesis, protein and lipid catabolism, and the body's resistance to stress. They reduce inflammation by inhibiting the migration of leukocytes and the production and release of cytokines, prostaglandins, leukotrienes, and other mediators of inflammation. They also stabilize lysosomal membranes and cause vasoconstriction.

■ Glucocorticoids are chiefly used as anti-inflammatory and immunosuppressive drugs in the treatment of a wide range of allergic, inflammatory, and autoimmune disorders. They are also used as replacement therapy in the treatment of primary adrenal insufficiency (Addison's disease) and congenital adrenal hyperplasia.

■ Glucocorticoids include short-acting drugs (cortisone and hydrocortisone), intermediate-acting drugs (methylprednisolone, prednisone, and triamcinolone), and long-acting drugs (betamethasone and dexamethasone).

■ In comparison with cortisol, most synthetic glucocorticoids have increased glucocorticoid potency and decreased mineralocorticoid potency.

■ Glucocorticoids are generally administered topically to treat skin, mucous membrane, and ocular disorders and by inhalation to treat allergic rhinitis and asthma.

■ Topical steroids for treating dermatologic conditions include desonide (low potency), triamcinolone and fluticasone (medium potency), desoximetasone (high potency), and clobetasol (very high potency).

■ In patients with acute allergic reactions, glucocorticoids are initially given in large doses. The doses are rapidly tapered and eventually discontinued. In patients with severe autoimmune and inflammatory diseases, large doses of prednisone or other glucocorticoids may be required for several months. Alternate-day therapy is preferred for their long-term administration.

■ Adverse effects of glucocorticoids include fat accumulation in the face and trunk, muscle wasting, skin changes, glucose intolerance, potassium depletion, osteoporosis, hypertension, and cataracts.

■ Aminoglutethimide, metyrapone, and ketoconazole inhibit various steps in corticosteroid biosynthesis and are occasionally used to diagnose and treat adrenal hyperplasia.

Review Questions

1. Which drug acts as an antagonist at glucocorticoid receptors?
   (A) ketoconazole
   (B) metyrapone
   (C) mifepristone
   (D) spironolactone
   (E) aminoglutethimide

2. How would prednisone be administered to treat acute allergic reactions, such as that caused by a wasp sting?
   (A) continuous high dose therapy for 4 to 6 weeks
   (B) continuous low dose therapy for 4 to 6 weeks
   (C) gradually increasing doses over several days
   (D) gradually decreasing doses over several days
   (E) intermittent every-other-day therapy until symptoms resolve

3. Which drug is the most potent mineralocorticoid drug and one that can be used as replacement therapy in persons with Addison's disease?
   (A) dexamethasone
   (B) fludrocortisone
   (C) triamcinolone
   (D) hydrocortisone
   (E) aldosterone

4. The long-term administration of large doses of prednisone will cause the least reduction in the secretion of which hormone?
   (A) cortisol
   (B) corticotropin
   (C) corticotropin-releasing hormone
   (D) aldosterone

5. Which of the following is an example of a very high-potency topical corticosteroid?
   (A) dexamethasone
   (B) prednisone
   (C) clobetasol
   (D) triamcinolone
   (E) hydrocortisone

Answers and Explanations

1. The answer is C: mifepristone. Mifepristone is an antagonist at both progesterone and glucocorticoid receptors. It has been investigated for use in the treatment of Cushing's syndrome.

2. The answer is D: gradually decreasing doses over several days. For the treatment of acute allergic reactions, the most effective regimens are those in which glucocorticoids are given in large doses initially and then gradually tapered over 5 to 7 days. This produces the most rapid improvement in symptoms while causing relatively little adrenal suppression.

3. The answer is B: fludrocortisone. Fludrocortisone is approximately 100 times more potent as a mineralocorticoid than is cortisol and is the most potent mineralocorticoid available for clinical use. Aldosterone, the primary endogenous mineralocorticoid, is not available as a drug.

4. The answer is D: aldosterone. Exogenous administration of glucocorticoid drugs causes feedback inhibition of the secretion of corticotropin-releasing hormone, corticotropin, cortisol, and cortisone. Secretion of the mineralocorticoid, aldosterone, is primarily under the influence of the renin-angiotensin axis and is not suppressed greatly by exogenous glucocorticoid administration.

5. The answer is C: clobetasol. Clobetasol is a very high-potency topical corticosteroid. Answers (A), dexamethasone, and (E), hydrocortisone, are low-potency topical corticosteroids. Answer (D), triamcinolone, is a medium-potency topical corticosteroid, whereas answer (B), prednisone, is not used topically.

SELECTED READINGS

Annane, D., E. Bellissant, P. E. Bollaert, et al. Corticosteroids for severe sepsis and septic shock: a systematic review and meta-analysis. BMJ 329:480, 2004.

Boguniewicz, M. Topical treatment of atopic dermatitis. Immunol Allergy Clin North Am 24:631–644, 2004.

Katz, J. A. Treatment of inflammatory bowel disease with corticosteroids. Gastroenterol Clin North Am 33:171–189, 2004.

Oren, D., I. Nulman, M. Makhija, et al. Using corticosteroids during pregnancy. Are topical, inhaled, or systemic agents associated with risk? Can Fam Physician 50:1083–1085, 2004.

Rowe, B. H., M. L. Edmonds, C. H. Spooner, et al. Corticosteroid therapy for acute asthma. Respir Med 98:275–284, 2004.

CHAPTER 34

Drugs Affecting Fertility and Reproduction

CLASSIFICATION OF DRUGS AFFECTING FERTILITY AND REPRODUCTION

Estrogens and Progestins
Estrogens
- Estradiol[a]
- Conjugated equine estrogens (PREMARIN)

Progestins
- Medroxyprogesterone (PROVERA)[b]
- Norethindrone[c]

Antiestrogens
- Clomiphene
- Raloxifene (EVISTA)
- Tamoxifen
- Anastrozole (ARIMIDEX)
- Letrozole (FEMARA)

Antiprogestins
- Mifepristone (MIFEPREX)

Androgens
- Danazol
- Testosterone
- Methyltestosterone

Antiandrogens
- Flutamide (EULEXIN)[d]
- Finasteride (PROPECIA, PROSCAR)

[a]also ethinyl estradiol, mestranol
[b]also hydroxyprogesterone, megestrol, progesterone
[c]also desogestrel, drospirenone, levonorgestrel,
  norethynodrel, norgestimate
[d]also bicalutamide and nilutamide

OVERVIEW

Human reproduction involves a cascade of hormonal secretions, beginning with the secretion of gonadotropin-releasing hormone (GnRH) from the hypothalamus. As described in Chapter 31, GnRH stimulates the pituitary to release two gonadotropins: follicle-stimulating hormone (FSH) and luteinizing hormone (LH). These gonadotropins then stimulate the production of **sex steroids** and gametes by the ovary in the female and by the testis in the male.

The three categories of sex steroids secreted by the gonads are (1) **estrogens,** which include **estradiol, estrone,** and **estriol;** (2) **progestins,** which include **progesterone;** and (3) **androgens,** which include **testosterone.** Estrogens, progesterone, and testosterone are produced in both males and females, but the relative amounts and patterns of secretion differ markedly between the sexes. Females primarily secrete estrogens and progesterone, whereas males primarily produce testosterone.

Biosynthesis of Sex Steroids

As shown in Fig. 34–1, **pregnenolone** is the precursor to progesterone. It is also the precursor to dehydroepiandrosterone and androstenedione (two androgens secreted by the adrenal gland and discussed in Chapter 33) and to testosterone (the major androgen in males). The adrenal and gonadal androgens are converted to estrogens by **aromatase,** an enzyme that forms the aromatic A-ring necessary for the selective high-affinity binding of estradiol, estrone, and estriol to **estrogen receptors.**

In females, ovarian **thecal cells** secrete small quantities of testosterone. In males, about 95% of testosterone is produced by **Leydig's cells** in the testes, and the remainder is derived from the **adrenal cortex.** Testosterone is synthesized in the testes by the same pathways as in the ovaries. Testosterone is subsequently converted to **dihydrotestosterone** (DHT) by **5α-reductase** in the prostate, hair follicles, and skin. In the plasma, testosterone is primarily bound to sex

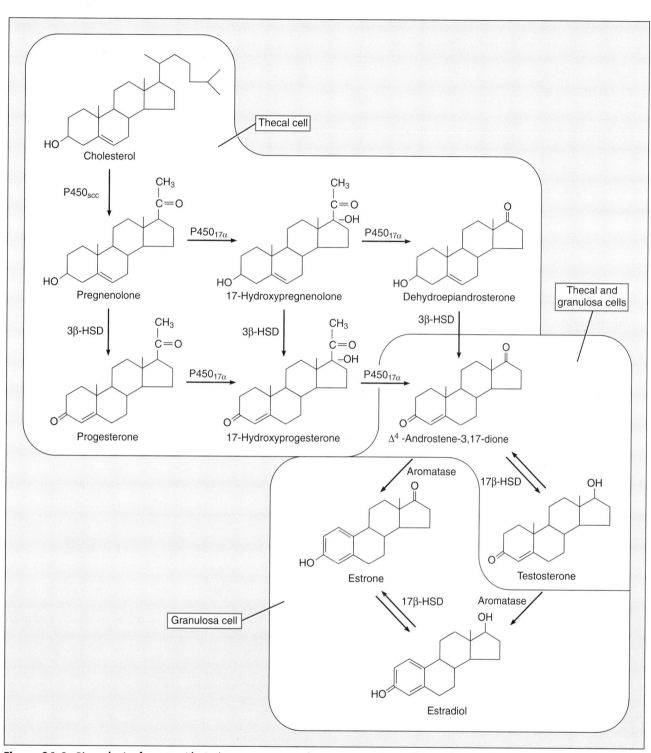

Figure 34–1. Biosynthesis of sex steroids. In the ovary, pregnenolone is converted to androstenedione and testosterone in thecal cells. These steroids are then converted to estrone and estradiol in granulosa cells. Enzymes involved in these steps include the cholesterol side-chain cleavage enzyme (P450$_{scc}$), steroid 17α-hydroxylase (P450$_{17α}$), 3β-hydroxysteroid dehydrogenase (3β-HSD), 17β-hydroxysteroid dehydrogenase (17β-HSD), and aromatase. Estrone and estradiol are partly converted to estriol by other enzymes. After ovulation, the major product of thecal cells is progesterone, owing to the development of a relative deficiency of 17α-hydroxylase activity.

steroid-binding globulin. In the liver, it is converted to androstenedione and other metabolites, including sulfate and glucuronide conjugates. About 90% of these metabolites are excreted in the urine.

Although both testosterone and DHT activate **androgen receptors,** DHT has greater receptor affinity and forms a more stable receptor-ligand complex than testosterone. If DHT formation is inhibited, this significantly reduces androgenic stimulation of the prostate gland and hair follicles. The androgen receptor located in the nuclei of target cells interacts with response elements in target genes and thereby stimulates protein synthesis in the same manner as other sex steroids.

Physiologic Actions of Estrogens and Progesterone

In males and females, estrogens are responsible for epiphyseal closure, which halts linear bone growth.

In females, estrogens and progesterone have multiple actions and interactions that are necessary for reproductive activity. Estrogens are formed in the **granulosa cells** of the ovary, whereas progesterone is primarily produced by the **corpus luteum** in response to LH secretion. Estrogens promote the development and growth of the fallopian tubes, uterus, and vagina, as well as secondary sex characteristics such as breast development, skeletal growth, and axillary and pubic hair patterns.

The pattern of hormonal changes occurring during the **menstrual cycle** is depicted in Fig. 34–2. During the **follicular phase** of the cycle, ovarian follicles are recruited and a dominant estrogen-secreting follicle develops. Estrogen levels gradually increase, whereas progesterone levels remain very low. A surge of LH is released at midcycle in response to positive estrogen feedback to the pituitary gland, and this LH surge triggers ovulation. During the **luteal phase** of the cycle, the follicle becomes the corpus luteum (yellow body) that secretes both estrogen and progesterone in response to LH. Together, these hormones prepare the uterus for implantation of a fertilized egg as the endometrium becomes more vascular and secretory. If pregnancy does not occur, the corpus luteum ceases to produce estrogen and progesterone, resulting in menstruation. If pregnancy occurs, the placenta produces human chorionic gonadotropin (hCG), which maintains the production of progesterone by the corpus luteum. After about 3 months, the placenta becomes the predominant source of progesterone. This hormone serves to maintain pregnancy and prevents endometrial sloughing and miscarriage.

Estrogens have a number of other actions that are important in reproduction and other bodily functions. They sensitize the myometrium to oxytocin at parturition, and this facilitates labor. They stimulate protein synthesis in the brain and may thereby affect mood and emotions. Estrogens influence the distribution of body fat and thereby contribute to the development of feminine body contours. They enhance blood coagulation by increasing the synthesis of clotting factors, and they prevent osteoporosis by inhibiting bone resorption.

Estrogens and progestins have different effects on serum lipoprotein levels. Estrogens decrease the levels of **low-density lipoprotein (LDL) cholesterol** and **lipoprotein(a)** while increasing the levels of **high-density lipoprotein (HDL) cholesterol.** In contrast, progestins produce a dose-related increase in LDL levels and a decrease in HDL levels.

Progesterone and other progestins increase basal body temperature by 0.5°C to 0.8°C (1.0°F to 1.5°F) at ovulation and throughout the luteal phase. They also affect the emotional state and have mild mineralocorticoid (salt-retaining) properties. Some of the synthetic progestins have other effects that are attributed to their androgenic activity (see below).

Physiologic Actions of Testosterone

Luteinizing hormone stimulates testosterone synthesis in **Leydig's cells,** whereas FSH promotes spermatogenesis by **Sertoli's cells** in the seminiferous tubules. These cells provide an environment rich in testosterone, which is necessary for germ cell development. Sertoli's cells also produce a protein called **inhibin,** which acts in concert with DHT as a feedback regulator of FSH secretion by the pituitary.

Testosterone is responsible for the development of secondary sex characteristics in males during puberty. These include growth of the larynx, thickening of the vocal cords, and growth of facial, axillary, and pubic hair. In addition to stimulating growth of the penis, scrotum, seminal vesicles, and prostate gland, testosterone stimulates and maintains sexual function in males. Testosterone and other androgens also do the following: increase lean body mass; stimulate skeletal growth; accelerate epiphyseal closure; increase sebaceous gland activity and sebum production, thereby contributing to the development of acne in both sexes; increase the production of erythropoietin in the kidneys; and decrease the levels of HDL cholesterol.

ESTROGENS AND PROGESTINS

An estrogen or progestin preparation can be used alone for the treatment of various disorders, or the two preparations can be used in combination for **hormone replacement therapy** (HRT) in postmenopausal women or for **contraception** in women of childbearing age.

Estrogens

Drug Properties

CHEMISTRY. The natural estrogens include **estradiol** and **conjugated estrogens.** Estradiol is an 18-carbon steroid with an aromatic A-ring that is hydroxylated in the 3 position (Fig. 34–3A). **Conjugated equine estrogens** are sulfate esters of **estrone** and **equilin** and can be obtained from the urine of pregnant mares. **Ethinyl estradiol** and **mestranol** are synthetic derivatives of estradiol.

PREPARATIONS. Micronized estradiol (ESTRACE) is an orally administered estradiol preparation that has good bioavailability. Also available are vaginal estradiol tablets (VAGIFEM) and a vaginal ring that slowly releases estradiol (ESTRING).

Ethinyl estradiol and **mestranol** have an ethinyl group at the C17 position of estradiol, which reduces first-pass

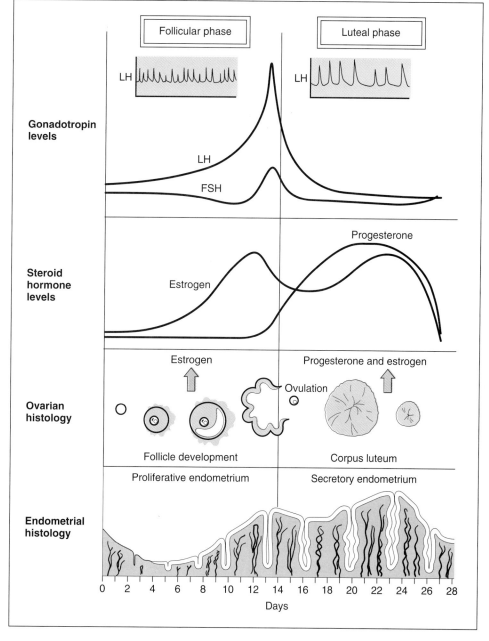

Figure 34–2. Hormone secretion during the human menstrual cycle. Luteinizing hormone (LH) and follicle-stimulating hormone (FSH) are released in a pulsatile manner from the pituitary gland in response to the pulsatile secretion of gonadotropin-releasing hormone (GnRH) from the hypothalamus. FSH stimulates ovarian follicle development and the secretion of estrogen during the follicular phase of the cycle. After ovulation, the corpus luteum produces both estrogen and progesterone during the luteal phase. Estrogen decreases FSH and LH secretion during most of the cycle (feedback inhibition) while provoking the midcycle LH and FSH surge that triggers ovulation. Progesterone decreases the frequency of hypothalamic GnRH pulses and the frequency of pulsatile LH and FSH secretion (inset in top panel). During the luteal phase, progesterone increases the amount of LH released (pulse amplitude). Estrogen stimulates the proliferation of the endometrium during the follicular phase, whereas progesterone causes the endometrium to become more vascular and secretory during the luteal phase.

metabolism, increases the half-life to about 20 hours, and results in greater oral potency compared with estradiol itself. These agents are primarily used in estrogen–progestin contraceptives. **Conjugated equine estrogens** (PREMARIN) are hydrolyzed to **estrone** and **equilin** before absorption from the gut. They undergo relatively little first-pass metabolism and are converted in the liver to sulfate and glucuronide conjugates that are primarily excreted in the urine. Estrone is also available in a rapidly absorbed formulation for intramuscular administration.

Several long-acting formulations of estradiol are available for transdermal or intramuscular administration. **Transdermal estradiol systems** (ALORA, CLIMARA, ESTRADERM, FEMPATCH, VIVELLE) slowly release the drug for absorption through the skin. These preparations are formulated for twice weekly or weekly application. **Estradiol cypionate** and **estradiol valerate** are long-acting esters of estradiol that are slowly absorbed following intramuscular administration and provide effective plasma concentrations of estradiol for several weeks.

Following their absorption, the natural estrogens are highly bound to sex steroid-binding globulin, are widely distributed, and are concentrated in fat. They undergo enterohepatic cycling, in which conjugated metabolites are excreted in the bile and converted to free estrogens by intestinal bacteria. The free estrogens are then reabsorbed into the circulation. As with estrone and equilin, estradiol is metabolized in the liver to sulfate and glucuronide conjugates, and these conjugates are primarily excreted in the urine, with small amounts excreted in the feces.

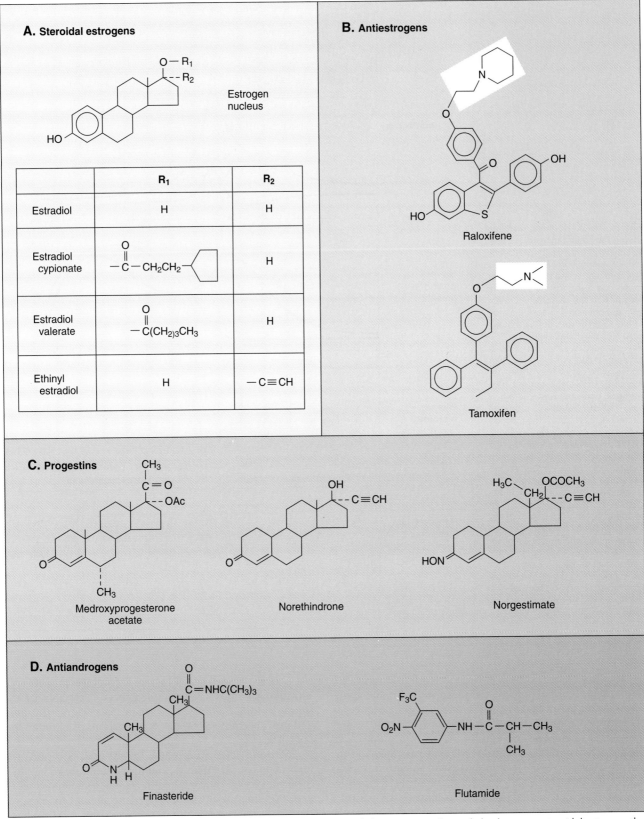

Figure 34–3. Structures of selected sex hormones and antagonists. (A) Estradiol cypionate and estradiol valerate are steroidal estrogens that are slowly hydrolyzed to estradiol following intramuscular administration. Ethinyl estradiol is a long-acting estradiol derivative that has good oral bioavailability. **(B)** Raloxifene and tamoxifen have estrogen antagonist and partial agonist activity. The antagonist activity is conferred by the unshaded moiety. **(C)** Medroxyprogesterone acetate is the acetate derivative of methylprogesterone (Ac denotes acetate), whereas norethindrone and norgestimate are derivatives of 19-nortestosterone. Norethindrone has an estrane nucleus, and norgestimate is a gonane derivative. **(D)** Finasteride is a 5α-reductase inhibitor, and flutamide is an androgen receptor antagonist.

INDICATIONS. Estrogen preparations are used in the treatment of **primary hypogonadism,** including cases caused by surgical oophorectomy, menopause, and other causes. Micronized estradiol, transdermal estradiol, and conjugated equine estrogens are primarily used for **hormone replacement therapy** (see below) in postmenopausal women. Combination estrogen–progestin preparations contain ethinyl estradiol or mestranol. These preparations are often used for **oral contraception** and for the treatment of **acne vulgaris** and **dysmenorrhea.**

ADVERSE EFFECTS. When used as hormone replacement to provide physiologic estrogen levels, estrogens occasionally cause breast tenderness, headache, edema, nausea, vomiting, anorexia, and changes in libido. Most of the minor side effects of estrogens can be managed by dosage reduction.

The more serious adverse effects of estrogens include **hypertension, thromboembolic disorders,** and **gallbladder disease.** The hypertensive effect of estrogens has been partly attributed to stimulation of angiotensinogen synthesis and subsequent formation of angiotensin II, whereas thromboembolic complications have been partly attributed to increased synthesis of clotting factors in the liver. Estrogens increase cholesterol excretion in the bile, and this accounts for their tendency to cause gallstones.

Estrogens are contraindicated during pregnancy and should be avoided in women with uterine fibroids. Estrogens should be used with great caution in women with hepatic diseases, endometriosis, thromboembolic diseases, or hypercalcemia.

Progesterone and Its Derivatives

Progesterone is the primary natural progestin in mammals. Progesterone undergoes extensive first-pass metabolism following oral administration and has a short plasma half-life. To extend the oral bioavailability and half-life, esters of progesterone have been developed. These include **megestrol, hydroxyprogesterone caproate,** and **medroxyprogesterone acetate** (see Fig. 34–3C). Megestrol is administered orally, whereas hydroxyprogesterone caproate is administered as a long-acting intramuscular preparation. Medroxyprogesterone acetate can be given either orally or intramuscularly. Following their absorption, the progesterone esters are bound to albumin in the circulation. The esters are converted to several hydroxylated metabolites and to pregnandiol glucuronide in the liver, and these metabolites are excreted in the urine.

Progesterone esters are used to suppress ovarian function in the treatment of **dysmenorrhea, endometriosis,** and **uterine bleeding.** In this setting, the progesterone derivatives produce feedback inhibition of gonadotropin secretion by the pituitary gland. In **hormone replacement therapy** (see below), the progesterone esters are often used in combination with estrogens to decrease the incidence of estrogen-induced irregular bleeding and to prevent uterine hyperplasia and endometrial cancer.

Synthetic Progestins

Synthetic progestins are primarily used as **oral contraceptives** (see below), but they are also used to treat **dysmenor-**rhea, **endometriosis,** and **uterine bleeding** in the same manner as the progesterone esters.

Most of the synthetic progestins are derivatives of 19-nortestosterone and have varying degrees of estrogenic, antiestrogenic, and androgenic activity. The drugs contain a C17 ethinyl substitution that increases their oral bioavailability and duration of action. Their half-lives range from 7 to 24 hours, whereas the half-life of progesterone is only about 5 minutes.

Two classes of 19-norprogestins have been developed: **estranes** and **gonanes.** The estranes include **norethindrone** and **norethynodrel,** whereas the gonanes include **levonorgestrel, desogestrel,** and **norgestimate** (see Fig. 34–3C). Desogestrel and norgestimate have improved progestational selectivity and lessened androgenic activity. **Drospirenone** is a spironolactone derivative with antiandrogenic effects (see below).

Hormone Replacement Therapy

Menopause refers to the cessation of menstruation that occurs in most women between the ages of 45 and 55. Before menopause, the supply of eggs in a woman's ovaries declines and ovulation becomes irregular. The ovarian follicles fail to develop and secrete normal amounts of estrogen. When estrogen levels are no longer sufficient to suppress FSH secretion by the pituitary gland, FSH levels rise. When FSH levels are above 40 mIU/mL, a woman is said to be in menopause.

Although estrogens can be used alone for HRT in women who have had a hysterectomy, an estrogen should be used in combination with a progestin for women with a uterus. This is because giving estrogen alone increases the risk of endometrial cancer in these women.

Therapeutic Effects

Studies consistently show that estrogens relieve symptoms of menopause in up to 90% of women. These symptoms include hot flashes or flushes that consist of alternating chills and sweating accompanied by nausea, dizziness, headache, tachycardia, and palpitations. Episodes of these symptoms often occur several times a day, but night sweats are particularly common. These symptoms occur in association with surges in GnRH and gonadotropins that result from the lack of estrogen feedback inhibition. The gonadotropin surges alter hypothalamic thermoregulatory centers, leading to the symptoms described above.

Estrogens also relieve other menopausal symptoms, including urogenital, vulvar, and vaginal atrophy. Estrogens may improve mood and reduce cognitive difficulties, possibly secondary to improved sleep.

Although some epidemiologic studies suggested that HRT reduced the risk of cardiovascular disease, recent clinical trials of estrogen replacement in postmenopausal women have reached the opposite conclusion. The **Nurses' Health Study** (NHS) was an observational study of a cohort of women that obtained information about the relationship between cardiovascular disease and lifestyle, lipid levels, and HRT. This study concluded that HRT decreased the risk of coronary artery disease and that women with the highest risk of cardiovascular disease obtained the greatest benefit from

HRT. This study has the same limitations as all cohort observational studies, and it has been postulated that the women who sought HRT were also more likely to adopt a healthy lifestyle that reduced their risk of heart disease.

The **Postmenopausal Estrogen/Progestin Interventions** (PEPI) study was a randomized, prospective trial of HRT in 875 women between the ages of 45 and 64. It demonstrated beneficial effects of HRT on risk factors for heart disease by showing that HRT reduced cholesterol and fibrinogen levels. The relatively short duration of the trial (3 years) was not sufficient to determine long-term effects of HRT on morbidity and mortality.

The **Heart and Estrogen-Progestin Replacement Study** (HERS) was the first trial to investigate the effects of HRT in postmenopausal women with existing heart disease. This study found a lack of benefit of HRT on fatal or nonfatal myocardial infarction (MI). In fact, the study found that women were at an increased risk of MI during the first year of HRT, although the risk of MI decreased in subsequent years. After an additional 3 years of study, no significant differences were noted in cardiovascular outcomes between women on HRT and those not receiving HRT. This trial has been criticized because women in the study were already receiving cardioprotective medications and were allowed to begin statin therapy or change therapy during the study. Also, the average age of women in the study was 67, which is well above the age when women enter menopause.

The **Women's Health Initiative** (WHI) provided additional data concerning HRT and cardiovascular disease in postmenopausal women. Part of this study was a randomized trial of more than 16,000 women who received **conjugated equine estrogen** plus **medroxyprogesterone acetate** or a placebo. After 5 years, the study was halted because the data showed that women receiving HRT had increased risk of **coronary artery disease, stroke,** and **pulmonary embolism.** HRT, however, reduced the risk of colorectal cancer and hip fractures. Another arm of this study looked at the effect of estrogen by itself in women without a uterus. This study was stopped when it was reported that estrogen increased the risk of stroke but did not affect the incidence of coronary artery disease in these women. The WHI study has been criticized in terms of the older age of the participants, the high drop-out rate, and the number of women who received HRT from their private physician. Furthermore, the method of analyzing the data in this study has been criticized with respect to confounding variables.

In summary, HRT produces physiologic effects that are both beneficial and detrimental. Long-term HRT does not appear to reduce the risk of coronary artery disease and may increase the risk of stroke. Although estrogens have beneficial effects on lipoprotein levels, these effects are impeded when a progestin is included in the regimen. Although estrogens prevent osteoporosis, other therapies are now available for this purpose. The most prudent approach to HRT appears to be the use of low-dose estrogen preparations to control menopausal symptoms, while using other medications to prevent osteoporosis and cardiovascular disease.

Treatment Considerations

Most women with an intact uterus should begin HRT with a combination of a progestin and a low-dose estrogen. Doses should be titrated to provide symptom relief without causing side effects such as headache, nausea, weight gain, breast tenderness, or vaginal bleeding. After 2 or 3 years of therapy, the dose of estrogen can be gradually reduced to the lowest level required to prevent hot flashes and other symptoms.

Estrogens can be administered using a wide variety of dosage forms and routes of administration, enabling women to try alternative preparations and determine which one is most effective and tolerable for them. Oral tablets are convenient and relatively inexpensive, whereas transdermal skin patches require less frequent administration. Women who suffer mainly vulvovaginal symptoms may prefer a vaginal cream, tablet, or ring. Other options include intramuscular injections and subcutaneously implanted pellets.

Hormone replacement therapy can be given as cyclic or continuous hormonal therapy. In cyclic therapy, estrogen is given for 25 days, a progestin (e.g., medroxyprogesterone) is given for the last 10 to 13 days of estrogen treatment, and then no therapy is given for 5 to 6 days. In continuous therapy, estrogen is given every day, and a progestin is added for the first 10 to 13 days of each month. The addition of a progestin suppresses endometrial hyperplasia and diminishes the risk of endometrial cancer.

CONTRACEPTIVES

Contraceptives are drugs or devices used to prevent conception (the onset of pregnancy, as indicated by the implantation of the blastocyst in the endometrium or the formation of a visible zygote). Some contraceptives act locally in the reproductive tract. These include agents that kill sperm (**spermicides**), devices that prevent sperm from reaching and fertilizing the ovum (**condoms and diaphragms),** and **intrauterine devices** (IUD) that prevent implantation of the blastocyst. Other contraceptives are administered orally or parenterally. **Oral contraceptives** contain female sex hormones that act primarily by preventing ovulation. Most of the oral contraceptives contain both an estrogen and a progestin, whereas two products contain only a progestin. Progestin-only contraceptives are also available for administration as **long-acting subdermal implants, intramuscular injections, or intrauterine devices.** Table 34–1 lists the estrogen and progestin components of selected hormonal contraceptive preparations.

Estrogen–Progestin Contraceptives

Drug Properties

CLASSIFICATION. The combination estrogen–progestin oral contraceptives are classified as monophasic, biphasic, or triphasic, based on their progestin content. **Monophasic contraceptives** contain the same amount of progestin throughout the administration cycle, whereas **biphasic and triphasic contraceptives** increase the amount after the first one third of the cycle (Fig. 34–4). The amount of progestin is increased in the biphasic and triphasic preparations to mimic the naturally occurring ratio of estrogen to progestin during the menstrual cycle. The estrogen content is constant in all monophasic and biphasic contraceptives and in most triphasic contraceptives.

TABLE 34–1. Estrogen and Progestin Components of Selected Hormonal Contraceptive Preparations

Preparations	Estrogen	Progestin
Monophasic oral contraceptives		
Brevicon, Genora 0.5/35, Loestrin, Norinyl, Norlestrin, Ovcon	Ethinyl estradiol	Norethindrone
Demulen	Ethinyl estradiol	Ethynodiol
Desogen, Ortho-Cept	Ethinyl estradiol	Desogestrel*
Yasmin	Ethinyl estradiol	Drospirenone
Lo/Ovral, Ovral	Ethinyl estradiol	Norgestrel
Levlen, Nordette, Seasonale	Ethinyl estradiol	Levonorgestrel
Ortho-Novum 1/50	Mestranol	Norethindrone
Biphasic oral contraceptives		
Mircette, Ortho-Novum 10/11	Ethinyl estradiol	Norethindrone
Triphasic oral contraceptives		
Ortho-Novum 7/7/7, Tri-Norinyl	Ethinyl estradiol	Norethindrone
Tri-Levlen, Triphasil	Ethinyl estradiol	Norgestrel
Ortho Tri-Cyclen	Ethinyl estradiol	Norgestimate
Progestin-only oral contraceptives		
Micronor, Nor-Q-D		Norethindrone
Contraceptive implant		
Norplant		Levonorgestrel
Intrauterine contraceptive		
Mirena		Levonorgestrel
Injectable contraceptives		
Lunelle	Estradiol cypionate	Medroxyprogesterone acetate
Depo-Provera		Medroxyprogesterone acetate
Transdermal contraceptive		
Ortho Evra	Ethinyl estradiol	Norelgestromin
Vaginal ring contraceptive		
Nuva-Ring	Ethinyl estradiol	Etonogestrel*
Emergency (postcoital) contraceptive		
Preven	Ethinyl estradiol	Levonorgestrel

*Etonogestrel is the active metabolite of desogestrel.

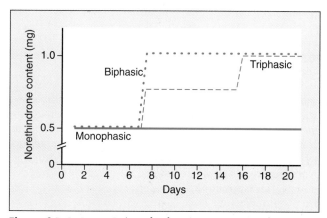

Figure 34–4. Progestin (norethindrone) content in typical monophasic, biphasic, and triphasic oral contraceptives. Monophasic preparations contain the same amount of progestin throughout the administration cycle. Biphasic and triphasic preparations increase the progestin content in a stepwise fashion after the initial part of the cycle. The amount of estrogen is constant in all monophasic and biphasic contraceptives and in most triphasic contraceptives. Some triphasic contraceptives contain a slightly greater amount of estrogen in the middle of the cycle.

MECHANISMS AND PHARMACOLOGIC EFFECTS. The estrogen–progestin contraceptives act primarily by feedback inhibition of gonadotropin-releasing hormone secretion from the hypothalamus, leading to decreased gonadotropin secretion and inhibition of ovulation. The estrogen component is believed to reduce FSH secretion and the selection and maturation of the dominant follicle, whereas the progestin component inhibits the midcycle LH surge required for ovulation. Neither the estrogen nor the progestin dose used in oral contraceptives is sufficient to prevent ovulation by itself, but used together they act synergistically to suppress ovulation. Other effects that contribute to contraception include delayed maturation of the endometrium, which prevents implantation of the blastocyst, and the development of viscous cervical mucus, which retards sperm motility. The actions on the endometrium and cervical mucus are believed to be the mechanisms of estrogen–progestin preparations used for emergency (postcoital) contraception.

ADMINISTRATION. Estrogen–progestin preparations for **oral contraception** are usually packaged as 21 tablets that are administered once a day, beginning on day 5 of the menstrual cycle. Some preparations also include 7 inert pills that can be taken for the remainder of the cycle. The tablets are packaged in a calendar format to facilitate proper utilization. An "extended-cycle" preparation is now available for continuous daily administration for 84 days followed by 7 days of inactive tablets. This preparation, SEASONALE, contains ethinyl estradiol and levonorgestrel, and allows for withdrawal bleeding only 4 times a year, whereas other estrogen–progestin oral contraceptives result in 13 withdrawal bleeding episodes a year. The extended-cycle preparation is as effective as 28-day cycle products. Whether the longer exposure to hormones could increase the risk of adverse effects (e.g., thromboembolism) has not been determined.

Estrogen–progestin preparations are also used to treat **acne vulgaris** and produce a significant improvement in facial acne lesions. They are also useful in managing **dysmenorrhea,** a condition characterized by episodic pain that is believed to result from a local increase in uterine prostaglandins. The release of prostaglandins is a reaction to the ischemia caused by vasoconstriction of small arteries in the uterine wall at the time of menstruation. For this condition, oral contraceptives are started a number of days before the onset of menstruation. Nonsteroidal anti-inflammatory drugs (e.g., ibuprofen and naproxen) can be used instead, especially by women desiring to maintain the ovulatory cycle. These drugs act by inhibiting prostaglandin synthesis (see Chapter 30).

A preparation containing ethinyl estradiol and levonorgestrel (PREVEN) is available for use as an emergency or **postcoital contraceptive** in women who have not been taking another contraceptive. A single dose of this preparation is taken within 72 hours of intercourse, followed by two doses 12 hours later. Use of an emergency contraceptive routinely causes nausea and vomiting and may require administration of an antiemetic agent (e.g., promethazine). It can also cause headache, dizziness, leg cramps, and abdominal cramps. The postcoital contraceptive is packaged with a urine pregnancy test that can be used to verify the prevention of pregnancy.

Other estrogen–progestin contraceptives include a transdermal skin patch (ORTHO EVRA) and a long-acting, injectable preparation containing estradiol cypionate and medroxyprogesterone acetate (LUNELLE).

ADVERSE EFFECTS. Table 34–2 lists the common adverse effects resulting from estrogen or progestin excess or deficiency. Less frequent effects of oral contraceptives include **hypertension, thromboembolic complications,** and **gallstones.**

Oral contraceptives have been associated with an increased risk of **stroke, myocardial infarction, deep vein thrombosis,** and other thromboembolic complications. The increased risk of thromboembolism in healthy women using preparations containing a low dose of estrogen (<50 μg of ethinyl estradiol) is extremely small. Smokers over 35 years of age have a greater risk of thromboembolic complications from oral contraceptives and should use other forms of contraception. Healthy nonsmokers who are 35 to 44 years old may continue to use oral contraceptives, according to the American College of Obstetricians and Gynecologists.

TABLE 34–2.	**Common Adverse Effects of Oral Contraceptives**

Effects of estrogen excess
Breast enlargement
Dizziness
Dysmenorrhea
Edema
Headache
Irritability
Nausea and vomiting
Weight gain (cyclic)

Effects of progestin excess
Acne
Depression
Fatigue
Hirsutism
Libido change
Oily skin
Weight gain (noncyclic)

Effects of estrogen deficiency
Atrophic vaginitis
Continuous bleeding
Early- or mid-cycle bleeding
Hypomenorrhea
Vasomotor symptoms

Effects of progestin deficiency
Dysmenorrhea
Hypermenorrhea
Late-cycle bleeding

Contraceptives containing estrogen should be used with caution in women with gallbladder disease. They are contraindicated in women with thromboembolic disease or a history of myocardial infarction or coronary artery disease. They are also contraindicated in women with active liver disease, breast cancer, or carcinoma of the reproductive tract. The relationship between oral contraceptive use and cancer remains controversial. Epidemiologic studies suggest that oral contraceptives decrease the incidence of **ovarian and endometrial cancer.** Although use of the high-dose estrogen preparations has been associated with an increased risk of **breast cancer,** the risk associated with newer low-dose preparations is much lower. Oral contraceptives have also been associated with a low risk of hepatic adenoma.

The progestin component of oral contraceptives can cause adverse effects that can be attributed to excessive androgenic activity. The androgenic side effects of progestins include **acne, hirsutism, increased libido,** and **oily skin. Norgestrel** is one of the most androgenic progestins, whereas **desogestrel** is one of the least androgenic. **Norethindrone** appears to have an intermediate androgenic potency. **Drospirenone** is a newer progestin that is derived from spironolactone (see Chapter 13). Drospirenone has no androgenic activity and exerts a weak **antiandrogenic effect.** As with its parent compound, it also acts as an aldosterone antagonist and causes a mild anti-mineralocorticoid effect, thereby reducing salt and water retention and lowering blood pressure in users of this progestin. It is available in combination with ethinyl estradiol in a product marketed as YASMIN.

INTERACTIONS. Barbiturates, carbamazepine, phenytoin, and other drugs that increase the hepatic metabolism of oral contraceptives may reduce the plasma levels of contraceptive steroids and lead to contraceptive failure. Antibiotics, including penicillins and tetracyclines, can eradicate intestinal flora involved in the enterohepatic cycling of contraceptive steroids and thereby diminish their effectiveness. This interaction is described in greater detail in Chapter 4. Estrogens can inhibit the metabolism and potentiate the effects of cyclosporine, imipramine and other antidepressants, and glucocorticoids. Estrogens increase the synthesis of vitamin K-dependent clotting factors and may thereby antagonize the effect of warfarin. Estrogens also appear to increase the hepatotoxicity of dantrolene.

Progestin-Only Contraceptives

The progestin-only contraceptives include **norethindrone** products that are administered orally (sometimes called minipills), subdermal implants and intrauterine devices that slowly release **levonorgestrel,** and long-acting intramuscular injections of **medroxyprogesterone acetate.**

The systemic progestin-only contraceptives may prevent pregnancy through several mechanisms. They act on the hypothalamus to decrease the frequency of the GnRH pulse generator and thereby blunt the midcycle LH surge that produces ovulation. Progestin-only pills thicken and decrease the amount of cervical mucus, making it more difficult for sperm to penetrate. Progestins also create a thin, atrophic endometrium that is hostile to implantation of the blastocyst. The IUD is believed to prevent pregnancy by producing localized effects on the endometrium.

The progestin-only contraceptives are particularly suited for women who smoke, older women, and women in whom an estrogen is contraindicated. The estimated failure rates, however, are slightly higher with perfect use of progestin-only contraceptives than with perfect use of estrogen–progestin products (rates of 0.5% and 0.1%, respectively). Progestin-only contraceptives are associated with frequent spotting and amenorrhea and with an increased risk of ectopic pregnancy. An irregular or unpredictable menstrual cycle is one of the most common reasons that women stop using these preparations. Unlike the estrogen–progestin preparations, the progestin-only preparations must be taken daily without interruption to prevent pregnancy.

Other Contraceptives

Other types of contraceptives are particularly useful for short-term contraception in women who cannot take oral contraceptives while breast-feeding or for other reasons. These nonhormonal contraceptives include spermicides and barrier devices (e.g., condoms and diaphragms).

Most spermicides contain nonoxynol-9, a detergent that disrupts the cell membrane of the sperm. Spermicides increase the contraceptive efficacy of condoms and other barrier methods. They are moderately effective and well tolerated, although they can cause local irritation in some women.

ANTIESTROGENS

Antiestrogens include the estrogen receptor antagonists and the estrogen synthesis inhibitors (aromatase inhibitors). The estrogen receptor antagonists are nonsteroidal drugs that bind to estrogen receptors and exert tissue-specific antagonist or partial agonist effects. Examples are clomiphene, raloxifene, and tamoxifen. These drugs contain the structural elements required for estrogen receptor binding and weak agonist activity, and they also possess a substituted ethylamine moiety that is responsible for their estrogen antagonist effect (see Fig. 34–3B).

Clomiphene

Drug Properties

PHARMACOKINETICS. Clomiphene is well absorbed after oral administration. It undergoes hepatic biotransformation and biliary excretion, and it is primarily eliminated in the feces. Its long elimination half-life of about 5 days is caused by extensive plasma protein binding, enterohepatic cycling, and accumulation in fatty tissues.

MECHANISMS AND INDICATIONS. Clomiphene is a weak estrogen agonist and a moderate estrogen antagonist. It is used to treat **anovulatory infertility,** including infertility associated with **polycystic ovary disease.** Clomiphene is believed to act by antagonizing estrogen receptors in the hypothalamic-pituitary-ovarian axis (Fig. 34–5). By blocking estrogen's negative feedback inhibition of gonadotropin secretion, clomiphene increases FSH and LH secretion and thereby induces ovarian follicle development and ovulation.

Suitable patients for clomiphene therapy often have an anovulatory disorder dating back to puberty but have a functional hypothalamic-pituitary-ovarian axis. Clomiphene is less successful in women who have reduced estrogen levels, and it is unlikely to benefit women with FSH levels at or above 40 mIU/mL or women with absent or resistant ovarian follicles.

Clomiphene treatment is usually begun on or about the fifth day of the cycle after the start of uterine bleeding and continues for 5 days. Ovulation is expected 5 to 10 days after the last dose of clomiphene and can be detected by monitoring basal body temperature, urinary LH secretion, plasma progesterone levels, or endometrial histology.

ADVERSE EFFECTS. From 5% to 12% of women treated with clomiphene have multiple births (twins in the vast majority of cases). The risk of multiple births is reduced if women are started on a lower dose of clomiphene. The dose can then be increased each cycle until ovulation occurs.

Tamoxifen

Drug Properties

PHARMACOKINETICS. Tamoxifen is administered orally, and it is well absorbed from the gut. It is then converted to a number of metabolites in the liver. Some of the minor metabolites (e.g., 4-hydroxytamoxifen) have greater affinity for the estrogen receptor than tamoxifen does. The terminal

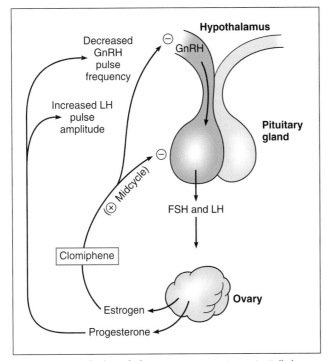

Figure 34–5. The hypothalamic-pituitary-ovarian axis. Follicle-stimulating hormone (FSH) and luteinizing hormone (LH) are released from the pituitary gland in response to gonadotropin-releasing hormone (GnRH) produced by hypothalamic neurons. During the follicular phase of the menstrual cycle, FSH stimulates the development of an ovarian follicle and the secretion of estrogen. Estrogen increases the synthesis of LH but inhibits its release until midcycle, when a surge in LH is accompanied by a smaller surge in FSH secretion, leading to ovulation. During the luteal phase, progesterone produced by the corpus luteum feeds back to the hypothalamus to decrease the frequency of GnRH pulses while acting on the pituitary to increase the amplitude of LH secretion. Together, these actions produce less-frequent LH pulses of greater amplitude. Clomiphene inhibits estrogen feedback and thereby increases gonadotropin secretion in anovulatory women.

elimination half-life of tamoxifen is about 7 days. Tamoxifen undergoes enterohepatic cycling and biliary excretion in the same manner as clomiphene.

MECHANISMS AND INDICATIONS. Tamoxifen has both estrogenic and antiestrogenic properties. In breast tissue, it acts as an estrogen receptor antagonist. It is primarily used to prevent or treat **breast cancer** in patients with tumor cells that are estrogen receptor-positive. In the treatment of breast cancer, it is typically used as adjuvant therapy in combination with surgery or other chemotherapy. Tamoxifen inhibits the proliferation of breast cancer cells and may thereby contribute to the eradication of micrometastases. In cases of advanced or metastatic breast cancer, tamoxifen can be used alone for palliative treatment.

ADVERSE EFFECTS. Tamoxifen can cause nausea, vomiting, hot flashes, vaginal bleeding, and menstrual irregularities. It can stimulate proliferation of endometrial cells, and some evidence suggests that it increases the risk of endometrial cancer.

Raloxifene

Raloxifene is a benzothiophene drug that is called a **selective estrogen receptor modulator** (SERM). Its structure is shown in Fig. 34–3B. Raloxifene acts in a manner similar to tamoxifen by producing estrogenlike effects on bone and lipid metabolism while antagonizing the effects of estrogen on breast tissue. Unlike tamoxifen, however, raloxifene also acts as an estrogen antagonist in uterine tissue.

Raloxifene is primarily indicated for the prevention of **osteoporosis** in postmenopausal women. The effect of raloxifene on total body bone mineral density is similar to that of conjugated estrogens or alendronate. The effect of raloxifene on bone mineral density of the lumbar spine, however, may be less than that of these other drugs. The effect of estrogens on bone metabolism is discussed in greater detail in Chapter 36.

The effect of raloxifene on serum lipoproteins differs from the effect of estrogens. Raloxifene decreases the levels of total cholesterol, LDL cholesterol, and lipoprotein(a). Unlike estrogens, raloxifene does not increase the level of HDL cholesterol. The effect of raloxifene on cardiovascular disease requires further evaluation.

Aromatase Inhibitors

Breast cancer is often hormonally responsive, including breast cancer classified as estrogen, progesterone, or both, receptor positive. This type of breast cancer has responded to a variety of efforts to decrease estrogen levels (e.g., ovariectomy) or to inhibit estrogen effects, such as with estrogen antagonists. These interventions lead to decreased tumor mass, delayed progression, and improved survival in many patients.

In postmenopausal women, estrogens are mainly derived from adrenal androgens, primarily testosterone and androstenedione, that are converted to estrogens in peripheral tissues and in cancer tissue itself by the enzyme aromatase (see Fig. 34–1). **Anastrozole** (ARIMIDEX) and letrozole (FEMARA) are nonsteroidal aromatase inhibitors that reduce circulating levels of estrogen and are indicated as first-line treatments for locally advanced or **metastatic breast cancer** in postmenopausal women. By lowering estrogen levels, these drugs may halt progression of estrogen-sensitive breast cancer. Anastrozole and letrozole are well absorbed after oral administration and have long half-lives of about 2 days. The aromatase inhibitors are well tolerated but can cause hot flashes, nausea, headache, vaginal bleeding, and back pain.

ANTIPROGESTINS

Mifepristone (MIFEPREX) is a synthetic steroid compound that acts as a progesterone receptor antagonist when progesterone is present. In the absence of progesterone, it acts as a partial agonist. It is also a competitive antagonist at the glucocorticoid receptor (see Chapter 33). Mifepristone is approved for **medical termination of pregnancy** through 49 days of gestation. It causes breakdown of the decidua (the endometrium of the pregnant uterus), leading to detachment of the blastocyst from the endometrium.

Mifepristone is administered as a single dose that is followed by a prostaglandin 48 hours later to stimulate uterine contractions (see Chapter 26). Mifepristone has good oral bioavailability. Following absorption, the drug is highly bound to plasma proteins, and this contributes to its long half-life of about 22 hours. Mifepristone is metabolized in the liver and excreted in the bile. It undergoes enterohepatic cycling and is primarily excreted in the feces.

The major adverse effects of mifepristone include anorexia, nausea, vomiting, abdominal pain, fatigue, and heavy uterine bleeding.

ANDROGENS

Several testosterone preparations and synthetic androgens are available for clinical use in the treatment of hypogonadism and a variety of other conditions.

Testosterone and Methyltestosterone

When given orally, testosterone undergoes extensive first-pass metabolism. It must, therefore, be given parenterally or transdermally instead. Testosterone and several long-acting esters of testosterone (e.g., testosterone cypionate) are available for intramuscular administration. The testosterone esters are slowly absorbed and provide effective plasma concentrations for several weeks.

Methyltestosterone is a derivative that is resistant to hepatic metabolism, has a longer half-life than testosterone, and is suitable for oral administration. Prolonged methyltestosterone use, however, is associated with hepatic damage and liver failure, so the drug is inappropriate for long-term treatment of hypogonadism.

Testosterone preparations are primarily used to treat **hypogonadism** caused by **primary testicular failure** or is secondary to **hypopituitarism.** In patients with hypopituitarism, testosterone should be given in combination with growth hormone to obtain a maximal effect on skeletal growth. In these patients, the androgen is added to the treatment regimen at the time of puberty, and the dosage is gradually increased. Either a long-acting injectable preparation or a transdermal testosterone patch can be used.

Testosterone is occasionally used in **gynecologic disorders.** It is sometimes combined with estrogens for **hormone replacement therapy** in postmenopausal women who experience endometrial bleeding when only an estrogen is used, and it has also been used to treat **osteoporosis.** A combination product containing esterified estrogens and methyltestosterone (ESTRATEST) is available for this purpose.

Anabolic Steroids

Testosterone and its derivatives can increase muscle mass and strength, particularly when used in a weight-training program. Anabolic steroids are synthetic derivatives of testosterone that have more anabolic than androgenic activity. The ratio of anabolic activity to androgenic activity for testosterone is 1:1, whereas the ratio for some synthetic androgens is as high as 3:1. Examples of androgenic steroids include oxandrolone and stanozolol. Tetrahydrogestrinone (THG) is a potent androgenic "designer drug" developed to escape detection in the urine. It is not approved by the US Food and Drug Administration (FDA) and cannot be legally marketed.

Anabolic steroids have been used by athletes to **increase body mass, strength, and physical performance.** This type of use has been banned by most sports organizations. The large doses of anabolic steroids often used for this purpose can lead to a number of adverse effects, including **tendon rupture,** hepatic dysfunction or failure, cholestatic jaundice, increased aggressiveness, psychotic symptoms, acne, decreased testicular size and function, and impotence. In adolescents, androgenic drugs can cause **closing of epiphyses** and premature cessation of growth. In women, excessive use of androgens can cause masculinization, hirsutism, deepening of the voice, and menstrual irregularities.

Danazol

Danazol, a derivative of 17-ethinyl testosterone, has antiestrogenic activity and weak androgenic and progestational activity.

Danazol is primarily used in the treatment of **endometriosis** because it causes atrophy of ectopic endometrial tissue and thereby relieves the symptoms of disease. It also decreases the growth rate of abnormal breast tissue, making it useful in the treatment of **fibrocystic breast disease.** Danazol works primarily by acting on the pituitary gland to reduce the secretion of FSH and LH. These actions indirectly lead to decreased estrogen production.

Danazol is also used to treat **hereditary angioedema,** a disorder caused by a deficiency of C1 esterase inhibitor, a serum inhibitor of the activated first component of complement. Danazol prevents attacks of hereditary angioedema in both males and females by increasing the circulating levels of C1 esterase inhibitor. The mechanisms by which the drug increases these levels are unknown.

Common adverse effects of danazol include mild hirsutism, oily skin, acne, and menstrual irregularities. The drug can also cause hypercholesterolemia, hepatotoxicity, and thromboembolic events, including stroke. Danazol is teratogenic and should not be given to pregnant women.

ANTIANDROGENS

Several types of androgen antagonists have been developed and used in the treatment of prostate disorders, male pattern baldness, and other conditions. These drugs act through a variety of mechanisms, including inhibition of LH secretion, testosterone synthesis, and DHT synthesis, and antagonism of androgen receptors.

Gonadotropin-Releasing Hormone Analogues

When a gonadotropin-releasing hormone analogue is administered in a continuous rather than a pulsatile fashion, it reduces LH secretion by the pituitary and thereby reduces testosterone production by the testes.

The GnRH analogues include **leuprolide,** an agent discussed in Chapter 31. Leuprolide has been successfully used in the treatment of inoperable **prostate cancer.** Because leuprolide increases the production of LH and testosterone when it is first administered, the drug is sometimes given in combination with an androgen receptor antagonist (e.g., flutamide). Combined androgen blockade with a GnRH analogue and an androgen receptor antagonist (see below) has been shown to significantly prolong the progression-free period and the length of survival in men with advanced prostate cancer.

Androgen Receptor Antagonists

Flutamide, bicalutamide, and nilutamide are nonsteroidal agents that compete with testosterone for the androgen receptor (Fig. 34–3D). These drugs are used in combination with a synthetic GnRH analogue to treat inoperable **prostate cancer.** Adverse effects of these drugs include nausea, gynecomastia, impotence, hot flashes, and hepatitis.

Cyproterone is a steroidal androgen receptor antagonist that has orphan drug status in the United States of America. It is being used to treat **hirsutism** in women and to reduce **excessive sex drive** in men.

5α-Reductase Inhibitors

Finasteride is a synthetic testosterone derivative that blocks 5α-reductase and thereby decreases the synthesis of DHT in the prostate gland, skin, and other target tissues. The drug is administered orally, undergoes hepatic metabolism, and is primarily eliminated in the feces. Finasteride has a half-life of about 8 hours, and it reduces DHT synthesis for about 24 hours.

Finasteride is primarily indicated for the treatment of **benign prostatic hyperplasia (BPH)** but has also been approved for the treatment of **male pattern baldness.** The drug reduces prostate volume and can prevent and retard the progression of BPH. In this setting, it improves urinary flow and decreases the risk of acute urinary retention. It is sometimes used in combination with an adrenergic α-receptor antagonist, such as tamsulosin (FLOMAX), for treating BPH (see Chapter 9).

The adverse effects of finasteride include impotence and decreased libido, but these effects occur in only a few men and tend to decrease over time.

SUMMARY OF IMPORTANT POINTS

■ Estradiol preparations include skin patches for transdermal administration, micronized estradiol for oral administration, and estradiol cypionate and estradiol valerate for intramuscular administration.

■ Conjugated equine estrogens are sulfate esters of estrone and equilin. They are used for hormone replacement therapy in postmenopausal women and to treat other forms of hypogonadism.

■ In menopausal women, estrogens relieve vasomotor symptoms and protect against osteoporosis. Recent clinical trials suggest that hormonal replacement therapy may increase the risk of stroke and that it does not protect against coronary artery disease.

■ Ethinyl derivatives of estradiol (ethinyl estradiol and mestranol) have higher oral bioavailability and longer half-lives than estradiol. They are used primarily in oral contraceptives.

■ Progesterone derivatives (e.g., medroxyprogesterone acetate) are primarily used in combination with estrogens in hormone replacement therapy to reduce endometrial hyperplasia and the risk of endometrial cancer. They are also used to suppress ovarian function in the treatment of dysmenorrhea, endometriosis, and uterine bleeding.

■ Synthetic progestins, including norethindrone, are primarily used in contraceptives, including combination estrogen–progestin contraceptives and progestin-only contraceptives.

■ Norgestrel is the most androgenic progestin, desogestrel is one of the least androgenic, and drospirenone has antiandrogenic and anti-mineralocorticoid activity.

■ Hormonal contraceptives act primarily by inhibiting gonadotropin secretion and ovulation. They also affect mucus viscosity, sperm transport, and endometrial histology.

■ Contraceptives have been associated with an increased risk of hypertension, thromboembolic disorders, and gallstones. The risk of thromboembolism is substantially reduced with preparations containing low doses of estrogen.

■ Some progestin-only contraceptives are administered as long-acting implants or injections, and others are given as oral tablets. Adverse effects include frequent spotting and amenorrhea.

■ Tamoxifen, an antiestrogen primarily used to treat breast cancer, is given in combination with surgery and other chemotherapy.

■ Anastrozole and letrozole, aromatase inhibitors that decrease estrogen synthesis, are used to treat breast cancer in postmenopausal women.

■ Clomiphene is an antiestrogen used to treat anovulatory infertility. By reducing estrogen feedback inhibition of gonadotropin secretion, clomiphene increases gonadotropin secretion and stimulates ovulation.

■ Raloxifene is a selective estrogen receptor modulator that acts as an estrogen antagonist in breast and uterine tissue. The drug produces estrogenlike effects on bone metabolism and reduces the risk of osteoporosis.

■ Mifepristone is an antiprogestin used for medical termination of intrauterine pregnancy.

■ Testosterone preparations are primarily used to treat hypogonadism.

■ Flutamide and other androgen receptor antagonists are used to treat prostate cancer, often in combination with a gonadotropin-releasing hormone agonist (e.g., leuprolide).

■ Finasteride is a 5α-reductase inhibitor that blocks the formation of dihydrotestosterone. It is used to treat benign prostatic hypertrophy and male pattern baldness.

Review Questions

1. Raloxifene produces estrogenlike effects in which tissue?
   (A) uterus
   (B) heart
   (C) bone
   (D) breast
   (E) hypothalamus

2. A progestin is included in regimens for hormone replacement therapy to prevent which of the following adverse effects?
   (A) breast cancer
   (B) endometrial cancer
   (C) myocardial infarction
   (D) stroke
   (E) elevated cholesterol levels

3. Which adverse effect occurs frequently in persons taking bicalutamide?
   (A) breast tenderness
   (B) alopecia
   (C) glaucoma
   (D) deep vein thrombosis
   (E) hot flashes

4. What is the primary mechanism by which the combination of ethinyl estradiol and norethindrone prevents conception?
   (A) decreased viscosity of cervical mucus
   (B) delayed maturation of the endometrium
   (C) reduced gonadotropin-releasing hormone secretion
   (D) cytotoxic effect on ovarian follicles
   (E) disruption of sperm cell membranes

5. Which progestin is most androgenic?
   (A) norgestrel
   (B) norethindrone
   (C) norethynodrel
   (D) desogestrel
   (E) drospirenone

Answers and Explanations

1. The answer is C: bone. Raloxifene acts as an estrogen antagonist in uterine, breast, and hypothalamic tissues. It reduces feedback inhibition of gonadotropin secretion and may thereby cause hot flashes. The drug is primarily used to prevent osteoporosis because it has estrogenlike effects in bone. It has also been used to prevent breast cancer in women with a high risk of this disease. It does not have significant effects on the heart.

2. The answer is B: endometrial cancer. Postmenopausal women receiving hormone replacement therapy should receive a progestin for 10 to 13 days each month to suppress endometrial hyperplasia that would otherwise be produced by unopposed estrogen therapy. A progestin is not required in women who have had a hysterectomy. Inclusion of a progestin will not prevent (A), breast cancer; (C), myocardial infarction; (D), stroke; or (E), elevated cholesterol levels.

3. The answer is E: hot flashes. Bicalutamide, an androgen receptor antagonist, prevents feedback inhibition of hypothalamic gonadotropin-releasing hormone (GnRH) secretion in men, leading to hot flashes. The drug does not cause (A), breast tenderness; (B), alopecia; (C) glaucoma; or (D), deep vein thrombosis.

4. The answer is C: reduced gonadotropin-releasing hormone secretion. Estrogen–progestin contraceptives cause feedback inhibition of GnRH secretion, leading to decreased LH and FSH secretion and inhibition of ovulation. Progestins can cause (A) increased viscosity of cervical mucus and (B) delayed maturation of the endometrium, but these are not the primary contraceptive mechanism of the estrogen–progestin preparations. None of the contraceptives cause (D), cytotoxic effect on ovarian follicles. Locally applied spermicides can cause (E), disruption of sperm cell membranes.

5. The answer is A: norgestrel. Norgestrel is the most androgenic progestin, whereas (D), desogestrel, is one of the least androgenic. Answer (B), norethindrone, has an intermediate level of androgenic effects, whereas (C), norethynodrel, has more estrogenic activity than other progestins. Answer (E), drospirenone, has antiandrogenic activity.

SELECTED READINGS

Andriole, G., N. Bruchovsky, L. W. Chung, et al. Dihydrotestosterone and the prostate: the scientific rationale for 5alpha-reductase inhibitors in the treatment of benign prostatic hyperplasia. J Urol 172:1399–1403, 2004.

Compston, J. E. The risks and benefits of HRT. J Musculoskel Neuronal Interact 4:187–190, 2004.

Grady, D., D. Herrington, V. Bittner, et al. Cardiovascular disease outcomes during 6.8 years of hormone therapy: Heart and Estrogen/progestin Replacement Study followup (HERS II). JAMA 288:49–57, 2002.

Eng-Wong, J., and J. A. Zujewski. Raloxifene and its role in breast cancer prevention. Expert Rev Anticancer Ther 4:523–532, 2004.

Sitruk-Ware, R. Pharmacological profile of progestins. Maturitas 47: 277–283, 2004.

Wassertheil-Smoller, S., S. L. Hendrix, M. Limacher, et al. Effect of estrogen plus progestin on stroke in postmenopausal women: the Women's Health Initiative: a randomized trial. JAMA 289:2673–2784, 2003.

CHAPTER 35

Drugs for Diabetes Mellitus

CLASSIFICATION OF DRUGS FOR DIABETES MELLITUS

Insulin Preparations
Short-acting Insulins
- Insulin lispro (HUMALOG)
- Insulin aspart (NOVOLOG)
- Regular insulin (HUMULIN R)

Intermediate-acting Insulins
- Insulin zinc suspension (lente insulin, HUMULIN L)
- Isophane insulin suspension (NPH insulin, HUMULIN N)
- Insulin glargine (LANTUS)

Long-acting Insulin
- Extended insulin zinc suspension (Ultralente insulin, Humulin U)

Oral Antidiabetic Drugs
Sulfonylurea Drugs
- Glimepiride (AMARYL)

- Glyburide (DIABETA, MICRONASE)
- Glipizide (GLUCOTROL)

Meglitinide Drugs
- Repaglinide (PRANDIN)
- Nateglinide (STARLIX)

Alpha-glucosidase Inhibitors
- Acarbose (PRECOSE)
- Miglitol (GLYSET)

Biguanide
- Metformin (GLUCOPHAGE)[a]

Thiazolidinediones
- Pioglitazone (ACTOS)
- Rosiglitazone (AVANDIA)

[a]also metformin + glyburide (GLUCOVANCE) and metformin + glipizide (METAGLIP).

OVERVIEW

Pancreatic Hormones

The hormones secreted by the endocrine pancreas are produced in clusters of cells called **islets of Langerhans.** These islets contain four types of cells: A (or alpha), B (or beta), D (or delta), and F cells.

The A cells produce **glucagon,** and the B cells secrete **insulin.** These two major hormones of the endocrine pancreas are primarily concerned with regulation of glucose metabolism and blood glucose concentration. Insulin promotes the uptake, utilization, and storage of glucose and thereby lowers the plasma glucose concentration, whereas glucagon increases the hepatic glucose output and blood glucose concentration. If insulin secretion or insulin activity is not sufficient to maintain normal blood glucose concentrations, diabetes mellitus (DM) results.

The D cells are the source of **somatostatin,** and the F cells produce **pancreatic peptide,** a peptide that appears to facil-

itate digestive processes. The pancreatic islets also produce **amylin,** a protein that appears to act on the brain to slow gastric churning and to decrease hepatic glucose output when digestion begins. Amylin is currently undergoing investigation as a potential adjunct to insulin therapy for DM.

Insulin

As shown in Box 35–1, **proinsulin** is converted to **insulin** and **C peptide.** Insulin consists of two peptide chains (the A chain and the B chain), which are linked by two disulfide bridges. Although both insulin and C peptide are released in response to rising glucose concentrations, the physiologic role of C peptide remains unknown.

Secretion

Insulin secretion has meal-stimulated and basal components. Insulin release is activated by the rise in blood glucose concentration that follows the digestion and absorption of

BOX 35-1. STRUCTURES OF PROINSULIN AND INSULIN MOLECULES

Preproinsulin is synthesized in the rough endoplasmic reticulum of pancreatic B cells, and proinsulin is formed by enzymatic cleavage of this precursor molecule. Proinsulin is then transported to the Golgi apparatus and converted to insulin and C peptide (connecting peptide) by the removal of four amino acids (dipeptide linkage). Insulin and C peptide are packaged in storage granules until released in equimolar amounts in response to rising glucose concentrations.

Insulin consists of a 21-amino-acid A chain and a 30-amino-acid B chain linked by two disulfide bridges.

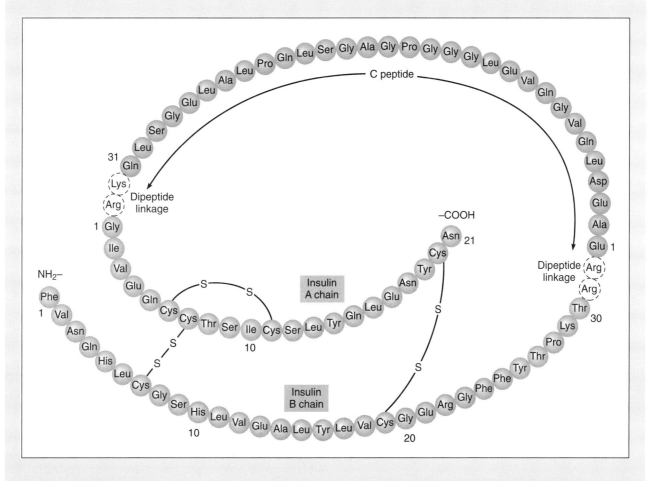

Species differences in the amino acid composition of insulin are shown in the following table. All other amino acids are identical in bovine, porcine, and human insulin. Insulin lispro is a recombinant insulin analogue that has the same structure as human insulin except for the transposition of proline and lysine at positions B28 and B29. Insulin aspart contains a single amino acid substitution of aspartic acid for proline at B28, which reduces aggregation of insulin aspart molecules and enables its rapid dissociation and absorption.

Type of Insulin	A Chain Position		B Chain Position		
	A8	A10	B28	B29	B30
Bovine insulin	Ala	Val	Pro	Lys	Ala
Porcine insulin	Thr	Ile	Pro	Lys	Ala
Human insulin	Thr	Ile	Pro	Lys	Thr
Insulin aspart	Thr	Ile	Asp	Lys	Thr
Insulin lispro	Thr	Ile	Lys	Pro	Thr

carbohydrates (Fig. 35–1A and 35–1B). The rate of release of insulin is 1 U/10 g of dietary carbohydrate, and it usually peaks within 1 hour of eating. The released insulin promotes the uptake and storage of glucose and other ingested nutrients, and the postprandial (postmeal) plasma concentrations of both insulin and glucose return to preprandial (premeal) levels within 2 hours. Basal secretion, which usually ranges from 0.5 to 1 U of insulin per hour, serves to retard hepatic glucose output during the postabsorptive state.

Physiologic Effects

Insulin is sometimes referred to as the storage hormone because it promotes anabolism and inhibits catabolism of carbohydrate, fatty acids, and protein.

Insulin has several important actions on the **liver,** the organ that normally serves as the major source of blood glucose to supply the brain in the fasting state. The liver provides blood glucose through the processes of gluconeogenesis (the formation of glucose from amino acids) and glycogenolysis (the breakdown of glycogen). Insulin stimulates the enzymes involved in glycogen synthesis while inhibiting glycogenolytic and gluconeogenetic enzymes. By these actions, insulin significantly inhibits glucose output by the liver.

Insulin promotes the uptake of glucose by **skeletal muscle** and **adipose tissue** via activation of a specific type of glucose transporter, called GLUT 4, which is located in muscle and adipose tissue. Skeletal muscle and adipose tissue are dependent on insulin for glucose uptake, whereas the brain can obtain glucose in the absence of insulin. By promoting glucose uptake, insulin facilitates the metabolism of glucose to provide energy for skeletal muscle contraction, and it stimulates glycogen synthesis. In adipose tissue, insulin stimulates the conversion of glucose to fatty acids for storage as triglyceride; promotes the uptake and esterification of fatty acids; and inhibits lipolysis (the conversion of triglyceride to fatty acids). In skeletal muscle, insulin inhibits protein catabolism and amino acid output.

Mechanisms of Action

Insulin binds to specific **insulin receptors** located in the plasma membrane of target cells, which are primarily cells of the liver, skeletal muscle, and adipose tissue. Stimulation of insulin receptors activates **tyrosine kinase** and leads to the phosphorylation of serine residues of target proteins. The phosphorylated proteins then alter the synthesis or activity of enzymes involved in gluconeogenesis, glycogenolysis, and other metabolic processes. Activation of tyrosine kinase also increases the insertion of glucose transporter molecules into cell membranes of muscle and fat tissue.

Glucagon

Glucagon is produced by A cells of the pancreas in response to decreased blood glucose concentrations. It activates glycogenolysis and gluconeogenesis and thereby increases hepatic glucose production. Patients with DM continue to produce glucagon, and the imbalance between glucagon and insulin is one factor that contributes to the metabolic derangements of this disease. Glucagon is available in a formulation for subcutaneous injection that is used to counteract hypoglycemic reactions in patients with DM.

Diabetes Mellitus

Classification

Diabetes mellitus, which is a disorder of glucose homeostasis characterized by the elevation of both basal and postprandial blood glucose concentrations, affects about 15 million people in the United States of America (USA). The two major forms of DM are type I and type II, with the latter accounting for about 85% of cases of DM.

Type I diabetes mellitus usually has its onset before the patient reaches 30 years of age, with a median onset of 12 years of age. It is believed to be an autoimmune disease that is triggered by a viral infection or other environmental factor. The resulting destruction of B cells leads to severe insulin deficiency and predisposes patients to **ketonemia** and **ketoacidosis.** Because patients with type I DM require exogenous insulin for survival, this type of disease is also called **insulin-dependent diabetes mellitus** (IDDM).

Type II diabetes mellitus is a heterogeneous disease that usually has its onset after the patient reaches 30 years of age and is often associated with a significant degree of **insulin resistance** and **obesity.** Insulin resistance can be caused by the presence of insulin antibodies or by defects in insulin receptors and signal transduction mechanisms in target organs. Patients with type II DM are not susceptible to developing ketonemia. Type II DM is also called **non–insulin-dependent diabetes mellitus** (NIDDM), but the term NIDDM is not always accurate. On the one hand, most patients with type II DM have normal or elevated concentrations of insulin and do not require exogenous insulin for survival. These patients can be effectively treated with oral antidiabetic medications in combination with dietary modifications and exercise. On the other hand, some patients with type II DM do require insulin treatment.

Additional forms of DM include **gestational diabetes**, which has its onset during pregnancy, and **secondary diabetes**, which occurs in association with other endocrine disorders or with exposure to drugs or chemical agents that are toxic to the pancreas.

Pathophysiology

The early manifestations of DM are primarily metabolic abnormalities resulting from the lack of insulin, whereas the long-term complications of DM are believed to result from the glycosylation of proteins. Type I DM is a serious disease that can quickly lead to ketoacidosis, coma, and death if exogenous insulin is not administered. Type II DM is usually less serious because patients can continue to secrete some amount of insulin.

The **acute metabolic abnormalities** that occur in untreated DM result from decreased glucose uptake by muscle and adipose tissue, increased hepatic output of glucose, increased catabolism of proteins in muscle tissue, and increased lipolysis and release of fatty acids from adipose tissue. A reduction in glucose utilization combined with an increase in hepatic glucose production leads to hyperglycemia. Hyperglycemia can then cause glycosuria

Figure 35-1. Time course of plasma glucose concentrations, endogenous insulin secretion, and exogenous insulin action. (A) Normal plasma glucose concentrations include a meal-stimulated component and a basal component. **(B)** In healthy individuals, insulin is secreted as the postprandial glucose concentration rises. This acts to increase glucose utilization and return the blood glucose concentration to its basal level. **(C, D, and E)** In patients with diabetes mellitus, insulin treatment seeks to mimic the natural secretion of insulin as closely as possible. Panels A, B, and C compare insulin concentrations obtained with three different treatment regimens. Panel C shows the results of two daily injections of regular insulin and neutral protamine Hagedorn (NPH) insulin. The first injection of each is given before breakfast, and the second injection of each is given before the evening meal. Panel D shows the results of treatment with one daily injection of ultralente insulin, which is given at bedtime, plus three daily injections of regular insulin, each of which is given before a meal. Panel E shows the results obtained with treatment via an insulin pump. The pump delivers a constant infusion of regular insulin to fulfill the basal insulin requirement, and the patient activates small bolus injections of insulin before meals, snacks, and bedtime.

(glucose in the urine), osmotic diuresis, polyuria (excessive urine formation), and polydipsia (excessive water intake). These derangements lead to dehydration and the loss of calories and weight. For these reasons, DM has been described as "starvation in the midst of plenty."

In patients with type I DM, the absence of insulin accelerates lipolysis, and this leads to increased production of ketones (acetoacetic acid, acetone, and β-hydroxybutyric acid) in the liver. When the body becomes unable to metabolize these ketones, the keto acids are excreted in the urine. These derangements ultimately lead to ketoacidosis, acetone breath, abnormal respiration, electrolyte depletion, vomiting, coma, and death. Insulin deficiency also leads to increased catabolism of proteins and increased loss of nitrogen in the urine.

The **long-term complications** of DM include microvascular complications, such as **nephropathy** and **retinopathy;** macrovascular complications, such as **cerebrovascular disease, coronary artery disease,** and **peripheral vascular disease;** and neuropathic complications, such as **sensory, motor, and autonomic neuropathic disorders.**

Although all of the complications of DM contribute significantly to morbidity, the most prevalent cause of death is coronary artery disease. Patients with DM often develop **hypertension** and **dyslipidemia** characterized by a decrease in the high-density lipoprotein cholesterol level and an increase in the triglyceride level. Furthermore, DM appears to be a risk factor for coronary artery disease that is independent of other risk factors such as smoking, hypertension, and dyslipidemia. For these reasons, patients with DM should exercise regularly, adhere closely to dietary guidelines, and comply with pharmacologic interventions to control hypertension and dyslipidemia and to achieve near-normal blood glucose concentrations.

INSULIN PREPARATIONS

Insulin preparations are used to treat all patients with type I DM and about one third of patients with type II DM. Insulin is also used to treat pregnant women with gestational diabetes. Many insulin preparations are available today. These preparations can be classified according to the source of insulin and to the onset and duration of action.

Sources

For many years, patients with DM were treated with **bovine and porcine insulin.** In recent years, **human insulin** has become available through recombinant DNA technology, and it is also produced by enzymatic modification of porcine insulin. Recombinant human insulin is produced by *Escherichia coli* strains that have been transfected with the human insulin gene.

Most diabetics now use human insulin because it has numerous advantages. Clinical studies have demonstrated that those using human insulin have diminished antibody production in comparison with those using animal insulin. Insulin antibodies can bind to insulin and contribute to insulin resistance. Patients with insulin resistance usually show a significant reduction in their insulin requirement when switched from animal insulin to human insulin. Insulin antibodies can also bind to and subsequently release insulin, thereby contributing to less predictable insulin activity. Human insulin is less likely to cause allergic reactions or to produce lipodystrophy (atrophy or hypertrophy of subcutaneous fat at the site of injection). For these reasons, authorities recommend that human insulin be used to treat patients with newly diagnosed type I DM, patients with insulin resistance or insulin allergy, patients with lipodystrophy, pregnant women who already have type II DM or acquire gestational diabetes during their pregnancy, and patients who have type II DM and require intermittent insulin administration, such as during surgery or infection.

Concentration and Purity

The concentration of insulin preparations is expressed as the number of units of insulin per milliliter of solution or suspension. The United States Pharmacopeia (USP) defines 1 U as the amount of insulin needed to decrease the blood glucose concentration by a defined amount in a fasting rabbit. Almost all insulin preparations used by diabetics contain 100 U/mL (U100 insulin). Regular insulin is also available in a concentrated preparation containing 500 U/mL (U 500 insulin). This concentrated preparation is used by persons with insulin resistance if they require more than 100 U as a single injection.

Human insulin preparations do not contain measurable amounts of proinsulin and are classified as highly purified by the US Food and Drug Administration (FDA).

Administration and Absorption

For the treatment of DM in ambulatory patients, insulin is usually injected subcutaneously or is administered by continuous subcutaneous infusion with an insulin pump. Several factors affect the rate of absorption of insulin from subcutaneous sites and thereby contribute to wide variations in the onset and duration of action of insulin preparations in individual patients. These factors include the technique and site of injection, the ambient temperature, the patient's level of exercise, whether the injection site is massaged, and whether subcutaneous lipodystrophy is present. Insulin absorption is fastest from an abdominal injection site and is progressively slower from sites on the arm, thigh, and buttock. Because repeated injections at the same site can contribute to tissue reactions that affect the rate of insulin absorption, patients should be taught to rotate injection sites within a particular anatomic area. The application of heat or massage can increase blood flow and thereby accelerate the rate of absorption of insulin and should generally be avoided.

Regular insulin, which is a clear solution, can also be injected intravenously in situations that require a more rapid response, such as in the treatment of diabetic ketoacidosis. The intermediate-acting and long-acting insulin preparations described below are suspensions of insulin particles that are usually administered subcutaneously and should never be injected intravenously.

TABLE 35–1.	Onset of Action, Peak Effect, and Duration of Action of Insulin Preparations Following Subcutaneous Administration		
Preparation	**Onset of Action**	**Peak Effect**	**Duration of Action**
Rapid-Acting Insulins			
Insulin aspart	15 minutes	1–3 hours	3–5 hours
Insulin lispro	15 minutes	30–90 minutes	6–8 hours
Regular insulin	30–60 minutes	1–5 hours	5–10 hours
Intermediate-Acting Insulins			
Lente insulin	1–2.5 hours	7–15 hours	24 hours
NPH (isophane) insulin	1–1.5 hours	4–12 hours	24 hours
Insulin glargine	1.1 hours	5 hours	24 hours*
Long-Acting Insulin			
Ultralente insulin	8 hours	10–30 hours	>36 hours

*Small amounts of insulin glargine are slowly released at a relatively constant rate.
NPH = neutral protamine Hagedorn.

Classification and Properties

Based on their onset and duration of action, insulin preparations are classified as short-acting, intermediate-acting, and long-acting. Table 35–1 compares the onset of action, peak effect, and duration of action of different insulin preparations.

Short-Acting Insulins

Three insulin preparations are now available for injection before meals to control postprandial glycemia: **insulin aspart, insulin lispro, and regular insulin** (insulin injection USP).

Regular insulin is a solution that contains insulin hexamers crystallized around a zinc molecule. After subcutaneous injection, the hexamers dissociate into dimers and monomers that are absorbed into the circulation. The dissociation of insulin hexamers occurs as the particles are diluted in body fluids when the insulin diffuses from the injection site into surrounding tissue. Because of the time required for this process, the onset of action of regular insulin occurs 30 to 60 minutes after an injection. The peak effect of regular insulin occurs between 1 and 5 hours after its administration, depending on the dose administered and other factors. Regular insulin should be injected about 30 minutes before eating to provide optimal control of postprandial glycemia.

Insulin lispro and insulin aspart are semisynthetic analogues of human insulin, with amino acid substitutions in the B-chain as shown in Box 35–1. These insulins have less capacity for self-association than regular insulin, and are more rapidly absorbed after subcutaneous injection. For this reason, the hypoglycemic effect of insulin lispro and insulin aspart begins about 15 minutes after subcutaneous injection and patients must eat within this time period. In comparison with the use of regular insulin, the use of insulin lispro and insulin aspart may enable patients to more easily coordinate insulin injection times and mealtimes. Except when administered by continuous injection with an insulin pump,

these insulins should be part of a regimen that includes an intermediate- or long-acting insulin.

Intermediate-Acting and Long-Acting Insulins

The intermediate- and long-acting insulin preparations are used to provide basal levels of insulin and to facilitate control of glycemia over an extended period of time. Because the plasma half-life of insulin is only about 5 to 7 minutes, these preparations have been formulated to slowly release the insulin for absorption into the circulation following a subcutaneous injection. The preparations contain suspensions of insulin particles prepared by (1) combining insulin with a large amount of zinc, as in the **insulin zinc suspensions** called **lente insulin** and **ultralente insulin,** or (2) combining insulin with protamine and a smaller amount of zinc, as in the **isophane insulin suspension** called **neutral protamine Hagedorn (NPH) insulin.** Protamine is a basic protein that readily complexes with insulin and zinc to form particles that slowly dissolve in body fluids.

Neutral protamine Hagedorn insulin (HUMULIN N) and lente insulin (HUMULIN L) are intermediate-acting preparations. Lente insulin is a mixture of two forms of insulin zinc suspension, the first of which is an amorphous form that dissolves rapidly in body fluids and is absorbed more quickly and the second of which is a crystalline form that is less soluble and is absorbed more slowly. The intermediate-acting insulins have an onset of action of 1 to 2.5 hours, a peak effect in 4 to 15 hours, and a duration of action of about 24 hours.

Insulin glargine (LANTUS) is a unique insulin preparation that contains an amino acid substitution at position A-21 and the addition of two arginine residues to the C-terminus of the B-chain. Insulin glargine is formulated to be slowly released and absorbed following subcutaneous injection. Insulin glargine is formulated as a solution at a pH of 4. At this pH, insulin glargine is completely soluble, but it is less soluble at neutral pH and it forms microprecipitates when injected subcutaneously. These precipitates release

TABLE 35–2. **Pharmacologic Properties of Oral Antidiabetic Drugs**

Drug	Hypoglycemia	Hyperinsulinemia	Lactic Acidosis	Gastrointestinal Symptoms
Acarbose	No	No	No	Yes (frequent)
Metformin	No	No	Yes (rare)	Yes (frequent)
Repaglinide	Yes	Yes	No	Yes (uncommon)
Sulfonylureas	Yes	Yes	No	Yes (rare)
Pioglitazone	No	No	No	No

small amounts of insulin glargine for absorption over a 24-hour period, thereby providing a relatively constant hypoglycemic effect over this time period. Insulin glargine is administered subcutaneously once daily at bedtime. It is used in combination with a short-acting insulin given at mealtimes to control postprandial glycemia.

Ultralente insulin (HUMULIN U) is the only long-acting insulin currently available in the USA. It consists entirely of crystalline insulin zinc particles that slowly dissolve in body fluids following a subcutaneous injection. Because ultralente insulin has a delayed onset and prolonged duration of action (see Table 35–1), it can be used to provide a basal insulin level that can be supplemented at mealtimes with a shorter-acting insulin.

Two other zinc-containing suspensions of insulin are no longer available in the USA: prompt insulin zinc suspension (semilente insulin) and protamine zinc insulin suspension (PZI).

Treatment Regimens

Regimens for the treatment of DM and its complications are discussed at the end of the chapter.

ORAL ANTIDIABETIC DRUGS

Oral antidiabetic drugs used to treat type II DM have no role in the treatment of type I DM. The purpose of these drugs is to maintain fasting and postprandial glucose concentrations in the normal range. These drugs can be divided into two major groups known as the hypoglycemic drugs and the antihyperglycemic drugs.

Hypoglycemic drugs act primarily by increasing insulin secretion. For this reason, excessive doses of these drugs can cause plasma glucose concentrations to fall below the normal range, whereas therapeutic doses serve to maintain blood glucose concentrations in the normal range in diabetic patients. The hypoglycemic drugs include the sulfonylurea compounds and the meglitinide drugs.

Antihyperglycemic drugs act to prevent or reduce hyperglycemia, but they do not cause hypoglycemia. This class of drugs includes the α-glucosidase inhibitors, the thiazolidinediones, and a biguanide drug called metformin.

The pharmacologic properties, metabolic effects, and therapeutic effects of oral antidiabetic drugs are shown in Table 35–2, Table 35–3, and Fig. 35–2.

Hypoglycemic Drugs

Sulfonylurea Drugs

The sulfonylurea drugs were the first oral antidiabetic agents. The original or first-generation sulfonylureas, including tolbutamide, chlorpropamide, and acetohexamide, are no longer used because of their lower potency and their greater tendency to cause side effects. These agents will not be discussed further in this chapter. The second-generation drugs, which are at least 100 times more potent than first-generation drugs, are widely used today. These agents include **glimepiride** (AMARYL), **glipizide** (GLUCOTROL), and **glyburide** (DIABETA, MICRONASE, GLYNASE).

CHEMISTRY AND PHARMACOKINETICS. The structures of two sulfonylurea drugs are shown in Fig. 35–3A. The sulfonylureas are administered orally and undergo varying degrees

TABLE 35–3. **Metabolic Effects of Oral Antidiabetic Drugs***

Drug	Glycemic Effects			Lipid Effects			Body Weight
	FPG	PPG	HbA$_{1c}$ (%)	LDL	HDL	TG	
Acarbose	→ or ↓	↓	↓0.3–1.0	→	→	↓	→ or ↓
Metformin	↓	↓	↓1.5–2.0	↓	↑	↓	→ or ↓
Repaglinide	→	↓	Unknown	→	→	→	→
Sulfonylureas	↓	↓	↓1.5–2.0	→	→	→ or ↓	↑
Pioglitazone	↓	↓	↓0.8–1.8	→	↑	↓	→

*FPG = fasting plasma glucose concentration; PPG = postprandial glucose concentration; HbA$_{1c}$ = glycosylated hemoglobin concentration; LDL = low-density lipoprotein cholesterol level; HDL = high-density lipoprotein cholesterol level; TG = triglyceride level; → = unchanged; ↓ = decreased; and ↑ = increased.

Figure 35–2. Therapeutic effects of diet, exercise, and oral drugs used in the treatment of patients with type II diabetes mellitus. If these treatment measures are not adequate, insulin can be used to control glycemia.

of hepatic metabolism followed by renal and biliary elimination of the metabolites.

MECHANISMS AND PHARMACOLOGIC EFFECTS. Sulfonylureas act primarily by increasing the secretion of insulin and secondarily by decreasing the secretion of glucagon.

Sulfonylureas increase the release of insulin from pancreatic B cells by inhibiting adenosine triphosphate-sensitive potassium channels in the plasma membrane. The potassium channel contains a pore-forming subunit through which potassium moves out of the cell. It also contains a subunit that functions as the receptor for sulfonylureas. When a sulfonylurea drug binds to this subunit, it closes the channel. This prevents potassium efflux and leads to depolarization of the B cell, influx of calcium, and activation of the secretory machinery that releases insulin. Sulfonylureas increase the pulsatile secretion of insulin but have no effect on the basal secretion. The drugs increase the amount of insulin secreted during each pulse, rather than by increasing the frequency of pulses.

The decrease in glucagon secretion appears to result from the increased secretion of insulin and pancreatic somatostatin evoked by sulfonylurea drugs. Both insulin and somatostatin are known to inhibit the release of glucagon from pancreatic A cells. This action tends to normalize the ratio of insulin to glucagon in diabetics. Sulfonylurea drugs also appear to increase insulin sensitivity in patients with type II diabetes.

In contrast to some of the antihyperglycemic drugs, sulfonylureas do not have beneficial effects on lipoprotein levels, and their use has been associated with weight gain.

INDICATIONS. A sulfonylurea drug can be used to treat type II DM that cannot be controlled with dietary restrictions, exercise, and body weight reduction. Therapy usually begins with a low dose, given once a day, and swallowed 30 minutes before breakfast to maximize absorption. The dose is then gradually increased until adequate glycemic control is achieved, side effects occur, or the maximal dose is reached. A sulfonylurea drug can be given in combination with metformin or a thiazolidinedione drug, and this type of drug combination may provide better control of blood glucose concentrations while causing fewer adverse reactions. The selection and use of oral antidiabetic drugs are described later in this chapter.

A. Hypoglycemic drugs

Glimepiride

Glyburide

B. Antihyperglycemic drugs

Metformin

Pioglitazone

Figure 35–3. Structures of oral antidiabetic drugs. (A) Most hypoglycemic drugs are sulfonylureas. The sulfonylurea moieties in glimepiride and glyburide are unshaded. **(B)** Metformin is a biguanide drug, and pioglitazone is a thiazolidinedione. The biguanide and thiazolidinedione moieties are unshaded.

ADVERSE EFFECTS. Hypoglycemia, the most common adverse effect of sulfonylurea drugs, can result from skipping or delaying meals, inadequate ingestion of carbohydrate, excessive doses, or renal or hepatic disease. Other adverse effects include skin rashes (which occur in up to 3% of patients), nausea, vomiting, and cholestasis. Less commonly, sulfonylureas cause hematologic reactions such as leukopenia, thrombocytopenia, and hemolytic anemia.

INTERACTIONS. Health care providers should be aware that sulfonylureas can interact with many other drugs. Although the clinical significance of many of these interactions is usually minimal, dosage adjustments may be required. Thiazide diuretics, corticosteroids, estrogens, thyroid hormones, phenytoin, and other drugs decrease the effectiveness of sulfonylureas and may necessitate a dosage increase.

Angiotensin-converting enzyme inhibitors, sulfonamides, salicylates and other nonsteroidal anti-inflammatory drugs, gemfibrozil, and alcohol (ethanol) are among the agents that can increase the hypoglycemic effect of sulfonylureas. Excessive ingestion of alcohol by patients treated with sulfonylureas or insulin can cause significant hypoglycemia. A disulfiram-like reaction can also result when alcohol is taken with sulfonylureas. Diabetics should be counseled to use alcohol moderately and to limit consumption to about 2 oz (60 mL) per day.

SPECIFIC DRUGS. The second-generation sulfonylurea drugs consist of glimepiride, glipizide, and glyburide. Glyburide is called glibenclamide in some countries.

The absorption of glipizide is slowed by food and it should be taken 30 minutes before breakfast. Glyburide and glimepiride can be taken with breakfast. Glyburide is available in a regular formulation and a micronized one. Because the micronized formulation provides higher plasma concentrations, the recommended doses of it are 60% of those of the regular formulation.

Glimepiride, glipizide, and glyburide have a duration of action of about 24 hours, which is considerably longer than their plasma half-life. Patients are started on lower doses of these drugs and then the dose is gradually increased every 1 to 2 weeks until glycemia is adequately controlled. Many patients require only a single daily dose of a sulfonylurea to control glycemia, but if larger doses are required they should be divided and given twice daily.

Clinical studies show that glimepiride, glipizide, and glyburide have similar efficacy in the treatment of type II DM. The use of these drugs in combination with other antidiabetic agents is described later in this chapter.

Meglitinide Drugs

Repaglinide (PRANDIN) and **nateglinide** (STARLIX) are meglitinide compounds that are rapidly absorbed and promptly produce a hypoglycemic effect. These drugs are intended to be taken before meals to control postprandial glycemia. Repaglinide and nateglinide increase the amount of insulin released by pancreatic B cells during and immediately after a meal by inhibiting adenosine triphosphate (ATP)-sensitive potassium channels in the same manner as do sulfonylurea compounds. This slows postprandial increases in blood glucose concentrations and causes an overall decline in the average blood glucose concentration over time and in glycosylated hemoglobin levels.

Repaglinide and nateglinide can be taken anytime from 30 minutes before a meal right up to mealtime. They achieve peak effectiveness in about 1 hour, which coincides with the time when postprandial glucose concentrations are rising toward their peak. Repaglinide and nateglinide are completely metabolized and inactivated by the liver in about 3 to 4 hours. For this reason, their duration of action is relatively short, and insulin concentrations return to basal levels before the next meal.

Repaglinide and nateglinide are indicated as first-line drugs to treat type II DM in conjunction with diet and exercise. They are particularly useful for patients whose meal schedules vary from day to day, a factor that increases their risk of hypoglycemic reactions to sulfonylureas. Repaglinide and nateglinide can also be used in combination with metformin when either agent alone does not adequately control blood glucose concentrations. They should not be used with other oral antidiabetic drugs or with insulin.

The primary adverse effect of meglitinide drugs is hypoglycemia. Hypoglycemic reactions are not often serious, but they have caused 1.4% of patients to discontinue their use of repaglinide. This is about half the rate of discontinued drug use attributed to hypoglycemic reactions in patients taking sulfonylureas. Mild hypoglycemia can be treated with oral glucose and severe hypoglycemia with intravenous D50W (50% dextrose in water) followed by a more dilute dextrose solution infusion.

Antihyperglycemic Drugs

Metformin

CHEMISTRY AND PHARMACOKINETICS. Metformin (GLU-COPHAGE) is the only **biguanide** type of oral antidiabetic medication currently available in the USA (see Fig. 35–3B). Another biguanide, **phenformin,** was removed from the market in the 1970s because of an unacceptable risk of fatal lactic acidosis (see below).

The immediate-release formulation of metformin is administered orally from two to three times a day and is eliminated by renal excretion of the parent compound. Its duration of action is about 18 hours. A sustained release metformin preparation (GLUCOPHAGE XR) is given as a single daily dose with the evening meal, starting at 500 mg/day and increasing at weekly intervals up to 2000 mg/day or 1000 mg twice daily.

MECHANISMS AND PHARMACOLOGIC EFFECTS. Metformin has several mechanisms of action that appear to result from increasing the number or affinity of insulin receptors in peripheral tissues. In patients with type II DM, it alleviates hyperglycemia partly by decreasing **hepatic glucose output**, resulting in increased glycogen stores. It also decreases glucose absorption from the gut and increases glucose uptake and utilization in skeletal muscle and adipose tissue. Unlike sulfonylureas, metformin does not stimulate insulin secretion or cause hypoglycemia and weight gain. Metformin often has a favorable effect on plasma lipid levels and can decrease body weight in some patients (see Table 35–3).

INDICATIONS. Metformin is now considered a first-line drug for the treatment of type II DM. It may be particularly appropriate for obese patients with insulin resistance and for patients with hyperlipidemia. It may also provide acceptable glycemic control in patients who do not adequately respond to a sulfonylurea drug. Metformin can be used alone, or it can be used in combination with a sulfonylurea for patients who fail to respond appropriately to single-drug therapy. For this purpose, metformin is available in combination products containing metformin and either glyburide (GLUCOV-ANCE) or glipizide (METAGLIP).

ADVERSE EFFECTS. The most common adverse effects of metformin are gastrointestinal disturbances. **Diarrhea** occurs in up to 30% of patients and causes about 4% of them to stop taking metformin. Unlike phenformin, metformin does not bind to mitochondria or interfere with glucose oxidation, and it causes **lactic acidosis** rarely (in only 3 cases per 100,000 patient years of use). Patients with renal or hepatic disease, alcoholism, or a predisposition to metabolic acidosis should not be treated with metformin, however, because they are at increased risk of lactic acidosis.

INTERACTIONS. Metformin has few drug interactions. Cimetidine can inhibit the drug's metabolism and elevate its plasma concentrations.

Thiazolidinediones

CHEMISTRY AND PHARMACOKINETICS. Pioglitazone (ACTOS) and rosiglitazone (AVANDIA) (see Fig. 35–3B) are members of the thiazolidinedione class of anti-hyperglycemic agents. The first drug in this class, troglitazone, was removed from the market because it caused a number of deaths from hepatic failure. Pioglitazone is taken once daily and rosiglitazone is taken once or twice daily. These drugs are well absorbed from the gut and can be taken with or without food. Both pioglitazone and rosiglitazone are almost entirely metabolized by the liver. Two metabolites of pioglitazone have pharmacologic activity but metabolites of rosiglitazone are inactive.

MECHANISMS AND PHARMACOLOGIC EFFECTS. The thiazolidinedione drugs act as agonists at the **peroxisome proliferator-activated receptor-gamma** (PPAR-γ), which is found in adipose tissue, skeletal muscle, and the liver. Hence, these drugs have a mechanism similar to the fibric acid drugs used to treat hyperlipidemia, which activate PPAR-α (see chapter 15).

Activation of PPAR-γ increases transcription of insulin-responsive genes that control glucose and lipid metabolism, leading to increased insulin sensitivity and decreased insulin resistance in patients with type II diabetes. These drugs appear to increase the sensitivity of peripheral tissues to insulin by about 60%. Specifically, thiazolidinediones increase the number of GLUT 4 glucose transporters in cell membranes of muscle and adipose tissue, which increases the uptake and utilization of glucose in these tissues. Pioglitazone and rosiglitazone also suppress hepatic glucose output.

The thiazolidinediones tend to lower serum triglyceride levels and increase high-density lipoprotein (HDL)-cholesterol levels. Rosiglitazone, however, may also increase low-density lipoprotein (LDL)-cholesterol and total cholesterol levels, and it may cause weight gain. Pioglitazone did not produce any consistent effect on LDL and total cholesterol levels.

INDICATIONS. Thiazolidinedione drugs are indicated as an adjunct to diet and exercise for the management of type II DM. They can be used in combination with metformin when diet, exercise, and metformin does not achieve glycemic control. Because they enhance insulin sensitivity, they are particularly useful in patients with insulin resistance. Clinical studies indicate that these drugs decrease plasma glucose concentrations by 40 to 80 mg/dL and decrease insulin requirements by 5% to 30%.

The glucose-lowering effects of pioglitazone and rosiglitazone do not occur quickly and their maximal effectiveness requires 4 to 6 weeks after initiating treatment or increasing doses.

ADVERSE EFFECTS. Pioglitazone and rosiglitazone can cause **edema** and plasma volume expansion, and are not recommended for persons with heart failure. These drugs have not been associated with hepatic failure, but **liver function tests** should be performed periodically as a precaution and the drugs should be discontinued if serum alanine aminotransferase (ALT) levels are two and a half to three times the upper limit of normal.

α-Glucosidase Inhibitors

MECHANISMS AND PHARMACOLOGIC EFFECTS. The digestion of dietary starch and disaccharides (e.g., sucrose) is dependent on the action of **α-glucosidase,** an enzyme located in the brush border of the intestinal tract that converts oligosaccharides and disaccharides to glucose and other monosaccharides. **Acarbose** (PRECOSE) and **miglitol** (GLYSET) competitively inhibit this enzyme and delay the digestion of starch and disaccharides such as sucrose. This action decreases the rate of glucose absorption and lowers postprandial blood glucose concentrations, thereby reducing postprandial hyperglycemia. Studies have shown that acarbose and miglitol reduce the glycosylated hemoglobin (HbA$_{1c}$) concentrations, although the reduction is usually less than that obtained with other oral antidiabetic drugs when used alone (see Table 35–3).

INDICATIONS AND PHARMACOKINETICS. Acarbose and miglitol are used in the treatment of type II DM, usually in combination with a sulfonylurea drug or other oral antidiabetic agent. Acarbose and miglitol should be administered with the first bite of a meal. Acarbose is not absorbed systemically and it is eliminated in the feces, whereas miglitol is partly absorbed from the gut. Both drugs, however, act locally to inhibit α-glucosidase in the gastrointestinal tract.

ADVERSE EFFECTS AND INTERACTIONS. The most common side effects of acarbose and miglitol are increased flatulence and abdominal bloating. These reactions probably result from the delivery of greater amounts of carbohydrate to the lower intestinal tract, where they exert an osmotic attraction for water and are metabolized by bacteria. These drugs do not inhibit lactase or cause lactose intolerance.

Acarbose can increase the oral bioavailability of metformin and cause a decrease in iron absorption. Miglitol can decrease absorption of ranitidine and propranolol.

If concurrent administration of insulin or a sulfonylurea drug results in hypoglycemia in patients taking acarbose, this complication should be treated with glucose (dextrose), rather than sucrose, because sucrose requires α-glucosidase activity for digestion.

MANAGEMENT OF DIABETES MELLITUS

Type I Diabetes Mellitus

All patients with type I DM require insulin therapy to achieve a high degree of glycemic control. In 1993, the Diabetes Control and Complications Trial Research Group showed that achieving and maintaining near-normal blood glucose concentrations in patients with type I DM reduced the incidence of nephropathy, neuropathy, and retinopathy. Although evidence indicates that poor glycemic control is associated with cardiovascular events, no study has yet shown that aggressive lowering of blood glucose concentrations reduces the incidence of cardiovascular disease.

Objectives of Insulin Therapy

The specific objectives of insulin therapy are to maintain the **fasting plasma glucose concentration** below 140 mg/dL (normal is <115 mg/dL); to maintain the **2-hour postprandial glucose concentration** below 175 mg/dL (normal is <140 mg/dL); and to maintain the **HbA$_{1c}$ concentration** below 8% (normal is 4% to 6%). The HbA$_{1c}$ concentration provides a cumulative indication of overall glycemic control and may directly relate to the extent to which glycosylation of tissue proteins contributes to the microvascular and other complications of DM.

Insulin Requirements and Dosing Schedules

In patients with type I DM, multiple daily injections of insulin are required to obtain acceptable control of glycemia without causing hypoglycemia. The total amount of insulin required by most of these patients is 0.5 to 1 U/kg/day. This amount, however, usually decreases during the "honeymoon phase" of DM (during the first several months after the initial episode of illness).

Although a number of different insulin treatment regimens are used, each of them seeks to mimic the natural secretion of insulin as closely as possible (see Fig. 35–1B). In most regimens, use of an **intermediate- or long-acting insulin preparation** is supplemented by use of a **short-acting insulin** at mealtimes in a dose that matches the quantity of ingested carbohydrate. Three examples of insulin dosing schedules that are used to treat type I DM are illustrated in Fig. 35–1.

One regimen consists of injecting an intermediate-acting insulin (NPH insulin, or lente insulin) plus a short-acting insulin (regular insulin) twice a day. Two thirds of the total daily dose is given in the morning 30 minutes before breakfast, and the remainder is given 30 minutes before the evening meal. The morning injection usually consists of a 2:1 or 70:30 ratio of intermediate-acting insulin to regular insulin, whereas the evening injection typically consists of a 50:50 ratio. The specific doses of intermediate-acting and regular insulin can be adjusted on the basis of self-monitored glucose readings taken at the time of the peak action of each insulin injection. If these blood glucose measurements are too high or too low, the subsequent doses of insulin can be adjusted appropriately.

Two mixtures of NPH and regular insulin are available for use in the abovementioned treatment regimen. One mixture contains NPH and regular insulin in a ratio of 70:30, and the other contains the two insulins in a ratio of 50:50. No premixed preparation of Lente and regular insulin is available; patients must mix these drugs immediately before administering them, because the mixture is not stable for long periods of time.

Other regimens for type I DM consist of a single daily injection of insulin glargine or ultralente insulin given at bedtime in combination with injections of a short-acting insulin before meals. Insulin glargine or ultralente insulin provides a basal level of insulin that controls hepatic glucose and the short-acting insulin controls postprandial glycemia.

Similar results can be obtained with an insulin pump. The insulin pump delivers a constant infusion of short-acting insulin to fulfill the basal insulin requirement, and the patient activates small bolus injections of insulin before meals and snacks. An insulin pump, theoretically, can provide greater glycemic control than other regimens, but its safe and effective use requires that patients be motivated to properly use and maintain the device.

Diabetic Ketoacidosis

Diabetic ketoacidosis is a common and life-threatening complication of type I DM, with a mortality rate as high as 6% to 10%. Therapy must be individualized, based on the clinical and laboratory status of the patient. Intravenous fluids are given to alleviate dehydration, and continuous intravenous infusion of insulin is given to decrease the plasma glucose concentration at a rate of at least 75 to 100 mg/dL/hour. Intravenous administration of potassium chloride is usually required to counteract hypokalemia that results from the correction of dehydration and acidosis. Dextrose (glucose) is often needed as therapy progresses, because hyperglycemia is usually corrected more rapidly than is acidosis. Insulin should be continued until acidosis is resolved. Bicarbonate is not routinely used and should be reserved for the treatment of patients who have severe acidosis after hypokalemia is corrected.

Type II Diabetes Mellitus

Treatment of type II DM rests on the foundation of a nutritious diet and appropriate exercise. Dietary recommendations should attempt to limit calories and saturated fat. Overweight patients should be encouraged to exercise and lose weight in an attempt to improve glycemic control, reduce insulin resistance, and lower plasma lipid levels. If nonpharmacologic measures are inadequate, as indicated by fasting blood glucose concentrations exceeding 140 mg/dL or HbA$_{1c}$ concentrations exceeding 8%, the next step is usually to add an oral antidiabetic medication.

Metformin and sulfonylureas are considered first-line drugs for type II DM. In obese patients with type II DM who have insulin resistance or hyperlipidemia, metformin is a logical choice to begin drug therapy, because it lowers elevated lipid levels and does not cause weight gain. Metformin and sulfonylurea drugs can be combined with each other and with an α-glucosidase inhibitor (e.g., acarbose) when a single drug does not adequately control blood glucose levels. Other useful drug combinations include a thiazolidinedione drug (e.g., pioglitazone) in combination with metformin or a sulfonylurea drug. These combinations can be tailored for individual patients based on their metabolic profiles and body weight,

Insulin can be used to treat type II DM when oral drugs are not effective or not tolerated. The insulin regimens used to treat type II DM are usually less complicated than those used to treat type I DM. Patients with type II disease are not susceptible to ketoacidosis, and most of them have significant endogenous insulin production. For these reasons, the initial insulin requirement is often less than 20 U/day. Insulin therapy is usually started with a single daily dose of intermediate- or long-acting insulin. Giving the single dose at bedtime may be adequate for patients who experience only early morning hyperglycemia. If multiple daily doses of insulin are needed or if insulin requirements are greater than 30 U/day, pioglitazone can be used in combination with insulin for management of type II diabetics and may improve insulin sensitivity in these patients.

SUMMARY OF IMPORTANT POINTS

■ All patients with type I DM require insulin. Most patients with type II DM can be managed with diet, exercise, and oral antidiabetic drugs. Oral antidiabetic drugs have no role in the treatment of type I DM.

■ Insulin increases glucose uptake by muscle and fat, decreases hepatic glucose output, and controls postprandial glycemia.

■ Insulin lispro, insulin aspart, and regular insulin are short-acting preparations; insulin glargine, lente insulin and isophane (NPH) insulin are intermediate-acting preparations; and ultralente insulin is a long-acting preparation.

■ Type I DM is often treated with an intermediate- or long-acting insulin in combination with a short-acting insulin. Alternatively, an insulin pump can be used to provide basal and mealtime injections of insulin.

■ Oral antidiabetic drugs include hypoglycemic agents (sulfonylureas and repaglinide) and antihyperglycemic agents (α-glucosidase inhibitors, metformin, and thiazolidinediones such as pioglitazone and rosiglitazone).

■ Sulfonylurea (glipizide, glyburide, and glimepiride) and meglitinide drugs (repaglinide and nateglinide) increase insulin release from pancreatic B cells. Hypoglycemia is the main side effect of these drugs.

■ Acarbose and miglitol inhibit α-glucosidase and slow digestion and absorption of glucose.

■ Metformin, pioglitazone, and rosiglitazone decrease hepatic glucose output and increase insulin sensitivity in muscle and fat.

■ Metformin, and sulfonylureas are first-line drugs for the treatment of type II DM and can be used alone or in combination with each other, with an α-glucosidase inhibitor, or with a thiazolidinedione.

Review Questions

1. Which insulin preparation is released and absorbed at a relatively constant rate over a 24-hour period after subcutaneous injection?
   (A) regular insulin
   (B) insulin lispro
   (C) ultralente insulin
   (D) insulin aspart
   (E) insulin glargine

2. Which drug is administered just before meals to increase insulin release and control postprandial glycemia?
   (A) miglitol
   (B) nateglinide
   (C) rosiglitazone
   (D) acarbose
   (E) metformin

3. Which drug activates the peroxisome proliferator-activated receptor-gamma and thereby increases insulin sensitivity?
   (A) glipizide
   (B) metformin
   (C) acarbose
   (D) pioglitazone
   (E) repaglinide

4. Which drug inhibits the digestion of sucrose and starch?
   (A) miglitol
   (B) nateglinide
   (C) glimepiride
   (D) rosiglitazone
   (E) metformin

5. Metformin primarily exerts which effect on glucose metabolism?
   (A) inhibits glycogenolysis
   (B) increases hepatic glucose uptake
   (C) decreases hepatic glucose output
   (D) increases glucose absorption from the gut
   (E) increases insulin secretion

Answers and Explanations

1. The answer is E: insulin glargine. Insulin glargine forms microprecipitates in subcutaneous tissue that release the drug for absorption at a relatively constant rate over a 24-hour period. Answer (A), regular insulin, answer (B), insulin lispro, and answer D, insulin aspart, are short-acting insulins with maximal durations of action of 5 to 10 hours. Answer (C), ultralente insulin, is a long-acting insulin with a delayed onset of action and peak effect, and a long duration of action.

2. The answer is B: nateglinide. Nateglinide is a meglitinide drug taken just before meals to increase insulin release and control postprandial glycemia. Answer (A), miglitol, and answer (D), acarbose, are α-glucosidase inhibitors taken before meals to inhibit digestion of starch and disaccharides. Answer (C), rosiglitazone, and answer (E), metformin, are anti-hyperglycemic agents that increase tissue responsiveness to insulin.

3. The answer is D: pioglitazone. Pioglitazone is a thiazolidinedione drug that activates the peroxisome proliferator-activated receptor-gamma. It increases transcription of genes encoding enzymes that mediate effects of insulin and thereby increase insulin sensitivity. Answer (B), metformin, increases responsiveness to insulin but by other mechanisms. Answer (A), glipizide, and answer (E), repaglinide, are hypoglycemic agents that increase insulin release. Answer (C), acarbose, inhibits α-glucosidase and the digestion of starch and disaccharides.

4. The answer is A: miglitol. Miglitol and acarbose are α-glucosidase inhibitors that reduce the conversion of starch and disaccharides to glucose, thereby reducing postprandial hyperglycemia. Answer (B), nateglinide, and answer (C), glimepiride, inhibit ATP-sensitive potassium channels in pancreatic B cells and thereby reduce insulin secretion. Answer (D), rosiglitazone, and answer (E), metformin, act by different mechanisms to increase insulin sensitivity.

5. The answer is C: decreases hepatic glucose output. Metformin increases insulin responsiveness and it decreases hepatic glucose output. Answer (A), inhibits glycogenolysis, is one of the metabolic effects of insulin. Answer (B), increases hepatic glucose uptake, and answer (D), increases glucose absorption from the gut, are effects not caused by any antidiabetic agent. Answer (E), increases insulin secretion, is caused by sulfonylurea and meglitinide drugs.

SELECTED READINGS

Del Prato, S., and P. Marchetti. Targeting insulin resistance and beta-cell dysfunction: the role of thiazolidinediones. Diabetes Technol Ther 6: 719–731, 2004.

Hirsch, I. B. Insulin analogues. N Engl J Med 352:174–183, 2005.

Patsouris, D., M. Muller, and S. Kersten. Peroxisome proliferator activated receptor ligands for the treatment of insulin resistance. Curr Opin Investig Drugs 5:104–1050, 2004.

Vivian, E. M., S. V. Olarte, and A. M. Gutierrez. Insulin strategies for type 2 diabetes mellitus. Ann Pharmacother 38:1916–1923, 2004.

Willett, L. L., and E. S. Albright. Achieving glycemic control in type 2 diabetes: a practical guide for clinicians on oral hypoglycemics. South Med J 97:1088–1092, 2004.

Drugs Affecting Calcium and Bone

OVERVIEW

Calcium and Bone Metabolism

The strength and the structure of bone depend on the presence of **calcium salts** deposited on bone matrix proteins. Normal bone is constantly undergoing remodeling via demineralization and mineralization processes. During remodeling, bone calcium is in a dynamic equilibrium with ionized calcium in extracellular fluid. Bone **mineralization** tends to increase as the extracellular calcium concentration rises, and **demineralization** tends to increase as this concentration falls. The proper extracellular calcium concentration is required for normal function of nerves and muscles, blood coagulation, enzyme activities, and other physiologic functions.

Control of the extracellular calcium concentration depends on hormonal regulation of the absorption and excretion of calcium, as well as on the exchange of ionized calcium with bone. As shown in Fig. 36–1, the hormones involved in regulation include **vitamin D, parathyroid hormone** (PTH), and **calcitonin.**

Vitamin D stimulates calcium absorption by increasing the synthesis of a calcium-binding protein that mediates the gastrointestinal absorption of calcium. Vitamin D also stimulates bone resorption and the closely coupled process of bone formation.

The PTH has four actions that increase the extracellular calcium concentration. First, it stimulates resorption of calcium by renal tubules. Second, it decreases resorption of phosphate by renal tubules. This decreases the extracellular phosphate concentration, which in turn tends to increase the extracellular calcium concentration. Third, PTH stimulates the hydroxylation of vitamin D in the kidneys (Fig. 36–2). Fourth, PTH increases bone resorption by stimulating osteoclast activity, which enables bone calcium to enter the extracellular pool. A recombinant form of PTH, teriparatide (FORTEO), has been developed for the treatment of **severe osteoporosis** (see later text).

Calcitonin is released in response to increased plasma calcium levels, and it acts to inhibit bone resorption and thereby decreases plasma calcium levels. The physiologic significance of calcitonin is unclear, because normal calcium

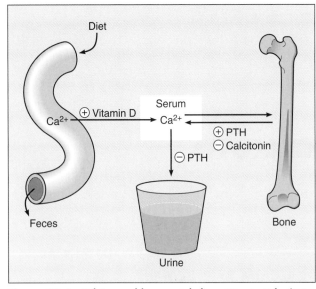

Figure 36–1. Calcium and bone metabolism. Vitamin D facilitates calcium absorption from the gut. Parathyroid hormone (PTH) decreases calcium excretion in the urine but increases phosphorus excretion (not shown). PTH also increases bone resorption, whereas calcitonin decreases bone resorption.

balance is maintained in the absence of calcitonin in persons who undergo thyroidectomy.

Bone remodeling consists of a sequence of events involving the dynamic interaction of **osteoclasts** (bone-resorbing cells) and **osteoblasts** (bone-forming cells). The recruitment and activation of osteoclasts, which are mediated by compounds released from osteoblasts and peripheral leukocytes, are called **bone cell cytokines.** The cytokines include **interleukins, tumor necrosis factor,** and **colony-stimulating factors.** After the osteoclasts are activated, they adhere to the bone surface and release hydrogen ions and proteases to break down the bone. The destroyed bone releases growth factors that increase osteoblast production and decrease osteoclast activity. The osteoblasts then lay down new bone in the cavity created by osteoclasts. The entire remodeling process takes about 100 days on average. Trabecular bone undergoes more remodeling than cortical bone (25% versus 3% annually).

The balance between **bone resorption** and **bone formation** is usually maintained until the third or fourth decade of life, when a slow, age-related imbalance begins and favors resorption over formation. Hormonal and nutritional deficiencies can also contribute to this imbalance.

Bone Disorders

Osteoporosis, the most common bone disorder, is characterized by a gradual reduction in bone mass that weakens the bone and leads to the occurrence of fractures with minimal trauma. The disorder is frequently classified as postmenopausal, senile, or secondary to other diseases. **Vertebral fractures** are the most frequent type of fractures seen in patients with **postmenopausal osteoporosis,** a disorder primarily caused by estrogen deficiency. **Hip, humerus, pelvis, and vertebral fractures** occur in patients with **senile osteoporosis,** a disorder primarily resulting from advanced age, and is a major cause of immobility, morbidity, and mor-

tality in the elderly. In the United States of America (USA), the annual cost of osteoporotic hip fractures alone is currently about $10 billion, and the cost is projected to rise to $240 billion by the year 2040 if more effective methods of prevention and treatment are not discovered and implemented.

Paget's disease of bone, or **osteitis deformans,** is the second most common bone disorder. Characterized by excessive bone turnover, it causes bone deformities, pain, and fractures. Its cause is unknown.

Osteomalacia is characterized by abnormal mineralization of new bone matrix. The condition has numerous causes, the most common of which include vitamin D deficiency, abnormal vitamin D metabolism, phosphate deficiency, and osteoblast dysfunction. In children, osteomalacia usually results from vitamin D deficiency and is called **rickets.** This disorder is uncommon today because of vitamin D-supplemented foods and sun exposure. In adults, factors such as aging, malabsorption, chronic renal impairment, and use of phenytoin or other anticonvulsant drugs can interfere with vitamin D absorption, metabolism, or target organ response and result in osteomalacia.

DRUGS

Calcium and Vitamin D Supplements

An adequate intake of calcium and vitamin D is essential for optimal bone formation in children and to prevent osteoporosis in adults.

In the USA, two thirds of women 18 to 30 years of age and three fourths of women over 30 years of age have an inadequate calcium intake, and this predisposes them to osteoporosis. All persons, regardless of age or gender, should

TABLE 36–1. **Clacium Intake Recommended by the National Institutes of Health Consensus Panel**

Age Group	Daily Calcium Intake (mg)
Infants	
0–6 months	400
7–12 months	600
Children	
1–5 years	800
6–10 years	800–1200
Adolescents and young adults	
11–24 years	1200–1500
Men	
25–65 years	1000
>65 years	1500
Women	
25–50 years	1000
>50 years (postmenopausal)	
Taking estrogens	1000
Not taking estrogens	1500
>65 years	1500
Pregnant and nursing	1200–1500

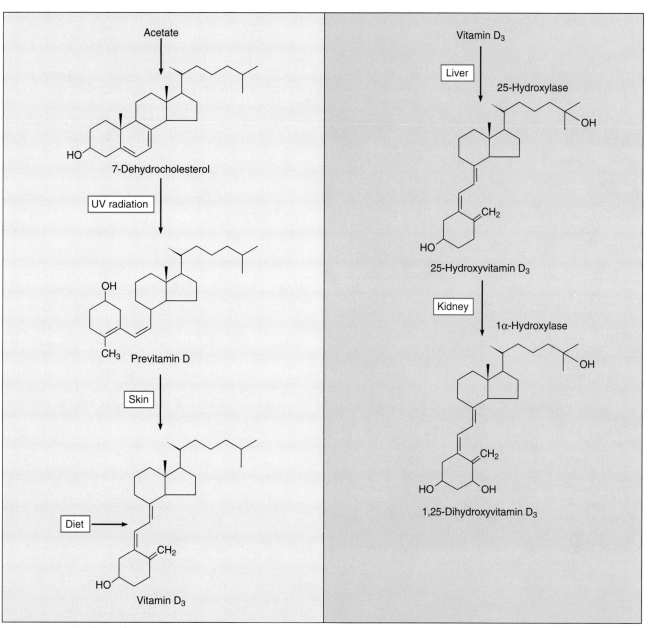

Figure 36–2. Synthesis of vitamin D. Vitamin D_3 (cholecalciferol) can be synthesized in the human body from acetate through a pathway that requires ultraviolet (UV) radiation. Diet and vitamin supplements also provide vitamin D_3, which is activated by specific hydroxylation steps in the liver and kidneys to form 1,25-dihydroxyvitamin D_3 (calcitriol).

meet the recommendations of the National Institutes of Health for daily calcium intake (Table 36–1). These recommendations can be met by ingesting calcium-rich foods, which are primarily dairy products, and taking oral calcium supplements if dietary intake is inadequate. By ingesting optimal amounts of calcium and vitamin D, young adults may be able to increase their bone mass, and older adults can decrease the rate of bone loss.

In one clinical study, nursing-home residents who were given 800 IU of vitamin D_3 and 1200 mg of calcium were found to have an increase in bone density and a decrease in the incidence of hip and nonvertebral fractures in comparison with nursing-home residents who were given placebos. In another study, administration of vitamin D_3 was found to decrease the incidence of vertebral and peripheral fractures in women with previous fractures.

Calcium

PHARMACOKINETICS. Calcium absorption from the gut is incomplete, even with consumption of adequate amounts of vitamin D. Only about 30% of calcium is absorbed from milk and other dairy products, and calcium absorption from supplements is often less than 30%. To enhance absorption, calcium tablets should be taken between meals.

The absorption of **calcium carbonate** requires stomach acid, whereas the absorption of **calcium citrate** does not. Because elderly persons can have decreased stomach acid secretion, they tend to benefit more from using calcium citrate.

INDICATIONS. In addition to their role in the prevention and treatment of **osteoporosis,** calcium and vitamin D are also the primary treatment for **hypocalcemia.** For this purpose, calcium can be given orally or intravenously.

ADVERSE EFFECTS AND INTERACTIONS. The most common adverse effect of calcium supplements is constipation. This is best managed by ingesting adequate amounts of fruits and vegetables. Calcium should not be taken with fiber laxatives, because they decrease calcium absorption. Calcium can decrease the absorption of ciprofloxacin, fluoride, phenytoin, and tetracycline, so calcium supplements should be taken at least 2 hours before or after taking these drugs.

Vitamin D

CHEMISTRY AND PHARMACOKINETICS. Vitamin D is a fat-soluble substance similar to cholesterol. The form of the vitamin that is obtained from the diet and can be synthesized in skin exposed to ultraviolet radiation is called **vitamin D_3** or **cholecalciferol.** It is a relatively inactive precursor of **1,25-dihydroxyvitamin D_3,** which is also called **calcitriol,** and is the most active form of the vitamin in the human body. The formation of calcitriol involves hydroxylation of vitamin D_3 at the 25 position in the liver to form **calcifediol** (25-hydroxycholecalciferol), which is then hydroxylated at the 1 position in the kidneys to form calcitriol (see Fig. 36–2). PTH stimulates the renal hydroxylation of vitamin D. The roles of PTH and vitamin D in calcium metabolism and homeostasis are described above.

VITAMIN D PREPARATIONS. Several Vitamin D preparations are available for use as nutritional supplements to prevent vitamin D deficiency. These preparations usually contain vitamin D obtained from fish oil. In addition to these preparations, specific vitamin D compounds are available to treat vitamin D deficiency and related disorders. These include calcifediol, calcitriol, and a form of the vitamin called **alfacalcidol** that is rapidly converted to calcitriol in the liver. Another preparation, **dihydrotachysterol,** which is a synthetic reduction product of **ergocalciferol,** is activated by 25-hydroxylation in the liver. Other vitamin D preparations include ergocalciferol and **paricalcitol.**

INDICATIONS. Vitamin D preparations are used for the following indications: to prevent and treat vitamin D deficiency and **vitamin D-dependent rickets,** to treat **familial hypophosphatemia** (vitamin D-resistant rickets), to treat **hypocalcemia** caused by **hypoparathyroidism,** to treat **postoperative and idiopathic tetany,** and to prevent vitamin D deficiency in persons with **chronic renal failure.** Persons, including the elderly, with inadequate dietary vitamin D intake and low sun exposure should take oral vitamin D supplements to develop and maintain skeletal mass and prevent osteoporosis. Patients with **chronic renal failure** must be treated with calcitriol because they lack the 1α-hydroxylase enzyme required to synthesize the active form of vitamin D (Fig. 36–2).

ADVERSE EFFECTS AND INTERACTIONS. Excessive doses of vitamin D can cause hypercalcemia and hypercalciuria. Cholestyramine inhibits vitamin D absorption, and phenytoin and barbiturates can induce enzymes that metabolize vitamin D and thereby lead to vitamin D deficiency.

Bisphosphonates

Several bisphosphonate compounds are used today to treat disorders of calcium metabolism and bone. These compounds include **alendronate** (FOSAMAX), **pamidronate** (AREDIA), **risedronate** (ACTONEL), and **tiludronate** (SKELID). Zoledronic acid (ZOMETA) is a similar compound used to treat hypercalcemia from to malignant tumors. The original bisphosphonate, **etidronate,** is no longer used extensively, because it is a less potent inhibitor of bone resorption than these newer compounds and because its long-term administration has been associated with the development of osteomalacia.

Drug Properties

CHEMISTRY. Bisphosphonate drugs are organic pyrophosphate compounds in which the P-O-P group is replaced with a nonhydrolyzable P-C-P moiety (Fig. 36–3).

PHARMACOKINETICS. Pamidronate is given intravenously, whereas alendronate, risedronate, and tiludronate are administered orally. Less than 5% of the oral drug is absorbed when taken on an empty stomach, and absorption is further reduced by food, certain drugs, and liquids other than water. Hence, patients should be advised to take alendronate, risedronate, or tiludronate with a full glass of water 30 minutes before ingesting anything else in the morning. Once absorbed, about half of the drug is deposited in bone, and the remainder is excreted in the urine.

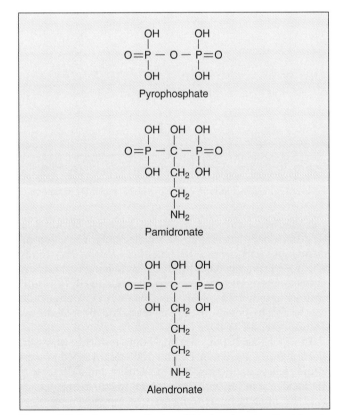

Figure 36–3. Structures of selected bisphosphonates. Pamidronate and alendronate are analogues of pyrophosphate.

The bisphosphonates adsorb to hydroxyapatite and become a permanent part of the bone structure. They are slowly released from bone during bone remodeling, and the terminal half-life in humans may be greater than 10 years.

MECHANISMS AND PHARMACOLOGIC EFFECTS. Bisphosphonates prevent bone resorption by inhibiting osteoclast activity through a variety of mechanisms. The most important mechanism appears to be prevention of the attachment of osteoclast precursor cells to bone. Bisphosphonates also decrease the metabolic activity of osteoclasts and their ability to resorb bone. Experimental evidence suggests that tiludronate inhibits tyrosine phosphatase activity in osteoclasts and thereby causes their detachment from bone surfaces. It can also inhibit the proton pump through which osteoclasts secrete hydrogen ions that participate in bone resorption.

INDICATIONS. Bisphosphonate compounds are used in the management of a variety of disorders, including **osteoporosis, Paget's disease of bone, hypercalcemia,** and **osteolytic bone lesions of metastatic cancer.** As discussed below, the various compounds have different uses.

ADVERSE EFFECTS. Orally administered bisphosphonates can cause esophageal erosion, but this can be prevented by advising the patient to remain upright after swallowing these drugs. The bisphosphonate compounds produce varying degrees of gastrointestinal distress. Pamidronate causes more gastric irritation than other bisphosphonates and is not currently available in an oral formulation. Alendronate and risedronate seldom cause gastric distress except when high doses are used to treat Paget's disease. Occasionally, alendronate causes mild and transient nausea, dyspepsia, constipation, or diarrhea. Unlike etidronate, alendronate does not cause osteomalacia during long-term use.

INTERACTIONS. The bisphosphonates have few interactions with other drugs. Calcium supplements and antacids decrease the bioavailability of alendronate and tiludronate and should be taken at least 2 hours before or after the bisphosphonate compound is taken.

Specific Drugs

Alendronate is the first bisphosphonate to be approved for the treatment of osteoporosis, and it appears to be effective in all forms of this disorder, including glucocorticoid-induced osteoporosis. Clinical trials in women with postmenopausal osteoporosis indicate that alendronate prevents bone loss and is more effective than calcium supplements or calcitonin therapy in producing a sustained increase in bone mass. A study of women with low bone mass and preexisting vertebral fractures has shown that alendronate treatment resulted in a 47% reduction in the risk of new vertebral fractures over a 3-year period. Alendronate is available as oral tablet formulations that can be administered once daily (5 or 10 mg) or once weekly (35 or 70 mg). The lower doses are indicated for prevention of osteoporosis and the higher doses are used for treatment of established osteoporosis.

Risedronate (ACTONEL) has also been approved to prevent and treat osteoporosis in postmenopausal women and **osteoporosis induced by corticosteroid therapy.** It is given as a single daily dose 30 minutes before breakfast in the same manner as is alendronate.

Alendronate, pamidronate, risedronate, and tiludronate are all approved for the treatment of **Paget's disease.** Before treatment, imaging and laboratory studies usually show evidence of increased bone turnover (remodeling), bone hypertrophy, and abnormal bone structure. By inhibiting abnormal osteoclast activity in patients with this disease, the bisphosphonates help to normalize biochemical indices of bone remodeling and restore normal bone structure. Patients who are symptomatic or who require orthopedic surgery are candidates for bisphosphonate therapy. Treatment should be initiated as early as possible to halt disease progression. Tiludronate given once daily is usually effective in 3 months, whereas other bisphosphonate compounds can require 6 months to be effective. If a relapse occurs, another course of treatment can be given after a 6-month interval.

In patients with cancer, bisphosphonates have been found to be useful in the management of hypercalcemia and metastatic bone disease. Intravenous administration of a bisphosphonate (e.g., pamidronate) is the most effective treatment for hypercalcemia associated with cancer. Bisphosphonate treatment has been found to inhibit bone resorption, reduce the tumor burden in bone, decrease bone pain, and reduce the risk of fractures in patients whose cancer has metastasized to the bone. For example, pamidronate was shown to significantly reduce the incidence and prolong the median time to skeletal complications in women who had stage IV breast cancer with bone metastases. In addition, monthly pamidronate infusions were found to significantly decrease the incidence of osteolytic bone lesions in women with metastatic breast cancer. In men, pamidronate was found to inhibit the adhesion of prostate carcinoma cells to bone, and this suggests a potential prophylactic role for bisphosphonate drugs in patients who have other forms of cancer that are known to metastasize preferentially to the bone.

Zoledronic acid (ZOMETA) is also indicated for treatment of hypercalcemia of malignancy, and it has been found to reduce bone loss associated with cancer therapy. For example, zoledronic acid was shown to prevent bone loss and increase bone mineral density in patients with prostate cancer with cancer treatment-induced bone loss (see Rosen, 2004).

Parathyroid Hormone and Related Drugs

Human parathyroid hormone (PTH) is an 84-amino acid hormone secreted by the parathyroid gland (see previous text). **Teriparatide** (FORTEO) is a recombinant form of human PTH containing the 34 biologically active N-terminal amino acids of the hormone. The skeletal effects of teriparatide depend on the dose and frequency of systemic administration. Once-daily subcutaneous administration of teriparatide stimulates new bone formation on trabecular and cortical bone surfaces by preferentially stimulating osteoblastic activity more than osteoclastic activity. In human studies, teriparatide increased markers of bone formation, skeletal mass, and bone strength. In contrast, continuous exposure to excessive amounts of PTH as occurs in hyperparathyroidism can stimulate bone resorption more than bone formation and have a detrimental effect on the skeleton.

Clinical trials of teriparatide in postmenopausal women and hypogonadal men with osteoporosis found that the drug increased vertebral and femoral neck bone mineral density, while reducing the risk of vertebral and nonvertebral fractures. Teriparatide is indicated for the treatment of **postmenopausal women** with osteoporosis who are at **high risk for bone fracture.** These include women with a history of osteoporotic fracture, women who have multiple risk factors for fracture, and women who are intolerant of other therapy. Teriparatide is also indicated to increase bone mass in **hypogonadal men** who are at high risk for fracture, such as those having gonadotropin-releasing hormone therapy for prostate cancer.

Teriparatide caused an increase in the incidence of **osteosarcoma** in rats and should not be prescribed for persons who are at increased risk of osteosarcoma, including those with Paget's disease of bone and those with unexplained elevations of serum alkaline phosphatase (a marker of bone turnover).

Cinacalcet (SENSIPAR) has been approved for treatment of hyperparathyroidism in adult patients with chronic kidney disease who are on dialysis, and for treatment of hypercalcemia in patients with parathyroid cancer. The drug acts to increase the sensitivity of calcium-sensing receptors in the parathyroid gland to extracellular calcium, leading to decreased secretion of PTH and lowering of serum calcium levels. It appears to be safe and effective for these conditions.

Other Agents for Calcium and Bone Disorders

Estrogen and Raloxifene

Estrogen is no longer considered a first-line therapy for the prevention of **osteoporosis** in postmenopausal women because of concerns about the increased risk of breast cancer and thromboembolic disease in women having hormone (estrogen) replacement therapy. The current consensus is that estrogen therapy for prevention of osteoporotic fractures should be restricted to women with menopausal symptoms, and to older women who are intolerant of other therapies and express a strong preference for estrogen treatment, despite being informed about potential adverse effects.

Estrogen reduces bone resorption by regulating various bone cell cytokines. Estrogen inhibits the production of interleukin-1, tumor necrosis factor, and granulocyte-macrophage colony-stimulating factor by peripheral blood monocytes, and the secretion of interleukin-6 and colony-stimulating factors by osteoblasts. These actions lead to a decrease in osteoclast differentiation and activation, which in turn slows the bone loss that occurs in postmenopausal women. The mechanisms by which estrogen exerts its beneficial effects remain a major area of research in the development of novel therapies for osteoporosis.

Raloxifene (EVISTA) is a **selective estrogen receptor modulator** (SERM) that mimics the effects of estrogen on bone but does not increase the risk of breast cancer or thromboembolic events. Raloxifene has been shown to increase bone mineral density in postmenopausal women and to lower the incidence of **vertebral fractures** in women with osteoporosis. Although raloxifene activates estrogen receptors in bone, it has antiestrogen effects in other tissues and can cause or intensify **hot flashes** and other symptoms of estrogen withdrawal in menopausal women. Estrogen preparations and raloxifene are discussed in greater detail in Chapter 34.

Calcitonin

CHEMISTRY AND PHARMACOKINETICS. Calcitonin is a peptide hormone secreted by the parafollicular cells of the thyroid gland. It is not reliably absorbed from the gut and must be administered parenterally or by nasal inhalation. **Salmon calcitonin** has been available for a number of years, and **recombinant human calcitonin** is also available. Salmon calcitonin is 50 to 100 times more potent than human calcitonin.

MECHANISMS AND EFFECTS. Calcitonin binds directly to receptors on osteoclasts and increases cyclic adenosine monophosphate (cAMP) levels. When given on a short-term basis, calcitonin inhibits osteoclast activity, decreases bone resorption, lowers serum calcium concentrations, and reduces bone pain. When given on a long-term basis, calcitonin also reduces the number of osteoclasts and decreases bone formation. The long-term effects of calcitonin on bone mass are uncertain.

INDICATIONS. Because of its ability to inhibit osteoclast activity and decrease bone turnover, calcitonin is used to treat **osteoporosis, Paget's disease of bone,** and **hypercalcemia.**

In patients with osteoporosis, calcitonin treatment has been shown to increase bone mass at multiple sites in the body during a period of up to 2 years, but some uncertainty exists about whether these changes are maintained over longer periods of time. Calcitonin treatment is usually reserved for women who cannot take estrogen and have been in menopause for more than 5 years. In these women, studies indicate that calcitonin increases the bone mineral density (BMD) in the spine but has variable effects on the BMD in the hips. Patients with osteoporosis can be treated with either subcutaneous or intranasal calcitonin. In those who have had fractures, treatment in the immediate postfracture period appears to be particularly useful because of the drug's analgesic effect. Patients taking calcitonin should be advised of the importance of adequate calcium and vitamin D intake.

In patients with Paget's disease, calcitonin is administered subcutaneously or intramuscularly every 1 to 3 days. The nasal spray is not used. When treatment inhibits osteoclast activity and slows the rate of bone turnover, this causes reductions in markers of abnormal bone turnover, such as serum alkaline phosphatase activity and urine hydroxyproline levels. Alleviation of bone pain usually occurs 2 to 8 weeks after calcitonin therapy has begun.

Hypercalcemia can be treated with subcutaneous or intramuscular injections of calcitonin. The injections are administered every 12 hours until a satisfactory response occurs.

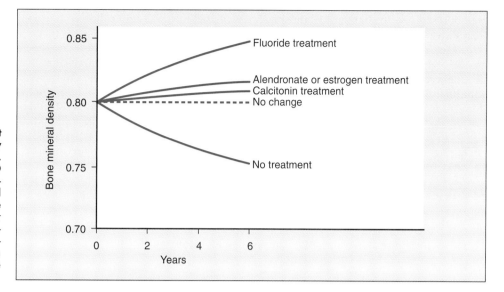

Figure 36–4. Effects of different treatments on bone mineral density (BMD) in postmenopausal women. In the absence of treatment, BMD steadily declines and may eventually reach the fracture threshold (0.70). Treatment with alendronate (a bisphosphonate), calcitonin, or estrogen can reduce bone resorption and increase BMD slightly. Fluoride increases bone formation and produces a greater and more sustained increase in BMD.

Fluoride

In some countries, fluoride is approved for the treatment of osteoporosis. In the USA, a sodium fluoride preparation is available but is approved only for the prevention of tooth decay. Fluoride is of considerable interest as a therapeutic agent for osteoporosis because it can stimulate new bone formation. All other substances currently used in the treatment of osteoporosis act by inhibiting bone resorption. Fig. 36–4 compares the effects that fluoride and other treatments have on BMD measurements over time.

MECHANISMS AND PHARMACOLOGIC EFFECTS. Fluoride, which is rapidly and almost completely absorbed from the gut, is primarily stored in bone and teeth. Fluoride replaces the hydroxyl group in the calcium phosphate salts (hydroxyapatite) of bone and teeth and thereby forms fluorapatite. Fluoride increases bone crystal size and decreases solubility to render bone more resistant to resorption. At the same time, fluoride prolongs the bone remodeling cycle by increasing the amount of time between new bone formation and subsequent mineralization. In this way, fluoride increases the BMD and can markedly increase bone mass.

INDICATIONS AND PHARMACOKINETICS. Fluoride is used to prevent **dental caries,** a condition in which localized destruction of calcified tissue on the tooth surface is followed by enzymatic lysis of organic material and by the subsequent development of cavities. Minerals deposited on the tooth surface as fluorapatite are more resistant to erosion than is hydroxyapatite.

Fluoride has been added to the drinking water supply in many localities as a method of caries prevention. It can also be administered orally as a liquid or chewable tablet, and it can be applied directly to the tooth surface as a dental gel or rinse. The oral liquid formulation (drops) is usually used to provide fluoride to infants and young children.

A sustained-release fluoride preparation is currently being evaluated by the US Food and Drug Administration for the treatment of **osteoporosis.** Monofluorophosphate products are also under development. The latter com-

pounds, which can be administered with calcium, may cause fewer adverse effects than other fluoride preparations.

ADVERSE EFFECTS. Sodium fluoride can cause considerable gastrointestinal distress, including nausea, vomiting, and bleeding. Skin rashes and arthralgia are also fairly common. These side effects can usually be prevented by using a lower dose or a sustained-release formulation and by taking the drug with food.

Excessive doses of fluoride can cause osteosclerosis (excessive hardness of bone) and mottling of tooth enamel.

Fluoride increases trabecular bone volume, but it can either decrease or have no effect on cortical bone volume. The use of lower doses and sustained-release fluoride products, along with the ingestion of sufficient calcium and vitamin D, may prevent the negative effect on cortical bone.

The type of bone formed in the presence of fluoride is more resistant to compressive forces but less resistant to torsional strain. Compressive strain tends to cause vertebral fractures, whereas torsional strain causes hip fractures. These factors probably explain why fluoride reduces vertebral fractures but can increase fractures at other sites. Intermittent fluoride regimens with a 2-month, drug-free interval may decrease some of the problems associated with continuous fluoride therapy.

INTERACTIONS. Fluoride forms a complex with calcium and magnesium and thereby reduces the absorption of these cations. Hence, calcium and magnesium supplements or antacids should not be taken at the same time as fluoride. Adequate calcium and vitamin D intake is essential in persons taking fluoride, however, because studies have shown that the use of fluoride without calcium supplementation can lead to osteomalacia.

Plicamycin

Plicamycin is a cytotoxic antibiotic that is a potent osteoclast inhibitor and may block the action of PTH. Plicamycin inhibits bone resorption and is used to treat **hypercalcemia** and **hypercalciuria** that are caused by malignant tumors and are not responsive to conventional therapy. It is also used to treat **Paget's disease of bone.**

Plicamycin is administered by intravenous infusion and causes numerous adverse effects, including myelosuppression, coagulation disorders, and frequent nausea and vomiting.

THE MANAGEMENT OF CALCIUM AND BONE DISORDERS

Osteoporosis

The prevention of osteoporosis rests on a foundation of lifelong calcium and vitamin D intake in an amount that is sufficient to maximize bone formation during development and to sustain bone mass during adulthood. Weight-bearing exercise reduces bone loss and helps improve strength and balance. Endogenous estrogen in women and testosterone in men also reduce bone resorption. After menopause, the absence of estrogen accelerates bone loss in women. Although all postmenopausal women are at risk of developing osteoporosis, BMD measurements are being used increasingly to identify those who are at greatest risk.

In most postmenopausal women, osteoporosis can be prevented by ensuring an adequate intake of calcium and vitamin D, exercising, and taking either estrogen replacement therapy or raloxifene. Other agents can be used in women who exhibit decreased or accelerated BMD measurements, women who have had fractures or other signs of osteoporosis, and women who are at an increased risk of developing osteoporosis because they require chronic corticosteroid therapy or because they had natural or surgical menopause at an early age. In these groups of women, alendronate can be used in place of or in addition to estrogen. Alendronate is a particularly attractive drug because it can be taken orally, is efficacious, and has a low incidence of adverse effects. Moreover, clinical trials comparing alendronate and calcitonin showed that only alendronate produced a sustained increase in bone mass in postmenopausal women with evidence of osteoporosis. The introduction of new fluoride preparations is anticipated and may provide another therapeutic modality for the prevention and treatment of osteoporosis.

Paget's Disease of Bone

The goals of treating patients with Paget's disease are to control bone pain and to prevent progressive bone deformity and other manifestations of the disease. Calcitonin is usually the first-line treatment, and it can be given alone or in combination with a bisphosphonate such as alendronate, pamidronate, or tiludronate. Alternatively, a bisphosphonate can be used alone. Plicamycin is reserved for the treatment of patients who fail to respond to other drugs.

Hypercalcemia

The treatment of hypercalcemia depends on the etiology and severity of the condition. The major causes of hypercalcemia are hyperparathyroidism and cancer.

Saline diuresis is usually the preferred method of managing hypercalcemia that is severe enough to cause symptoms. A saline infusion is used for this purpose, which serves to increase renal calcium excretion and to counteract the dehydration that often accompanies hypercalcemia. A loop diuretic (e.g., furosemide) can be added to the saline infusion, and this will further enhance calcium excretion.

Pamidronate and other bisphosphonates are useful in the treatment of hypercalcemia associated with cancer. Calcitonin is usually used to supplement other treatments for hypercalcemia, and plicamycin is useful if other therapeutic agents and procedures fail. As a last resort, intravenous phosphate infusions can be used to control hypercalcemia, but these infusions place the patient at considerable risk for acute hypocalcemia, hypotension, renal failure, and tissue calcification.

SUMMARY OF IMPORTANT POINTS

■ The extracellular calcium concentration is regulated by vitamin D, parathyroid hormone (PTH), and calcitonin. Vitamin D increases calcium absorption from the gut; PTH increases calcium reabsorption from renal tubules and increases bone resorption; and calcitonin decreases bone resorption.

■ Vitamin D is converted to its most active form, 1,25-dihydroxyvitamin D_3 (calcitriol), by hydroxylation in the liver and kidneys. This active form must be supplied to patients with renal impairment. Dietary vitamin D is essential to prevent rickets in children.

■ Osteoporosis, the most common bone disorder, is characterized by a gradual loss of bone mass that leads to skeletal weakness and increased fractures.

■ In most postmenopausal women, osteoporosis can be prevented by ensuring an adequate intake of calcium and vitamin D, exercising, and taking either estrogen replacement therapy or raloxifene.

■ Osteoporosis can be treated with alendronate (a bisphosphonate), calcitonin, or fluoride (not yet approved for this indication in the USA). Alendronate reduces osteoclast activity and can increase bone mass and reduce fractures in postmenopausal women. It is taken orally and is effective and well tolerated.

■ In addition to alendronate, the bisphosphonate compounds include pamidronate and tiludronate. These agents are used to treat Paget's disease of bone, hypercalcemia, and osteolytic bone lesions associated with cancer.

■ Calcitonin is also used to treat Paget's disease and hypercalcemia.

Review Questions

For each numbered drug description, select the corresponding drug from the lettered choices.

1. This drug reduces vertebral fractures in postmenopausal women with osteoporosis but can increase the severity of hot flashes.

2. This drug is only used to prevent bone loss and counteract hypercalcemia in persons with malignant diseases.

3. This drug is a recombinant hormone that acts to preferentially increase osteoblastic activity; it is used to prevent fractures in men and women at high risk of osteoporotic fractures.

4. This drug adsorbs to hydroxyapatite and inhibits osteoclastic activity; it is used for prevention of osteoporosis.

5. This drug is administered subcutaneously for the treatment of Paget's disease of bone.

(A) zoledronic acid
(B) teriparatide
(C) calcitonin
(D) risedronate
(E) raloxifene

Answers and Explanations

1. The answer is E: raloxifene. Raloxifene stimulates estrogen receptors in bone and is reduces osteoporotic fractures. It acts as an estrogen antagonist in breast and other tissues and can increase the incidence and severity of estrogen withdrawal symptoms such as hot flashes.

2. The answer is A: zoledronic acid. Zoledronic acid is a newer bisphosphonate drug that prevents bone loss and reduces hypercalcemia in persons with malignancies.

3. The answer is B: teriparatide. Teriparatide is a recombinant form of human parathyroid hormone. When administered as a single daily dose, it acts to preferentially increase osteoblastic activity and bone mass while reducing fractures. It is indicated for treating persons at high risk of osteoporotic fractures.

4. The answer is D: risedronate. Risedronate and alendronate are bisphosphonate drugs used to prevent and treat osteoporosis. These drugs bind to hydroxyapatite in bone and reduce osteoclastic activity, leading to increased bone mineral density and reduced fractures.

5. The answer is C: calcitonin. Calcitonin is a hormone that inhibits osteoclastic activity and decreases bone resorption and bone turnover. It is usually considered the primary treatment for persons with Paget's disease of bone.

SELECTED READINGS

Badenhop-Stevens, N., and V. Matkovic. Calcium needs in children. Orthoped Nurs 4:228–232, 2004.

Quattrocchi, E., and H. Kourlas. Teriparatide: a review. Clin Ther 26:841–854, 2004.

Rodan, G., A. Reszka, E. Golub, et al. Bone safety of long-term bisphosphonate treatment. Curr Med Res Opin 20:1291–1300, 2004.

Rosen, L. S. New generation of bisphosphonates: broad clinical utility in breast and prostate cancer. Oncology (Huntingt) 18(5 Suppl 3):26–32, 2004.

Saag, K. G. Prevention of glucocorticoid-induced osteoporosis. South Med J 97:555–558, 2004.

Zizic, T. M. Pharmacologic prevention of osteoporotic fractures. Am Fam Physician 70:1219–1220, 2004.

CHEMOTHERAPY

CHAPTER 37

Principles of Antimicrobial Chemotherapy

ANTIBIOTICS AND CHEMOTHERAPY

Overview

Chemotherapy can be defined as the use of drugs to eradicate pathogenic organisms or neoplastic cells in the treatment of infectious diseases or cancer. Chemotherapy is based on the principle of **selective toxicity.** According to this principle, chemotherapeutic drugs inhibit functions in invading organisms or neoplastic cells that differ qualitatively or quantitatively from functions in normal host cells. The chemotherapeutic drugs include antimicrobial drugs (introduced in this chapter and discussed further in Chapters 38 through 43), antiparasitic drugs (discussed in Chapter 44), and antineoplastic drugs (discussed in Chapter 45).

The **antimicrobial drugs** can be subclassified as **antibacterial, antifungal, and antiviral agents.** These agents include natural compounds, called antibiotics, as well as synthetic compounds produced in laboratories. An **antibiotic** is a substance that is produced by one microbe and inhibits the growth or viability of other microbes. The earliest use of antibiotics was probably in the treatment of skin infections with **moldy bean curd** by the ancient Chinese. The development of modern antibiotics can be traced to the work of **Louis Pasteur,** who observed that the in vitro growth of one microbe was inhibited when another microbe was added to the culture. Pasteur called this phenomenon **antibiosis** and predicted that substances derived from microbes would someday be used to treat infectious diseases.

Several decades later, **Alexander Fleming** observed that the growth of his staphylococcal cultures was inhibited by a *Penicillium* contaminant. Fleming postulated that the fungus produced a substance, which he called **penicillin,** and that this substance inhibited the growth of staphylococci. His observations eventually led to the isolation and use of penicillin for treating bacterial infections. The discovery of penicillin stimulated the discovery and development of a large number of other antibiotics, the use of which has revolutionized the treatment of infectious diseases.

Synthetic drugs have also provided major advances in the treatment of infectious diseases and cancer. During the Renaissance, **Paracelsus** used **mercury compounds** for the treatment of syphilis. In the late 19th and early 20th centuries, **Paul Ehrlich** pioneered the search for selectively toxic compounds. After many failed attempts, he discovered **arsphenamine (Salvarsan),** an arsenical compound for the treatment of syphilis. Ehrlich, who became known as the father of chemotherapy, also studied bacterial stains as potential antimicrobial agents. He reasoned that a stain's selective affinity for bacteria could be coupled with an inhibitory action to halt microbial metabolism and thereby destroy invading organisms. This concept led to the discovery of **sulfonamides,** drugs that were originally derived from a bacterial stain called **Prontosil.** The sulfonamides were the first effective drugs for the treatment of systemic bacterial infections, and their development accelerated the search for other antimicrobial agents.

Classification of Antimicrobial Drugs

Antimicrobial drugs are usually classified on the basis of their site and mechanism of action and are subclassified on the basis of their chemical structure. The antimicrobial drugs include **cell wall synthesis inhibitors, protein synthesis inhibitors, metabolic and nucleic acid inhibitors,** and **cell membrane inhibitors.** The sites of action of these drugs are depicted in Fig. 37–1, and their mechanisms of action, pharmacologic properties, and clinical uses are described in subsequent chapters.

ANTIMICROBIAL ACTIVITY

The antimicrobial activity of a drug can be characterized in terms of its bactericidal or bacteriostatic effect, its spectrum of activity against important groups of pathogens, and its concentration- and time-dependent effects on sensitive organisms.

Bactericidal or Bacteriostatic Effect

A **bactericidal drug** kills sensitive organisms so that the number of viable organisms falls rapidly after exposure to the drug (Fig. 37–2). In contrast, a **bacteriostatic drug** inhibits the growth of bacteria but does not kill them. For

Figure 37-1. Sites of action of antimicrobial drugs. Antimicrobial drugs include cell wall synthesis inhibitors, protein synthesis inhibitors, metabolic and nucleic acid inhibitors (e.g., inhibitors of folate synthesis, DNA gyrase, and RNA polymerase), and cell membrane inhibitors.

Figure 37-2. In vitro effects of bactericidal and bacteriostatic drugs. In the absence of an antimicrobial drug, bacteria exhibit logarithmic growth in a broth culture. The addition of a bacteriostatic drug (tetracycline) inhibits further growth but does not reduce the number of bacteria. The addition of a bactericidal drug (penicillin) reduces the number of viable bacteria.

this reason, the number of bacteria remains relatively constant in the presence of a bacteriostatic drug, and immunologic mechanisms are required to eliminate organisms during treatment of an infection with this type of drug. (The same principle applies to a drug that kills or inhibits the growth of fungi and is referred to as a **fungicidal drug** or a **fungistatic drug,** respectively.)

A bactericidal drug is usually preferable to a bacteriostatic drug for the treatment of most bacterial infections. This is because bactericidal drugs usually produce more rapid microbiologic response and clinical improvement and are less likely to elicit microbial resistance. Bactericidal drugs have actions that induce lethal changes in microbial metabolism or block activities that are essential for microbial viability. For example, drugs that inhibit the synthesis of the bacterial cell wall (e.g., **penicillins**) prevent the formation of a structure that is required for the survival of bacteria. At the same time, penicillins activate autolytic enzymes that destroy bacteria. In contrast to bactericidal drugs, bacteriostatic drugs usually inhibit a metabolic reaction that is needed for bacterial growth but is not necessary for cell viability. For example, **sulfonamides** block the synthesis of folic acid, which is a cofactor for enzymes that synthesize DNA components and amino acids.

Drugs that reversibly inhibit bacterial protein synthesis (e.g., **tetracyclines**) are also bacteriostatic, whereas drugs that irreversibly inhibit protein synthesis (e.g., **streptomycin**) are usually bactericidal.

Some drugs can be either bactericidal or bacteriostatic, depending on their concentration and the bacterial species against which they are used.

Antimicrobial Spectrum

The spectrum of antimicrobial activity of a drug is the primary determinant of its clinical use. Antimicrobial agents that are active against a single species or a limited group of pathogens (e.g., gram-positive bacteria) are called **narrow-spectrum drugs,** whereas agents that are active against a wide range of pathogens are called **broad-spectrum drugs.** Agents that have an intermediate range of activity are sometimes called **extended-spectrum drugs.**

If the specific pathogen that is responsible for an infection is known, a narrow-spectrum drug is the logical choice to treat the infection. This is because a broad-spectrum drug is more likely to cause superinfection by eradicating organisms that make up the normal flora of the gut or respiratory tract. In cases in which an infection is serious and the responsible pathogen is not yet known, however, a broad-spectrum bactericidal drug (e.g., imipenem) is often used for initial treatment.

Concentration- and Time-Dependent Effects

Antimicrobial drugs exhibit various concentration- and time-dependent effects that influence their clinical efficacy, dosage, and frequency of administration. Examples of these effects are the **minimal inhibitory concentration** (MIC), the

concentration-dependent killing rate (CDKR), and the **postantibiotic effect** (PAE).

The MIC is the lowest concentration of a drug that inhibits bacterial growth. Based on the MIC, a particular strain of bacteria can be classified as susceptible or resistant to a particular drug (see below).

An example of a CDKR is shown in Fig. 37–3A. Some **aminoglycosides** (e.g., tobramycin) and some **fluoro-**

Figure 37-3. Concentration- and time-dependent effects of antimicrobial drugs. **(A)** When an aminoglycoside (e.g., tobramycin) is added to a culture of a gram-negative bacterium (e.g., *Escherichia coli*) it will exhibit a concentration-dependent killing rate. In this example, 10^6 bacteria were incubated with different concentrations of tobramycin, ranging from one to four times the minimal inhibitory concentration (MIC). **(B)** When tobramycin is removed from the culture, bacterial growth continues to be inhibited for several hours.

quinolones (e.g., ciprofloxacin) exhibit a CDKR against a large group of gram-negative bacteria, including *Pseudomonas aeruginosa* and members of the family Enterobacteriaceae. In contrast, **penicillins and other beta-lactam antibiotics** usually do not exhibit a CDKR.

After an antibacterial drug is removed from a bacterial culture, evidence of a persistent effect on bacterial growth may exist. This effect (see Fig. 37–3B) is called the PAE. Most bactericidal antibiotics exhibit a PAE against susceptible pathogens. For example, penicillins show a PAE against gram-positive cocci, and aminoglycosides show a PAE against gram-negative bacilli. Because aminoglycosides exhibit both a CDKR and a PAE, treatment regimens have been developed in which the entire daily dose of an aminoglycoside is given at one time. Theoretically, the high rate of bacterial killing produced by these regimens would more rapidly eliminate bacteria, and the PAE would prevent any remaining bacteria from replicating for several hours after the drug has been eliminated from the body.

MICROBIAL SENSITIVITY AND RESISTANCE

Laboratory Tests for Microbial Sensitivity

Microbial sensitivity to drugs can be determined by various means, including the **broth dilution test,** the **disk diffusion method (Kirby-Bauer test),** and the **Etest method.** These laboratory procedures are described in Box 37–1.

Either the broth dilution test or the Etest method can be used to determine the MIC of a drug, which is the lowest drug concentration that prevents visible growth of bacteria. On the basis of the MIC, the organism is classified as having **susceptibility, intermediate sensitivity,** or **resistance** to the drug tested. These categories are based on the relationship between the MIC and the peak serum concentration of the drug after administration of typical doses. In general, the peak serum concentration of a drug should be 4 to 10 times greater than the MIC in order for a pathogen to be susceptible to a drug (see below). Pathogens with intermediate sensitivity may respond to treatment with maximal doses of an antimicrobial drug.

Microbial Resistance to Drugs

Origin of Resistance

Resistance can be innate or acquired. Acquired drug resistance arises from mutation and selection or from the transfer of plasmids that confer drug resistance.

MUTATION AND SELECTION. Microbes can spontaneously mutate to a form that is resistant to a particular antimicrobial drug. These mutations occur at a relatively constant rate, such as 1 in 10^{12} organisms per unit of time. If the organisms are exposed to an antimicrobial drug during this time

---

BOX 37–1. LABORATORY DETERMINATION OF MICROBIAL SENSITIVITY TO ANTIBIOTICS

Microbial sensitivity to drugs can be determined by various means, including the broth dilution test, the disk diffusion method, and the Etest method.

Broth Dilution Test

Tubes that contain a nutrient broth are inoculated with equal numbers of bacteria and serially diluted concentrations of an antibiotic. After incubation, the minimal inhibitory concentration (MIC) is identified as the lowest antibiotic concentration that prevents visible growth of bacteria. On the basis of the MIC, the organism is classified as having susceptibility, intermediate sensitivity, or resistance to the drug tested. In the following example, the MIC is 1 μg/mL, and the organism is susceptible to the drug.

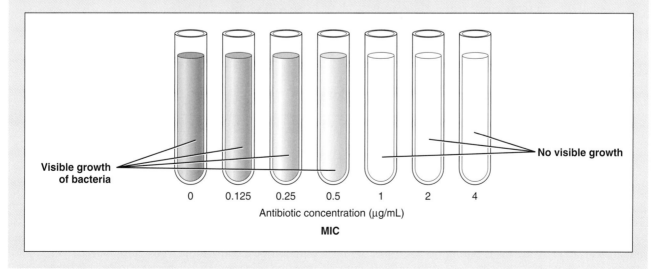

Visible growth of bacteria — No visible growth

0   0.125   0.25   0.5   1   2   4

Antibiotic concentration (μg/mL)

MIC

Continued

BOX 37–1. LABORATORY DETERMINATION OF MICROBIAL SENSITIVITY TO ANTIBIOTICS—cont'd

Disk Diffusion Method (Kirby-Bauer Test)

Each disk used in the disk diffusion method is impregnated with a different antibiotic. The disks are placed on agar plates seeded with the test organism. During the incubation period, the antibiotic diffuses from the disk and inhibits bacterial growth. After incubation, the zone inhibited by each antibiotic is measured. The zone diameter for each antibiotic is compared with standard values for that particular antibiotic. The organism is thereby determined to be susceptible, intermediate, or resistant to the various antibiotics tested.

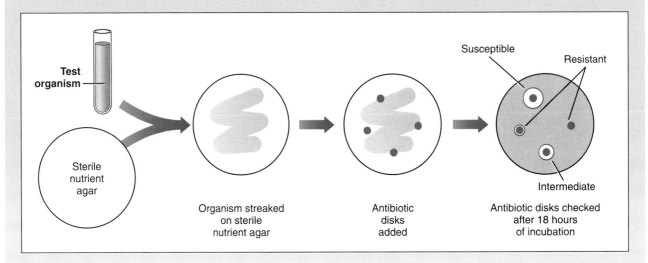

Etest Method

The Etest strip is a proprietary device that uses a diffusion method to determine the MIC of an organism. The device is a plastic strip that is impregnated with a gradient of antibiotic concentrations. After the strip is placed on an agar culture of the organism, the culture is incubated. During incubation, a tear-shaped zone of inhibition is formed. The point of intersection between the zone of inhibition and the scale displayed on the strip is the MIC. In the following example, the MIC is 0.125 μg/mL.

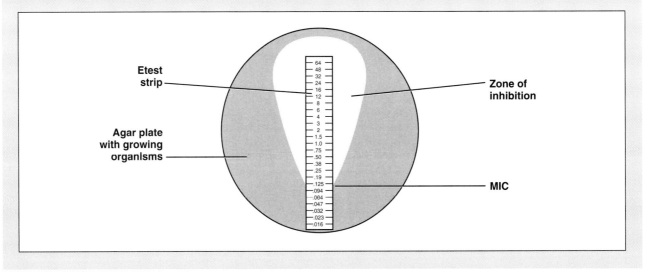

period, the sensitive organisms may be eradicated, enabling the resistant mutant to multiply and become the dominant strain (Fig. 37–4A).

The probability that mutation and selection of a resistant mutant will occur is increased during the exposure of an organism to suboptimal concentrations of an antibiotic, and it is also increased during prolonged exposure to an antibiotic. This observation has obvious implications for antimicrobial therapy. Laboratory tests should be used to guide the selection of an antimicrobial drug, and the dosage and duration of therapy should be appropriate for the type of infection being treated. Whenever possible, the bacteriologic

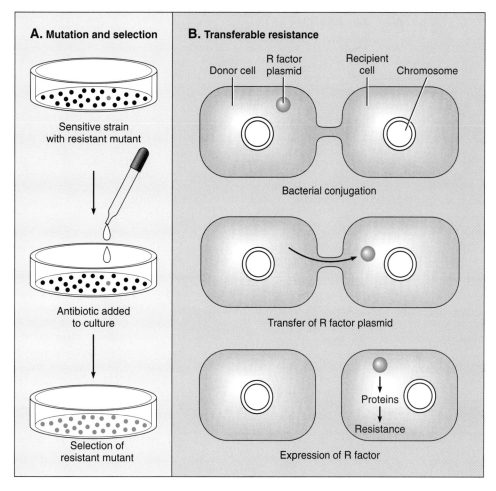

Figure 37–4. Acquired resistance to antimicrobial drugs can arise by mutation and selection or by transferable resistance. (A) Exposure of an organism to an antibiotic can result in the selection of a resistant mutant. (B) The most common mechanism of transferable resistance is bacterial conjugation and exchange of plasmids containing resistance factors (R factors).

response to drug therapy should be verified by culturing samples of appropriate body fluids.

TRANSFERABLE RESISTANCE. Transferable resistance usually results from bacterial conjugation and the transfer of plasmids (extrachromosomal DNA) that confer drug resistance (see Fig. 37–4B). Transferable resistance, however, can also be mediated by transformation (uptake of naked DNA) or transduction (transfer of bacterial DNA by a bacteriophage). Bacterial conjugation enables a bacterium to donate a plasmid containing genes that encode proteins responsible for resistance to an antibiotic. These genes are called **resistance factors (R factors)**. The R factors can be transferred both within a particular species and also between different species, so they often confer **multidrug resistance.** The various species need not all be present during the period in which the antibiotic is administered. Studies have shown that resident microflora of the human body can serve as reservoirs for resistance genes, allowing the transfer of these genes to organisms that later invade and colonize the host.

Several genes responsible for drug resistance have been cloned, and the factors that control their expression are being studied. In the future, drugs that block the expression of these genes may find use as adjunct therapy for infectious diseases. For example, it may be possible to develop antisense nucleotides that block the transcription or translation of genes that encode proteins responsible for drug resistance.

Mechanisms of Resistance

The three primary mechanisms of microbial resistance to an antibiotic are (1) inactivation of the drug by microbial enzymes, (2) decreased accumulation of the drug by the microbe, and (3) reduced affinity of the target macromolecule for the drug. Examples of drugs affected by these mechanisms are provided in Table 37–1.

Inactivation of the drug by enzymes is an important mechanism of resistance to β-lactam antibiotics, including the penicillins. This form of resistance results from bacterial elaboration of β-lactamase enzymes that destroy the β-lactam ring. Resistance to aminoglycosides (e.g., gentamicin) is partly caused by the elaboration of drug-inactivating enzymes that acetylate, adenylate, or phosphorylate these antibiotics.

Decreased accumulation of an antibiotic can result from **increased efflux** or **decreased uptake** of the drug. Both of these mechanisms contribute to the resistance of microbes to tetracyclines and fluoroquinolones. Increased drug efflux is often mediated by membrane proteins that transport antimicrobial drugs out of bacterial cells. Some of these

Table 37-1. **Mechanisms of Microbial Resistance**

Mechanism	Examples
Inactivation of the drug by microbial enzymes	Inactivation of aminoglycosides by acetylase, adenylase, and phosphorylase enzymes Inactivation of penicillins and other β-lactam antibiotics by β-lactamase enzymes
Decreased accumulation of the drug by the microbe	Decreased uptake of β-lactam antibiotics due to altered porins in gram-negative bacteria Decreased uptake and increased efflux of fluoroquinolones Decreaed uptake and increased efflux of tetracyclines
Reduced affinity of the target macromolecule for the drug	Reduced affinity of DNA gyrase for fluoroquinolones Reduced affinity of folate synthesis enzymes for sulfonamides and trimethoprim Reduced affinity of ribosomes for aminoglycosides, chloramphenicol, clindamycin, macrolides, or tetracyclines Reduced affinity of RNA polymerase for rifampin Reduced affinity of transpeptidase and other penicillin-binding proteins for penicillins and other β-lactam antibiotics

transport proteins are similar to or indistinguishable from human **P-glycoprotein,** a glycoprotein that transports antineoplastic drugs out of human cancer cells and thereby confers resistance to the drugs (see Chapter 45). Compounds that inhibit these transport proteins are being investigated as potential therapeutic agents to reduce drug resistance. Decreased uptake of antimicrobial drugs can result from altered bacterial **porins.** Porins are membrane proteins containing channels through which drugs and other compounds enter bacteria. Resistance to penicillins by gram-negative bacilli is partly caused by altered porin channels that do not permit penicillin entry.

Reduced affinity of target macromolecules for antimicrobial drugs is a common mechanism of drug resistance. It is partly responsible for resistance to cell wall synthesis inhibitors, protein synthesis inhibitors, DNA gyrase inhibitors, and RNA polymerase inhibitors (see Table 37–1). This type of drug resistance often results because of bacterial mutation followed by the selection of resistant mutants during exposure to an antimicrobial drug. Altered target affinity has been the most difficult form of drug resistance to counteract by pharmacologic agents.

SELECTION OF ANTIMICROBIAL DRUGS

The selection of an antimicrobial agent for the treatment of a particular infection is based on the type of infection, the status of the patient, and the pharmacologic properties of the available drugs.

Host Factors

Host factors that influence the choice of a drug include pregnancy, drug allergies, age and immune status, and the presence of renal impairment, hepatic insufficiency, abscesses, or indwelling catheters and similar devices.

Most antimicrobial drugs cross the placenta and can thereby affect the fetus. For example, administering tetracyclines to a woman during **pregnancy** can cause permanent staining of her offspring's teeth. Penicillins and cephalosporins, however, cause very little fetal toxicity and can be safely administered to pregnant women who are not allergic to these drugs.

Many individuals are allergic to one or more antimicrobial drugs. Penicillins are the most common cause of drug allergy (see Chapter 38).

The patient's **immune status** is an important factor determining the success of antimicrobial therapy. **Advanced age, diabetes, cancer chemotherapy,** and **human immunodeficiency virus (HIV) infection** are among the more common causes of impaired immunity. Immunocompromised individuals should be treated with larger doses of bactericidal drugs and may require a longer duration of therapy than do immunocompetent individuals.

Antibiotic access to **abscesses** is poor, so the concentration of an antibiotic in an abscess is usually lower than normal. Moreover, immune responses to abscesses are impaired. For these reasons, abscesses must be surgically drained before they can be cured.

Foreign bodies, such as **indwelling catheters,** provide sites where microbes can become covered with a glycocalyx coating that protects them from antibiotics and immunologic destruction.

Many antibiotics are excreted unchanged by the kidneys, and lower doses must be used if the patient has significant **renal impairment.** Less commonly, **hepatic insufficiency** may require dosage adjustment for antimicrobial drugs that are extensively metabolized in the liver. For example, neonates cannot metabolize chloramphenicol, so their dosage of this drug per kilogram of body weight must be lower than the dosage given to older children or adults.

Antimicrobial Activity

Antimicrobial agents can be selected on the basis of laboratory test results (described earlier) or knowledge of the most common organisms causing various types of infections and the drugs of choice for these organisms (empiric considerations). Empiric therapy is often used initially to treat serious infections until test results are available. Empiric therapy is also used to treat minor upper respiratory tract infections and urinary tract infections because of the predictability of causative organisms and their sensitivity to drugs. In these situations, the cost of microbial culture and drug sensitivity testing is not usually justified.

The current drugs of choice for the treatment of infections caused by specific bacterial pathogens are listed in Table 37–2.

TABLE 37-2. **Antimicrobial Drugs Most Often Used for the Treatment of Infections Caused by Selected Bacteria**

Bacteria	Antimicrobial Drugs
Gram-positive cocci	
Enterococcus species	Penicillin G or ampicillin plus gentamicin; vancomycin plus gentamicin; quinupristin + dalfopristin, linezolid, daptomycin
Staphylococcus aureus	Penicillin G (if sensitive), nafcillin, oxacillin, vancomycin, quinupristin + dalfopristin, linezolid, daptomycin
Streptococcus pyogenes	Penicillin G or V, a cephalosporin, a macrolide, clindamycin
Viridans group streptococci	Penicillin G + gentamicin; vancomycin
Streptococcus pneumoniae	Penicillin G (if sensitive), a cephalosporin II or III, amoxicillin + clavulanate, an advanced fluoroquinolone, azithromycin, telithromycin
Gram-positive bacilli	
Bacillus anthracis (anthrax)	Ciprofloxacin ± clindamycin and rifampin; doxycycline
Clostridium difficile (diarrhea, pseudomembranous colitis)	Metronidazole, oral vancomycin
Clostridium perfringens, C. tetani	Penicillin G
Corynebacterium diphtheriae	A macrolide, penicillin G
Listeria monocytogenes	Ampicillin, gentamicin
Gram-negative cocci	
Moraxella catarrhalis	Amoxicillin + clavulanate, a cephalosporin II or III, a macrolide
Neisseria gonorrhoeae	Ceftriaxone, spectinomycin, a fluoroquinolone
Neisseria meningitides	Penicillin G, a cephalosporin II or III, chloramphenicol
Gram-negative bacilli	
Bacteroides species (anaerobes)	Metronidazole, penicillin + β-lactamase inhibitor, clindamycin, chloramphenicol, penicillin G (oropharyngeal strains)
Bordetella pertussis (whooping cough)	A macrolide, trimethoprim-sulfamethoxazole
Helicobacter pylori (peptic ulcer disease)	Tetracycline, clarithromycin, amoxicillin, metronidazole, bismuth compounds, proton pump inhibitors
Haemophilus influenzae	Amoxicillin + clavulanate, a cephalosporin II or III, azithromycin, a fluoroquinolone
Pseudomonas aeruginosa	An aminoglycoside, ceftazidime, a fluoroquinolone, aztreonam, a carbapenem, piperacillin + tazobactam
Most *Enterobacteriaceae* (*E. coli*; *Klebsiella, Proteus, Serratia, Enterobacter, Citrobacter, Providencia* species and others)	A cephalosporin II or III, an aminoglycoside, piperacillin + tazobactam, a carbapenem, aztreonam, a fluoroquinolone, trimethoprim + sulfamethoxazole (urinary tract infections)
Salmonella and *Shigella* species, *Campylobacter jejuni* (bacterial diarrhea)	A fluoroquinolone, ceftriaxone (Salmonella), ampicillin + sulbactam (Shigella)
Yersinia pestis (plague); *Francisella tularensis* (tularemia)	Streptomycin, a tetracycline, chloramphenicol
Actinomycetes	
Nocardia asteroides, N. brasiliensis	Trimethoprim-sulfamethoxazole
Chlamydiae, Ehrlichia, Rickettsiae	
Spirochetes	A macrolide or a tetracycline antibiotic
Borrelia burgdorferi (Lyme disease)	Doxycycline, amoxicillin, a cephalosporin II or III
Borrelia recurrentis (relapsing fever)	A tetracycline, penicillin G
Treponema pallidum (syphilis, yaws)	Penicillin, a tetracycline

Pharmacokinetic Properties

The pharmacokinetic parameters of antibiotics that influence their selection for a particular use include their oral bioavailability, peak serum concentration, distribution to particular sites of infection, routes of elimination, and elimination half-life. An ideal antimicrobial drug for ambulatory patients would have good oral bioavailability and a long plasma half-life so that it would need to be taken only once or twice a day.

As described previously, the peak serum concentration of an antimicrobial drug should be several times greater than the MIC of the pathogenic organism for the drug to eliminate the organism. This is partly because the tissue concen-

trations of a drug are often lower than the plasma concentration. The relationship between the plasma concentration of a typical antimicrobial drug and the drug's MIC for several organisms is shown in Fig. 37–5. The urine concentration of an antimicrobial drug can be 10 to 50 times the peak serum concentration. For this reason, infections of the urinary tract can be easier to treat than are infections at other sites.

Sites of infection that are not readily penetrated by many antimicrobial drugs include the central nervous system, bone, prostate gland, and ocular tissues. The treatment of meningitis requires that drugs achieve adequate concentrations in the cerebrospinal fluid (CSF). Some antibiotics (e.g., penicillin G) penetrate the blood–CSF barrier when the meninges are inflamed, but the aminoglycosides do not. For

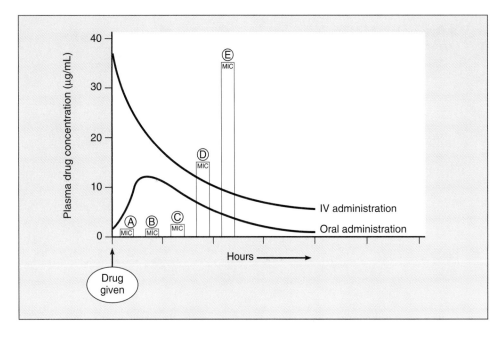

Figure 37–5. Relationship between the plasma concentration of a typical antimicrobial drug and the drug's minimal inhibitory concentration (MIC) for five bacterial organisms. The curves represent typical plasma concentrations over time after intravenous (IV) or oral administration of the drug. Each bar represents the MIC of a particular organism: *Streptococcus pneumoniae*, *Staphylococcus aureus*, and *Escherichia coli* (shown as A, B, and C, respectively, in this example) are susceptible to the drug; *Enterobacter* species (shown as D) are intermediate in sensitivity; and *Pseudomonas aeruginosa* (shown as E) is resistant.

this reason, aminoglycosides can be given intrathecally for the treatment of meningitis. Because antimicrobial drug concentrations are low in bone, patients with osteomyelitis must usually be treated with antibiotics for several weeks to produce a cure. The prostate gland restricts the entry of some antimicrobial drugs because the drugs have difficulty crossing the prostatic epithelium and because prostatic fluid has a low pH. These characteristics favor the entry and accumulation of weak bases (e.g., trimethoprim) and tend to exclude the entry of weak acids (e.g., penicillin).

The route of elimination affects both the selection and the use of antimicrobial drugs. Drugs that are eliminated by renal excretion are more effective for urinary tract infections than are drugs that are largely metabolized or undergo biliary excretion. Antibiotics that are eliminated by the kidneys (e.g., the aminoglycosides) can accumulate in patients whose renal function is compromised, however, so their dosage must be reduced in these patients.

Adverse Effect Profile

Any antimicrobial drug can cause mild to severe adverse effects, but the incidence of these effects varies greatly among different classes of drugs. For this reason, it is important to consider the probable risk-to-benefit ratio when selecting drugs for treatment. The β-lactam and macrolide antibiotics cause a relatively low incidence of organ system toxicity and are often used to treat minor infections, including infections in pregnant women. In contrast, the aminoglycosides cause a relatively high incidence of severe adverse effects and are usually reserved for the treatment of serious or life-threatening infections.

COMBINATION DRUG THERAPY

When antimicrobial drugs are given in combination, they can exhibit antagonistic, additive, synergistic, or indifferent effects against a particular microbe (Fig. 37–6). The relationship between two drugs and their combined effect is as follows: **antagonistic** if the combined effect is less than the effect of either drug alone; **additive** if the combined effect is equal to the sum of the independent effects; **synergistic** if the combined effect is greater than the sum of the independent effects; and **indifferent** if the combined effect is similar to the greatest effect produced by either drug alone.

Treatment of Infections Caused by a Single Species

Some bacteriostatic drugs (e.g., chloramphenicol or tetracycline) are antagonistic to bactericidal drugs. Bactericidal drugs are usually more effective against rapidly dividing bacteria, and their effect is reduced if bacterial growth is slowed by a bacteriostatic drug.

Most infections caused by a single microbial species are treated with a single drug. This is because monotherapy usually is less expensive, equally or more effective, and less toxic than is combination therapy. As discussed below, however, a few situations occur in which combination therapy is preferable.

If two bactericidal drugs that act by two different mechanisms are given in combination, they tend to exhibit additive or synergistic effects against susceptible bacteria (Table 37–3). For example, penicillins, which are cell wall synthesis inhibitors, often show additive or synergistic effects with aminoglycosides, which are protein synthesis inhibitors, when they are used in combination against a gram-negative bacillus such as *P. aeruginosa*. These drugs also show additive or synergistic effects against many enterococci and staphylococci.

A few antimicrobial agents exhibit synergistic activity against some or all of the bacteria that are sensitive to the drugs. For example, sulfamethoxazole and trimethoprim inhibit sequential steps in bacterial folate synthesis and

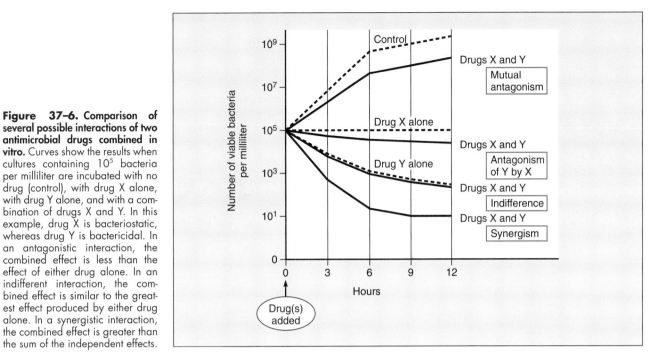

Figure 37–6. Comparison of several possible interactions of two antimicrobial drugs combined in vitro. Curves show the results when cultures containing 10^5 bacteria per milliliter are incubated with no drug (control), with drug X alone, with drug Y alone, and with a combination of drugs X and Y. In this example, drug X is bacteriostatic, whereas drug Y is bactericidal. In an antagonistic interaction, the combined effect is less than the effect of either drug alone. In an indifferent interaction, the combined effect is similar to the greatest effect produced by either drug alone. In a synergistic interaction, the combined effect is greater than the sum of the independent effects.

TABLE 37–3 · **In Vitro Activity of Antimicrobial Drug Combinations**

Synergistic combinations
- Aminoglycoside plus ampicillin used against enterococci
- Aminoglycoside plus penicillin G used against enterococci
- Aminoglycoside plus broad-spectrum penicillin used against gram-negative bacilli
- Aminoglycoside plus cephalosporin used against gram-negative bacilli
- Amphotericin B plus flucytosine used against *Cryptococcus neoformans*
- Antistaphylococcal penicillin plus aminoglycoside used against staphylococci
- Antistaphylococcal penicillin plus rifampin used against staphylococci
- Reverse transcriptase inhibitor plus protease inhibitor used against human immunodeficiency virus

Antagonistic combinations
- Aminoglycoside plus chloramphenicol used against members of the family Enterobacteriaceae
- Broad-spectrum penicillin plus chloramphenicol used against *Streptococcus pneumoniae*
- Broad-spectrum penicillin plus imipenem used against gram-negative bacilli

exhibit synergistic activity against many strains of organisms that are resistant to either drug alone.

Treatment of Mixed Infections

Mixed infections (i.e., infections caused by more than one microbial species) are usually treated with more than one drug. For example, an intra-abdominal infection can be caused by the combination of an aerobic gram-negative bacillus and an anaerobic gram-negative bacillus, such as *Escherichia coli* and *Bacteroides fragilis,* respectively. This type of infection can be treated with an aminoglycoside (active against aerobic bacilli) plus either metronidazole or clindamycin (active against anaerobic bacilli). Urethritis caused by a mixed infection with *Neisseria gonorrhoeae* and *Chlamydia trachomatis* can be treated with a cephalosporin such as ceftriaxone (active against gonococci) plus a tetracycline (active against chlamydiae).

Empiric Treatment of Serious Infections

More than one antibiotic is often used to treat patients with a serious infection until the causative organism can be identified and its sensitivity to antimicrobial drugs can be determined. For example, the initial treatment of serious nosocomial (hospital-acquired) infections can include the use of penicillin or vancomycin (active against staphylococci) in combination with an aminoglycoside or a cephalosporin (active against gram-negative bacilli).

Prevention of Antibiotic Resistance

As discussed in Chapter 40, tuberculosis is always treated with more than one drug. This is because about 1 in 10^6 *Mycobacterium tuberculosis* organisms will mutate to a resistant form during treatment with a single drug. The rate of mutation to a form that is resistant to two drugs is the product of the individual drug resistant rates, or about 1 in 10^{12} organisms. Because fewer than 10^{12} organisms are usually present in a patient with tuberculosis, it is unlikely that a resistant mutant will emerge during combination therapy.

Table 37-4. Prophylactic Use of Antimicrobial Drugs

Prevention of infection during invasive procedures

- To prevent **endocarditis** in persons with a history of valvular heart disease, administer amoxicillin or other antibiotic prior to dental, oral, or upper respiratory tract procedures.
- To prevent **wound and tissue infections** in persons who will undergo surgery, administer a single dose of cefazolin (active against staphylococci and oral anaerobic organisms) or a single dose of cefoxitin or cefotetan (active against aerobic or anaerobic enteric bacilli).

Prevention of disease transmission in persons at increased risk

- To prevent **influenza type A,** give amantadine or rimantadine.
- To prevent **malaria,** give chloroquine or mefloquine.
- To prevent **meningococcal disease,** give rifampin.
- To prevent **tuberculosis,** give isoniazid.

PROPHYLACTIC THERAPY

The prevention of infections requires the sterilization of diagnostic and surgical instruments, the use of disinfectants to reduce environmental pathogens in hospitals and clinics, and the disinfection of skin and mucous membranes before invasive procedures. In some cases, antimicrobial drugs are also administered prophylactically either to reduce the incidence of infections associated with surgical and other invasive procedures or to prevent disease transmission to close contacts of infected persons. Recommendations for prophylaxis are summarized in Table 37–4.

Prevention of Infection Caused by Invasive Procedures

Antibiotics are used to prevent **endocarditis** in persons with a history of valvular heart disease, such as mitral valve prolapse and rheumatic heart disease. These individuals are at risk of developing acute bacterial endocarditis caused by viridans and other streptococci that can be acquired during dental, oral, or upper respiratory tract procedures and surgery. Amoxicillin is currently considered the drug of choice, but endocarditis can be prevented by using an alternative drug (e.g., clindamycin, cephalexin, azithromycin, or clarithromycin).

Antibiotics are routinely used to prevent **wound and tissue infections** that can be acquired during a wide range of surgical procedures. The choice of antibiotic depends on the most likely sources of bacterial pathogens during a particular procedure. The skin is the most common source of pathogens, especially staphylococci, during most types of surgery. The gastrointestinal tract is also an important source of pathogens when surgical procedures involve the gastrointestinal system. Surgery to repair contaminated wounds (e.g., gunshot or knife wounds) presents the most severe requirements for prophylaxis because of the greater number and variety of bacteria that are often associated with this type of trauma.

Prevention of Disease Transmission

Antimicrobial drugs are occasionally used to prevent the transmission of a highly contagious disease, such as **meningococcal infection,** from an infected person or insect vector to an exposed individual. Drugs are also used to prevent **malaria** in persons who are traveling to regions of the world where malaria is endemic and to prevent **influenza type A** and **tuberculosis** in certain groups at increased risk for these diseases. Prophylactic drugs are discussed more thoroughly in subsequent chapters.

SUMMARY OF IMPORTANT POINTS

- Antibiotics, which are substances produced by one microbe, are capable of inhibiting the growth or viability of other microbes. Antimicrobial drugs include cell wall synthesis inhibitors, protein synthesis inhibitors, metabolic and nucleic acid inhibitors, and cell membrane inhibitors.

- Antimicrobial drugs can be characterized as bactericidal (able to kill microbes) or bacteriostatic (able to slow the growth of microbes). They can also be characterized as narrow-spectrum, broad-spectrum, or extended-spectrum, based on their range of antimicrobial activity.

- Laboratory tests used to determine microbial sensitivity to drugs include the disk diffusion method (Kirby-Bauer test) and the broth dilution test. The latter test is used to determine the minimal inhibitory concentration (MIC), which is the lowest drug concentration that inhibits microbial growth in vitro.

- Acquired microbial resistance arises by mutation and selection or by transfer of genes encoding resistance factors (R factors). The most common mechanism of transferable resistance is bacterial conjugation and exchange of plasmids containing R factors.

- The mechanisms responsible for microbial resistance to a drug include inactivation of the drug by microbial enzymes, decreased accumulation of the drug by the microbe, and reduced affinity of the target macromolecule for the drug.

- The selection of an antimicrobial drug for treating a particular infection requires consideration of host factors (pregnancy, drug allergies, age and immune status, and the presence of concomitant diseases) and drug characteristics (antimicrobial activity, pharmacokinetic properties, adverse effect profile, cost, and convenience).

- Combination drug therapy is generally used for the treatment of mixed infections, the empiric treatment of serious infections, and the prevention of antibiotic resistance. In some cases, combination therapy with synergistic drugs is used for the treatment of infections caused by a single microbial species.

- Antibiotic prophylaxis is used to prevent infections during surgical and other invasive procedures and to prevent the transmission of infectious diseases to persons at increased risk.

Review Questions

For each numbered description, select the corresponding term from the lettered choices.

1. Cell membrane protein that transports chemotherapeutic drugs out of the cell.

2. Continued suppression of bacterial growth after an antibiotic is eliminated from the body.

3. An antibiotic that inhibits bacterial growth but does not kill the bacteria.

4. Most frequent mechanism of transferable drug resistance.

5. An antibiotic diffusion device for determining the minimal inhibitory concentration of an antibiotic against a strain of bacteria.

   (A) Etest strip
   (B) postantibiotic effect
   (C) synergistic effect
   (D) bacterial conjugation
   (E) P-glycoprotein
   (F) selective toxicity
   (G) bacteriostatic

Answers and Explanations

1. The answer is E: P-glycoprotein. The P-glycoprotein is a cell membrane protein that pumps antibiotics and other drugs out of mammalian and microbial cells. It prevents accumulation of drugs in target cells and is one of the mechanisms that confer resistance to chemotherapeutic agents.

2. The answer is B: postantibiotic effect (PAE). The PAE refers to a period of time during which bacterial growth continues to be inhibited after an antibiotic has been removed from a bacterial culture or eliminated from the body. The PAE increases the effective duration of action of antimicrobial agents and enables less-frequent dosing of some antibiotics.

3. The answer is G: bacteriostatic. Some antimicrobial agents (e.g., tetracyclines) slow the growth of microbes but do not kill the organisms. Hence, treatment with a bacteriostatic drug requires that the host immune system destroy the pathogen in order to effect a cure. Bactericidal drugs (e.g., penicillins) kill microbes and are not as dependent on host immune mechanisms to cure the infection. Bactericidal drugs, however, work in concert with the immune system and are much less effective in immunocompromised hosts.

4. The answer is D: bacterial conjugation. Transferable drug resistance refers to the acquisition of genes conferring resistance from other bacteria. Most commonly, this occurs by bacterial conjugation and exchange of plasmids containing resistance (R) factors. Transformation and transduction are less common mechanisms of transferring drug resistance.

5. The answer is A: Etest strip. The Etest strip is a semi-quantitative antibiotic diffusion device for determining the minimal inhibitory concentration (MIC) of an antibiotic. It is based on visualization of the point of intersection between the zone of bacterial growth inhibition and the concentration scale on the test trip. The Etest method is more convenient and economical than broth dilution methods.

SELECTED READINGS

Drew, R. H. Key references in infectious diseases pharmacotherapy. Pharmacotherapy 24:1586–1593, 2004.

Livermore, D. M. The need for new antibiotics. Clin Microbiol Infect 10(Suppl 4):1–9, 2004.

Nathan, C. Antibiotics at the crossroads. Nature 431:899–902, 2004.

Schwartz, R. S. Paul Ehrlich's magic bullets. N Engl J Med 350:1079–1080, 2004.

Wright, G. D. Mechanisms of resistance to antibiotics. Curr Opin Chem Biol 7:563–569, 2003.

CHAPTER 38

Inhibitors of Bacterial Cell Wall Synthesis

CLASSIFICATION OF INHIBITORS OF BACTERIAL CELL WALL SYNTHESIS

β-Lactam Antibiotics
Narrow-spectrum Penicillins
- Penicillin G
- Penicillin V

Penicillinase-resistant Penicillins
- Nafcillin[a]

Extended-spectrum Penicillins
- Amoxicillin
- Ampicillin
- Piperacillin
- Ticarcillin

β-Lactamase Inhibitors
- Clavulanate[b]

First-generation Cephalosporins
- Cefazolin
- Cephalexin (KEFLEX)

Second-generation Cephalosporins
- Cefprozil (CEFZIL)[c]
- Cefotetan (CEFOTAN)
- Cefuroxime (CEFTIN, ZINACEF)[d]

Third-generation Cephalosporins
- Ceftriaxone (ROCEPHIN)[e]
- Cefdinir (OMNICEF)[f]

Fourth-generation Cephalosporin
- Cefepime (MAXIPIME)

Monobactams
- Aztreonam

Carbapenems
- Imipenem, meropenem, and
- ertapenem

Other Bacterial Cell Wall Synthesis Inhibitors
- Bacitracin
- Fosfomycin
- Vancomycin

[a]also oxacillin, cloxacillin, dicloxacillin
[b]also sulbactam, tazobactam
[c]also cefaclor (CECLOR)
[d]also cefoxitin, cefonicid, cefmetazole
[e]also cefotaxime, ceftazidime, ceftizoxime
[f]also cefpodoxime (VANTIN)

OVERVIEW

A large group of antimicrobial drugs, including the penicillins and other β-lactam antibiotics, act by inhibiting the synthesis of the bacterial cell wall. The penicillins were the first true antibiotics to be discovered, and their development inaugurated the modern era of antimicrobial chemotherapy.

Cell Envelope

Two components of the cell envelope that are found in both gram-positive and gram-negative bacteria are the **cytoplasmic membrane** and the **cell wall.** The cell wall is much thicker in gram-positive bacteria than it is in gram-negative bacteria. The envelope of each gram-negative bacterium also has an **outer membrane** that is not found in other types of bacteria. The cell envelope components are illustrated in Fig. 38–1.

Cytoplasmic and Outer Membranes

The cytoplasmic membrane is a trilaminar membrane. It contains various types of **transport proteins,** which facilitate the uptake of a wide variety of substrates used by bacteria, and it also contains several enzymes required for the synthesis of the cell wall. These enzymes, whose functions are described below, are collectively known as **penicillin-binding proteins** (PBP).

The outer membrane of gram-negative bacteria is also a trilaminar membrane. It contains species-specific forms of a

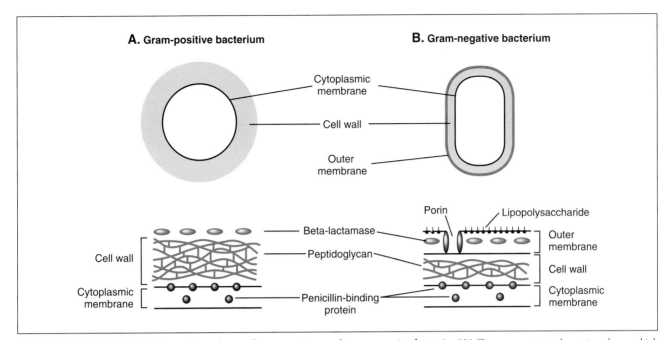

Figure 38–1. Comparison of the cell envelopes of gram-positive and gram-negative bacteria. (A) The gram-positive bacterium has a thick cell wall but does not have an outer membrane. β-Lactamases are located in the outer portion of the cell wall. Penicillin-binding proteins are found in the cytoplasmic membrane. **(B)** The gram-negative bacterium has a thin cell wall. It also has an outer membrane that contains lipopolysaccharide and protein channels called porins.

complex **lipopolysaccharide** (LPS) and various types of protein channels called **porins.** One portion of LPS (the lipid A portion) is the **endotoxin** responsible for gram-negative sepsis. This endotoxin activates immunologic mechanisms that lead to fever, platelet aggregation, increased vascular permeability, and other adverse effects on tissues. Porins allow ions and other small hydrophilic molecules to pass through the outer membrane, and they are responsible for the entry of several types of antibiotics. Acquired alterations in porin structure can lead to microbial resistance to antibiotics, such as is the case with resistance to imipenem.

The bacterial cytoplasmic membrane is the target of two peptide antibiotics, **daptomycin** and **polymyxin.** These drugs act directly on the cell membranes to increase membrane permeability and thereby cause the cytoplasmic contents to leak out of the cell. The properties and uses of these antibiotics are discussed in Chapter 40.

Cell Wall

The cell wall consists primarily of **peptidoglycan,** a polymer constructed from repeating disaccharide units of *N*-**acetylglucosamine** (GlcNAc) and *N*-**acetylmuramic acid** (MurNAc). Each disaccharide is attached to others through glycosidic bonds. Each molecule of MurNAc has a peptide containing two molecules of D-alanine and a pentaglycine side chain (Fig. 38–2). The strands of peptidoglycan in the cell wall are cross-linked by a transpeptidase reaction in which the glycine pentapeptide of one strand is attached to the penultimate D-alanine molecule of another strand. During this reaction, the terminal D-alanine is removed.

The cell wall maintains the shape of the bacterium and protects it from osmotic lysis if it is placed in a hypotonic

medium. Without a cell wall, the bacterium is unprotected. This is why inhibition of cell wall synthesis by antimicrobial drugs is usually bactericidal. Because a cell wall is not found in higher organisms, antimicrobial drugs can inhibit its formation without harming host cells. The cell wall is synthesized during bacterial replication, and drugs that inhibit cell wall synthesis are more active against rapidly dividing bacteria than they are against bacteria in the resting or stationary phase. For the same reason, the effectiveness of cell wall inhibitors is usually reduced by concurrent administration of bacteriostatic antibiotics that slow the growth of bacteria.

Sites of Drug Action

β-Lactam Drugs

The β-lactam antibiotics bind to a diverse group of bacterial enzymes known as the **penicillin-binding proteins.** These enzymes are anchored in the cytoplasmic membrane and extend into the periplasmic space. The PBP are responsible for the assembly, maintenance, and regulation of the peptidoglycan portion of the bacterial cell wall. Some of the PBP have transpeptidase activity, whereas others have carboxypeptidase and transglycosylase activity.

Table 38–1 outlines the functions of the three major types of PBP: PBP-1, PBP-2, and PBP-3. The β-lactam antibiotics form a covalent bond with PBP and thereby inhibit the catalytic activity of these enzymes. Inhibition of some PBP prevents **cross-linking of peptidoglycan** (see Fig. 38–2), whereas inhibition of other PBP leads to the bacterium's **autolysis** or to its change to a **spheroplast** or a **filamentous form.**

Figure 38–2. Sites of action of bacterial cell wall synthesis inhibitors. The bacterial cell wall consists primarily of peptidoglycan, a polymer constructed from repeating disaccharide units of *N*-acetylglucosamine (GlcNAc) and *N*-acetylmuramic acid (MurNAc). Numbers indicate the steps involved in the synthesis of the cell wall. In step 1, bactoprenol pyrophosphate (bactoprenol-P-P) is dephosphorylated to regenerate the carrier molecule, bactoprenol phosphate (bactoprenol-P). In step 2, uridine diphosphate-MurNAc (UDP-MurNAc) is added. Uridine monophosphate (UMP) is a by-product. In steps 3 and 4, UDP-GlcNAc and a glycine pentapeptide (5-Gly-tRNA) are added. In step 5, the disaccharide peptide is transferred to the peptidoglycan growth point. In step 6, the cross-linking of peptidoglycan strands is catalyzed by transpeptidase, a type of penicillin-binding protein. In this reaction, a glycine in one strand forms a new peptide bond with a D-alanine in the adjacent strand, and the terminal D-alanine is released from the adjacent strand. Bacitracin blocks step 1 and β-lactam antibiotics and vancomycin block step 6 by different mechanisms. Fosfomycin (not shown) inhibits enolpyruvyl transferase, the enzyme that catalyzes the condensation of UDP-GlcNAc with phosphoenolpyruvate to synthesize UDP-MurNAc.

TABLE 38-1.	**Major Types of Penicillin-Binding Proteins (PBPs)**	
Type	**Function**	**Effect of PBP Inhibition on Bacterium**
PBP-1	Elongation of bacterial cell wall	Rapid autolysis of bacterium
PBP-2	Maintenance of rod shape of bacterium	Change of bacterium to a spheroplast
PBP-3	Formation of septa	Change of bacterium to a filamentous form

Bacterial species have different types of PBP, and specific β-lactam antibiotics selectively bind to the different types. This partly accounts for the variation in the sensitivity of different organisms to β-lactam antibiotics.

Other Drugs

Bacitracin and **fosfomycin** inhibit cell wall peptidoglycan synthesis by blocking specific steps in the formation of the disaccharide precursor, MurNAc-GlcNAc. As shown in Fig. 38–2, bacitracin inhibits the dephosphorylation of bactoprenol pyrophosphate, which is the carrier lipid required for regeneration of bactoprenol phosphate, the active carrier of the disaccharide precursor. Fosfomycin inhibits enolpyruvyl transferase, the enzyme that catalyzes the condensation of uridine diphosphate-GlcNAc (UDP-GlcNAc) with phosphoenolpyruvate to synthesize UDP-MurNAc. **Vancomycin** binds tightly to the D-alanyl-D-alanine portion of the peptidoglycan precursor and prevents bonding of the penultimate D-alanine to the pentaglycine peptide during cross-linking of peptidoglycan strands.

β-LACTAM ANTIBIOTICS

The β-lactam drugs include penicillins, β-lactamase inhibitors, cephalosporins, monobactams, and carbapenems.

Penicillins

The penicillins were the first antibiotics to be isolated from microorganisms and used to treat systemic bacterial infections. Alexander Fleming is credited with the discovery of penicillin, but he was unable to isolate the substance in sufficient purity and quantity for clinical use. Later, E. B. Chain and H. W. Florey, working in England, obtained enough penicillin to establish its clinical effectiveness. The production of sufficient quantities of penicillin for widespread use around the world was made possible by advances in microbial fermentation technology in the United States of America.

Classification

The penicillins can be grouped according to their antimicrobial spectrum of activity. Narrow-spectrum penicillins include **penicillin G** and **penicillin V**. Penicillinase-resistant penicillins include **dicloxacillin** and **nafcillin**. Extended-spectrum penicillins include **amoxicillin, ampicillin, piperacillin,** and **ticarcillin**.

Drug Properties

CHEMISTRY. The penicillins consist of a β-lactam ring fused to a thiazolidine ring, with an R group that is unique for each drug (Fig. 38–3). The **original (natural) penicillins,** isolated from strains of *Penicillium,* were assigned letter designations because their chemical structures could not be identified at that time. Of the original penicillins, only penicillin G and penicillin V are still used today, and they are classified as narrow-spectrum drugs. The **semisynthetic penicillins** are produced from 6-aminopenicillanic acid, a building block obtained by removing the R group of a natural penicillin. A different R group is then substituted to prepare each of the various penicillinase-resistant and extended-spectrum penicillins that are available today. The penicillinase-resistant penicillins have a large, bulky R group that protects them from hydrolysis by staphylococcal β-lactamase.

PHARMACOKINETICS. The route of administration of penicillins depends on the stability of the drugs in gastric acid. **Acid-stable penicillins,** which include amoxicillin, dicloxacillin, and penicillin V, are effective when given orally. In contrast, **acid-labile penicillins,** which include piperacillin and ticarcillin, must be administered parenterally. Penicillin G has intermediate sensitivity to gastric acid and can be given orally in large doses, but penicillin V has better acid stability and oral bioavailability, so it is usually preferable when an oral narrow-spectrum penicillin is indicated.

The penicillins are widely distributed to organs and tissues except the central nervous system. Because penicillins readily penetrate the cerebrospinal fluid when the meninges are inflamed (Fig. 38–4A), they can be administered intravenously for the treatment of meningitis.

Most penicillins are eliminated primarily by active renal tubular secretion and have short half-lives of about 0.5 to 1.3 hours (Table 38–2). A few penicillins (e.g., ampicillin and nafcillin) are excreted primarily in the bile. The renal tubular secretion of penicillins is inhibited by **probenecid,** a drug that competes with penicillins for the organic acid transporter located in the proximal tubule. Probenecid has been used to slow the excretion and prolong the half-life of penicillin G (see Fig. 38–4B).

Penicillin G is available in two long-acting forms for intramuscular administration, **procaine penicillin G** and **benzathine penicillin G.** Penicillin G is slowly released from these two preparations for absorption into the circulation following an intramuscular injection. Benzathine penicillin G is hydrolyzed slowly over a period of several weeks and provides low plasma concentrations of the drug for an extended period of time. In contrast, procaine penicillin G is hydrolyzed more rapidly and produces significant plasma concentrations of penicillin for about 24 hours (see Fig. 38–4B).

SPECTRUM AND INDICATIONS. Table 38–3 outlines the spectrum and major clinical uses of penicillins.

The **narrow-spectrum penicillins,** penicillins G and V, are used to treat infections caused by sensitive strains of streptococci (including pneumococci), meningococci, and spirochetes (e.g., *Treponema pallidum*). For example, penicillin G is used to treat group A streptococcal infections and to treat syphilis. Penicillin G is also active against *Clostridium perfringens,* the cause of gas gangrene, and other pathogens. Most staphylococci and gonococci, and some strains of pneumococci are now resistant to penicillin G.

The **penicillinase-resistant penicillins** (e.g., dicloxacillin and nafcillin) were developed to treat penicillin-resistant strains of staphylococci that elaborate penicillinase (β-lactamase). The penicillinase-resistant penicillins are not active against most other species of penicillinase-producing bacteria. Oxacillin is a member of the isoxazol group of penicillins, which also includes dicloxacillin and cloxacillin. Dicloxacillin can be used when an orally administered drug is needed, whereas nafcillin is usually preferred when parenteral administration is required.

The penicillinase-resistant drugs are used to treat serious staphylococcal infections, such as acute endocarditis and osteomyelitis, as well as skin and soft tissue infections caused by susceptible staphylococci. Staphylococci that are resistant to these penicillins are often designated **methicillin-resistant *Staphylococcus aureus*** (MRSA) because methicillin was the original drug in this class. Methicillin is seldom used today, however, because of its greater toxicity and tendency to cause interstitial nephritis. Bacteria that are resistant to methicillin are also cross-resistant to nafcillin and all

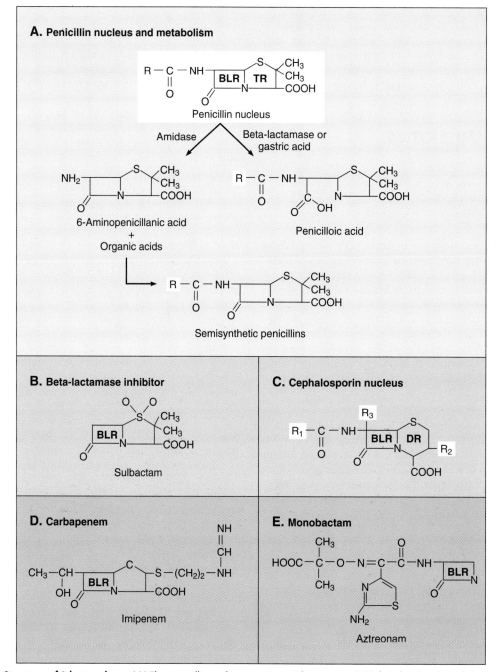

Figure 38–3. Structures of β-lactam drugs. (A) The penicillin nucleus contains a β-lactam ring (BLR) fused with a thiazolidine ring (TR). Amidase enzymatically removes the R group from penicillins and thereby forms 6-aminopenicillanic acid, the building block for semisynthetic penicillins. β-Lactamases hydrolyze the β-lactam ring and thereby inactivate penicillins and other β-lactam drugs. Some penicillins are also degraded by gastric acid. **(B)** β-Lactamase inhibitors (e.g., sulbactam) contain a β-lactam ring. **(C)** The cephalosporin nucleus contains a BLR fused with a dihydrothiazine ring (DR). **(D)** Aztreonam, a monocyclic β-lactam (monobactam) antibiotic, has a BLR that is not attached to another ring structure.

other penicillinase-resistant penicillins. Most strains of MRSA are also resistant to cephalosporins.

The **extended-spectrum penicillins** can be subdivided into the **aminopenicillins** (amoxicillin and ampicillin) and the **antipseudomonal penicillins** (piperacillin, ticarcillin, and others).

The aminopenicillins are active against many streptococci, some strains of enterococci, and a limited number of gram-negative bacilli. Amoxicillin and ampicillin are often combined with a β-lactamase inhibitor (described below), and drug products containing amoxicillin and **clavulanate** (AUGMENTIN) or ampicillin and **sulbactam** (UNASYN) are widely used to treat infections caused by β-lactamase-producing bacteria.

Amoxicillin can be used alone to treat respiratory tract infections caused by sensitive bacteria, including **otitis**

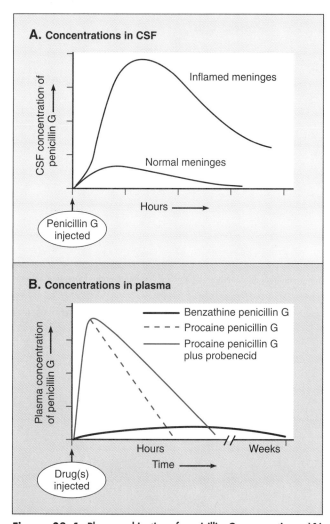

Figure 38–4. Pharmacokinetics of penicillin G preparations. (A) When penicillin G is administered to patients with normal meninges, the concentration in cerebrospinal fluid (CSF) remains low. When it is administered to patients with meningitis, the concentration increases. This is because meningitis increases the permeability of meninges to penicillin G. **(B)** Administration of benzathine penicillin G produces low plasma concentrations of the drug for several weeks. Administration of procaine penicillin G produces therapeutic plasma concentrations for about 24 hours. Probenecid inhibits the renal excretion of penicillin G, prolongs its half-life, and increases its plasma concentrations.

media, **sinusitis, bronchitis,** and community-acquired **pneumonia.** Many strains of *Haemophilus influenzae* and *Moraxella catarrhalis,* however, produce penicillinase, and infections caused by these organisms should be treated with amoxicillin-clavulanate. In addition, many strains of *Streptococcus pneumoniae* (pneumococci) have become increasingly resistant to amoxicillin, necessitating the use of larger doses to treat upper respiratory infections caused by this organism. For this reason, two formulations of amoxicillin-clavulanate have been developed to provide higher plasma levels of these drugs for longer periods of time. A sustained release tablet containing 1000 and 62.5 mg of amoxicillin and clavulanate, respectively, is available as AUGMENTIN XR. It is given twice daily and is intended for treatment of **adult respiratory tract infections** caused by drug-resistant pneu-

mococci, *H. influenzae,* or *M. catarrhalis.* A liquid suspension suitable for administering 90 and 6.4 mg/kg/day of amoxicillin-clavulanate in two divided doses to pediatric patients is available as AUGMENTIN ES-600. It is used to treat **otitis media** in places where resistant strains of pneumococci, *H. influenzae,* or *M. catarrhalis* are prevalent. For infections not caused by resistant organisms, the usual dose of amoxicillin has been 30 to 45 mg/kg/day in two divided doses.

Amoxicillin-clavulanate is also indicated for treating **bite wound infections** because it is active against the common pathogens causing bite wounds, including *Pasteurella multocida* and *Staphylococcus aureus.* Amoxicillin alone is used for prophylaxis of bacterial endocarditis in persons with heart valve defects.

Ampicillin is active against *Listeria monocytogenes* and is used to treat meningitis and other infections caused by this organism. It is also used in combination with **sulbactam** (a β-lactamase inhibitor) to treat infections caused by penicillinase-producing strains of bacteria, including bite wounds and diabetic foot ulcers. Ampicillin can be combined with an **aminoglycoside** (e.g., gentamicin) for the treatment of serious enterococcal infections, such as enterococcal endocarditis. Other uses for ampicillin and amoxicillin are listed in Table 38–3.

The **antipseudomonal penicillins** (e.g., **piperacillin**) are active against infections caused by *Pseudomonas aeruginosa* and a number of other aerobic gram-negative bacilli, including *Serratia* and *Citrobacter* species. In some cases, they are given in combination with an aminoglycoside. Piperacillin is usually combined with a β-lactamase inhibitor, tazobactam to treat mixed infections, such as nosocomial pneumonia involving gram-positive and anaerobic organisms. Other uses for these drugs are listed in Table 38–3.

BACTERIAL RESISTANCE. As shown in Table 38–4, there are three primary mechanisms by which bacteria exert resistance to penicillins and other β-lactam antibiotics: inactivation of the drugs by β-**lactamase** enzymes, reduced affinity of PBP for the antibiotics, and decreased entry of the drugs into bacteria through outer membrane **porins.** In some bacteria, resistance can be caused by a combination of these effects.

The production of β-lactamases (BLM) is the predominant cause of bacterial resistance to penicillins and other β-lactam antibiotics. These enzymes cleave the amide bond in the β-lactam ring and thereby inactivate the antibiotic (Fig. 38–3). β-Lactamases are expressed by both chromosomal and plasmid genes. Some BLM are constitutive, whereas others can be induced by β-lactam antibiotics. In gram-positive bacteria, BLM are secreted as exoenzymes and act extracellularly. BLM remain in the periplasmic space in gram-negative bacteria where they attack the antibiotic before it can bind to PBP.

The BLM are classified in two ways. The **functional or biochemical classification** of Bush-Jacoby-Medeiros contains four groups of BLM (groups 1 to 4). The **molecular classification** based on amino acid sequences includes classes A through D, with A and C occurring most frequently in bacteria. Functional **group 1 BLM** are enzymes that hydrolyze cephalosporins (cephalosporinases) and correspond to molecular **class C. Group 2 BLM** enzymes corre-

TABLE 38-2. **Pharmacokinetic Properties of Selected Bacterial Cell Wall Synthesis Inhibitors***

Drug	Route of Administration	Elimination Half-Life (Hours)	Primary Route of Elimination
β-lactam antibiotics			
Narrow-spectrum penicillins			
— Penicillin G	Oral or parenteral	0.5	Renal (TS)
— Penicillin V	Oral	1.0	Renal (TS)
Penicillinase-resistant penicillins			
— Dicloxacillin	Oral	0.6	Renal (TS)
— Nafcillin	Oral or parenteral	0.5	Biliary
Extended-spectrum penicillins			
— Amoxicillin	Oral	1.0	Renal (TS)
— Ampicillin	Oral or parenteral	1.0	Renal (TS) and biliary
— Piperacillin	Parenteral	1.3	Renal (TS)
— Ticarcillin	Parenteral	1.2	Renal (TS)
First-generation cephalosporins			
— Cefazolin	Parenteral	2.0	Renal (TS)
— Cephalexin	Oral	0.5	Renal (TS)
Second-generation cephalosporins			
— Cefotetan	Parenteral	4.0	Renal (TS)
— Cefoxitin	Parenteral	0.8	Renal (TS)
— Cefprozil	Oral	1.3	Renal (TS)
— Cefuroxime	Oral or parenteral	1.7	Renal (TS)
Third-generation cephalosporins			
— Cefdinir	Oral	1.7	Renal (TS)
— Cefotaxime	Parenteral	1.6[†]	Renal (TS)
— Ceftazidime	Parenteral	1.8	Renal (GF)
— Ceftriaxone	Parenteral	8.0	Biliary
Fourth-generation cephalosporins			
— Cefepime	Parenteral	2.0	Metabolized
Monobactams			
— Aztreonam	Parenteral	1.7	Metabolized
Carbapenems			
— Imipenem	Parenteral	1.0	Renal (TS)
— Meropenem	Parenteral	1.2	Renal (TS)
Other bacterial cell wall synthesis inhibitors			
— Bacitracin	Topical	NA	NA
— Fosfomycin	Oral	6.0	Renal (GF)
— Vancomycin	Oral or parenteral	6.0	Renal (GF)

*Values shown are the mean of values reported in the literature. TS = tubular secretion; GF = glomerular filtration; and NA = not applicable.
[†]For cefotaxime, the value shown is the half-life of the metabolite.

spond to molecular **classes A and D** and includes penicillinases, cephalosporinases, and carbapenemases. These enzymes are derived from the original BLM genes called TEM and SHV. Class A enzymes are the only BLM that are inhibited by **clavulanic acid, sulbactam,** or **tazobactam.**

Group 3 BLM are metallo (zinc) enzymes that correspond to molecular **class B.** Group 3 enzymes hydrolyze most penicillins, cephalosporins, and carbapenems (but not monobactams), and are not inhibited by clavulanate. **Group 4 BLM** are penicillinases that are not inhibited by clavulanate. These BLM do not yet have a molecular classification.

The staphylococci were the first major group of bacterial pathogens to acquire β-lactamases that rendered them resistant to penicillin G. Later, many gonococci and other gram-negative bacteria acquired BLM. Resistance of *H. influenzae* to amoxicillin and other penicillins is primarily caused by

the presence of these enzymes. Many strains of Enterobacteriaceae, including *E. coli* and *Klebsiella pneumoniae*, have acquired plasmid-mediated TEM and SHV BLM. In recent years, **extended spectrum β-lactamases** (ESBL) have emerged and spread globally. ESBL are derivatives of common TEM and SHV genes whose amino acid substitutions enable them to hydrolyze a wider range of substrates including the third-generation cephalosporins, cefotaxime, ceftriaxone, and ceftazidime.

Resistance caused by decreased affinity of PBP for β-lactam drugs is also a growing problem. Gram-positive bacteria are innately resistant to aztreonam because their PBP do not bind to this drug. Resistance of other bacteria to penicillins can be acquired when the structure of PBP is altered in a manner that reduces the affinity of PBP for the drugs. This mechanism has been responsible for the emergence of pneumococci that are resistant to penicillin G and of staphylococci that are resistant to methicillin.

TABLE 38-3. Major Clinical Uses of Selected Bacterial Cell Wall Synthesis Inhibitors

Drug	Infections	Major Pathogens
Penicillins		
Penicillin G	Syphilis	*Treponema pallidum*
	Endocarditis	Viridans streptococci, enterococci
	Meningitis	Meningococci
	Pneumonia	Pneumococci
Penicillin V	Various	Streptococci
	Pharyngitis	*Streptococcus pyogenes*
Nafcillin, oxacillin	Osteomyelitis, endocarditis, pneumonia, skin/soft tissue	*Staphylococcus aureus*
Amoxicillin ± clavulanate		Pneumococci, streptococci,
Ampicillin ± sulbactam	Otitis, upper respiratory tract, pneumonia, skin/soft tissue, urinary tract	staphylococci, *Haemophilus influenzae, Moraxella catarrhalis, E. coli, Pasteurella multocida*
	Meningitis	*Listeria monocytogenes*
	Decubitus and diabetic foot ulcers	Gram-positive and anaerobic organisms
Piperacillin ± tazobactam	Endocarditis	Streptococci, enterococci
	Lyme disease	*Borrelia burgdorferi*
	Intra-abdominal, skin/soft tissue, pneumonia and other	Aerobic and anaerobic organisms, including *Pseudomonas aeruginosa*
Cephalosporins		
Cephalexin	Skin and soft tissue infections	Streptococci, staphylococci
Cefazolin	Perioperative prophylaxis	Staphylococci, *E. coli*
Cefotetan	Intra-abdominal, gynecologic, biliary tract	Aerobic and anaerobic bacilli
	Respiratory tract, skin/soft tissue	Pneumococci, *Haemophilus influenzae, Moraxella catarrhalis*
Cefdinir, cefprozil, cefuroxime axetil	Gonorrhea[1], urinary tract, otitis, meningitis, pneumonia, Lyme disease	Gonococci, pneumococci, meningococci, *Borrelia burgdorferi, H. influenzae,* other gram-negative bacilli
Ceftriaxone	Urinary tract, pneumonia, others	*Pseudomonas aeruginosa*
	Intra-abdominal, urinary tract, pneumonia, skin/soft tissue	Drug-resistant gram-negative bacilli, including *Citrobacter* and *Enterobacter* species
Ceftazidime		
Cefepime		
Carbapenems	Intra-abdominal, meningitis, febrile neutropenia	Aerobic, anaerobic, and drug-resistant gram-negative bacilli
Monobactam (aztreonam)	Urinary tract, gynecologic, intra-abdominal, skin, lungs and others	Aerobic, gram-negative bacilli
Vancomycin	Bone and joint, skin and soft tissue, pneumonia, septicemia, endocarditis and others	Methicillin-resistant staphylococci, enterococci, and others
Bacitracin	Skin and eye	Staphylococci, streptococci
Fosfomycin	Lower urinary tract	*E. coli, Enterococcus faecalis,* others

[1]Also cefpodoxime as a single oral dose.

Many gram-negative bacteria are innately resistant to penicillins because porins in their outer membrane are impermeable to these drugs. This is also an important mechanism of acquired resistance to penicillins, as in the case of *P. aeruginosa* resistance to imipenem.

ADVERSE EFFECTS. The penicillins are the most common cause of **drug-induced hypersensitivity reactions.** Hypersensitivity reactions are evoked when penicillin in the body is degraded to penicilloic acid and other compounds. These compounds subsequently combine with body proteins to form antigens that elicit antibody formation.

Immediate hypersensitivity reactions, which are a type of reaction mediated by immunoglobulin E (IgE), can lead to urticaria (hives) or anaphylactic shock. Other types of hypersensitivity reaction can lead to serum sickness, interstitial nephritis, hepatitis, and various skin rashes. Hepatitis is more common with antistaphylococcal and extended-spectrum penicillins and is usually reversible when use of the drug is discontinued. Ampicillin is particularly likely to cause a maculopapular skin rash in patients with certain viral infections, such as mononucleosis. This reaction is mediated by sensitized lymphocytes, and its incidence in ampicillin-treated patients with mononucleosis is over 90%.

TABLE 38-4. Bacterial Resistance to β-Lactam Antibiotics

Mechanism	Examples
Inactivation of the drug by β-lactamase enzymes	Resistance of gonococci and staphylococci to penicillin G
	Resistance of gram-negative bacteria to carbapenems, extended-spectrum penicillins, cefoxitin, and other cephalosporins
	Resistance of *Haemophilus influenzae* to amoxicillin and other penicillins
Reduced affinity of penicillin-binding proteins (PBPs) for the drug	Resistance of enterococci to cephalosporins
	Resistance of gram-positive bacteria to aztreonam
	Resistance of meningococci, pneumococci, and streptococci to penicillin G
	Resistance of staphylococci to methicillin
Decreased entry of the drug into bacteria through outer membrane porins	Resistance of gram-negative bacteria to various β-lactam antibiotics
	Resistance of *Pseudomonas aeruginosa* to imipenem

Penicillin allergy can be confirmed by the use of commercial preparations of penicillin antigens. These preparations contain the major and minor antigenic determinants of penicillin that are formed in the body during penicillin degradation. These preparations are injected intradermally and will cause erythema at the injection site if allergy is present. The preparations should be administered only by personnel who are prepared to provide treatment for anaphylactic shock in the event that the patient develops a severe hypersensitivity reaction following the injection.

Except for hypersensitivity reactions, the penicillins are remarkably nontoxic to the human body and produce very few other adverse effects. High concentrations of penicillins can be irritating to the central nervous system and elicit seizures in patients who have received very large doses of these drugs. As with other antibiotics, penicillins can disturb the normal flora of the gut and produce diarrhea and superinfections with penicillin-resistant organisms, such as staphylococci and *Clostridium difficile*. Pseudomembranous colitis can occur in association with *C. difficile* superinfections.

β-Lactamase Inhibitors

Clavulanate, sulbactam (Fig. 38–3), and **tazobactam** are β-lactam drugs that inhibit molecular class A β-lactamases. When one of these drugs is given alone, it has no antimicrobial activity. When it is given in combination with a penicillin antibiotic, it will act as a suicide inhibitor of these BLM enzymes by serving as a surrogate substrate for them. The

current BLM inhibitors do not inhibit class B, C, and D β-lactamases, but broad-spectrum BLM inhibitors are now being developed.

Currently available drug combinations and their routes of administration are as follows: **amoxicillin plus clavulanate** (AUGMENTIN) is given orally; **ampicillin plus sulbactam** (UNASYN) is given parenterally; **piperacillin plus tazobactam** (ZOSYN) is given parenterally; and **ticarcillin plus clavulanate** (TIMENTIN) is given parenterally. The major uses of these combinations are listed in Table 38–3.

Cephalosporins

Classification

The cephalosporins are one of the largest and most widely used groups of antibiotics. Based on differences in their antimicrobial spectrum, they have been divided into four generations. Table 38–2 lists examples of each. The first-generation cephalosporins are primarily active against gram-positive cocci and a limited number of gram-negative bacilli. Subsequent generations of cephalosporins have increased activity against gram-negative bacilli and less activity against some species of gram-positive cocci. With the large number of cephalosporin drugs that are available, it is important to recognize that the members of each generation share many common characteristics.

Drug Properties

CHEMISTRY. The cephalosporins comprise a large group of semisynthetic drugs, most of which are derived from cephalosporin C, a substance obtained from a species of *Cephalosporium* discovered near a sewage outlet off the coast of Sardinia. Cephalosporins have a β-lactam ring and a dihydrothiazine ring (Fig. 38–3). Unlike the penicillins, the cephalosporins have at least two R groups attached to the molecule, thereby enabling the synthesis of a greater number of derivatives with potentially useful properties. In **cephamycins**, a subcategory of cephalosporins that includes **cefotetan** and **cefoxitin**, there is a third R group that is attached to the β-lactam ring. By manipulating the structure of cephalosporins, it has been possible to obtain drugs with greater resistance to bacterial BLM and with a wider range of antimicrobial activity.

PHARMACOKINETICS. In comparison with penicillins, the cephalosporins are more stable when administered to patients and are less likely to form antigens that evoke hypersensitivity reactions.

The route of administration depends on the particular cephalosporin being used. Some of the cephalosporins are given only orally; others are given only parenterally. **Cefuroxime** is one of the few cephalosporins available for use by both routes (as cefuroxime axetil for oral administration and cefuroxime sodium for parenteral administration). Some of the parenterally administered cephalosporins are used only intravenously; others are given either intravenously or intramuscularly. **Ceftriaxone,** for example, is administered as a single intramuscular injection for the treatment of gonococcal infections.

The orally administered cephalosporins are well absorbed from the gut, and their bioavailability usually is not significantly affected by food.

Most cephalosporins are excreted primarily by renal tubular secretion. Ceftriaxone is excreted primarily in the bile and has a much longer half-life than other cephalosporins.

SPECTRUM AND INDICATIONS. Table 38–3 outlines the spectrum and major clinical uses of cephalosporins.

The **first-generation cephalosporins** have good activity against most streptococci and methicillin-sensitive staphylococci. They are also active against a few gram-negative enteric bacilli, including *E. coli* and *Klebsiella pneumoniae.* The orally administered drugs (e.g., **cephalexin**) are primarily used to treat skin and soft tissue infections caused by gram-positive cocci and to treat uncomplicated urinary tract infections caused by susceptible organisms. Many strains of *E. coli* are now resistant to cephalexin. The parenterally administered drugs (e.g., **cefazolin**) are used to treat more serious infections caused by these organisms. Cefazolin is also widely used for surgical prophylaxis of infections caused by staphylococci and aerobic gram-negative enteric bacilli.

In comparison with first-generation cephalosporins, the **second-generation cephalosporins** have similar activity against gram-positive cocci while demonstrating increased activity against gram-negative bacilli. In addition, the second-generation drugs are active against many strains of *H. influenzae* and have been used to treat respiratory tract and other infections caused by this organism. Oral second-generation drugs, including **cefprozil** and **cefuroxime axetil,** are used to treat otitis media, particularly when it is caused by *H. influenzae* strains that are resistant to amoxicillin and other drugs. **Cefuroxime sodium,** a parenteral preparation, has been used as empiric therapy for patients with community-acquired pneumonia. **Cefotetan** is active against both aerobic and anaerobic gram-negative bacilli, including *Bacteroides fragilis,* and it is used to treat intra-abdominal, gynecologic, and biliary tract infections caused by these organisms. **Cefoxitin** has activity similar to that of cefotetan and is used for surgical prophylaxis of infections caused by gram-negative bacteria.

In comparison with second-generation cephalosporins, the **third-generation cephalosporins** have greater activity against a wider range of gram-negative organisms, including enteric gram-negative bacilli (Enterobacteriaceae), *H. influenzae,* and *M. catarrhalis.* In addition, **ceftazidime** is active against *P. aeruginosa.* Several third-generation drugs, including **cefpodoxime** (VANTIN), **cefotaxime,** and **ceftriaxone,** are active against gonococci and have been used as a single-dose treatment for gonorrhea. Other clinical indications for third-generation drugs include otitis media, pneumonia, meningitis, intra-abdominal or urinary tract infections, and advanced Lyme disease.

Cefepime (MAXIPIME) is more resistant to hydrolysis by β-lactamases than third-generation cephalosporins, and some authorities have classified it as a **fourth-generation cephalosporin.** Cefepime is resistant to plasmid-encoded BLM, including TEM-1, TEM-2, and SHV-1, and it is relatively resistant to inducible chromosomally encoded BLM.

Cefepime penetrates rapidly into gram-negative bacteria and targets multiple penicillin-binding proteins. For these reasons, cefepime is effective in treating infections caused by many Enterobacteriaceae, including *Citrobacter freundii* and *Enterobacter cloacae* that are resistant to other cephalosporins. The activity of cefepime against gram-positive organisms is similar to that of third-generation cephalosporins. It is not active, however, against methicillin-resistant staphylococci, penicillin-resistant pneumococci and most strains of enterococci. Cefepime has been used in treating a variety of systemic infections, including intra-abdominal and urinary tract, infections and pneumonia.

BACTERIAL RESISTANCE. Bacteria acquire resistance to cephalosporins through the same three mechanisms by which they acquire resistance to penicillins (see Table 38–4). The cephalosporins are more resistant to beta-lactamases-BLM than are the penicillins, and resistance to gram-negative BLM increases with successive generations of cephalosporins. Many cephalosporins, however, are susceptible to the extended spectrum BLM (see previous text). Some cephalosporins induce certain BLM.

ADVERSE EFFECTS. The cephalosporins cause little toxicity to the host and have an excellent safety record. Although they can elicit hypersensitivity reactions, the incidence of this is lower for cephalosporins than for most penicillins. Cephalosporins exhibit some **cross-sensitivity** with penicillins. On the one hand, a person who has had a mild hypersensitivity reaction to a penicillin will usually not cross-react to a cephalosporin. On the other hand, a person who has had a severe hypersensitivity reaction to a penicillin (e.g., an anaphylactic reaction) has a greater risk of cross-reacting and should usually not be given a cephalosporin.

A few cephalosporins can cause **platelet dysfunction and bleeding,** including cefotetan, cefmetazole, cefamandole, and cefoperazone. These cephalosporins can potentiate the effects of anticoagulants and antiplatelet drugs and thereby increase the risk of bleeding. These same cephalosporins can also produce a disulfiram-like reaction if they are taken with alcohol.

Monobactams

Aztreonam is a monocyclic β-lactam (monobactam) antibiotic (see Fig. 38–3). It is active against many aerobic gram-negative bacilli, including strains of *Enterobacter, Citrobacter, Klebsiella,* and *Proteus* species as well as *P. aeruginosa.* Aztreonam is used to treat serious infections caused by susceptible organisms and is particularly useful for infections caused by multidrug-resistant strains of *these organisms.* The drug is administered intravenously and is extensively metabolized before undergoing renal excretion. Aztreonam can cause hypersensitivity reactions and thrombophlebitis. It only rarely shows cross-sensitivity with penicillins and cephalosporins, however, and can usually be used in persons allergic to other β-lactam antibiotics.

Carbapenems

Imipenem, meropenem, and **ertapenem** are penicillin-like antibiotics in which the sulfur atom of the thiazolidine ring is replaced with a carbon atom (see Fig. 38–3). These antibiotics, called carbapenems, are bactericidal to a wide range of gram-positive and gram-negative bacteria, including many aerobic and anaerobic gram-negative bacilli. Imipenem has high affinity for PBP-2, whereas meropenem binds to both PBP-2 and PBP-3. The greater affinity of meropenem for PBP-3 appears to account for its superior activity against many Enterobacteriaceae, *P. aeruginosa,* and other gram-negative organisms. For example, they are drugs of choice to treat infections caused by *Serratia marcescens.* Imipenem and meropenem are used to treat a wide range of systemic infections, including endocarditis, pneumonia, urinary tract, pelvic, skin and soft tissue, and intra-abdominal infections. They are particularly useful for infections caused by multidrug-resistant organisms, and for mixed infections caused by aerobic and anaerobic enteric bacilli.

Imipenem and meropenem are administered intravenously. Unlike meropenem and ertapenem, imipenem is rapidly inactivated by renal dehydropeptidase. For this reason, imipenem is combined with a dehydropeptidase inhibitor called **cilastatin** in a product called PRIMAXIM. Imipenem and meropenem are primarily eliminated in the urine by the process of renal tubular secretion. Dosage adjustments are required when either drug is given to persons with renal impairment. Probenecid interacts with imipenem and meropenem, causing inhibition of their renal excretion.

The carbapenems exhibit cross-sensitivity with penicillins, cephalosporins, and other β-lactam antibiotics and should not be administered to patients who are allergic to these drugs. The carbapenems are generally well tolerated, but they can cause seizures in patients with epilepsy, so they should be used cautiously in these patients. Imipenem and meropenem sometimes cause hematologic reactions, including anemia, leukopenia, thrombocytopenia, and altered bleeding time.

OTHER BACTERIAL CELL WALL SYNTHESIS INHIBITORS

Vancomycin

Vancomycin is a glycopeptide antibiotic. Because it has activity against various **gram-positive cocci and bacilli,** including some strains that are resistant to penicillin, it is often used to treat staphylococcal or enterococcal endocarditis, staphylococcal osteomyelitis, streptococcal necrotizing fasciitis, and other serious infections caused by penicillin-resistant organisms. Nevertheless, some strains of staphylococci and enterococci have acquired resistance to vancomycin. This resistance is conferred by mutations which alter the amino acid sequence of the cell wall pentapeptide component containing D-alanine.

Vancomycin is also active against some *Bacillus, Clostridium,* and *Corynebacterium* species. Although it is occasionally used to treat diarrhea and **pseudomembranous colitis** caused by *C. difficile,* metronidazole is usually preferred for this indication because of its much lower cost.

Vancomycin is poorly absorbed from the gut and must be administered parenterally to treat systemic infections. It is administered orally, however, to treat gastrointestinal *C. difficile* infections. Vancomycin is distributed to most body fluids and tissues, and it is excreted in the urine by the process of glomerular filtration. The half-life of vancomycin is normally about 6 hours (see Table 38–2), but the half-life is markedly prolonged in patients with renal failure.

Improvements in the manufacturing of vancomycin preparations have reduced the incidence of **nephrotoxicity** and **ototoxicity** associated with their use. Vancomycin, however, should be used cautiously with other nephrotoxic drugs, including aminoglycosides and amphotericin B. Ototoxic effects of vancomycin can include both **vestibular dysfunction** (ataxia, vertigo, nystagmus, and nausea) and **cochlear dysfunction** (tinnitus and hearing loss). Ototoxicity is usually caused by excessive serum concentrations and is reversible when these concentrations are reduced.

If vancomycin is infused at an excessive rate, it can cause an **erythematous rash** on the face and upper body known as the **red neck** or **red man syndrome.**

Bacitracin

Bacitracin is an antibiotic derived from a *Bacillus subtilis* strain isolated from a girl named Tracy. The drug inhibits cell wall peptidoglycan synthesis by blocking the regeneration of bactoprenol phosphate, the lipid carrier molecule (see Fig. 38–2). Bacitracin is active against gram-positive cocci, including staphylococci and streptococci, and it is primarily used for the topical treatment of minor skin and ocular infections. It is often combined with polymyxin or neomycin in ointments and creams. Bacitracin is very nephrotoxic and is not used systemically.

Fosfomycin

Fosfomycin is a unique antibiotic that blocks one of the first steps in cell wall peptidoglycan synthesis, the formation of UDP-MurNAc. Fosfomycin is structurally similar to phosphoenolpyruvate. By irreversibly inhibiting the enzyme enolpyruvyl transferase, fosfomycin blocks the addition of phosphoenolpyruvate to UDP-GlcNAc and thereby prevents the synthesis of UDP-MurNAc.

Fosfomycin is active against enterococci and many gram-negative enteric bacilli, including *E. coli, Citrobacter* species, *Klebsiella* species, *Proteus* species, and *Serratia marcescens.* The drug is specifically approved for the treatment of uncomplicated urinary tract infections caused by *E. coli* or *Enterococcus faecalis.* For this purpose, fosfomycin is administered orally as a single dose. The drug is excreted unchanged in the urine and feces and has a half-life of about 6 hours. Fosfomycin sometimes causes diarrhea but is otherwise well tolerated and is associated with few adverse effects.

SUMMARY OF IMPORTANT POINTS

■ β-Lactam antibiotics, vancomycin, bacitracin, and fosfomycin are drugs that inhibit bacterial cell wall synthesis.

■ The β-lactam antibiotics inhibit the transpeptidase reaction that cross-links the peptidoglycan component of the cell wall. These antibiotics include penicillins, cephalosporins, monobactams, and carbapenems.

■ A β-lactamase inhibitor (e.g., clavulanate, sulbactam, or tazobactam) is administered in combination with a β-lactam antibiotic to prevent degradation of the antibiotic by bacteria.

■ Narrow-spectrum penicillins (e.g., penicillin G) are primarily active against gram-positive cocci and spirochetes; penicillinase-resistant penicillins (e.g., dicloxacillin and nafcillin) are used to treat staphylococcal infections; and extended-spectrum penicillins (e.g., amoxicillin and ticarcillin) are active against various gram-negative bacilli.

■ Acid-stable penicillins (e.g., penicillin V, amoxicillin, and dicloxacillin) can be given orally, whereas acid-labile drugs (e.g., piperacillin and ticarcillin) must be given parenterally.

■ Most penicillins are eliminated primarily by renal tubular secretion, a process that is inhibited by probenecid. Two long-acting forms of penicillin G (procaine and benzathine penicillin G) are available for intramuscular administration.

■ Penicillins can elicit any of the four types of hypersensitivity reactions, including anaphylactic shock and other immediate hypersensitivity reactions mediated by IgE.

■ Cephalosporins are semisynthetic antibiotics that are subdivided into four generations on the basis of their antimicrobial spectrum. The activity against gram-negative organisms increases from the first to the fourth generation.

■ Some cephalosporins (e.g., cefazolin) are eliminated by renal tubular secretion, whereas others (e.g., ceftriaxone) are eliminated in the bile. Ceftriaxone has a much longer half-life than other cephalosporins, enabling it to be used as single-dose treatment for certain infections, including gonorrhea.

■ Carbapenems (e.g., imipenem and meropenem) are active against a broad spectrum of bacteria including many strains resistant to other antibiotics. Aztreonam is a monobactam active against aerobic gram-negative bacilli. It does not cross-react with other β-lactam drugs.

■ Vancomycin is a glycopeptide antibiotic that is active against gram-positive organisms, including methicillin-sensitive and methicillin-resistant staphylococci, enterococci, and *Clostridium difficile.*

■ Bacitracin is used topically for infections caused by gram-positive cocci. Fosfomycin is administered as a single-dose treatment for uncomplicated urinary tract infections caused by *E. coli* or enterococci.

Review Questions

For each numbered drug described, select the corresponding drug from the lettered choices.

1. It is active against most strains of methicillin-resistant staphylococci and penicillin-resistant enterococci.

2. It is an orally effective third-generation cephalosporin that can be given as a single dose to treat gonorrhea.

3. This drug's resistance to plasmid and chromosomally encoded β-lactamases confers greater activity against Enterobacteriaceae than have other cephalosporins.

4. It is used to treat *Pseudomonas aeruginosa* infections in persons who are allergic to other β-lactam drugs.

5. A single oral dose of this non–β-lactam antibiotic can be used to treat lower urinary tract infections.

   (A) ceftriaxone
   (B) vancomycin
   (C) fosfomycin
   (D) cefotetan
   (E) cefpodoxime
   (F) aztreonam
   (G) cefepime

Answers and Explanations

1. The answer is B: vancomycin. Vancomycin is a unique peptide antibiotic that does not exhibit cross-resistance with β-lactam antibiotics. It is active against gram-positive organisms including methicillin-resistant staphylococci and penicillin-resistant enterococci.

2. The answer is E: cefpodoxime. Cefpodoxime is an orally administered third-generation cephalosporin that is used to treat respiratory tract infections and can be given as a single dose to treat uncomplicated gonorrhea.

3. The answer is G: cefepime. Cefepime is a fourth-generation cephalosporin that exhibits greater resistance to β-lactamase enzymes than third-generation cephalosporins. It is used to treat a variety of serious infections caused by drug-resistance gram-negative bacilli.

4. The answer is F: aztreonam. Aztreonam is a monobactam antibiotic that is only active against aerobic gram-negative bacilli, including *Pseudomonas aeruginosa.* Because it rarely exhibits cross-sensitivity with other β-lactam drugs, it can be used to treat infections in persons allergic to penicillins or cephalosporins.

5. The answer is C: fosfomycin. Fosfomycin is a unique antibiotic that is only used to treat acute uncomplicated lower urinary tract (bladder) infections caused by susceptible organisms.

SELECTED READINGS

Oliver, R., G. J. Roberts, and L. Hooper. Penicillins for the prophylaxis of bacterial endocarditis in dentistry. Cochrane Database of Syst Rev (2):CD003813, 2004.

Pichichero, M. E., and J. R. Casey. Acute otitis media disease management. Minerva Pediat 55:415–438, 2003.

Poole, K. Resistance to beta-lactam antibiotics. Cell Mol Life Sci 61:2200–2223, 2004.

Schito, G. C. Why fosfomycin trometamol as first line therapy for uncomplicated UTI? Int J Antimicrob Agents 22:79–83, 2003.

Thethi, A. K., and R. G. Van Dellen. Dilemmas and controversies in penicillin allergy. Immunol Allergy Clin N Am 24:445–461, 2004.

White, A. R., C. Kaye, J. Poupard, et al. Augmentin (amoxicillin/clavulanate) in the treatment of community-acquired respiratory tract infection: a review of the continuing development of an innovative antimicrobial agent. J Antimicrob Chemother 53(Suppl 1):13–20, 2004.

CHAPTER 39

Inhibitors of Bacterial Protein Synthesis

OVERVIEW

After the introduction of penicillin, scientists began an extensive search for antibiotics that could inhibit penicillin-resistant bacteria. A number of *Streptomyces* species were isolated from soil samples collected from all over the world, and these species eventually yielded several new classes of antibiotics, including the aminoglycosides, tetracyclines, and macrolides. Streptomycin, an aminoglycoside, was the first new antibiotic to be introduced through these efforts.

Bacterial Protein Synthesis

Several classes of antibiotics act by selectively blocking one or more steps in the protein synthesis of bacteria (prokaryotes) while having relatively little effect on the protein synthesis of humans and other eukaryotes. The selectivity for bacterial protein synthesis is caused by differences in the structure and function of ribosomes in prokaryotic versus eukaryotic organisms.

Each ribosome has two subunits. The **ribosome in prokaryotes** is composed of a 30S subunit and a 50S subunit (with S denoting the Svedberg unit of flotation, which forms the basis for the separation and isolation of ribosomal subunits from cell homogenates). In contrast, the **ribosome in eukaryotes** is composed of a 40S and a 60S subunit, and the proteins that initiate and carry out translation of messenger RNA (mRNA) in eukaryotic systems are more complex and function differently than the proteins of bacterial systems.

The basic steps in bacterial protein synthesis are illustrated in Fig. 39–1. These steps include the binding of aminoacyl transfer RNA (tRNA) to the ribosome, the for-

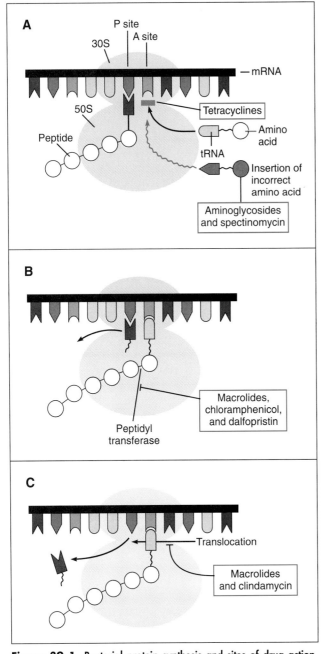

Figure 39–1. Bacterial protein synthesis and sites of drug action. The bacterial ribosome is composed of a 30S subunit and a 50S subunit. The steps in protein synthesis and translation of messenger RNA (mRNA) include the binding of aminoacyl transfer RNA (tRNA) to the ribosome, the formation of a peptide bond, and translocation. **(A)** Under normal circumstances, the nascent peptide is attached to the ribosome at the peptidyl site (P site), and the next aminoacyl tRNA binds to the acceptor or aminoacyl site (A site). Tetracyclines block aminoacyl tRNA from binding to the A site. Aminoglycosides and spectinomycin cause misreading of the genetic code, which leads to binding of the wrong aminoacyl tRNA and insertion of the wrong amino acid into the nascent peptide. **(B)** Macrolides, chloramphenicol, and dalfopristin block peptidyl transferase, the enzyme that catalyzes the formation of a peptide bond between the nascent peptide and the amino acid attached to the A site. **(C)** Macrolides and clindamycin block the translocation step in which the nascent peptide is transferred from the A site to the P site following the formation of a new peptide bond.

mation of a peptide bond, and translocation. Aminoacyl tRNA binds to the 30S ribosomal subunit, whereas peptide bond formation and translocation involve components of the 50S ribosomal subunit.

Sites of Drug Action

As shown in Fig. 39–1, each type of antibiotic discussed in this chapter acts at a specific site on the ribosome to inhibit one or more particular steps in protein synthesis. Tetracyclines, aminoglycosides, and spectinomycin act at the **30S ribosomal subunit.** Macrolides, chloramphenicol, dalfopristin, and clindamycin act at the **50S ribosomal subunit.**

Tetracyclines competitively block binding of tRNA to the 30S subunit and thereby prevent the addition of new amino acids to the growing peptide chain. This reversible effect is responsible for the bacteriostatic action of tetracyclines.

Aminoglycosides and **spectinomycin** bind primarily to the 30S subunit, where they interfere with the initiation of protein synthesis. They also cause misreading of the genetic code so that the wrong amino acid is inserted into the protein structure. These irreversible actions account for the bactericidal effects of aminoglycosides and spectinomycin.

Macrolides, chloramphenicol, and **dalfopristin** block peptidyl transferase, the enzyme that catalyzes the formation of a peptide bond between the new amino acid and the nascent peptide. **Macrolides** and **clindamycin** prevent translocation of the nascent peptide from the acceptor or aminoacyl site (A site) to the peptidyl site (P site) on the ribosome which, in turn, prevents binding of the next aminoacyl tRNA to the ribosome.

DRUGS THAT AFFECT THE 30S RIBOSOMAL SUBUNIT

Aminoglycosides

The aminoglycosides include **amikacin, gentamicin, neomycin, streptomycin,** and **tobramycin.** The properties and major clinical uses of these drugs are compared in Tables 39–1 and 39–2.

Drug Properties

CHEMISTRY AND PHARMACOKINETICS. All aminoglycosides are composed of amino sugars linked through glycosidic bonds (Fig. 39–2A). The amino groups are highly basic and become extensively protonated and ionized in body fluids. Their highly ionized structure determines many of their pharmacokinetic properties, including their absorption, distribution, and excretion.

The aminoglycosides are poorly absorbed from the gut and must be administered parenterally for the treatment of systemic infections. Occasionally, they are administered orally to treat gastrointestinal infections such as neonatal necrotizing enterocolitis. They are also administered topically to treat infections of the skin, mucous membranes, and ocular tissues.

Because of their highly ionized nature, aminoglycosides do not penetrate body cells. As a result, their volumes of dis-

TABLE 39-1.　**Pharmacokinetic Properties of Bacterial Protein Synthesis Inhibitors***

Drug	Route of Administration	Oral Bioavail-ability	Elimination Half-Life (Hours)	Primary Route of Elimination
Drugs that affect the 30S ribosomal subunit				
Aminoglycosides				
— Amikacin	IV	NA	2.5	Renal excretion
— Gentamicin	IV or topical	NA	1.5	Renal excretion
— Neomycin	Topical	NA	NA	NA
— Streptomycin	IM	NA	2.0	Renal excretion
— Tobramycin	IV or topical	NA	2.5	Renal excretion
Tetracyclines				
— Doxycycline	Oral or IV	90%	20.0	Fecal and renal excretion
— Minocycline	Oral or IV	95%	20.0	Biliary and renal excretion
— Tetracycline	Oral or IV	70%	10.0	Renal excretion
Other antibiotics				
— Spectinomycin	IM	NA	2.0	Renal excretion
Drugs that affect the 50S ribosomal subunit				
Macrolides and Ketolides				
— Azithromycin	Oral or IV	37%	12.0	Biliary excretion
— Clarithromycin	Oral	62%	5.0	Biliary and renal excretion
— Telithromycin	Oral	60%	10.0	Biliary and renal excretion
— Erythromycin	Oral, IV, or topical	35% ± 25%	2.0	Biliary excretion
Other antibiotics				
— Chloramphenicol	Oral, IV, or topical	95%	3.0	Hepatic metabolism; renal excretion
— Clindamycin	Oral, IV, or topical	95%	2.5	Hepatic metabolism; renal, biliary, and fecal excretion
— Quinupristin-dalforpristin	IV	NA	0.8/0.4[†]	Hepatic metabolism; biliary excretion
Other bacterial protein synthesis inhibitors				
Mupirocin	Topical	NA	NA	NA
Linezolid	Oral or IV	100%	6	Hepatic metabolism; renal excretion

*Values shown are the mean of values reported in the literature. IV = intravenous; IM = intramuscular; and NA = not applicable.
[†]The half-lives for quinupristin and dalfopristin are 0.8 and 0.4 hours, respectively. The drugs are given in combination.

tribution are similar to the extracellular fluid volume. Aminoglycosides do not penetrate the meninges very well, even when the meninges are inflamed, so intrathecal administration may be required to treat meningitis.

The aminoglycosides are not metabolized. They are excreted primarily by the process of renal glomerular filtration, with little tubular reabsorption. The renal clearance of aminoglycosides is approximately equal to the creatinine clearance, because creatinine is also filtered at the glomerulus but is not secreted or reabsorbed significantly by the tubules. Because the clearance of aminoglycosides is proportional to the glomerular filtration rate, the dosage of aminoglycosides must be reduced in patients with renal impairment. In most cases, this is accomplished by increasing the interval between doses.

The plasma concentrations of aminoglycosides are routinely measured to ensure adequate dosage and to minimize toxicity. The peak concentration is usually found about 30 minutes after completing an intravenous infusion of an aminoglycoside, whereas the trough concentration is found before administration of the next dose. Optimal peak and trough concentrations have been established and can be used to guide dosage adjustments for individuals receiving the

standard regimen of three daily doses given at 8-hour intervals. For example, therapeutic concentrations of gentamicin and tobramycin are usually between 4 and 8 mg/L. A peak concentration above 12 mg/L or a trough concentration above 2 mg/L is considered toxic and indicates the need to reduce the dosage of gentamicin or tobramycin. Therapeutic concentrations of amikacin are between 16 and 32 mg/L, and the toxic peak and trough concentrations are above 35 mg/L and above 10 mg/L, respectively.

SPECTRUM AND INDICATIONS. In comparison with other classes of antibiotics, the aminoglycosides have greater activity against **aerobic gram-negative bacilli** but are often more toxic. Although the less toxic classes of drugs are preferred for the treatment of patients whenever possible, aminoglycosides continue to be extensively used for prophylaxis and treatment of serious infections. As is discussed later, the specific aminoglycoside drugs differ in terms of their antimicrobial spectrum.

BACTERIAL RESISTANCE. Resistance to aminoglycosides is primarily caused by inactivation of the drugs by bacterial acetylase, adenylase, and phosphorylase enzymes (Table 39–3).

TABLE 39-2. **Major Clinical Uses of Selected Bacterial Protein Synthesis Inhibitors**

Drug	Infections
Aminoglycosides Streptomycin	Plague, tularemia, drug-resistant tuberculosis
Gentamicin, tobramycin, and amikacin	Serious infections due to aerobic gram-negative bacilli, including *Pseudomonas aeruginosa* and many *Enterobacteriaceae* species
Tetracycline antibiotics	Lyme disease, Rocky Mountain spotted fever, ehrlichiosis, granuloma inguinale, brucellosis, cholera, relapsing fever, peptic ulcer disease due to *H. pylori*, chlamydial urethritis, acne
Macrolides and Ketolide Erythromycin	Respiratory tract infections due to streptococci, pneumococci, *Legionella pneumophila, Mycoplasma pneumoniae,* or *Chlamydia pneumoniae*
Azithromycin, clarithromycin, telithromycin	Respiratory tract infections due to organisms sensitive to erythromycin, *Haemophilus influenzae,* or *Moraxella catarrhalis*
Azithromycin, clarithromycin	*Mycobacterium avium-intracellulare* infections
Clarithromycin	Peptic ulcer disease due to *Helicobacter pylori*
Chloramphenicol	Meningitis, brain abscess
Clindamycin	Streptococcal infections, anaerobic infections
Quinupristin-dalfopristin	Infections due to vancomycin-resistant *Enterococcus faecium*
Linezolid	Infections due to vancomycin-resistant *Enterococcus faecium,* streptococci and staphylococci
Mupirocin	Impetigo due to streptococci, staphylococci Eradication of nasal colonization of methicillin-resistant staphylococci

These enzymes attach acetyl, adenyl, or phosphoryl moieties to the amino groups on the antibiotics, thereby preventing inhibition of bacterial protein synthesis. Resistance to aminoglycosides can also be caused by decreased binding of the drugs to the 30S ribosomal subunit or to decreased uptake of the drugs via porins in bacterial membranes. Both plasmid and chromosomal genes can be involved in resistance caused by enzymatic inactivation of the antibiotics, whereas only chromosomal genes are involved in resistance caused by decreased binding or decreased uptake.

ADVERSE EFFECTS. The major adverse effects of aminoglycosides are **nephrotoxicity** and **ototoxicity**. The risk of toxicity is related to the dosage and duration of treatment and varies with the specific drug. Irreversible toxicity can occur, even after use of the drug is discontinued, but serious toxicity is less likely if the offending drug is discontinued at the earliest sign of dysfunction.

Aminoglycosides are the most common cause of drug-induced renal failure. When the drugs accumulate in proximal tubule cells, they can cause **acute tubular necrosis.** This reduces the level of renal function and leads to a rise in plasma concentrations of the aminoglycosides. The elevated drug concentrations can further impair renal function and contribute to ototoxicity. For this reason, it is important to monitor renal function and plasma aminoglycoside concentrations and to adjust the aminoglycoside dosage accordingly.

Ototoxicity is associated with the accumulation of aminoglycosides in the **labyrinth** and in the **hair cells of the cochlea.** Patients can suffer from both **vestibular and cochlear toxicity.** Manifestations of vestibular toxicity include dizziness, impaired vision, nystagmus, vertigo, nausea, vomiting, and problems with postural balance and walking. Cochlear toxicity is characterized by tinnitus and hearing impairment and can lead to irreversible deafness. Often, a delay occurs between the beginning of drug administration and the onset of symptoms, so many hospitalized patients are ambulatory before signs of toxicity appear.

Specific Drugs

The aminoglycosides differ in their potential to cause toxicity and in their antimicrobial activity.

Of the five aminoglycosides listed in Table 39–2, streptomycin is the least toxic, but it is also the least active against *Pseudomonas aeruginosa* and other gram-negative bacilli. Streptomycin is primarily used to treat multidrug-resistant tuberculosis and infections caused by *Yersinia pestis* (plague) and *Francisella tularensis* (tularemia).

Amikacin, gentamicin, and tobramycin have superior activity against most members of the family Enterobacteriaceae and against *P. aeruginosa.* Tobramycin is the most active aminoglycoside against many strains of *P. aeruginosa.* Gentamicin is usually more active against members of the family *Enterobacteriaceae.* Gentamicin is also used in combination with a penicillin or other appropriate antibiotic to

A. Aminoglycosides

Tobramycin

B. Tetracyclines

	R₁	**R₂**	**R₃**
Doxycycline*	—H	—CH₃	—OH
Minocycline	—N(CH₃)₂	—H	—H
Tetracycline	—H	—CH₃	—H
* There is no —OH on the carbon attached to R₂			

C. Macrolides

	R₁	**R₂**
Azithromycin	CH₃ | —N—CH₂—	—OH
Clarithromycin	O ‖ —C—	—OCH₃
Erythromycin	O ‖ —C—	—OH

Figure 39–2. Structures of selected inhibitors of bacterial protein synthesis. Aminoglycosides **(A)** and tetracyclines **(B)** are drugs that affect the 30S ribosomal subunit. Macrolides **(C)** bind to the 50S ribosomal subunit. G = glycosidic bond.

TABLE 39–3. Bacterial Resistance to Protein Synthesis Inhibitors

Mechanism	Examples
Inactivation of the drug by bacterial enzymes	Inactivation of aminoglycosides by acetylase, adenylase, and phosphorylase enzymes Inactivation of chloramphenicol by acetyltransferase
Decreased binding of the drug	Decreased binding of aminoglycosides to the 30S ribosomal subunit Decreased binding of macrolides and clindamycin to the 50S ribosomal subunit
Decreased accumulation of the drug by bacteria	Active removal of macrolides from bacteria via membrane proteins Decreased uptake of aminoglycosides via porins in bacterial membranes Decreased uptake of tetracyclines via porins in bacterial membranes

treat serious enterococcal, staphylococcal, or viridans group streptococcal infections. Amikacin is more resistant to inactivation by acetylases, adenylases, and phosphorylases than are gentamicin and tobramycin, so it can be used to treat infections caused by organisms that are resistant to these drugs. Because amikacin is the most expensive aminoglycoside, it is generally reserved for use against organisms that are resistant to other aminoglycosides.

The aminoglycosides vary in their propensity to cause cochlear or vestibular toxicity. Amikacin produces more cochlear toxicity (deafness), whereas gentamicin and streptomycin cause more vestibular toxicity. Tobramycin appears to cause similar degrees of cochlear and vestibular toxicity.

Neomycin is the most nephrotoxic aminoglycoside, so its use is limited to topical treatment of superficial infections. Neomycin is available in ointments and creams and is usually combined with bacitracin and polymyxin in **triple antibiotic preparations** such as NEOSPORIN. Bacitracin provides gram-positive coverage, polymyxin provides gram-negative coverage, and neomycin is active against both gram-positive and gram-negative organisms. Neomycin can elicit hypersensitivity reactions, especially with long-term topical administration. Partly for this reason, products containing only bacitracin and polymyxin (e.g., POLYSPORIN) are also available and can be used by individuals who are allergic to neomycin.

Tetracyclines

The tetracyclines include **doxycycline, minocycline,** and **tetracycline.** The properties and major clinical uses of these drugs are outlined in Tables 39–1 and 39–2.

Drug Properties

CHEMISTRY AND PHARMACOKINETICS. Tetracycline antibiotics are anthracene derivatives, some of which are produced by various *Streptomyces* species. Doxycycline, minocycline, and tetracycline (see Fig. 39–2B) are semisynthetic derivatives of two older tetracycline antibiotics, chlortetracycline and oxytetracycline. As is discussed below, the various drugs in the tetracycline class are primarily distinguished by their pharmacokinetic properties.

SPECTRUM AND INDICATIONS. The tetracyclines are broad-spectrum, bacteriostatic drugs that have similar antimicrobial activities and inhibit the growth of many gram-positive and gram-negative organisms, rickettsiae, spirochetes, mycoplasmas, and chlamydiae.

Tetracyclines are the drugs of choice for **Rocky Mountain spotted fever** and other infections caused by *Rickettsia* species. They are also the drugs of choice for the treatment of two spirochetal infections, **Lyme disease** and relapsing fever, which are caused by *Borrelia burgdorferi* and *Borrelia recurrentis,* respectively. Tetracyclines can be used as alternatives to macrolides to treat infections caused by *Mycoplasma pneumoniae.* For most genital infections caused by *Chlamydia trachomatis,* the Centers for Disease Control and Prevention recommends a 7-day course of oral doxycycline. For pelvic inflammatory disease caused by chlamydiae, intravenous doxycycline may be necessary.

Tetracyclines (especially minocycline) are used in the management of **acne vulgaris** and are usually the most effective drugs for the treatment of moderately severe acne. Tetracyclines and other antibiotics are used to treat acne because they suppress the growth of *Propionibacterium acnes,* an organism found on the skin that can infect sebaceous glands. This organism converts sebum triglycerides to fatty acids, which then cause skin irritation and contribute to sebaceous gland inflammation and the formation of comedones.

Tetracyclines are used in the treatment of **brucellosis, ehrlichiosis,** and **granuloma inguinale.** Whereas oral rehydration therapy is the most important treatment modality for persons suffering from severe diarrhea caused by *Vibrio cholerae,* a tetracycline can be used to shorten the course of **cholera** and reduce the risk of disease transmission to other persons. A tetracycline is included in some regimens to treat **peptic ulcers** caused by *Helicobacter pylori.*

Although tetracyclines continue to inhibit the growth of a wide range of bacteria, they are infrequently used today to treat infections caused by many gram-positive cocci and gram-negative bacilli because strains of these organisms have become resistant.

BACTERIAL RESISTANCE. Resistance to tetracyclines, which is widespread, is caused by the transmission of plasmids containing R (resistance) factors by bacterial conjugation. The R factors usually confer resistance to tetracyclines via altered bacterial porins that prevent bacterial uptake of the drugs. The practice of including tetracyclines in **animal feeds** to promote weight gain probably contributed significantly to the development and transmission of tetracycline resistance around the world. Resistance to tetracyclines can also result from increased drug efflux, altered target binding, and enzymatic inactivation.

ADVERSE EFFECTS. Tetracyclines can cause many adverse effects, including several that are potentially life-threatening. These effects, however, can be avoided in most cases by careful screening of patients before the drugs are administered.

Tetracyclines are concentrated in growing teeth and bone. Their use by pregnant women or children under 8 years of age can cause **discoloration of the teeth** and hypoplasia of the enamel. In affected children, yellow-brown or gray mottling of a significant portion of the enamel of the front teeth occurs and is cosmetically unattractive.

Tetracyclines can cause potentially severe **nephrotoxicity** and **hepatotoxicity** in the form of fatty degeneration. Both of these reactions are rare, but the fact that pregnant women are at increased risk of hepatotoxicity is another reason for not administering tetracyclines to this population. Use of tetracyclines potentiates the nephrotoxicity of aminoglycosides and other nephrotoxic drugs and should be avoided in patients having treatment with these other drugs. Tetracyclines are slowly degraded in pharmaceutical preparations to products that are more nephrotoxic than the parent drug. For this reason, tetracycline preparations must be used or discarded by their expiration date.

Tetracyclines sometimes cause **photosensitivity** in individuals who are exposed to the sun during therapy. This adverse effect appears to result from the absorption of ultraviolet radiation by the tetracycline following its accumulation in the skin. The activated drug then emits energy at a lower frequency that damages skin tissue, leads to erythema, and either exacerbates sunburn or causes a reaction that appears similar to sunburn.

Specific Drugs

Doxycycline, minocycline, and tetracycline have similar chemical structures, spectrums, and uses. They are primarily distinguished by their pharmacokinetic properties.

The oral bioavailability of the drugs varies from about 70% for tetracycline to 90% or more for doxycycline and minocycline. All tetracyclines bind divalent and trivalent cations, including calcium, aluminum, and iron. For this reason, their oral bioavailability is reduced if they are taken with foods or drugs containing these cations. **Dairy products** reduce the oral bioavailability of tetracycline but have little effect on the bioavailability of doxycycline and minocycline. None of the tetracyclines, however, should be taken with antacids or iron supplements containing these cations.

The tetracycline drugs undergo minimal biotransformation and are excreted primarily in the urine and feces. Unlike most other tetracyclines, doxycycline is not dependent on renal elimination, and doses do not need to be adjusted in persons with renal insufficiency. It is therefore the preferred tetracycline for patients with renal failure. Minocycline is more lipophilic than are other tetracyclines, and it reaches higher concentrations in the central nervous system. This is why minocycline occasionally causes mild **vestibular toxicity,** an adverse effect usually manifested as dizziness and ataxia. Elderly persons appear to be more susceptible to this effect than are younger individuals. Doxycycline is more frequently associated with photosensitivity than are tetracycline and minocycline.

In general, minocycline and doxycycline exhibit pharmacokinetic properties that are superior to those of tetracycline, so they are often preferred for the treatment of infections. Minocycline is preferred for the treatment of **acne** because of its excellent penetration of the skin.

Other Antibiotics

Spectinomycin has an aminocyclitol structure that is similar to but chemically distinct from the structure of aminoglycoside drugs. As with the aminoglycosides, spectinomycin acts at the 30S ribosomal subunit. Although spectinomycin can be used to treat **gonorrhea** caused by **penicillinase-producing gonococci,** this type of infection is usually treated with ceftriaxone or another third-generation cephalosporin. Spectinomycin can cause nausea and produce pain at the site of injection.

DRUGS THAT AFFECT THE 50S RIBOSOMAL SUBUNIT

Macrolides

The macrolides include **azithromycin, clarithromycin,** and **erythromycin.** The properties and major clinical uses of these drugs are compared in Tables 39–1 and 39–2.

Drug Properties

CHEMISTRY AND PHARMACOKINETICS. Each macrolide antibiotic consists of a large, 14-atom lactone ring with two sugars attached to the ring (see Fig. 39–2C). Erythromycin is produced by *Saccharopolyspora erythraea* (formerly *Streptomyces erythreus*). The newer macrolides (e.g., azithromycin and clarithromycin) are semisynthetic derivatives of erythromycin. As is discussed below, the derivatives offer considerably improved pharmacokinetic properties.

SPECTRUM AND INDICATIONS. The macrolides are active against several bacteria that cause upper **respiratory tract infections** and pneumonia. They are most active against group A streptococci, pneumococci, chlamydiae, *M. pneumoniae,* and *Legionella pneumophila.* They are less active against gram-negative bacteria, such as *Klebsiella pneumoniae,* which most often cause pneumonia in neonates, elderly individuals, and chronic alcoholics.

The newer macrolides are also active against important pathogens responsible for sinusitis, otitis media, bronchitis, and other infections, and this significantly extends their clinical use. Erythromycin and azithromycin are available in intravenous formulations for the treatment of patients with severe infections.

BACTERIAL RESISTANCE. Bacterial resistance to macrolide antibiotics has gradually increased over several decades. Acquired resistance to macrolides can result from decreased binding to the 50S ribosomal subunit, enzymatic inactivation, and increased **bacterial efflux.** Most strains of staphylococci have been sensitive to macrolides, but many strains of staphylococci are now resistant. Pneumococci are increasingly resistant to macrolides. A study of over 3000 pneumococcal isolates from around the world found that 31% were resistant to erythromycin and a similar percentage was resistant to azithromycin and clarithromycin. Pneumococci expressing the **macrolide efflux (mef) A transporter** are increasingly prevalent.

ADVERSE EFFECTS. The macrolides are largely devoid of serious toxicity. Their most common adverse effects are stomatitis, heartburn, nausea, anorexia, abdominal discomfort, and diarrhea. Erythromycin binds to receptors for motilin, a gastric hormone that activates duodenal and jejunal receptors to initiate peristalsis. Activation of these receptors by erythromycin causes uncoordinated peristalsis leading to anorexia, nausea, and vomiting. Azithromycin and clarithromycin have less affinity for motilin receptors and, therefore, cause less gastrointestinal distress than does erythromycin.

Large intravenous doses of erythromycin cause ototoxicity in the form of **tinnitus** or **impaired hearing.** The ototoxic effects usually subside when use of the macrolide is discontinued. Intravenously administered erythromycin is irritating to veins and can cause thrombophlebitis. Rarely, use of a macrolide causes cholestatic hepatitis, which is probably a form of hypersensitivity and is reversible. The estolate form of erythromycin causes this reaction more frequently than do other esters or erythromycin base.

Specific Drugs

The macrolide antibiotics are usually administered orally. Erythromycin and azithromycin are also available as intravenous formulations to treat serious infections, and erythromycin can be administered topically to treat acne.

When given orally, erythromycin has a relatively low and highly variable degree of bioavailability (see Table 39–1), whereas azithromycin and clarithromycin are more reliably absorbed from the gut, have a greater degree of bioavailability, and achieve higher tissue concentrations.

Erythromycin has a shorter half-life than the newer macrolides and is administered two to four times a day. Clarithromycin is administered twice a day, and azithromycin is given once a day. The macrolides undergo variable degrees of hepatic metabolism and are primarily excreted in the bile and urine. Erythromycin and clarithromycin inhibit **cytochrome P450 isozyme 3A4** (CYP3A4) and, thereby, can elevate the plasma concentration of a large number of drugs metabolized by this isozyme. For example, concurrent administration of erythromycin or clarithromycin with carbamazepine can lead to serious, life-threatening carbamazepine toxicity, and this combination should usually be avoided. Erythromycin and clarithromycin also inhibit the metabolism of lovastatin and simvastatin, and concurrent administration of these macrolide and statin drugs can lead to elevated statin levels and rhabdomyolysis. In contrast, azithromycin has little effect on P450 drug metabolism and may be the preferred macrolide antibiotic for persons taking other drugs metabolized by CYP3A4.

As shown in Table 39–2, several macrolides are active against chlamydiae and are effective in treating pneumonia and genitourinary tract infections caused by *Chlamydia pneumoniae* and *C. trachomatis*, respectively. Indeed, azithromycin is an effective single-dose treatment for uncomplicated **chlamydial urethritis.** Azithromycin also has good activity against *Haemophilus influenzae* and can be used to treat **otitis media, sinusitis** and other respiratory tract infections caused by this organism. Either azithromycin or clarithromycin can be used to treat *Mycobacterium avium-intracellulare* infections, such as those occurring in patients with acquired immunodeficiency syndrome (AIDS). Clarithromycin is the most active macrolide against *H. pylori*, an organism that is frequently associated with **peptic ulcer disease.** As discussed in Chapter 28, clarithromycin is used in combination with amoxicillin and a gastric acid inhibitor to treat this condition.

Ketolides

Telithromycin (KETEK) is the first member of a new class of ketolide antibiotics that are structurally similar to macrolide antibiotics. As with the macrolide antibiotics, telithromycin binds to the 50S ribosomal subunit. It differs from erythromycin by ketone- and methoxy-group substitutions that make it more stable to stomach acid and that increase the drug's ribosomal binding affinity. Telithromycin is also less susceptible to bacterial export pumps than are the macrolide antibiotics.

Telithromycin has good activity against community-acquired respiratory pathogens, including multidrug-resistant strains of *Streptococcus pneumoniae*. It is also active against *Legionella* and *Chlamydia* species as well as *Haemophilus influenzae* and *Moraxella catarrhalis*. It has been approved for the treatment of acute bacterial **sinusitis,** acute exacerbations of chronic **bronchitis,** and mild-to-moderate **community-acquired pneumonia.** Clinical trials found that it has similar efficacy in these infections as amoxicillin-clavulanate and cefuroxime axetil.

Telithromycin is administered orally without regard to food and has an absolute oral bioavailability of nearly 60%. Because of its relatively long half-life (10 hours), it is given once daily for 5 to 10 days for most infections. Telithromycin is generally well tolerated, with the most common adverse effects being diarrhea and nausea. A small percentage of patients receiving the drug have exhibited elevated serum levels of hepatic enzymes and a small fraction of these persons have developed reversible hepatitis. The drug prolongs the **QT interval** of the electrocardiogram slightly and should not be taken with antiarrhythmic or other drugs that prolong the QT interval or by persons with a congenitally prolonged QT interval. Telithromycin can cause increased weakness in persons with myasthenia gravis, and it can impair visual accommodation in any person taking the drug.

Other Antibiotics

Clindamycin

Clindamycin is a semisynthetic derivative of lincomycin, an antibiotic that was isolated from a *Streptomyces* species found in soil near Lincoln, Nebraska. The two drugs are amino-sugar compounds that are structurally unrelated to other antibiotics. Because lincomycin is less active than clindamycin against most bacteria, it is no longer used.

Clindamycin is primarily active against gram-positive cocci and anaerobic organisms, such as *Bacteroides fragilis* and *Clostridium perfringens,* the cause of gas gangrene. It has gained importance as a treatment for infections caused by penicillin-resistant streptococci, including necrotizing fasciitis caused by *Streptococcus pyogenes.*

Clindamycin can be administered orally, parenterally, or topically. It is generally well tolerated, but the use of clindamycin is associated with a higher incidence of gastrointestinal superinfections caused by *Clostridium difficile* than is the use of other antibiotics. These superinfections can lead to severe diarrhea and life-threatening **pseudomembranous colitis.** In affected patients, the pseudomembrane can be observed during proctoscopic examination and consists of mucous, desquamated epithelial cells, and inflammatory cells. Persons who develop diarrhea during clindamycin therapy should discontinue use of the drug and be closely monitored for superinfection and colitis.

Chloramphenicol

CHEMISTRY. Chloramphenicol is a nitrobenzene derivative structurally unrelated to other antibiotics.

PHARMACOKINETICS AND ADVERSE EFFECTS. Because chloramphenicol is highly lipophilic, it is well absorbed from the gut and achieves high concentrations in the central nervous system, even in the absence of inflamed meninges. This property contributes to the drug's effectiveness in the treatment of meningitis.

Chloramphenicol is metabolized partly by glucuronate conjugation, and the parent drug and metabolites are excreted in the urine. In neonates, the ability to conjugate the drug is decreased because of low levels of glucuronosyltransferase. If doses of chloramphenicol are not reduced in neonates, plasma drug concentrations become excessive, and this leads to "gray baby" syndrome. The syndrome is characterized by ashen gray cyanosis, weakness, respiratory depression, hypotension, and shock.

Other adverse effects of chloramphenicol include two distinct forms of anemia. One form is a reversible, dose-dependent anemia caused by blockade of iron incorporation into heme. The blockade occurs when high plasma concentrations of the drug are reached and the activity of the enzyme **ferrochelatase** is inhibited. Another form of anemia is a potentially fatal **aplastic anemia.** This form of anemia is rare, affecting 1 of 20,000 to 40,000 individuals who are exposed to the drug. Although the exact mechanism responsible for the anemia is unknown, a hypersensitivity mechanism is suspected. Epidemiologic evidence indicates that prolonged or repeated exposure to the drug increases the incidence of chloramphenicol-induced aplastic anemia, so such exposure should be avoided. In addition, clinical reports indicate that aplastic anemia can occur after only a single topical ocular administration of chloramphenicol. Because safer antibiotics are now available, little justification exists for the use of chloramphenicol for most infections.

SPECTRUM AND INDICATIONS. Chloramphenicol is a broad-spectrum antibiotic that is active against pneumococci, meningococci, and *H. influenzae,* which are the most common pathogens causing meningitis. Chloramphenicol has also been used to treat *Salmonella* and *Bacteroides* infections. The drug can be either bacteriostatic or bactericidal, depending on the organisms and the drug concentration. Today, chloramphenicol treatment is usually reserved for treating meningitis and other infections caused by organisms that are resistant to other drugs and for infections in persons who are allergic to other, less toxic antibiotics.

Quinupristin-Dalfopristin

CHEMISTRY AND PHARMACOKINETICS. Quinupristin and dalfopristin are combined in a drug product called SYNERCID. They are members of a new class of antibacterial agents called **streptogramins.** Both of these antibiotics are semisynthetic derivatives of pristinamycin. Dalfopristin is designated a group A streptogramin, whereas quinupristin is designated a group B streptogramin. These drugs are administered intravenously, are partly converted to active metabolites, and are extensively distributed to tissues except those in the central nervous system. About 75% of the drugs is excreted in the bile.

Quinupristin and dalfopristin act synergistically to inhibit bacterial protein synthesis when they are administered in a ratio of 30 parts of quinupristin to 70 parts of dalfopristin. Quinupristin and dalfopristin bind to separate sites on the 50S ribosomal subunit and form a ternary complex with the ribosome. Quinupristin prevents the addition of new amino acids to the nascent peptide chain, partly by inhibiting the synthesis of tRNA. Dalfopristin directly blocks peptide bond formation by inhibiting peptidyl transferase in the same manner as chloramphenicol and erythromycin inhibit this enzyme.

SPECTRUM AND INDICATIONS. Quinupristin and dalfopristin are bactericidal against susceptible strains of staphylococci and streptococci, but they are usually bacteriostatic against *Enterococcus faecium.* They do not appear to exhibit synergism with β-lactam or aminoglycoside antibiotics against most strains of bacteria.

The combination quinupristin and dalfopristin is active against a wide range of gram-positive bacteria, including staphylococci that are resistant to methicillin, quinolones, and vancomycin; pneumococci that are resistant to penicillin; and *E. faecium* strains that are resistant to vancomycin. The combination has been used primarily to treat bacteremia, pneumonia, and skin and soft tissue infections caused by drug-resistant, gram-positive cocci. For example, it has been successfully used in cases of bacteremia,

peritonitis, endocarditis, or aortic graft infections that are caused by vancomycin-resistant organisms.

ADVERSE EFFECTS. Quinupristin-dalfopristin is generally well tolerated but can cause inflammation of veins, arthralgia, myalgia, diarrhea, and nausea. A few cases of elevated serum transaminase levels have been reported.

Linezolid

Linezolid (ZYVOX) is the first member of a new class of synthetic antibacterial agents called **oxazolidinediones.** Linezolid inhibits bacterial protein synthesis through a mechanism of action different from that of other antibacterial agents. It binds to a site on the bacterial 23S ribosomal RNA of the 50S subunit, and it prevents the formation of a functional 70S initiation complex, which is an essential component of the bacterial translation process. Because of its unique mechanism of action, cross-resistance between linezolid and other classes of antibiotics is unlikely.

Linezolid is active against many aerobic gram-positive bacteria, including methicillin-resistant staphylococci and vancomycin-resistant *E. faecium.* It also exhibits activity against many streptococci, including penicillin-susceptible *S. pneumoniae* and *S. pyogenes.* Bacterial time-kill studies have shown that linezolid is bacteriostatic against enterococci and staphylococci, and that it is bactericidal against most strains of streptococci.

Linezolid is indicated for the treatment of infections caused by **vancomycin-resistant *E. faecium,*** pneumonia caused by methicillin-sensitive and **methicillin-resistant *Staphylococcus aureus,*** and skin and soft tissue infections caused by methicillin-sensitive or methicillin-resistant staphylococci, *S. pyogenes,* or *S. agalactiae.* The drug is administered intravenously for serious infections and can be given orally for mild to moderate infections. Its oral bioavailability is approximately 100% and it is well distributed to highly perfused tissues. About 70% of linezolid is metabolized and the remainder is excreted unchanged in the urine.

OTHER BACTERIAL PROTEIN SYNTHESIS INHIBITORS

Mupirocin, an antibiotic obtained from *Pseudomonas fluorescens,* is structurally unrelated to all other antibiotics.

Mupirocin contains an epoxide side chain that is similar in structure to isoleucine. The drug competes with isoleucine for binding to bacterial isoleucyl tRNA synthetase, an enzyme that catalyzes the formation of isoleucyl tRNA from isoleucine and tRNA. In this manner, mupirocin prevents the addition of isoleucine to nascent peptides during protein synthesis. Because of its unique mechanism of action, it does not exhibit cross-resistance with other antimicrobial drugs.

Mupirocin is active against most staphylococci, including many strains that are resistant to methicillin. It inhibits most β-hemolytic streptococci, including most strains of *S. pyogenes.* Mupirocin is the first effective topical therapy for **impetigo** caused by streptococci or staphylococci. In cases of impetigo, it is applied as a cream to affected areas three times a day for 5 days. Mupirocin is also used to eradicate **nasal** colonization of methicillin-resistant staphylococci in infected adult patients and in health care workers. This reduces the risk of spreading infection during institutional outbreaks of this pathogen.

SUMMARY OF IMPORTANT POINTS

■ Inhibitors of bacterial protein synthesis act by selectively binding to components of the 30S or 50S ribosomal subunits. Aminoglycosides, tetracyclines, and spectinomycin inhibit 30S ribosomal function. Macrolides, clindamycin, chloramphenicol, and dalfopristin inhibit 50S ribosomal function.

■ Aminoglycosides exist as positively charged cations in body fluids. They are poorly absorbed from the gut and do not penetrate the central nervous system. They are excreted unchanged in the urine. Aminoglycosides are active against many aerobic gram-negative bacilli, including *P. aeruginosa*.

■ Tetracyclines are broad-spectrum, bacteriostatic drugs primarily used to treat infections caused by rickettsiae, chlamydiae, and mycoplasmas. They are concentrated in growing teeth and bone and can cause permanent staining of teeth if administered during pregnancy or in children under 8 years of age.

■ Most tetracyclines are excreted primarily in the urine, but doxycycline is excreted by other routes and can be used without dosage adjustment in patients with renal failure.

■ Macrolides, which are active against most pathogens causing respiratory tract infections, are used to treat otitis media and pneumonia caused by pneumococci, chlamydiae, *M. pneumoniae*, and *L. pneumophila*. Azithromycin is particularly effective against *H. influenzae*, whereas clarithromycin is active against *H. pylori* and can be used in the treatment of peptic ulcer disease.

■ Telithromycin is a ketolide antibiotic active against pathogens causing respiratory tract infections.

■ Clindamycin, which is active against gram-positive cocci, is useful in treating infections caused by gram-positive cocci and anaerobes that are resistant to penicillin and other drugs. It causes a higher incidence of pseudomembranous colitis than do other antibiotics.

■ Chloramphenicol is used to treat meningitis when other antibiotics cannot be used. It rarely causes aplastic anemia.

■ Quinupristin-dalfopristin and linezolid are active against gram-positive cocci, including methicillin and vancomycin-resistant staphylococci and vancomycin-resistant enterococci.

■ Mupirocin is active against streptococci and staphylococci. It is administered topically to treat impetigo and to eradicate nasal carriers of methicillin-resistant staphylococci.

Review Questions

For each numbered antimicrobial agent described, select the corresponding drug from the lettered choices.

1. This drug's relatively high oral bioavailability, long elimination half-life, and high tissue levels enable it to be given once daily for 5 days to treat upper respiratory tract infections.

2. It is the preferred drug for treating most rickettsial infections, including Rocky Mountain spotted fever.

3. It provides an effective topical therapy for superficial streptococcal and staphylococcal infections.

4. It is active against many Enterobacteriaceae and some strains of *Pseudomonas aeruginosa*, but lacks activity against anaerobic bacteria.

5. It can be administered orally or intravenously to treat infections caused by drug-resistant, gram-positive cocci.

  (A) tobramycin
  (B) telithromycin
  (C) azithromycin
  (D) doxycycline
  (E) clindamycin
  (F) mupirocin
  (G) doxycycline
  (H) linezolid

Answers and Explanations

1. The answer is C: azithromycin. Macrolides are active against most pathogens causing respiratory tract infections, although some pneumococcal resistance has emerged. Azithromycin has good oral bioavailability, a long half-life, and achieves high levels in respiratory tract tissues and secretions. For these reasons, it is often used to treat upper respiratory tract infections.

2. The answer is G: doxycycline. Tetracyclines such as doxycycline are used to treat ricketsial infections as well as infections caused by *Ehrlichia* species (which are related to *Rickettsia*). Other infections treated with tetracyclines include brucellosis, cholera, and Lyme disease.

3. The answer is F: mupirocin. Mupirocin is the first topical treatment for impetigo, which is usually caused by streptococcal or staphylococcal species. Systemically administered antibiotics for this infection include cloxacillin and dicloxacillin.

4. The answer is A: tobramycin. Aminoglycoside antibiotics (e.g., gentamicin and tobramycin) are active against a wide range of aerobic gram-negative bacilli but are not active against anaerobes. This is because aminoglycosides use an oxygen-dependent transport system to enter bacteria.

5. The answer is H: linezolid. Linezolid is an oxazolidinone drug that has activity against drug-resistant staphylococci and enterococci. It has nearly 100% oral bioavailability and can be given orally or intravenously. Other drugs for treating infections caused by resistant gram-positive

organisms include quinupristin-dalfopristin and dapto-mycin (Chapter 40).

SELECTED READINGS

Kauffman, C. A. Therapeutic and preventative options for the management of vancomycin-resistant enterococcal infections. J Antimicrob Chemother 51(Suppl)S3:iii23–iii30, 2003.

Southern, K. W., and P. M. Barker. Azithromycin for cystic fibrosis. Eur Resp J 24:834–838, 2004.

Wellington, K., and S. Noble. Telithromycin. Drugs 64:1683–1694, 2004.

Zhanel, G. G., T. Hisanaga, K. Nichol, et al. Ketolides: an emerging treatment for macrolide-resistant respiratory infections, focusing on S. pneumoniae. Expert Opin Emerging Drugs 8:297–321, 2003.

CHAPTER 40

Quinolones, Antifolate Drugs, and Other Antimicrobial Agents

CLASSIFICATION OF QUINOLONES, ANTIFOLATE DRUGS, AND OTHER ANTIMICROBIAL AGENTS

Antifolate Drugs
- Sulfamethoxazole[a]
- Trimethoprim
- Trimethoprim-sulfamethoxazole (BACTRIM, SEPTRA)

Fluoroquinolones
- Ciprofloxacin (CIPRO)[b]
- Levofloxacin (LEVAQUIN)[c]

Other Antibacterial Agents
- Nitrofurantoin (MACRODANTIN)
- Daptomycin (CUBICIN)
- Polymyxin B
- Rifaximin (XIFAXAN)

[a]also sulfacetamide, sulfisoxazole, sulfadiazine.
[b]also norfloxacin, ofloxacin, sparfloxacin.
[c]also gatifloxacin (TEQUIN), gemifloxacin (FACTIVE), moxifloxacin (AVELOX).

ANTIFOLATE DRUGS

There are two basic groups of antifolate drugs. Members of the first group, the **sulfonamides,** selectively inhibit the synthesis of dihydrofolate. Members of the second group, the **folate reductase inhibitors,** block the action of dihydrofolate reductase and the formation of tetrahydrofolate in various organisms. This second group includes the following: **pyrimethamine,** which inhibits folate reduction in some protozoa, is primarily used to treat toxoplasmosis and malaria, and is discussed in Chapter 44; **methotrexate,** which inhibits folate reduction in mammalian cells, is used in the treatment of neoplastic and autoimmune diseases, and is discussed in Chapter 45; and **trimethoprim,** which selectively blocks folate reduction in bacteria and is discussed later.

Mechanisms of Action

Bacterial synthesis of folate begins with the fusion of pteridine and *p*-aminobenzoic acid (PABA) to form **dihydrofolate.** This step involves the enzyme **dihydropteroate synthase.** Dihydrofolate is then converted to **tetrahydrofolate** in a reaction involving **folate reductase.**

In bacteria, the sulfonamides and trimethoprim inhibit sequential steps in the synthesis of folate (Fig. 40–1). The

sulfonamides are structural analogues of PABA. They act by competitively inhibiting dihydropteroate synthase, and their effects can be counteracted by the administration of PABA. Trimethoprim acts by inhibiting folate reductase.

In mammalian cells, dihydrofolate synthesis does not occur, so humans must obtain folic acid as a vitamin in food. As discussed in Chapter 17, however, folate reduction is a necessary step in the formation of active folate derivatives (methyl, formyl, and methylene tetrahydrofolate) that donate single-carbon atoms during the synthesis of purine bases and other components of DNA. Although folate reductase is found in microbial and mammalian cells, the affinity of trimethoprim for the enzyme in bacteria is about 100,000 times greater than the affinity of the drug for the enzyme in mammalian cells.

Trimethoprim is often administered in combination with sulfamethoxazole. One reason is that their inhibition of sequential steps in bacterial folate synthesis produces a synergistic effect against susceptible organisms. Another reason is that together the drugs sometimes exhibit bactericidal activity against organisms that are not susceptible to either drug when given alone.

Sulfonamides

In the 1930s, sulfanilamide was found to be the active metabolite of Prontosil, a dye that had been developed in the

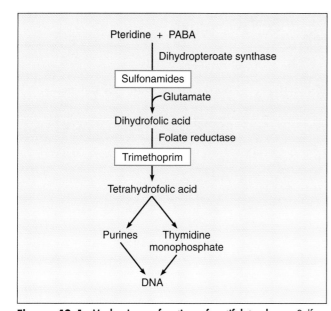

Figure 40–1. Mechanisms of action of antifolate drugs. Sulfonamides inhibit the action of dihydropteroate synthase and thereby block the synthesis of dihydrofolate. Trimethoprim inhibits the action of dihydrofolate reductase and thereby blocks the formation of tetrahydrofolate. PABA = p-aminobenzoic acid.

Figure 40–2. Structures of selected sulfonamides (A) and a fluoroquinolone (B). The sulfonamides are analogues of p-aminobenzoic acid (PABA). Sulfamethoxazole (a sulfonamide) is often given in combination with trimethoprim (a folate reductase inhibitor). The fluoroquinolone moiety of ciprofloxacin is unshaded.

search for bacterial stains with antimicrobial properties. This discovery led to the synthesis and development of a large number of sulfonamide compounds that are used to treat human infections. Examples include **sulfacetamide**, **sulfamethoxazole**, and **sulfisoxazole**.

Drug Properties

CHEMISTRY AND PHARMACOKINETICS. The structures of several sulfonamides are shown in Fig. 40–2A. Each drug is a substituted benzene sulfonic acid amide derivative.

Some sulfonamides are available in topical ocular preparations, and others are administered orally or parenterally. Most oral compounds are adequately absorbed from the gut and are widely distributed to tissues and fluids throughout the body, including the cerebrospinal fluid. The half-lives of sulfonamides vary greatly (Table 40–1), but the most widely used compounds for treating human infections have half-lives ranging from 6 to 10 hours.

Sulfonamides are converted to inactive compounds by N-acetylation, and the parent drug and its metabolites are excreted in the urine. The acetylated metabolites are less soluble than the parent compound in urine, and they can precipitate in the renal tubules, causing **crystalluria**. Therefore, it is important for patients who are being treated with a sulfonamide to consume adequate quantities of water.

SPECTRUM, INDICATIONS, AND BACTERIAL RESISTANCE. The sulfonamides were the first drugs used in the treatment of systemic bacterial infections. They were once active against a wide variety of organisms, including streptococci, gonococci, meningococci, many gram-negative bacilli, and chlamydiae. Over the years, however, significant resistance to sulfonamides has developed in many species, and the effective clinical spectrum of these drugs has been greatly curtailed. Today, sulfonamides are primarily used to prevent or treat urinary tract infections. (Table 40–2).

ADVERSE EFFECTS. In some patients, sulfonamides cause skin rashes, which are hypersensitivity reactions that can remain mild or progress to a serious or life-threatening form, such as erythema multiforme or Stevens-Johnson syndrome. Other adverse effects of sulfonamides include crystalluria (discussed previously), gastrointestinal reactions, headaches, hepatitis, and hematopoietic toxicity. In persons with glucose-6-phosphate dehydrogenase deficiency, sulfonamides can cause hemolytic anemia.

TABLE 40–1. **Pharmacokinetic Properties of Selected Antifolate Drugs, Fluoroquinolones, and Other Agents***

Drug	Route of Administration	Oral Bioavailability (%)	Elimination Half-Life (Hours)	Routes of Elimination
Antifolate drugs				
Sulfacetamide	Topical	NA	10	Metabolism; renal excretion
Sulfamethoxazole	Oral	≈100	10	Metabolism; renal excretion
Sulfisoxazole	Oral	≈100	6	Metabolism; renal excretion
Trimethoprim	Oral	≈100	10	Metabolism; renal excretion
Trimethoprim-sulfamethoxazole	Oral or IV	≈100	10	Metabolism; renal excretion
Fluoroquinolones				
Ciprofloxacin	Oral, IV, or topical	75	4	Metabolism; renal excretion
Levofloxacin	Oral or IV	99	8	Metabolism; renal excretion
Norfloxacin	Oral	35	3.5	Metabolism; renal excretion
Moxifloxacin	Oral	90	12	Metabolism; renal excretion
Gatifloxacin	Oral	96	7.5	Metabolism; renal excretion
Other antibacterial drugs				
Nitrofurantoin	Oral	87	0.5	Metabolism; renal excretion
Polymyxin B	IV or topical	NA	5	NA
Daptomycin	IV	NA	9	Renal excretion

*Values shown are the mean of values reported in the literature. IV = intravenous; and NA = not applicable.

TABLE 40–2. **Major Clinical Uses of Selected Fluoroquinolones, Antifolate Drugs, and Other Antibacterial Drugs**

Drug	Major Clinical Uses
Fluoroquinolones	
Ciprofloxacin	Bacterial diarrhea; intra-abdominal infections; infections of the urinary tract, prostate, bone and joints, skin, and eye; anthrax exposure
Levofloxacin	Bronchitis and community-acquired pneumonia; infections of the urinary tract, prostate, skin, and eye
Gatifloxacin, gemifloxacin, moxifloxacin	Community-acquired pneumonia, sinusitis, bronchitis
Norfloxacin	Urinary tract infections
Antifolate Drugs	
Trimethoprim-sulfamethoxazole	Urinary tract and prostatic infections; pulmonary infections caused by *Pneumocystis jiroveci (carinii)* and *Nocardia* species
Silver sulfadiazine	Burn infections, other skin infections
Sulfacetamide	Ocular infections
Other antibacterial drugs	
Nitrofurantoin	Lower urinary tract (bladder) infections
Polymyxin B	Superficial infections of skin and mucous membranes
Daptomycin	Infections due to methicillin- or vancomycin-resistant staphylococci or vancomycin-resistant enterococci

Specific Drugs

Sulfisoxazole or sulfamethoxazole can be used to prevent urinary tract infections or to treat uncomplicated infections of the urinary tract caused by susceptible organisms. Sulfamethoxazole is usually administered in combination with trimethoprim (see later text).

Sulfadiazine is available in the form of **silver sulfadiazine** ointment to prevent or treat **burn infections** and other superficial skin infections. The silver ions in this preparation have antibacterial activity and contribute to its utility in these infections.

Sulfacetamide is administered topically to treat blepharitis and conjunctivitis, **ocular infections** that are common throughout the world. It is also effective in treating **trachoma,** a highly contagious ocular infection that is caused by *Chlamydia trachomatis* and is prevalent in Asia and the Middle East.

Folate Reductase Inhibitors

Trimethoprim

Trimethoprim is a synthetic aminopyrimidine drug. It is well absorbed from the gut and is widely distributed to tissues. After it undergoes extensive hepatic metabolism, the parent compound and metabolites are excreted in the urine.

Trimethoprim is a weak base. It is concentrated in prostatic tissues and vaginal fluids because they are more acidic than plasma. This makes trimethoprim useful in the treatment of bacterial prostatitis and vaginitis.

Trimethoprim is active against a wide variety of aerobic gram-negative bacilli and a few gram-positive organisms. It is usually administered in combination with sulfamethoxazole to prevent or treat urinary tract infections (see later text), but it can be used alone for these purposes.

The adverse effects of trimethoprim include nausea, vomiting, and epigastric distress; rashes and other hypersensitivity reactions; hepatitis; and thrombocytopenia, leukopenia, and other hematologic disorders.

Trimethoprim-Sulfamethoxazole

PHARMACOKINETICS. Sulfamethoxazole is the sulfonamide commonly used in combination with trimethoprim because it has a similar half life (10 hours). In vitro tests have shown that the maximal synergistic activity of the two drugs against microbes occurs when the concentration of sulfamethoxazole is 20 times greater than the concentration of trimethoprim. To obtain plasma drug concentrations in a ratio of 20 : 1, the drugs are administered in a ratio of 5 parts of sulfamethoxazole to 1 part of trimethoprim. The 5 : 1 dose ratio produces a 20 : 1 plasma concentration ratio because trimethoprim has a greater volume of distribution than does sulfamethoxazole.

SPECTRUM AND INDICATIONS. Trimethoprim-sulfamethoxazole (TMP-SMX) is active against some members of the family **Enterobacteriaceae,** including some strains of *Escherichia coli, Klebsiella pneumoniae, Proteus* species, and *Enterobacter* species. TMP-SMX is often used to prevent or treat **urinary tract and prostate infections** caused by these organisms. Because of increased bacterial resistance to TMP-SMX, it is not recommended for the empiric treatment of urinary tract infections in locations where greater than 30% of *E. coli* isolates are resistant to TMP-SMX. In these locations, fosfomycin, nitrofurantoin, or a fluoroquinolone drug can be used to treat these infections. TMP-SMX is not active against *Pseudomonas aeruginosa,* a common cause of urinary tract infections in hospitalized patients.

TMP-SMX is the drug of choice for treating pulmonary infections caused by **Pneumocystis jiroveci (carinii)** and **Nocardia asteroides,** which most often occur in immunocompromised patients. TMP-SMX is active against *Burkholderia cepacia* and some strains of *Haemophilus* influenzae and *Moraxella catarrhalis.*

TMP-SMX is active against some strains of *Salmonella* and *Shigella,* but other strains are resistant. Currently, a fluoroquinolone (see below) is usually preferred to treat most infections caused by these organisms.

ADVERSE EFFECTS. The adverse effects of TMP-SMX are similar to those of the individual drugs. TMP-SMX can cause megaloblastic anemia in persons who have a low dietary intake of folic acid, but this adverse effect is uncommon.

FLUOROQUINOLONES

The original quinolone antibacterial drug, nalidixic acid, has limited activity against gram-negative bacteria. Successive modifications of the structure of nalidixic acid led to the development of a number of fluoroquinolone drugs with improved antimicrobial activity and pharmacokinetic properties.

The fluoroquinolone drugs can be subdivided into two groups. The **original fluoroquinolones** (e.g., **ciprofloxacin**) have excellent activity against a wide range of gram-negative bacteria but limited activity against many gram-positive cocci, including pneumococci. The **advanced generation fluoroquinolones,** including **levofloxacin, moxifloxacin, gatifloxacin** and **gemifloxacin,** have good active against pnuemococci while retaining activity against gram-negative organisms.

Drug Properties

CHEMISTRY AND MECHANISMS. The structure of a representative fluoroquinolone, ciprofloxacin, is depicted in Fig. 40–2B. The fluorine moiety increases its antibacterial potency and binding affinity for DNA gyrase.

Fluoroquinolones act by inhibiting two types of bacterial **DNA topoisomerase: type II topoisomerase,** which is also called **DNA gyrase,** and **type IV topoisomerase.** The topoisomerase enzymes are essential for maintaining DNA in a stable and biologically active form. DNA gyrase introduces **negative supercoils** (superhelical twists) into closed circular bacterial DNA. These negative supercoils eliminate the **positive supercoils** that occur ahead of the DNA replication fork during DNA replication. DNA replication cannot proceed without DNA gyrase activity. As shown in Fig. 40–3, DNA gyrase produces supercoiling by breaking doubled-stranded DNA, moving another section of double-stranded DNA through the break, and then resealing the broken strands of DNA. DNA gyrase is a tetramer composed of two A and two B subunits. Fluoroquinolones selectively bind to the A subunits, which contain the catalytic site of the breaking and resealing reactions.

Type IV topoisomerase is responsible for separating the DNA of daughter chromosomes once DNA replication is completed. This process is called **decatenation.** In general, DNA gyrase is the primary target of fluoroquinolones in gram-negative bacteria, whereas topoisomerase IV is the primary target in gram-positive organisms.

PHARMACOKINETICS. Fluoroquinolones have attractive pharmacokinetic properties and can be given orally to treat infections that formerly required parenteral therapy with other antibacterial drugs (see Table 40–2). Some fluoroquinolones (e.g., ciprofloxacin and levofloxacin) can also be administered intravenously, and topical formulations of these and other fluoroquinolones are available to treat **ocular infections.**

When given orally, fluoroquinolones are well absorbed from the gut and are widely distributed to tissues. In addition to being available for oral use, some fluoroquinolones

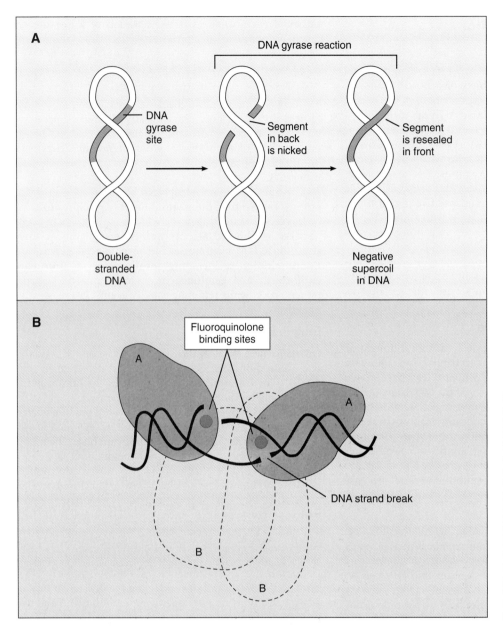

Figure 40–3. Effect of fluoroquinolones on DNA gyrase. **(A)** In the absence of fluoroquinolones, DNA gyrase catalyzes the formation of negative supercoils in the double-stranded DNA of bacteria. After both strands of one segment are nicked, the broken strands are passed across the other strands of DNA and then are resealed. This reaction requires energy in the form of adenosine triphosphate (ATP). **(B)** DNA gyrase is a tetramer composed of two A subunits and two B subunits. Fluoroquinolones inhibit DNA gyrase by binding to the catalytic sites on the A subunits. ATP binds to the B subunits.

are available for intravenous or topical ocular administration. Fluoroquinolone concentrations in many tissues, including the lungs, kidneys, liver, gallbladder, prostate, endometrium, fallopian tubes, and ovaries, are greater than concentrations in the plasma. For example, levofloxacin concentrations in lung tissue are two to five times greater than those in the plasma. Fluoroquinolones have relatively long elimination half-lives and a long **postantibiotic effect,** with some organisms failing to resume growth for 2 to 6 hours after drug levels are no longer detectable. For these reasons, they are usually administered once or twice a day.

As with the tetracyclines, the fluoroquinolones chelate **divalent and trivalent cations,** including calcium, iron, magnesium, and zinc. Therefore, fluoroquinolones should be taken 2 hours before or 2 hours after ingesting dairy products, drugs, or nutritional supplements containing these cations.

Fluoroquinolones undergo varying degrees of hepatic biotransformation, and they are excreted unchanged in the urine, along with their metabolites. Some metabolites have low levels of antimicrobial activity, but these metabolites probably do not contribute significantly to the clinical efficacy of the drugs. Fluoroquinolones inhibit the hepatic metabolism of caffeine and theophylline and can thereby increase their serum levels (see later text).

SPECTRUM AND INDICATIONS. Fluoroquinolones show **bactericidal activity** against a broad spectrum of aerobic gram-positive and gram-negative bacteria, and acid-fast bacilli. These drugs also exhibit **concentration-dependent killing,** and higher peak serum concentrations result in more rapid and complete killing of susceptible organisms. It appears that maximal bacterial killing occurs when the ratio of the peak serum drug level to the organism's minimal inhibitory concentration (MIC) is at least 10. A peak drug level to MIC ratio of 10 is also required to prevent emergence of bacterial resistance.

The fluoroquinolones are highly effective in eradicating organisms that cause **urinary tract infections and prostatitis,** including *P. aeruginosa* and many members of the family **Enterobacteriaceae.** Some fluoroquinolones are also active against enterococci. Fluoroquinolones can kill several bacterial species that cause **bacterial diarrhea,** including *Campylobacter, Salmonella,* and *Shigella* species, as well as *Yersinia enterocolitica.* The drugs are also effective in treating traveler's diarrhea, which is often caused by enterotoxigenic strains of *E. coli.* Fluoroquinolones are used in combination with other drugs to treat patients with intra-abdominal infections, bone and joint infections, skin infections, and patients with febrile neutropenia. Ciprofloxacin is also indicated to treat **anthrax** and for postexposure prophylaxis of inhalational anthrax, such as might occur in a **bioterrorism event.**

Advanced fluoroquinolones, including **levofloxacin, moxifloxacin, gatifloxacin,** and **gemifloxacin,** have had a growing role in the treatment of respiratory tract infections. They are used to treat sinusitis and bronchitis caused by pneumococci, *H. influenzae,* or *M. catarrhalis.* They are also approved for the treatment of **community-acquired pneumonia** caused by pneumococci, *Chlamydia pneumoniae, K. pneumoniae, Mycoplasma pneumoniae,* and *Legionella pneumophila.* They are also active against mycobacteria and are used in the treatment of *Mycobacterium avium-intracellulare* infections (see Chapter 41). Fluoroquinolones achieve high concentrations in neutrophils, and this contributes to their effectiveness in patients with mycobacterial infections. Advanced fluoroquinolones are also indicated for treating **ocular infections.**

BACTERIAL RESISTANCE. Resistance to fluoroquinolone drugs develops through two primary mechanisms: alterations in the target enzymes (topoisomerases) and alterations in drug access to the target enzymes. Alterations in bacterial DNA gyrase occur most commonly in gram-negative bacteria, whereas alterations in type IV topoisomerase are more prevalent in gram-positive organisms. Resistance by DNA gyrase mutations is usually caused by decreased affinity of the A subunit of DNA gyrase for the drugs, but B subunit mutations can also lead to resistance. Topoisomerase IV mutations also lead to reduced fluoroquinolone binding affinity.

Resistance to fluoroquinolones can also occur through expression of membrane transport proteins or **efflux pumps** that actively transport a number of antibacterial agents out of bacterial cells, and thereby confer **multidrug resistance.** In addition, some gram-negative bacteria have decreased levels of **porins** in their outer membrane, resulting in decreased fluoroquinolone uptake by these bacteria.

ADVERSE EFFECTS AND INTERACTIONS. Fluoroquinolones are generally well tolerated. Because they have been found to cause **arthropathy** and **osteochondrosis** in juvenile animals, the drugs are usually not administered to persons less than 18 years of age. The drugs have been used safely, however, to treat serious *P. aeruginosa* infections in children with cystic fibrosis.

Fluoroquinolones inhibit the metabolism of caffeine and theophylline. In a few cases, seizures have occurred in persons who consumed large quantities of caffeine while taking a fluoroquinolone. Patients having fluoroquinolone therapy should be advised to reduce their intake of caffeine to avoid excessive central nervous system stimulation. Because serum levels of theophylline can rise during fluoroquinolone therapy, doses of theophylline may need to be reduced.

Specific Drugs

The individual fluoroquinolone drugs differ in their antimicrobial activity and pharmacokinetic profile (see Table 40–1).

Norfloxacin has a relatively short half-life and is rapidly excreted in the urine. It is indicated only for the treatment of urinary tract infections. Ciprofloxacin has a half-life of 4 hours and is usually administered every 12 hours. Advanced fluoroquinolones (e.g., levofloxacin, gatifloxacin, gemifloxacin, and moxifloxacin) have half-lives ranging from 7 to 12 hours and are given once every 24 hours to treat most infections.

OTHER ANTIBACTERIAL DRUGS

Nitrofurantoin

As with norfloxacin (a fluoroquinolone discussed above), nitrofurantoin (MACRODANTIN) is an example of a **urinary tract antiseptic.** The antibacterial activity of these antiseptics is localized to the urinary bladder.

Nitrofurantoin is a synthetic nitrofuran derivative. It is administered orally, and ingesting it with food enhances its absorption and reduces the risk of gastrointestinal irritation. Once absorbed from the gut, the drug is rapidly excreted in the urine.

Nitrofurantoin is bactericidal against gram-positive and gram-negative bacteria that commonly cause acute lower urinary tract infections, including *E. coli, Enterococcus faecalis, K. pneumoniae,* and *Staphylococcus saprophyticus.* Nitrofurantoin, however, is not active against *Proteus* species, *Serratia* species, or *P. aeruginosa.* Acquired microbial resistance to nitrofurantoin has generally not been a significant clinical problem.

Nitrofurantoin is usually well tolerated, but it can cause gastrointestinal irritation, nausea, vomiting, and diarrhea. To avoid these adverse effects, a **macrocrystalline formulation** of the drug is usually administered. The large crystals of drug in this formulation dissolve slowly in the gut, producing less gastrointestinal distress than do other formulations. Less common adverse effects of nitrofurantoin include pulmonary fibrosis, hepatitis, and hematologic toxicity.

Daptomycin

Daptomycin (CUBICIN), a **cyclic lipopeptide,** is the first antibiotic in its class. Daptomycin exerts its rapid bactericidal effect by disrupting **plasma membrane function** without penetrating into the cytoplasm. This antibiotic has received much interest because of its activity against **drug-resistant, gram-positive bacteria** such as methicillin-resistant

Staphylococcus aureus, vancomycin intermediate and resistant *S. aureus,* and vancomycin-resistant enterococci. Daptomycin has been approved for the treatment of skin and skin-structure infections that are a complication of surgery, diabetic foot ulcers, and burns. The use of daptomycin in treating systemic infections is currently under investigation. Other agents used to treat infections caused by drug-resistant, gram-positive organisms include quinupristin-dalfopristin and linezolid (Chapter 39).

Daptomycin is administered intravenously once a day. Its adverse effects appear to be minimal and manageable.

Polymyxin B

Polymyxin B is a drug often found in creams or ointments containing bacitracin, neomycin, or trimethoprim. The preparations are applied topically for skin and ocular infections.

Polymyxin B is a polypeptide antibiotic that interacts with the phospholipid component of bacterial cell membranes to disrupt cell membrane integrity and permit cytoplasmic components to leak out of the cell. Polymyxin is active against most gram-negative bacilli except *Proteus* species, but it produces considerable nephrotoxicity when given parenterally. Although the drug has been used to treat systemic infections caused by these organisms, safer drugs are now available for parenteral use.

Rifaximin

Rifaximin (XIFAXAN) is a nonabsorbed, oral antibiotic derived from rifampin (see Chapter 41). It is used to treat **travelers' diarrhea** in patients 12 years of age or older. Travelers' diarrhea is usually a self-limited illness lasting several days that is acquired by drinking water or eating foods contaminated with various intestinal bacteria. The most common causes are enterotoxigenic or enteroaggregative strains of *E. coli.* Less commonly, strains of *Salmonella, Shigella, Campylobacter,* or other species are responsible. For mild to moderate travelers' diarrhea, nonprescription loperamide (IMODIUM) or bismuth subsalicylate (PEPTOBISMOL) usually relieve symptoms in less than 24 hours.

Rifaximin is active against noninvasive strains of *E. coli* and some *Salmonella* and *Shigella* species, but it is much less active against *Campylobacter jejuni* and *Yersinia enterocolitica.* The results of clinical trials indicate that rifaximin is about as effective as ciprofloxacin for travelers' diarrhea caused by *E. coli* but that it is not effective in patients with fever or blood in the stool, or in persons infected with *C. jejuni.* Rifaximin produces few adverse effects, but it is not currently recommended for pregnant women.

SUMMARY OF IMPORTANT POINTS

■ Sulfonamides and trimethoprim inhibit sequential steps in bacterial folic acid synthesis. Sulfonamides inhibit dihydropteroate synthase and the synthesis of dihydrofolate, whereas trimethoprim inhibits folate reductase and the formation of tetrahydrofolate.

■ The combination of sulfamethoxazole and trimethoprim (TMP-SMX) is primarily used to treat urinary tract infections, upper respiratory tract infections, and infections caused by *P. carinii* or *N. asteroides.*

■ Fluoroquinolones inhibit DNA gyrase and have bactericidal activity against a wide range of pathogens. Many fluoroquinolones, including ciprofloxacin, are used to treat a variety of infections, including urinary tract and gastrointestinal tract infections, bone and joint infections, skin infections, and anthrax exposure.

■ Advanced fluoroquinolones (e.g., levofloxacin) are also used to treat community-acquired pneumonia.

■ Because of the risk of arthropathy and osteochondrosis, fluoroquinolones are usually not used in children.

■ Nitrofurantoin is a urinary tract antiseptic that is effective in the treatment of uncomplicated urinary tract infections.

■ Polymyxin B is primarily used in combination with other drugs to treat superficial ocular and skin infections.

■ Daptomycin, a unique lipopeptide antibiotic, is used to treat infections caused by methicillin and vancomycin-resistant staphylococci and vancomycin-resistant enterococci.

Review Questions

1. Which drug is most often used to treat pneumonia caused by *Pneumocystis jiroveci* or *Nocardia asteroides?*
   (A) daptomycin
   (B) ciprofloxacin
   (C) nitrofurantoin
   (D) trimethoprim-sulfamethoxazole
   (E) polymyxin B

2. Which antimicrobial agent is active against many strains of vancomycin-resistant enterococci?
   (A) polymyxin B
   (B) daptomycin
   (C) trimethoprim-sulfamethoxazole
   (D) nitrofurantoin
   (E) ciprofloxacin

3. Which antimicrobial agent would most likely be effective in treating a urinary tract infection caused by *Pseudomonas aeruginosa?*
   (A) trimethoprim
   (B) nitrofurantoin
   (C) daptomycin
   (D) levofloxacin
   (E) sulfamethoxazole

4. Concurrent administration of iron or zinc preparations can interfere with the absorption of which drug?
   (A) ciprofloxacin
   (B) sulfamethoxazole
   (C) daptomycin
   (D) polymyxin B
   (E) nitrofurantoin

Answers and Explanations

1. The answer is D: trimethoprim-sulfamethoxazole. Pneumonia caused by *Nocardia asteroides* or *Pneumocystis jiroveci (carinii)* is most likely to occur in immunocompromised persons, and is often treated with trimethoprim-sulfamethoxazole. Treatment of these infections can require several weeks to several months of drug administration.

2. The answer is B: daptomycin. Daptomycin is a unique lipopeptide antibiotic that is active against many drug-resistant strains of gram-positive cocci, including methicillin-resistant staphylococci and vancomycin-resistant enterococci.

3. The answer is D: levofloxacin. Fluoroquinolones such as levofloxacin are active against many strains of *Pseudomonas aeruginosa*, whereas sulfonamides, trimethoprim, nitrofurantoin, and daptomycin are not active against this pathogen.

4. The answer is A: ciprofloxacin. Fluoroquinolones such as ciprofloxacin bind to cations in the gut. Concurrent administration of fluoroquinolones with antacids, iron salts, bismuth preparations, and zinc salts decreases the absorption of fluoroquinolones.

SELECTED READINGS

Blondeau, J. M. Fluoroquinolones: mechanism of action, classification, and development of resistance. Surv Ophthalmol 49(Suppl 2):S73–S78, 2004.

Mofenson, L. M., J. Oleske, L. Serchuck, et al. Treating opportunistic infections among HIV infected children. MMWR 53(RR14):1–63, 2004.

O'Donnell, J. A., and S. P. Gelone. The newer fluoroquinolones. Infect Dis Clin N Am 18:691–716, 2004.

CHAPTER 41

Antimycobacterial Drugs

CLASSIFICATION OF ANTIMYCOBACTERIAL DRUGS*

Drugs for Tuberculosis
- Isoniazid
- Rifampin[a]
- Ethambutol
- Pyrazinamide
- Streptomycin
- Amikacin

Drugs for *Mycobacterium avium-intracellulare* Infections
- Azithromycin[b]

Drugs for Leprosy
- Dapsone
- Rifampin
- Clofazimine
- Thalidomide

[a]also rifabutin and rifapentine.
[b]also clarithromycin, ciprofloxacin, ethambutol, rifabutin, and amikacin.

MYCOBACTERIAL INFECTIONS

Mycobacteria are acid-fast bacilli that cause a variety of diseases, including tuberculosis, leprosy, and localized or disseminated *Mycobacterium avium-intracellulare* infections.

Tuberculosis is caused by *Mycobacterium tuberculosis.* Atypical mycobacteria (e.g., *Mycobacterium kansasii* and members of the *M. avium-intracellulare* complex [MAC]) can cause infections resembling tuberculosis. It is estimated that about one third of the world's population is infected with *M. tuberculosis*. In the United States of America (USA), the incidence of tuberculosis underwent a steady decline from the 1960s through the mid 1980s, owing to public health measures and the availability of effective drug therapy. This trend was reversed temporarily during the late 1980s partly because the incidence of acquired immunodeficiency syndrome (AIDS) was rising and tuberculosis was frequently found in patients with AIDS. At the same time, an increased incidence of tuberculosis occurred among economically disadvantaged persons and immigrants, and this increase was associated with the development of increased drug resistance by tubercular organisms.

Although the incidence of tuberculosis has declined in this decade, the treatment of tuberculosis poses a greater challenge to clinicians than it did a few decades ago. The treatment of active tuberculosis requires at least 6 months of **multidrug therapy** to eradicate the pathogen and prevent the emergence of resistant strains. Isolation of patients with tuberculosis in single-person rooms is essential until sputum cultures are negative, and extended isolation may be required to prevent the spread of drug-resistant strains. Because of the long duration of treatment and difficulties with patient compliance, **directly observed therapy** (DOT) has been used in treating some patients with tuberculosis. In DOT programs, a health care provider observes each drug administration to ensure compliance with the treatment regimen.

M. avium-intracellulare infections are seen most frequently in immunocompromised patients (e.g., those with AIDS) and often take the form of **pulmonary disease, lymphadenitis,** or **bacteremia.** In immunocompetent persons with chronic bronchitis or emphysema, exposure to *M. avium-intracellulare* can also result in pulmonary infections.

Leprosy is relatively common in many parts of the world. Also called **Hansen's disease,** leprosy results from infection of the skin and peripheral nervous system with *Mycobacterium leprae*. Because *M. leprae* grows so slowly, the disease exhibits a slow, progressive course over several decades. Contrary to popular opinion, leprosy is not highly contagious, and transmission of infection usually requires prolonged close contact with an infected individual. The disease occurs in two primary forms, **lepromatous leprosy** and **tuberculoid leprosy,** each of which has a characteristic pathophysiology and clinical presentation. If leprosy is not treated, it ultimately causes severe deformities and disabilities. Treatment of leprosy can require years of therapy with antimycobacterial agents, although the introduction of newer drugs has enabled the use of shorter courses of therapy for many patients.

DRUGS FOR MYCOBACTERIAL INFECTIONS

Drugs for Tuberculosis

Drugs initially used to treat most patients with tuberculosis are referred to as **first-line drugs.** They include the following: **isoniazid, ethambutol,** and **pyrazinamide** (which are synthetic drugs); **rifampin** (which is a semisynthetic derivative of the antibiotic rifamycin); and **streptomycin or amikacin** (which are antibiotics). The first-line drugs are discussed below, and some of their properties and structures are shown in Table 41–1.

The **second-line drugs** are usually reserved to treat patients who are infected with organisms that are resistant to first-line drugs. Drug resistance is more likely to develop in patients who do not take their medicine as directed or are not treated for long enough.

The second-line drugs include the following: **rifabutin** and **rifapentine** (which, as with rifampin are derivatives of rifamycin); **fluoroquinolone drugs, cycloserine, capreomycin, ethionamide,** and **aminosalicylic acid.** Most of the second-line drugs are not discussed further in this chapter.

Isoniazid

After in vitro studies showed that nicotinic acid had a weak antitubercular effect, investigators began to synthesize and test many nicotinic acid derivatives. Isoniazid, also known as **isonicotinic acid hydrazide** (INH), was found to be the most active derivative and subsequently became available for clinical use. Isoniazid is often considered the premier drug for the management of tuberculosis. The introduction of isoniazid in the early 1960s revolutionized the treatment of this disease.

CHEMISTRY AND MECHANISMS. The structures of isoniazid and its metabolites are shown in Fig. 41–1.

Isoniazid acts by inhibiting the synthesis of **mycolic acid.** This acid is the mycobacterial cell wall component responsible for the acid-fast staining property of mycobacteria.

Isoniazid is activated by mycobacterial **catalase-peroxidase,** an enzyme encoded by the *kat*G **gene.** The hydrazine moiety of isoniazid reduces the ferric component of catalase-peroxidase, and the reduced (ferrous) enzyme

Figure 41–1. Structures of isoniazid and its metabolites. Isoniazid conjugates with acetyl CoA and is converted to acetylisoniazid in a reaction catalyzed by acetyltransferase. A small amount of acetylisoniazid is hydrolyzed to isonicotinic acid and acetylhydrazine.

TABLE 41-1. **Pharmacokinetic Properties of Antimycobacterial Drugs***

Drug	Route of Administration	Oral Bioavailability	Elimination Half-Life	Routes of Elimination
Azithromycin	Oral	37%	12 hours	Biliary excretion
Ciprofloxacin	Oral or IV	75%	4 hours	Metabolism; renal excretion
Clarithromycin	Oral	62%	5 hours	Biliary and renal excretion
Clofazimine	Oral	55%	70 days	Biliary and fecal excretion
Dapsone	Oral	≈100%	28 hours[†]	Metabolism; renal excretion
Ethambutol	Oral	≈100%	3.5 hours	Metabolism; renal and fecal excretion
Isoniazid	Oral or IM	≈100%	2.5 hours[†]	Metabolism; renal excretion
Pyrazinamide	Oral	≈100%	9.5 hours	Metabolism; renal excretion
Rifabutin	Oral	16%	45 hours	Metabolism; renal and biliary excretion
Rifampin	Oral or IV	≈100%	2.75 hours	Metabolism; renal and biliary excretion
Streptomycin	IM	NA	2 hours	Renal excretion
Thalidomide	Oral	≈90%	6 hours	Metabolism; renal excretion

*Values shown are the mean of values reported in the literature. IM = intramuscular; IV = intravenous; and NA = not applicable.
[†]The half-lives of dapsone and isoniazid exhibit genetic variation.

combines with oxygen to form an oxyferrous enzyme complex. This complex ultimately interacts with the target enzyme, a long-chain enoyl reductase involved in the **synthesis of mycolic acid.**

PHARMACOKINETICS. Although isoniazid is available for oral and intramuscular administration, it is usually given orally and is well absorbed from the gut. The drug is widely distributed to tissues and reaches intracellular concentrations sufficiently high to act effectively against organisms inside cells and caseous lesions.

Isoniazid is extensively metabolized. The primary metabolite, acetylisoniazid, is formed by conjugation of acetyl CoA with isoniazid (see Fig. 41–1). The reaction is catalyzed by acetyltransferase, an enzyme whose rate of activity is genetically determined. Slow acetylation is an autosomal recessive trait, and persons with the slow phenotype are homozygous for the slow allele. Persons with the fast phenotype are either heterozygous or autosomal dominant. The prevalence of phenotypes varies from population to population. The slow phenotype predominates in some Middle Eastern populations, whereas the fast phenotype predominates in Japanese populations. In the United States of America, about half the population exhibits each phenotype. Because of the different rates of acetylation of isoniazid, persons with the fast phenotype have lower plasma isoniazid concentrations than do persons with the slow phenotype (Fig. 41–2).

A small amount of acetylisoniazid is converted to isonicotinic acid and acetylhydrazine (see Fig. 41–1). Investigators believe that acetylhydrazine is responsible for the hepatic toxicity of the drug.

Isoniazid and its metabolites are excreted in the urine.

SPECTRUM AND INDICATIONS. Isoniazid is active against sensitive strains of *M. tuberculosis* and sensitive strains of some atypical mycobacteria, such as *M. kansasii.* It has little activity against *M. avium-intracellulare.* It is not active against *M. leprae* or against most other bacteria, and its use is limited to the prevention and treatment of tuberculosis.

Isoniazid is given to treat **latent tuberculosis** (formerly called prophylaxis) in persons with a positive reaction to the tuberculin skin test (TST) and who meet one of the following criteria: human immunodeficiency virus (HIV) positive; recently infected (conversion from a negative to a positive TST in the past 2 years); chest x-ray study showing nonprogressive tuberculous disease; predisposing conditions including illicit injected drug use, diabetes mellitus, immunosuppression, or certain diseases. The preferred duration of treatment for latent tuberculosis is 9 months but 6 months may be sufficient in some cases. Rifampin can be used for prophylaxis if isoniazid is contraindicated or if the mycobacterial strain is known to be resistant to isoniazid (Table 41–2) .

Isoniazid is also given to prevent tuberculosis in neonates and children who have had close contact with persons in whom active tuberculosis was recently diagnosed.

Isoniazid is used to treat persons with newly diagnosed tuberculosis unless they are known to be infected with a strain that is resistant to the drug. In persons who have had a relapse of tuberculosis after earlier treatment, the choice of drugs is guided by in vitro susceptibility of the infecting mycobacterial strain.

BACTERIAL RESISTANCE. Resistance to isoniazid is increasingly prevalent. In some cases, immigrants have tuberculosis and harbor organisms that are resistant to isoniazid and other first-line drugs. Resistance to isoniazid appears to be mediated primarily by mutations of the *kat*G gene, which result in loss of the catalase-peroxidase enzyme required for activation of isoniazid in bacteria.

ADVERSE EFFECTS. Isoniazid is well tolerated by most patients. It causes elevation of serum transaminase levels and potentially life-threatening **hepatitis** in some individuals, however. The risk of developing hepatitis during isoniazid therapy is low in persons under 35 years of age, is moderate in persons between 35 and 50 years of age, and is highest in persons over 50 years of age. Isoniazid treatment of latent tuberculosis (formerly called prophylaxis), however, appears to have a positive risk-benefit ratio in patients over 35 years of age if they are monitored appropriately for hepatotoxicity. Patients who have tuberculosis and are being treated with isoniazid should have their serum transaminase levels monitored periodically and should be told to inform their health care provider if they develop symptoms of hepatitis.

Isoniazid can also cause **peripheral neuritis,** with symptoms including paresthesias and numbness of the fingers and toes. This adverse effect is more likely to occur in individuals with the slow acetylator phenotype, because they have higher plasma concentrations of isoniazid. Peripheral neuritis is caused by a **pyridoxine (vitamin B$_6$) deficiency** resulting from inactivation of pyridoxine by the drug. It can be prevented or treated by administering pyridoxine supplements to patients who are taking isoniazid.

In rare circumstances, isoniazid causes toxic encephalopathy or seizures. Hematologic abnormalities, such as granulocytosis, anemia, or thrombocytopenia, can occur.

Figure 41–2. Bimodal distribution of plasma isoniazid concentrations. Plasma concentrations of isoniazid were measured 2 hours after the administration of a single 300-mg dose of isoniazid to each member of a general population of human subjects. Subjects with the fast acetylation phenotype showed lower plasma drug concentrations than did subjects with the slow acetylation phenotype.

TABLE 41–2. **Regimens for Treating Mycobacterial Infections***

Situation	Preferred Therapy	Alternative Therapy
Prevention of tuberculosis in neonates and children <5 years of age who are exposed to tuberculosis	Isoniazid 10 mg/kg/day for 3 months	
Latent tuberculosis (formerly called prophylaxis)	Isoniazid for 9 months (adults: 5 mg/kg/day; children: 10 mg/kg/day)	Rifampin for 4 months (for isoniazid-resistant strains)
Active tuberculosis		
Isoniazid resistance <4%	Isoniazid, rifampin, pyrazinamide, and ethambutol for 6 months (up to 9 months for HIV-positive)	Isoniazid, rifampin, ethambutol for 9 months
Isoniazid resistance >4%	Rifampin, pyrazinamide, ethambutol ± a fluoroquinolone for 6 months	
Rifampin resistance	Isoniazid, ethambutol, and a fluoroquinolone for 18–24 months, with pyrazinamide for 2 months	
Isoniazid and rifampin resistance	A fluoroquinolone, pyrazinamide, ethambutol, and amikacin for 18–24 months	
Mycobacterium avium-intracellulare prophylaxis	Azithromycin weekly or clarithromycin twice daily	Rifabutin or azithromycin
M. avium-intracellulare treatment	Clarithromycin or azithromycin + ethambutol + rifabutin	Preferred therapy + ciprofloxacin and/or amikacin
Leprosy		
Tuberculoid	Dapsone + rifampin	
Lepromatous	Dapsone + rifampin + clofazimine	

*HIV = human immunodeficiency virus.

Ethambutol

Ethambutol is a butanol derivative that has bacteriostatic activity against mycobacterial organisms. As shown in Table 41–2, it is used in combination with other drugs to treat tuberculosis or *M. avium-intracellulare* infections.

Ethambutol is administered orally, undergoes hepatic biotransformation, and is excreted in the urine and feces. The drug is generally well tolerated, but it can produce dose-dependent **optic neuritis** and **impaired red-green color discrimination.** It can also cause hyperuricemia, gout, hepatitis, and thrombocytopenia.

Pyrazinamide

Pyrazinamide is a nicotinamide derivative that is converted to pyrazinoic acid by susceptible mycobacteria. Pyrazinoic acid inhibits the growth of *M. tuberculosis*, partly by lowering the ambient pH to a level at which the organism can no longer grow.

Pyrazinamide was considered a second-line drug until investigators found that giving it in combination with other antimycobacterial drugs made it possible to reduce the treatment duration for tuberculosis to 6 months. Pyrazinamide is usually given in combination with isoniazid, rifampin, and ethambutol (see Table 41–2).

Pyrazinamide is given orally, is widely distributed to tissues, and is largely converted to pyrazinoic acid in the liver. A small amount of the drug is excreted unchanged in the urine, along with its metabolite.

Adverse reactions to pyrazinamide include hyperuricemia, **gout,** hematologic toxicity, fever, **hepatitis,** and an increase in the serum iron concentration.

Rifampin

CHEMISTRY AND PHARMACOKINETICS. Rifampin is a rifamycin derivative. Also called **rifampicin,** rifampin is rapidly absorbed after oral administration and is converted in the liver to an active metabolite, desacetylrifampin. The drug and its metabolite are widely distributed to tissues and fluids, including lung tissue, saliva, and peritoneal and pleural fluids. Rifampin undergoes significant enterohepatic cycling. It is primarily excreted in the feces via biliary elimination, but up to 30% is excreted in the urine. The half-life of rifampin decreases with long-term administration, owing to increased biliary excretion.

MECHANISMS, SPECTRUM, AND INDICATIONS. Rifampin is a broad-spectrum antibiotic that has significant activity against many gram-positive, gram-negative, and acid-fast bacilli, including *M. tuberculosis, M. avium-intracellulare, M. kansasii,* and *M. leprae*. The drug acts by binding to the β subunit of DNA-dependent RNA polymerase. This prevents the enzyme from binding to DNA and thereby prevents subsequent DNA transcription. The drug does not bind to the RNA polymerase of eukaryotic cells.

Rifampin is given prophylactically to prevent several types of diseases. It is used as an alternative to isoniazid for latent tuberculosis when resistance to isoniazid is known or suspected. It is used to prevent meningococcal disease in individuals who have had close contact with a *Neisseria meningitidis*-infected person or an asymptomatic meningococcal carrier. It is also given to individuals who have been exposed to *Haemophilus influenzae* type b (Hib) and are at risk of transmitting infection to children 4 years of age or younger.

Rifampin is usually combined with isoniazid, ethambutol, and pyrazinamide to treat active tuberculosis, and it can be combined with a sulfone (e.g., dapsone) or with clofazimine to treat leprosy (see below). Rifampin penetrates inflamed meninges and reaches levels in the cerebrospinal fluid that are 10% to 20% of levels in the serum. Hence, it can be used in the treatment of tubercular meningitis.

Rifampin is used in combination with vancomycin and gentamicin to treat staphylococcal endocarditis. It is occasionally used to treat *Legionella pneumophila* infections, usually in combination with a macrolide or a quinolone drug.

BACTERIAL RESISTANCE. The major drawback of rifampin is the tendency for microbes to acquire resistance during exposure to the drug. Resistance is usually caused by the decreased affinity of RNA polymerase for rifampin. Because of the potential for the emergence of resistance during treatment, rifampin is never used alone to treat active infections.

ADVERSE EFFECTS AND INTERACTIONS. The adverse effects of rifampin are usually mild, but the drug can impair liver function, elevate serum bilirubin and transaminase levels, and cause **hepatitis.** Liver function tests should be conducted every 2 to 4 weeks during treatment, and rifampin should be discontinued if signs or symptoms of hepatic dysfunction become evident.

A hypersensitivity reaction, manifested as a flulike illness with chills, fever, fatigue, and headache, develops in as many as 50% of persons taking rifampin. This reaction is more common in those who take large doses once or twice a week than in those who take smaller doses every day. High-dose intermittent therapy can also cause renal disease, leukopenia, and thrombocytopenia. Rifampin should be discontinued if purpura develops in persons taking the drug.

The consumption of alcohol by individuals who are taking rifampin appears to increase the risk of hepatitis. Rifampin can cause a reddish-orange to reddish-brown discoloration of saliva, tears, and urine. It can also cause permanent staining of soft contact lenses. Patients should be informed of these potential reactions.

Rifampin induces cytochrome P450 isozymes CYP1A2, CYP2C9, and CYP3A4 and can thereby accelerate the metabolism of other drugs and reduce their serum concentrations and therapeutic effectiveness. The affected drugs include macrolide antibiotics, benzodiazepines, calcium channel blockers, digoxin, estrogens, sulfonylureas, theophylline, and warfarin.

Rifabutin

As with rifampin, rifabutin inhibits DNA-dependent RNA polymerase in susceptible *Mycobacteria*. The drug is active against *M. avium-intracellulare* and most strains of *M. tuberculosis*.

Rifabutin is primarily used to prevent or treat *M. avium-intracellulare* disease in individuals who are HIV-positive or immunosuppressed. For the treatment of *M. avium-intracellulare* infections, rifabutin is administered in combination with azithromycin or clarithromycin plus ethambutol for a period of at least 16 weeks. Rifabutin is administered orally once a day with food to reduce gastrointestinal irritation. The drug is highly lipophilic, is widely distributed to tissues, and reaches substantial intracellular concentrations. Rifabutin undergoes hydroxylation and deacetylation to active metabolites that contribute about 10% of the drug's antimicrobial activity.

Streptomycin and Amikacin

Streptomycin and amikacin are aminoglycoside antibiotics used to treat tuberculosis in cases where resistance to other drugs is known or suspected. Amikacin is more active than streptomycin against some strains of *M. tuberculosis*. These drugs must be administered parenterally and are not as convenient as other drugs in the treatment of tuberculosis.

R207910

R207910 is the code name for diarylquinoline drug now in clinical trials for treatment of tuberculosis. If successful, it will be the first new type of drug for tuberculosis in four decades. R207910 is especially attractive because of its very long half-life and its extremely rapid bactericidal effect. For these reasons, it is believed that it might shorten the duration of tuberculosis treatment significantly. It also appears to be very well tolerated and it is active against multidrug resistant strains of *M. tuberculosis*.

Drugs for Mycobacterium avium-intracellulare Infections

Drugs that are active against *M. avium-intracellulare* include **ethambutol** and **rifabutin** (described above); **azithromycin** and **clarithromycin** (described in Chapter 39); **ciprofloxacin** and other fluoroquinolones (described in Chapter 40); and **clofazimine** (described later).

Azithromycin, clarithromycin, or rifabutin can be used to prevent *M. avium-intracellulare* diseases in HIV-positive or immunosuppressed patients.

Multiple-drug therapy involving various combinations of azithromycin, ciprofloxacin, clarithromycin, ethambutol, amikacin, and rifabutin are used to treat *M. avium-intracellulare* disease. Clofazimine has been used as an alternative drug in regimens for HIV-positive or immunosuppressed patients with *M. avium-intracellulare* diseases.

Drugs for Leprosy

The treatment of leprosy requires the administration of antimycobacterial drugs for long periods of time, ranging from several months to a person's lifetime. The World Health Organization now recommends multidrug therapy for most persons with leprosy. Multidrug therapy has been shown to hasten the eradication of bacteria, to reduce the duration of active disease, and to prevent worsening of disabilities in persons with leprosy. In addition, multidrug therapy appears to reduce overall costs, increase patient compliance, and increase the motivation and availability of leprosy workers.

Sulfones

The sulfones have served as the foundation of drug therapy for leprosy for several decades. These compounds are structurally related to the sulfonamides and have a similar mechanism of action. They inhibit the synthesis of folic acid by *M. leprae,* and they exhibit a bacteriostatic action against this organism.

Dapsone, or **diaminodiphenylsulfone,** is the sulfone that is most commonly used in the treatment of leprosy. It is given orally in combination with other drugs (see Table 41–2), is metabolized by acetylation, and is excreted in the urine. Adverse reactions are usually minimal, but dapsone can cause gastrointestinal disturbances, peripheral neuropathy, optic neuritis and blurred vision, proteinuria and nephrotic syndrome, lupus erythematosuslike syndrome, and hematologic toxicity. Individuals who have **glucose-6-phosphate dehydrogenase deficiency** may exhibit **hemolytic anemia** resulting from the oxidation of erythrocyte membranes by dapsone.

Rifampin

Rifampin (described previously) is the drug that exhibits the greatest bactericidal activity against *M. leprae.* For the treatment of leprosy, rifampin is usually combined with dapsone or with dapsone plus clofazimine. It is never used alone, because of the probability that organisms will become resistant to it during treatment.

Clofazimine

Clofazimine is a phenazine dye that has antimycobacterial and anti-inflammatory effects. The drug is bactericidal against *M. tuberculosis,* is bacteriostatic against *M. leprae,* and is active against *M. avium-intracellulare.* Clofazimine has little activity against other bacteria. In addition to its antimicrobial effects, the drug enhances the phagocytic activity of neutrophils and macrophages while reducing the motility of neutrophils and the ability of lymphocytes to transform.

The anti-inflammatory and immunologic effects of clofazimine may contribute to the drug's efficacy in the prevention and treatment of **erythema nodosum leprosum,** a type II hypersensitivity reaction sometimes seen during or after the treatment of patients with lepromatous leprosy. This reaction is characterized by tender erythematous skin nodules that occur with inflammation of subcutaneous fat and acute vasculitis. Clofazimine appears to reduce the incidence of the reaction.

In patients with lepromatous leprosy, clofazimine is approved for use in combination with dapsone and rifampin. Clofazimine is usually combined with corticosteroids to treat leprosy that is complicated by erythema nodosum leprosum.

Clofazimine is slowly and incompletely absorbed from the gut, with an average bioavailability of about 55%. The highly lipophilic drug is primarily distributed to adipose tissue and reticuloendothelial cells, but it is accumulated by macrophages and can also concentrate in the liver, lungs,

lymph nodes, spleen, and other tissues. The drug has a long half-life (about 70 days), and some of it remains in the body for years after therapy is discontinued. It is primarily excreted unchanged in the feces following biliary excretion.

Adverse effects of clofazimine include various forms of gastrointestinal distress (e.g., anorexia, nausea, vomiting, abdominal pain, and diarrhea); photosensitivity; skin discoloration or other dermatologic reactions; and discoloration of body secretions (sweat, tears, sputum, feces, and urine) during therapy. Because clofazimine can elevate hepatic enzyme levels and cause hepatitis, use of the drug is generally avoided in persons with hepatic disease.

Thalidomide

Thalidomide is a drug that was once banned because it caused phocomelia (congenital abnormalities of the limbs) in the offspring of women who took it during pregnancy. Subsequent investigations have shown that the drug has immunomodulating actions (see Chapter 45) that are beneficial in the management of several conditions. Thalidomide currently has orphan drug status in the USA and can be used to treat tuberculosis, leprosy, or erythema nodosum leprosum. The drug is often effective in alleviating the manifestations of erythema nodosum leprosum, possibly because of its ability to stimulate human T cells (particularly the CD8+ cell subset of T cells).

SUMMARY OF IMPORTANT POINTS

■ Tuberculosis and leprosy are chronic mycobacterial infections that often require treatment with multiple drugs for months or years. Combination drug therapy accelerates the eradication of bacteria and reduces the emergence of microbial drug resistance during therapy.

■ Most patients with tuberculosis are initially treated with a combination of isoniazid, rifampin, ethambutol, and pyrazinamide. If patients are suspected or known to be infected with drug-resistant organisms, streptomycin, amikacin, or a fluoroquinolone can be substituted.

■ Most patients with leprosy are treated with a combination of dapsone and rifampin or a combination of dapsone, rifampin, and clofazimine.

■ Isoniazid (isonicotinic acid hydrazide, or INH) acts partly by inhibiting mycolic acid synthesis. The rate of acetylation of the drug exhibits genetic polymorphism, with some persons showing fast acetylation and some showing slow acetylation.

■ Isoniazid sometimes causes hepatitis; the risk is age-related. The drug can also cause peripheral neuritis, an effect that results from drug-induced pyridoxine deficiency that can be prevented or treated with pyridoxine supplementation.

■ Rifampin is a semisynthetic antibiotic with broad-spectrum activity. It is used in the treatment of tuberculosis and leprosy, in the prevention of meningococcal and *H. influenzae* type b infections, and in the treatment of serious staphylococcal and *L. pneumophila* infections.

Adverse effects of rifampin include hepatitis and discoloration of body fluids.

■ Pyrazinamide is a synthetic drug that shortens the total duration of therapy for patients with tuberculosis.

■ Rifabutin, a semisynthetic antibiotic, is primarily used for the prevention and treatment of *M. avium-intracellulare* diseases in individuals who are infected with human immunodeficiency virus (HIV) or are immunosuppressed. Rifabutin is usually given in combination with azithromycin or clarithromycin and ethambutol.

■ Dapsone is a sulfone drug that forms the foundation of therapy for leprosy. It is used in combination with other drugs, such as rifampin and clofazimine.

■ Clofazimine is a synthetic dye that has antimycobacterial and anti-inflammatory activity. As with rifampin, it can discolor body fluids.

Review Questions

1. Which of the following is recommended for treatment of latent tuberculosis?
   (A) rifampin for 6 months
   (B) isoniazid for 9 months
   (C) isoniazid and rifampin for 6 months
   (D) ethambutol for 6 months
   (E) isoniazid, rifampin, and ethambutol for 9 months

2. Which antitubercular drug can contribute an orange-red color to urine?
   (A) pyrazinamide
   (B) streptomycin
   (C) ethambutol
   (D) isoniazid
   (E) rifampin

3. A patient being treated for tuberculosis has impaired red-green color discrimination. Which drug is most likely responsible?
   (A) rifabutin
   (B) pyrazinamide
   (C) ethambutol
   (D) isoniazid
   (E) ciprofloxacin

4. Bacterial resistance to which drug can result from mutations in the gene for RNA polymerase?
   (A) amikacin
   (B) pyrazinamide
   (C) isoniazid
   (D) rifampin
   (E) ethambutol

5. Persons with a fast drug acetylation phenotype will have comparatively lower plasma levels of which drug?
   (A) isoniazid
   (B) rifabutin
   (C) amikacin
   (D) ethambutol
   (E) pyrazinamide

Answers and Explanations

1. The answer is B: isoniazid for 9 months. Isoniazid is recommended for treating all persons with latent tuberculosis. If isoniazid is not tolerated, rifampin can be given for 4 months.

2. The answer is E: rifampin. Rifampin is a semisynthetic antibiotic that has an intense orange-red color. Rifampin is widely distributed and can impart an orange-red color to tears, saliva, and urine.

3. The answer is C: ethambutol. Ethambutol, particularly at higher doses above 15 mg/kg/day, can cause optic neuritis leading to impaired red-green color discrimination. This adverse effect is reversible if the drug is discontinued.

4. The answer is D: rifampin. Rifampin acts by inhibiting bacterial RNA polymerase and RNA synthesis. Mutations in the gene for RNA polymerase can lead to reduced affinity of the enzyme for rifampin and bacterial resistance. Rifampin should never be used alone for the treatment of an active infection. It can be used alone, however, for latent tuberculosis and prophylaxis of meningitis in close contacts of an active case.

5. The answer is A: isoniazid. Isoniazid is initially metabolized by conjugation with acetate catalyzed by acetyltransferase. Genetic polymorphisms confer differences in the catalytic rate of this enzyme, giving rise to slow and fast acetylation phenotypes. Persons with the fast phenotype act to acetylate isoniazid and other drugs (e.g., hydralazine) more rapidly and, therefore, such persons have lower levels of unmetabolized isoniazid.

SELECTED READINGS

Cohen, J. Medicine. New TB drug promises shorter, simpler treatment. Science 306:1872, 2004.

Volmink, J., and P. Garner. Directly observed therapy for treating tuberculosis. Cochrane Database Syst Rev 1:CD003343, 2003.

CHAPTER 42

Antifungal Drugs

CLASSIFICATION OF ANTIFUNGAL DRUGS

Polyene Antibiotics
- Amphotericin B[a]

Azole Derivatives
- Clotrimazole (LOTRIMIN, MYCELEX)[b]
- Fluconazole (DIFLUCAN)
- Itraconazole (SPORANOX)
- Ketoconazole (NIZORAL)
- Voriconazole (VFEND)

Allylamine Drugs
- Terbinafine (LAMISIL)[c]

Echinocandin Drugs
- Caspofungin (CANCIDAS)[d]

Other Antifungal Drugs
- Ciclopirox
- Flucytosine
- Griseofulvin
- Tolnaftate (TINACTIN)

[a]also nystatin, natamycin
[b]also econazole
[c]also naftifine, butenafine
[d]also micafungin, anidulafungin

OVERVIEW

Fungal Infections

Fungal infections can be divided into three groups: systemic mycoses, subcutaneous mycoses, and superficial mycoses.

Patients with **systemic mycoses** can present with signs and symptoms of **soft tissue infection, urinary tract infection, pneumonia, meningitis,** or **septicemia.** The diseases can be chronic and indolent or invasive and life-threatening. The systemic mycoses are most commonly caused by members of the genera *Aspergillus, Blastomyces, Candida, Coccidioides, Cryptococcus,* and *Histoplasma.* Some infections (e.g., **blastomycosis, coccidioidomycosis,** and **histoplasmosis**), which are endemic to certain geographic regions, are found in both immunocompetent and immunocompromised individuals. Other infections (e.g., **aspergillosis, candidiasis, cryptococcosis,** and **mucormycosis**) are more likely to occur in immunocompromised or debilitated patients, such as those receiving immunosuppressive drugs, those with indwelling catheters or prostheses, or those with acquired immunodeficiency syndrome (AIDS), diabetes, or chronic renal, hepatic, or cardiac diseases. These conditions either suppress cellular immunity or facilitate colonization and infection by fungi. For example, an increased incidence is seen of invasive infections caused by *Aspergillus, Scedosporium,* and *Fusarium* species among recipients of hematopoietic stem cell transplants in the past decade.

Subcutaneous mycoses are often caused by puncture wounds contaminated with soil fungi. Examples of these infections are **chromomycosis, pseudallescheriasis,** and **sporotrichosis.**

Superficial mycoses are infections of the nails, skin, and mucous membranes, which are usually caused by dermatophytes or yeasts. The most common dermatophytes are *Epidermophyton, Microsporum,* and *Trichophyton.* Dermatophyte infections of the nails are referred to as **tinea unguium** or **onychomycosis.** Other dermatophyte infections include **tinea pedis** (athlete's foot), **tinea capitis** (ringworm of the scalp), **tinea corporis** (ringworm of the body), and **tinea cruris** ("jock itch"). These infections usually present as a rash with pruritus (itching) and erythema. **Ringworm** is described as an annular, scaling rash with a clear center.

The most common yeasts causing superficial mycoses are *Candida albicans* and other *Candida* species. Affected patients may present with **thrush** (oral candidiasis), **vaginal candidiasis,** or *Candida* **infections of the axilla, groin, and gluteal folds** (including **diaper rash** in infants). Less common yeasts causing superficial mycoses include *Malassezia furfur* (also called *Pityrosporum orbiculare*) and *Malassezia ovalis* (also called *Pityrosporum ovale*). *M. furfur* causes **tinea versicolor** or **pityriasis versicolor,** a skin infection characterized by hypo- and hyperpigmented macules, typically in the shoulder girdle area. *P. ovale and M. furfur* cause **seborrheic dermatitis,** characterized by scaling and erythema on the ears, eyebrows, nose, and chest.

Clinical Uses and Mechanisms of Antifungal Drugs

Fungi are eukaryotic organisms whose growth is not inhibited by antibacterial drugs. Drugs that are selectively toxic to fungi have been discovered, however, and they are used to treat fungal infections in humans.

As shown in Table 42–1, drugs used in the treatment of systemic and subcutaneous mycoses include a polyene antibiotic (amphotericin B), several azole derivatives (fluconazole, itraconazole, ketoconazole, and voriconazole), an echinocandin drug (caspofungin), and flucytosine. The other drugs listed are used in the treatment of superficial mycoses. Amphotericin B tends to be used for treating severe mycoses, whereas the azoles are used for less severe forms of these infections. Newer antifungal agents (e.g., voriconazole and caspofungin) can be used to treat invasive *Candida* and *Aspergillus* infections. Flucytosine is usually administered in combination with amphotericin B for the treatment of systemic *Cryptococcus* or *Candida* infections.

Many antifungal drugs act by impairing **plasma membrane function** in fungal cells. The selective toxicity of these drugs is caused by the difference in the sterols found in fungal and mammalian cell membranes. Fungal cell membranes contain **ergosterol,** whereas mammalian cell membranes contain **cholesterol.** Some antifungal drugs bind to ergosterol and thereby increase plasma membrane permeability, whereas other drugs inhibit the synthesis of ergosterol (Fig. 42–1 and Table 42–1).

Polyene antibiotics selectively bind to ergosterol in fungal membranes. This action increases fungal plasma membrane permeability and allows the cytoplasmic contents to escape from the cell. The polyene drugs can also bind to cholesterol in mammalian cells, and this may account for their ability to produce kidney damage. **Ciclopirox** increases fungal cell membrane permeability by a different mechanism. It prevents amino acid transport into fungal cells, thereby altering membrane structure and allowing the escape of intracellular material.

The **allylamine drugs** and the **azole derivatives** block distinct steps in ergosterol biosynthesis, but these groups of drugs have little effect on cholesterol biosynthesis in humans. The allylamine drugs inhibit **squalene monooxygenase,** which converts squalene to squalene-2,3-oxide, the immediate precursor of lanosterol. The azoles inhibit **14-α-demethylase,** a cytochrome P450 enzyme that converts lanosterol to ergosterol.

The **echinocandin drugs** (e.g., caspofungin) represent a new class of antifungal agents that inhibit the synthesis of a **fungal cell wall** component, β-1,3-D-glucan. The fungal cell wall surrounds the plasma membrane and protects the cell from osmotic and mechanical stress.

Flucytosine, a pyrimidine antimetabolite, is the only antifungal drug that affects nucleic acid. Flucytosine is converted to **5-fluorouracil** (5-FU) in fungal cells by cytosine deaminase, an enzyme not found in mammalian cells. 5-FU

TABLE 42–1. Clinical Uses and Mechanisms of Antifungal Drugs

Drug	**CLINICAL USES**			
	Systemic and Subcutaneous Mycoses	Dermatophyte Infections	Superficial *Candida* Infections	Mechanisms
Polyene antibiotics				
Amphotericin B	Yes	No	Yes	Binds ergosterol in fungal cell membrane; increases membrane permeability
Natamycin	No	No	Yes	Same as amphotericin B
Nystatin	No	No	Yes	Same as amphotericin B
Azole derivatives				
Clotrimazole	No	Yes	Yes	Inhibits ergosterol synthesis
Econazole	No	Yes	Yes	Same as clotrimazole
Fluconazole	Yes	No	Yes	Same as clotrimazole
Itraconazole	Yes	Yes	Yes	Same as clotrimazole
Ketoconazole	No	Yes	Yes	Same as clotrimazole
Voriconazole	Yes	No	No	Same as clotrimazole
Allylamine drugs				
Naftifine	No	Yes	No*	Inhibits ergosterol biosynthesis
Terbinafine	No	Yes	No*	Same as naftifine
Other antifungal drugs				
Caspofungin	Yes	No	No	Inhibits fungal cell wall synthesis
Ciclopirox	No	Yes	Yes	Increases fungal cell membrane permeability
Flucytosine	Yes	No	No	Inhibits nucleic acid synthesis
Griseofulvin	No	Yes	No	Inhibits microtubule function and mitosis
Tolnaftate	No	Yes	No	Unknown

*Naftifine and terbinafine have fungistatic activity against *Candida* but are not approved for the treatment of candidiasis.

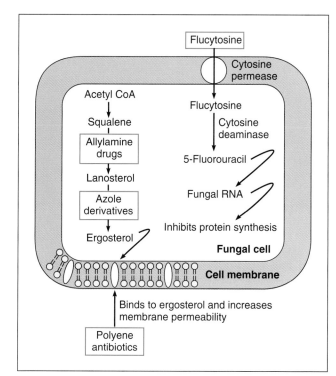

Figure 42-1. Mechanisms of action of antifungal drugs. The synthesis of ergosterol is inhibited by allylamine drugs and by azole derivatives. Amphotericin B and other polyene antibiotics bind to ergosterol in fungal cell membranes and increase membrane permeability. Ciclopirox increases membrane permeability by another mechanism (not shown). Flucytosine is accumulated by fungal cells and converted to 5-fluorouracil (5-FU). When 5-FU is incorporated into fungal RNA, protein synthesis is inhibited. Griseofulvin interferes with microtubule function and blocks mitosis (not shown). Caspofungin inhibits fungal cell wall synthesis (not shown).

is then incorporated into fungal RNA, and this inhibits fungal protein synthesis.

Griseofulvin acts by binding to fungal microtubules and thereby inhibiting microtubule function and mitosis. The mechanism of action of **tolnaftate** is unknown.

DRUGS

Polyene Antibiotics

The polyene antibiotics are produced by various soil organisms of the family *Streptomycetaceae*. Examples are amphotericin A and B, natamycin, and nystatin. Each of these compounds consists of a macrolide (lactone) ring containing conjugated double bonds (polyene), with acidic and basic side groups. Because the acidic group and basic group are capable of donating or accepting a proton, respectively, the polyene drugs are **amphoteric.**

Amphotericin B has greater antifungal activity than does amphotericin A, which is not used clinically. Amphotericin B is the only polyene drug used to treat systemic and subcutaneous mycoses. The other polyene drugs are limited to topical application for the treatment of superficial mycoses.

Amphotericin B

Chemistry and Pharmacokinetics. The structure and pharmacokinetic properties of amphotericin B are shown in Fig. 42-2A and Table 42-2.

Because amphotericin B is not absorbed from the gut, it is not available in oral formulations. It is available in parenteral formulations for the treatment of systemic or subcutaneous infections: a deoxycholate complex and three

TABLE 42-2. **Pharmacokinetic Properties of Antifungal Drugs***

Drug	Route of Administration	Oral Bioavailability	Elimination Half-Life	Routes of Elimination
Polyene antibiotics				
Amphotericin B	Topical, IV, intrathecal, or intraventricular	NA	24 hours or 15 days[†]	Metabolism; renal excretion
Natamycin	Topical ocular	NA	NA	NA
Nystatin	Oral or topical	None	NA	NA
Azole derivatives				
Clotrimazole	Topical	NA	NA	NA
Econazole	Topical	NA	NA	NA
Fluconazole	Oral or IV	95%	35 hours	Renal excretion
Itraconazole	Oral	55%	60 hours	Biliary, fecal, and renal excretion
Ketoconazole	Oral or topical	Highly variable	8 hours	Biliary and fecal excretion
Voriconazole	Oral or IV	96%	Dose dependent	Metabolism, renal excretion
Caspofungin	IV	NA	11 hours	Metabolism
Allylamine drugs				
Naftifine	Topical	NA	2.5 days	Renal and fecal excretion
Terbinafine	Oral or topical	40%	12.5 days	Metabolism; renal excretion
Other antifungal drugs				
Ciclopirox	Topical	NA	NA	NA
Flucytosine	Oral	82%	3.5 hours	Renal excretion
Griseofulvin	Oral	Variable	16 hours	Metabolism; renal excretion
Tolnaftate	Topical	NA	NA	NA

*Values shown are the mean of values reported in the literature. IV = intravenous; and NA = not applicable.
[†]For amphotericin B, the values represent the initial and terminal half-life, respectively.

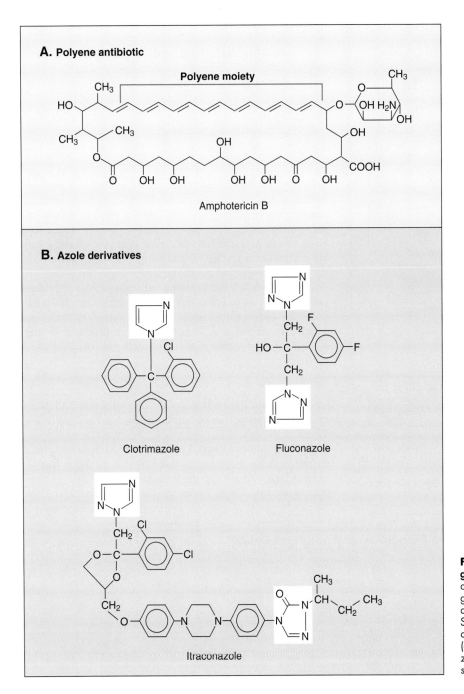

A. Polyene antibiotic

Polyene moiety

Amphotericin B

B. Azole derivatives

Clotrimazole

Fluconazole

Itraconazole

Figure 42–2. Structures of selected antifungal drugs. **(A)** Polyene antibiotics consist of a macrolide (lactone) ring containing conjugated double bonds (polyene), with acidic and basic (amphoteric) side groups. **(B)** Some azole derivatives (e.g., clotrimazole) are diazole (imidazole) compounds. Others (e.g., fluconazole and itraconazole) are triazole congeners. The diazole and triazole structures are unshaded.

lipid-based formulations. The **amphotericin B lipid formulation** appears to protect the kidney and other organs from the drug's toxicity while retaining its antifungal activity. The drug is also available in topical preparations for the treatment of superficial infections.

The dosage and route of parenteral treatment depend on the site and severity of the infection and on the immune status of the patient. In general, higher doses of amphotericin B are used to treat infections with more resistant fungi, especially *Aspergillus* species, and lower doses are used to treat esophageal and urinary tract infections. Concentrations of the drug in cerebrospinal fluid are only 2% to 3% of those in plasma, reflecting that amphotericin B does not

penetrate the blood–brain barrier very well. Nevertheless, the drug is usually administered intravenously to treat fungal meningitis and other systemic mycoses. Intrathecal administration or intraventricular administration with an Ommaya reservoir is generally reserved for extremely ill patients and those who do not respond to intravenous therapy.

Amphotericin B is extensively metabolized in the liver, and the metabolites are slowly excreted in the urine. The biotransformation pathways are not well understood. Amphotericin B has a biphasic half-life, with an initial half-life of about 24 hours and a terminal half-life of about 15 days.

SPECTRUM AND INDICATIONS. Amphotericin B is active against a wide variety of fungi (Table 42–3). In addition, it is active against *Naegleria fowleri,* a freshwater ameba that causes a rare but often fatal form of meningoencephalitis (see Chapter 44).

FUNGAL RESISTANCE. Although polyene antibiotics have been used to treat fungal infections for nearly 50 years, a few reports have been issued of fungal resistance to these drugs. Fungi that do become resistant to polyenes have a reduced content of ergosterol in their cell membranes.

ADVERSE EFFECTS. Amphotericin B is often called "amphoter-rible" and is probably the most toxic antibiotic in use today. It has been reported to cause some degree of renal toxicity in about 80% of patients who are treated with it, although the incidence appears to be reduced when the lipid complex formulation of amphotericin B is used. Renal toxicity reduces the glomerular filtration rate and contributes to azotemia (accumulation of nitrogenous compounds in the blood), hypokalemia, and hypomagnesemia. Therefore, electrolytes (especially sodium, potassium, and magnesium) should be monitored weekly during treatment with amphotericin B, and replacements should be administered as needed.

Lipid-based formulations of amphotericin B cause less renal toxicity and should be used in persons with renal impairment and those who are intolerant of the traditional deoxycholate formulation. These preparations include amphotericin B cholesteryl complex (AMPHOTEC), amphotericin B lipid complex (ABELCET), and amphotericin B liposomal complex (AMBISOME). The lipid formulations have unique pharmacokinetic characteristics that reduce renal drug concentrations and toxicity. Following intravenous administration, the lipid-based formulations are sequestered by cells of the reticuloendothelial system in the liver and spleen, which slowly release amphotericin B into the circulation over several days.

In addition to causing nephrotoxicity, amphotericin B can cause acute liver failure, cardiac arrhythmias, and hematopoietic disorders such as anemia, leukopenia, and thrombocytopenia. The drug frequently causes less severe but unpleasant effects, including chills, fever, headache, nausea, and vomiting. The severity of these minor adverse effects can be lessened by pretreatment with corticosteroids, antipyretic drugs (e.g., acetaminophen), and antihistamine drugs.

Nystatin and Natamycin

Nystatin, which is active against *Candida* species, is available in various formulations, including the following: creams, ointments, and powders for mucocutaneous candidiasis; lozenges (troches) for oral candidiasis; orally administered tablets and suspensions for intestinal candidiasis; and vaginal tablets for vaginal candidiasis.

Natamycin is active against *Aspergillus, Candida, Fusarium,* and *Penicillium* species and is available as an ophthalmic suspension for the treatment of fungal blepharitis, conjunctivitis, or keratitis.

Azole Derivatives

The azole derivatives are synthetic drugs used in the treatment of various mycoses (see Table 42–1). One group, the diazole (imidazole) compounds, includes **clotrimazole, econazole,** and **ketoconazole.** Another group, the triazole congeners, includes **fluconazole, itraconazole, and voriconazole.**

Drug Properties

CHEMISTRY AND PHARMACOKINETICS. Representative structures of azole derivatives are shown in Fig. 42–2B, and pharmacokinetic properties are compared in Table 42–2.

Some azoles are applied topically to treat superficial fungal infections, whereas others are given orally to treat the

---

TABLE 42–3. Causes and Management of Selected Systemic and Subcutaneous Mycoses

Mycosis	Pathogens	Treatments
Aspergillosis	*Aspergillus fumigatus*	Voriconazole, caspofungin, or both; amphotericin B
Blastomycosis	*Blastomyces dermatitidis*	Itraconazole or amphotericin B
Candidiasis	*Candida albicans, C. glabrata, C. parapsilosis, C. tropicalis, C. krusei*	Fluconazole, voriconazole, amphotericin B ± flucytosine, or caspofungin
Coccidioidomycosis*	*Coccidioides immitis*	Itraconazole or fluconazole (mild to moderate disease); amphotericin B (severe disease); fluconazole for meningitis
Cryptococcosis	*Cryptococcus neoformans*	Amphotericin B + flucytosine followed by fluconazole for meningitis; fluconazole or amphotericin B for nonmeningeal infections
Fusariosis	*Fusaria* species	Voriconazole
Histoplasmosis	*Histoplasma capsulatum*	Itraconazole for moderate disease; amphotericin B for severe disease and meningitis
Mucormycosis	*Absidia, Rhizopus,* and *Rhizomucor* species	Amphotericin B
Pseudallescheriasis	*Pseudallescheria boydii*	Voriconazole, itraconazole, or miconazole, with surgery
Sporotrichosis	*Sporothrix schenckii*	Itraconazole, fluconazole, or saturated potassium iodide solution

*No treatment needed for uncomplicated pulmonary infection in normal host (valley fever).

more stubborn superficial mycoses (e.g., onychomycosis). Several of the azole drugs are given orally to treat systemic or subcutaneous mycoses. Fluconazole, itraconazole, and voriconazole can also be administered intravenously to treat serious infections.

Most azole drugs are well absorbed from the gut. The absorption of ketoconazole and itraconazole requires the presence of gastric acid, so other drugs that reduce gastric acid should not be administered concurrently. Azoles are widely distributed to tissues and body fluids, but only fluconazole achieves significant concentrations in the cerebrospinal fluid (about 50% of concentrations in the plasma). For this reason, only fluconazole is used in the prophylaxis and treatment of fungal meningitis.

The azole derivatives undergo considerable hepatic biotransformation, and the parent compound and metabolites are excreted in the urine and feces. Itraconazole has an active metabolite, hydroxyitraconazole.

SPECTRUM AND INDICATIONS. Azole drugs can be either fungistatic or fungicidal, depending on the particular organism and the drug concentration. The drugs are active against a wide range of fungi that cause systemic and subcutaneous mycoses (see Table 42–3) and frequently serve as alternatives to amphotericin B for the treatment of these mycoses. Azoles are active against most dermatophytes that cause tinea infections, including *Epidermophyton floccosum*, *Microsporum canis*, *Microsporum gypseum*, *Trichophyton mentagrophytes*, *Trichophyton rubrum*, and *Trichophyton tonsurans*. Azoles also inhibit the growth of yeasts, including *Candida* and *Malassezia* species.

FUNGAL RESISTANCE. Resistance to azoles has emerged during treatment of systemic candidiasis with fluconazole, but the mechanisms have not been clearly defined.

ADVERSE EFFECTS AND INTERACTIONS. Azole derivatives are usually well tolerated, but systemic administration can cause skin rash, elevated hepatic enzyme levels, hepatic injury, hematopoietic toxicity, or gastrointestinal distress (nausea, vomiting, and diarrhea). Because azoles inhibit CYP3A4, a cytochrome P450 isozyme, their concurrent use with other drugs sometimes results in drug interactions. Ketoconazole is the most potent cytochrome inhibitor, and it can interfere with the biotransformation of other drugs and with the biosynthesis of testosterone. In fact, ketoconazole has been used to suppress testosterone synthesis in the treatment of prostate cancer and other conditions. Drugs whose metabolism is inhibited by the azoles include 3-hydroxy-3-methylglutaryl coenzyme A (HMG-CoA) reductase inhibitors, some benzodiazepines, quinidine, and warfarin. The dosage of these drugs may need to be reduced during concurrent azole therapy.

Specific Drugs

Itraconazole (SPORANOX) is particularly useful in the treatment of blastomycosis and histoplasmosis, and it is widely used to treat **onychomycosis** (fungal infection of the nails). For onychomycosis, the drug is often administered orally three times a week. This procedure is called pulse dosing.

Fluconazole (DIFLUCAN) achieves excellent penetration of the cerebrospinal fluid. It is useful in the prevention of **cryptococcal meningitis** in patients with acquired immunodeficiency syndrome (AIDS), and it is effective as follow-up therapy in patients whose cryptococcal meningitis has been successfully treated with amphotericin B. Based on the results of clinical studies, fluconazole is probably the drug of choice to prevent the relapse of cryptococcal meningitis. Fluconazole is also used to treat mucocutaneous (oropharyngeal and esophageal) and disseminated **candidiasis**. Because the drug is excreted in the urine, it is effective in patients with urinary tract infections caused by *Candida species*. A single dose of fluconazole can eradicate acute **vaginal candidiasis**.

Voriconazole (VFEND) is a fluconazole derivative that has been called a **second-generation conazole** because of its enhanced activity against *Aspergillus* and *Candida* species. Against *Candida* species, voriconazole is 60 to 100 times more potent than fluconazole and it is active against nonalbicans *Candida* species that are inherently resistant to fluconazole, such as *C. krusei*. In one study, voriconazole demonstrated better fungicidal activity against *Aspergillus fumigatus* than did amphotericin B, and voriconazole is active against some *Aspergillus* species that are inherently resistant to amphotericin B (see Boucher et al., 2004). Voriconazole has also demonstrated clinical efficacy in a wide variety of systemic fungal infections including **invasive aspergillosis**, and **esophageal and invasive candidiasis**. It has also been used to treat infections caused by *Cryptococcus*, *Fusaria*, *Coccidioides*, and *Pseudallescheria* species. Moreover, voriconazole appears to have additive activity with caspofungin (see later) in the treatment of invasive aspergillosis.

Although voriconazole is administered intravenously to treat serious fungal infections, patients can be easily switched to oral voriconazole as they improve because the oral bioavailability of the drug is approximately 96%.

Voriconazole is usually well tolerated, especially in comparison to amphotericin B. The most common adverse effects have been **visual disturbances** such as altered perception of light, abnormally colored vision (chromatopsia), and photophobia. These events were usually mild and transitory. Elevated serum levels of hepatic enzymes, primarily alanine aminotransferase and aspartate aminotransferase, occurred in 12% to 20% of patients treated with voriconazole and are the dose-limiting adverse effect of this drug. These elevations are usually transitory and reversible, but a few cases of **hepatic failure** and death have been reported. Hence, hepatic enzymes should be routinely monitored during voriconazole therapy.

Ketoconazole (NIZORAL) is available in oral and topical formulations. The oral drug is less widely used than itraconazole or fluconazole, because it has a greater potential for drug interactions, does not effectively penetrate the cerebrospinal fluid, and has lower activity against most fungi. Topical formulations are useful for treating **seborrheic dermatitis**.

Clotrimazole (LOTRIMIN, MYCELEX) is available in topical formulations for treatment of the following: *Candida* **infections** of the mouth, throat, vagina, and vulva; *M. furfur* infection of the skin (tinea versicolor); and **dermatophyte**

infections of the skin (e.g., tinea pedis and tinea cruris). Econazole is also available in topical formulations for the treatment of *Candida* and dermatophyte infections of the skin. These and other topical drugs are not effective for the treatment of dermatophyte infections of the scalp (tinea capitis) or nails (tinea unguium, or onychomycosis).

Several other azole derivatives not discussed in this chapter are available for the treatment of vaginal candidiasis and other superficial fungal infections.

Allylamine Drugs

Naftifine and **terbinafine** (LAMISIL) are allylamines that inhibit ergosterol synthesis (see Fig. 42–1). Although they are primarily used to treat superficial dermatophyte infections, they are also fungistatic against *Candida* species.

Both drugs are available in topical formulations, and terbinafine is also available for oral administration. Terbinafine is often administered orally once a day to treat **onychomycosis**. Fingernail infections usually require 6 weeks of therapy, whereas toenail infections can require 12 weeks of treatment.

Naftifine and terbinafine are well tolerated and rarely cause serious adverse effects.

Echinocandin drugs

The echinocandin drugs are a new class of large, cyclic hexapeptide compounds with lipid side-chains that inhibit **fungal cell wall synthesis**. The fungal cell wall is a rigid structure located just outside the plasma membrane that protects fungal cells from osmotic and mechanical stress. The fungal cell wall is composed of chitin and various glucans and glycoproteins. The echinocandin drugs inhibit the synthesis of the cell wall component known as β-(1,3)-D-glucan by noncompetitive inhibition of the β-(1,3)-D-glucan synthase enzyme complex. Inhibition of glucan synthesis leads to disruption of the fungal cell wall and cell death. Mammalians do not have cell walls and inhibition of glucan synthesis has no direct effect on human hosts.

Caspofungin (CANCIDAS) is the first echinocandin drug to be approved in the United States. It is a semisynthetic derivative of pneumocandin, a fermentation product of *Glarea lozoyensis*. Caspofungin has excellent activity against ***Candida* species** and good activity against ***Aspergillus* species**. It is highly active against *Candida albicans*, *C. glabrata*, *C. tropicalis*, and *C. krusei*, including strains that are resistant to azole compounds. Clinical trials have shown that caspofungin is very effective in treating esophageal, oropharyngeal, and invasive candidiasis (74% to 96% response rate). In one study, caspofungin was moderately effective in treating invasive aspergillosis (45% response rate). Most patients in this study, however, had failed treatment with amphotericin B or azole drugs.

Caspofungin produces few adverse effects. The most common problems have been headache, fever, phlebitis at the site of drug administration, and abnormal liver function tests. Compared with amphotericin B, caspofungin has been very well tolerated. Because of its poor oral bioavailability, it must be administered intravenously. Caspofungin has a long half-life and is administered once daily.

Other echinocandin drugs now being developed include **micafungin** and **anidulafungin**.

Other Antifungal Drugs

Flucytosine

Flucytosine is a fluorinated pyrimidine analogue that is used orally to treat severe fungal infections. The drug is accumulated by fungal cells and is converted to its active metabolite, 5-fluorouracil, by cytosine deaminase. The metabolite is incorporated into fungal RNA, and this interferes with fungal protein synthesis (see Fig. 42–1). Unlike fungal cells, human cells lack cytosine deaminase and are unable to activate the drug.

Fungal resistance to flucytosine can result from mutations in genes encoding cytosine deaminase, cytosine permease, or enzymes that incorporate 5-FU into fungal RNA. Because drug resistance develops rapidly when flucytosine is given alone, the drug is usually administered in combination with amphotericin B. This combination produces a synergistic effect against *Candida* and *Cryptococcus* species and is effective in the treatment of pneumonia, meningitis, endocarditis, or septicemia caused by these organisms.

The adverse effects of flucytosine are usually mild. In some patients, however, hematologic toxicity and cardiopulmonary arrest have occurred.

Griseofulvin

Griseofulvin is an antibiotic derived from *Penicillium griseofulvum*. The antibiotic has fungistatic activity against numerous dermatophytes, including *E. floccosum*, *Microsporum audouinii*, *M. canis*, *M. gypseum*, *T. rubrum*, *T. tonsurans*, and *Trichophyton verrucosum*, but it is not active against *Candida* or other fungi.

Griseofulvin is a lipophilic drug that is not very soluble in water. To enhance its dissolution in the gut, a microcrystalline form of the drug is used in pharmaceutical preparations. Because of the drug's high lipid solubility, its absorption is increased when it is taken with a high-fat meal. The drug is deposited in keratin precursor cells of the skin, hair, and nails, where it disrupts microtubule function and inhibits the mitosis of susceptible dermatophytes. The cells are gradually exfoliated and replaced by noninfected tissue. After being metabolized in the liver, griseofulvin is excreted in the urine as inactive metabolites. Mild infections usually respond to griseofulvin therapy in 2 to 8 weeks, but persistent nail infections may require 3 to 6 months of treatment.

Griseofulvin is usually well tolerated, but it can cause dizziness, headache, insomnia, gastrointestinal bleeding, hepatitis, skin rash, or leukopenia. Griseofulvin **induces the CYP3A4 isozyme of cytochrome P450** and, thereby, can reduce the plasma concentrations of warfarin, oral contraceptives, and barbiturates that are taken concurrently. As a result, griseofulvin may reduce the anticoagulant effect of warfarin. The clinical significance of the other drug interactions has not been established.

Ciclopirox

Ciclopirox is an *N*-hydroxy-pyridinone compound that is active against dermatophytes, *C. albicans,* and *M. furfur.* It is applied topically twice a day to treat skin infections caused by these organisms. A lacquer formulation (nail polish) is available for topical treatment of mild onychomycosis.

Tolnaftate

Tolnaftate is a nonprescription thiocarbamate drug used to treat tinea versicolor and mild dermatophyte infections of the skin. The drug is usually applied twice daily to the affected areas for 2 to 6 weeks. As with most other topical antifungal drugs, tolnaftate is not reliable for treating infections of the scalp or nail beds.

SUMMARY OF IMPORTANT POINTS

■ Polyene antibiotics (amphotericin B, nystatin) and ciclopirox increase the permeability of the fungal cell membrane. Azole derivatives and allylamine drugs inhibit synthesis of plasma membrane ergosterol, and caspofungin inhibits cell wall glucan synthesis.

■ Flucytosine is converted to 5-fluorouracil by fungal cells and is then incorporated into fungal RNA, where it inhibits protein synthesis. Flucytosine is used in combination with amphotericin B for cryptococcal meningitis and candidiasis.

■ Amphotericin B is used to treat severe systemic and subcutaneous mycoses, but it often causes chills, fever, nephrotoxicity, and other adverse effects. Lipid formulations have less toxicity and similar efficacy as nonlipid formulations.

■ Several azole derivatives are used to treat systemic mycoses. Itraconazole can be used to treat blastomycosis, coccidioidomycosis, histoplasmosis, and sporotrichosis. Fluconazole is used to treat candidiasis and cryptococcosis.

■ Voriconazole and caspofungin are used to treat invasive candidiasis and aspergillosis. Caspofungin inhibits the synthesis of a fungal cell wall component, β-(1,3)-D-glucan.

■ Superficial *Candida* infections can be treated with nystatin, azole derivatives, or ciclopirox.

■ Dermatophyte infections can be treated by topical or oral administration of an azole derivative or terbinafine; by oral administration of griseofulvin; or by topical administration of ciclopirox, naftifine, or tolnaftate.

■ Itraconazole or terbinafine is given orally to treat onychomycosis.

■ Griseofulvin interferes with microtubule function and blocks mitosis. It is used orally in treating dermatophyte infections.

Review Questions

Questions 1–5. For each numbered drug description, select the corresponding drug from the lettered choices.

(A) griseofulvin
(B) voriconazole
(C) fluconazole
(D) terbinafine
(E) caspofungin
(F) amphotericin B
(G) ciclopirox

1. It achieves high levels in the cerebrospinal fluid and is used as follow-up therapy for cryptococcal meningitis.

2. It inhibits the synthesis of a fungal cell wall glucan.

3. It inhibits ergosterol synthesis by blocking squalene monooxygenase.

4. It frequently causes chills, fever, and electrolyte abnormalities.

5. It inhibits a fungal cytochrome P450 enzyme and is active against *Aspergillus* species that are inherently resistant to amphotericin B.

Answers and Explanations

1. The answer is C: fluconazole. Fluconazole achieves effective levels in the cerebrospinal fluid and is used to treat fungal meningitis. For cryptococcal meningitis, it is sometimes used as follow-up therapy after initial treatment of the disease with amphotericin B and flucytosine.

2. The answer is E: caspofungin. Caspofungin is a echinocandin drug that inhibits the synthesis of β-(1,3)-D-glucan, an integral component of the fungal cell wall. This action produces a fungicidal effect on susceptible strains of *Candida* and *Aspergillus* species.

3. The answer is D: terbinafine. Allylamine and azole drugs inhibit unique steps in fungal membrane ergosterol synthesis. Terbinafine and other allylamine drugs block squalene monooxygenase, which converts squalene to squalene-2,3-oxide. The azole antifungal agents inhibit the cytochrome P450 enzyme that converts lanosterol to ergosterol.

4. The answer is F: amphotericin B. Amphotericin B is one of the most toxic antibiotics used in treating human infections. It usually causes chills and fever during intravenous administration of the drug, and many patients experience some degree of nephrotoxicity leading to electrolyte imbalances (e.g., hypokalemia and hypomagnesemia). Lipid-based formulations cause less renal toxicity.

5. The answer is B: voriconazole. Both caspofungin and voriconazole are active against some *Candida* and *Aspergillus* species that are inherently resistant to other antifungal drugs. Voriconazole acts by inhibiting a cytochrome P450 enzyme involved in fungal membrane ergosterol synthesis, whereas caspofungin inhibits cell wall glucan synthesis.

SELECTED READINGS

Boucher, H. W., A. H. Groll, C. C. Chiou, et al. Newer systemic antifungal agents: pharmacokinetics, safety, and efficacy. Drugs 64:1997–2020, 2004.

Denning, D. W. Echinocandin antifungal drugs. Lancet 362:1142–1151, 2003.

Goldman, R. D., and G. Koren. Amphotericin B nephrotoxicity in children. J Pediatr Hematol Oncol 26:421–426, 2004.

Rapp, R. P. Changing strategies for the management of invasive fungal infections. Pharmacotherapy 24(2 Pt 2):4S–28S, 2004.

Veerareddy, P. R., and V. Vobalaboina. Lipid-based formulations of amphotericin B. Drugs Today (Barc) 40:133–245, 2004.

CHAPTER 43

Antiviral Drugs

CLASSIFICATION OF ANTIVIRAL DRUGS*

Drugs for Herpesvirus Infections
Nucleoside Analogues
- Acyclovir (ZOVIRAX)[a]
- Ganciclovir and cidofovir
- Trifluridine (VIROPTIC)

Other drugs
- Foscarnet

Drugs for Human Immunodeficiency Virus Infection
Nucleoside Reverse Transcriptase Inhibitors
- Zidovudine (RETROVIR)[b]
- Lamivudine (EPIVIR)
- Emtricitabine (EMTRIVA)

Nonnucleoside Reverse Transcriptase Inhibitors
- Efavirenz (SUSTIVA)
- Nevirapine (VIRAMUNE)

Nucleotide Reverse Transcriptase Inhibitor
- Tenofovir (VIREAD)

Protease Inhibitors
- Lopinavir and ritonavir (KALETRA)
- Atazanavir[c]

Fusion Inhibitor
- Enfuvirtide (FUZEON)

Drugs for Influenza
- Amantadine and rimantadine
- Oseltamivir (TAMIFLU) and zanamivir (RELENZA)

Drugs for Other Viral Infections
- Ribavirin (VIRAZOLE)
- Interferon alfa

[a]also famciclovir, penciclovir, valacyclovir
[b]also abacavir, didanosine, stavudine
[c]also fosamprenavir, indinavir, nelfinavir, saquinavir

OVERVIEW

Viruses are obligate intracellular parasites that use the host cell's metabolic pathways for reproduction. This limits the number of potential sites for antiviral drug action. Furthermore, antibacterial and antifungal drugs have little or no effect on viruses. Despite these obstacles, effective antiviral compounds have been developed for the treatment of some viral infections. These include herpesvirus infections, human immunodeficiency virus (HIV) infection, influenza, and hepatitis.

Most antiviral drugs, which are antimetabolites of endogenous nucleosides, prevent the replication of viral nucleic acid. Other antiviral drugs inhibit the entry, uncoating, or release and spread of the virus. Other targets for antiviral therapy are currently being investigated.

DRUGS FOR HERPESVIRUS INFECTIONS

All herpesviruses are DNA viruses. The most common examples are **herpes simplex virus** (HSV), **varicella-zoster virus** (VZV), and **cytomegalovirus** (CMV).

HSV frequently causes **herpes genitalis** (genital herpes infection), **herpes labialis** (infection of the lips and mouth), or **herpetic keratoconjunctivitis** (infection of the cornea and conjunctiva). Less commonly, it causes **herpetic encephalitis,** a potentially fatal disease.

Varicella-zoster virus is the cause of **chickenpox (varicella)** and **shingles (herpes zoster).** Chickenpox occurs primarily in young children. Shingles, which is reported more frequently in the elderly, results from activation of

468

latent VZV in nerve root ganglia. In patients with shingles, pain and skin lesions occur in areas where the virus travels peripherally along sensory nerves to the corresponding cutaneous or mucosal surfaces. The skin lesions eventually heal but can leave residual scars. Postherpetic neuralgia is a common and disabling complication of shingles.

Cytomegalovirus infections in immunocompetent individuals are usually asymptomatic. Symptomatic **CMV diseases,** such as **retinitis, esophagitis,** and **colitis,** are seen most often in immunocompromised patients, including those with HIV infection or acquired immunodeficiency syndrome (AIDS).

Numerous drugs are available to treat herpesvirus infections. With the exception of foscarnet, all of the drugs are nucleoside analogues.

Nucleoside Analogues

Drug Properties

CHEMISTRY. Most of the nucleoside analogues used to treat herpesvirus infections contain a naturally occurring purine or pyrimidine base that is coupled to a unique carbohydrate moiety (Fig. 43–1A).

MECHANISMS. The nucleoside analogues are prodrugs that are phosphorylated by viral and host cell kinases to form active triphosphate metabolites (Fig. 43–2). In this process, the nucleoside analogues are initially converted to monophosphate metabolites by a virus-encoded thymidine kinase. The conversion occurs only in infected host cells, thereby contributing to the selective toxicity of the analogues. Host cell kinases subsequently convert the monophosphates to active triphosphate metabolites. The active metabolites then compete with endogenous nucleoside triphosphates and competitively inhibit viral DNA polymerase which, in turn, prevents the synthesis of viral DNA. Some nucleoside analogues (e.g., acyclovir) are incorporated into nascent viral DNA and cause DNA chain termination because they lack the 3′-hydroxyl group required for attachment of the next nucleoside (see Fig. 43–2). Other analogues (e.g., ganciclovir and penciclovir) inhibit viral DNA polymerase but do not cause DNA chain termination.

PHARMACOKINETICS, SPECTRUM, AND INDICATIONS. The properties and clinical uses of individual drugs for herpesvirus infections are compared in Tables 43–1 and 43–2 and discussed in greater detail below.

VIRAL RESISTANCE. The incidence of resistance to the nucleoside analogues varies with the drug and viral pathogen.

Resistance of HSV and VZV to acyclovir is not common, and resistant strains are usually less infective than are sensitive strains. Furthermore, most acyclovir-resistant HSV and VZV strains are not resistant to other nucleoside analogues or to foscarnet. Most acyclovir-resistant strains have been recovered from immunocompromised patients. Loss of thymidine kinase activity is the major cause of innate and acquired resistance to acyclovir.

Resistance of CMV to ganciclovir is a more serious clinical problem than is HSV resistance, but most ganciclo-

Figure 43–1. Structures of selected drugs for herpesvirus infections (A) and other viral infections (B). Acyclovir and ganciclovir are nucleoside analogues. These analogues contains a naturally occurring purine or pyrimidine base, which is coupled to a unique carbohydrate moiety (unshaded area). Unlike the other drugs, foscarnet is a pyrophosphate derivative. Amantadine is a tricyclic amine compound.

vir-resistant CMV strains are sensitive to cidofovir and foscarnet. Loss of a virus-specific protein kinase is the major cause of resistance to ganciclovir.

Acyclovir, Famciclovir, and Valacyclovir

Acyclovir, famciclovir, and valacyclovir are nucleoside analogues that are effective in the treatment of various HSV and VZV infections (see Table 43–2). These drugs are not sufficiently active against CMV to be effective in treating CMV infections, but acyclovir and valacyclovir can be used for **prophylaxis of CMV infections** such as in bone marrow and organ transplant recipients, and in persons with HIV infec-

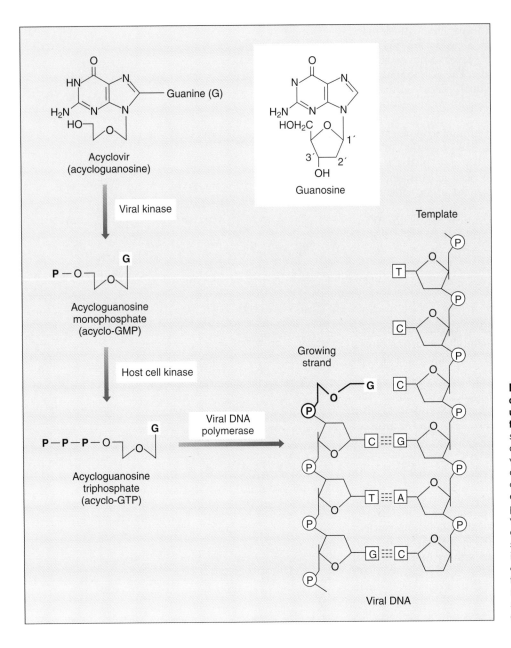

Figure 43–2. Mechanisms of action of nucleoside analogues used in the treatment of viral infections. Acyclovir and other nucleoside analogues are converted to active nucleoside triphosphates by viral and host cell kinases. These active nucleoside triphosphates compete with the corresponding endogenous nucleoside triphosphates and competitively inhibit viral DNA polymerase. Acyclovir and the nucleoside reverse transcriptase inhibitors (NRTI) are incorporated into viral DNA and cause chain termination because they lack the 3'-hydroxyl group required to attach the next nucleoside. Ganciclovir and penciclovir do not cause chain termination.

tion. All three drugs are available for oral use. In addition, acyclovir is available for intravenous and topical use.

The intravenous form of acyclovir is the most effective treatment for serious herpesvirus infections, including herpetic encephalitis and severe HSV and VZV infections in immunocompromised patients.

The topical form of acyclovir can be used to treat herpes genitalis and mild mucocutaneous infections in immunocompromised patients. In cases of herpes genitalis, however, the topical form is less effective than the oral form of acyclovir.

In its oral form, acyclovir has a relatively low bioavailability (22%). Valacyclovir, which was developed later than acyclovir, is a prodrug that is rapidly converted to acyclovir by intestinal and hepatic enzymes and is more completely absorbed than acyclovir. Because of its greater bioavailability (55%), valacyclovir requires less frequent administration

than acyclovir. Famciclovir has the greatest bioavailability (80%) and is rapidly hydrolyzed to penciclovir following its absorption.

When acyclovir, famciclovir, or valacyclovir is given orally for the treatment of herpes genitalis, it prevents the replication of HSV and thereby reduces pain and other symptoms of acute infection. It also shortens the time to healing of lesions and reduces the amount of viral shedding. It does not eliminate the virus, however, so recurrent episodes of infection are common. Shorter courses of therapy are usually sufficient for these episodes, because recurrent infections are usually milder than the initial infection. Severe herpes genitalis may require intravenous acyclovir therapy.

When acyclovir, famciclovir, or valacyclovir is given orally for the treatment of shingles, it shortens the duration of acute illness and pain, and the duration of postherpetic pain (neuralgia). In patients with shingles, famciclovir and vala-

TABLE 43-1. **Pharmacokinetic Properties of Antiviral Drugs***

Drug	Route of Administration	Oral Bioavailability (%)	Elimination Half-Life (Hours)	Routes of Elimination
Drugs for herpesvirus infections				
Nucleoside analogues				
Acyclovir	Oral, IV, or topical	22	3	Renal excretion
Cidofovir	IV	NA	2.5	Renal excretion
Famciclovir	Oral	80	2	Metabolism; renal and fecal excretion
Ganciclovir	Oral or IV	8	4	Renal excretion
Penciclovir	Topical	NA	NA	NA
Trifluridine	Topical ocular	NA	NA	NA
Valacyclovir	Oral	55	3	Renal excretion
Other drugs				
Foscarnet	IV	NA	5	Renal excretion
Drugs for human immunodeficiency virus infection				
NRTI				
Didanosine	Oral	30	2	Metabolism; renal excretion
Lamivudine	Oral	85	6	Renal excretion
Stavudine	Oral	85	3.5	Renal excretion
Zidovudine	Oral or IV	65	1	Metabolism; renal excretion
NNRTI				
Efavirenz	Oral	50	65	Metabolism; fecal excretion
Nevirapine	Oral	92	30	Metabolism; fecal excretion
Protease inhibitors				
Indinavir	Oral	80	2	Metabolism; fecal excretion
Nelfinavir	Oral	50	4.5	Metabolism; fecal excretion
Ritonavir	Oral	80	4	Metabolism; fecal excretion
Saquinavir	Oral	12	12	Metabolism; fecal excretion
Lopinauir	Oral	80	6	Metabolism; fecal excretion
Fusion inhibitor				
Enfuvirtide	Subcutaneous	NA	3	Metabolism
Drugs for influenza				
Amantadine	Oral	75	24	Renal excretion
Rimantadine	Oral	90	25	Metabolism; renal excretion
Oseltamivir	Oral	75	8	Metabolism; renal excretion
Zanamivir	Nasal	NA	U	Metabolism; renal excretion
Drugs for other viral infections				
Interferon alfa	Subcutaneous	NA	7	Metabolism
Peginterferon alfa-2b	Subcutaneous	NA	40	Metabolism
Ribavirin	Inhalation or IV	NA	9.5	Metabolism; renal excretion

*Values shown are the mean of values reported in the literature. IV = intravenous; IM = intramuscular; NA = not applicable; U = unknown; NRTIs = nucleoside reverse transcriptase inhibitors; and NNRTIs = nonnucleoside reverse transcriptase inhibitors.

TABLE 43-2. **Clinical Uses of Drugs for Herpesvirus Infections**

Drug	Herpes Genitalis	Herpes Labialis	Herpetic Keratoconjunctivitis	Herpetic Encephalitis	Chickenpox	Shingles	Cytomegalovirus Diseases
Acyclovir	Yes	Yes	No	Yes	Yes	Yes	No
Cidofovir	No	No	No	No	No	No	Yes*
Famciclovir	Yes	No	No	No	No	Yes	No
Foscarnet	Yes*	No	No	No	No	Yes*	Yes
Ganciclovir	No	No	No	No	No	No	Yes
Penciclovir	No	Yes	No	No	No	No	No
Trifluridine	No	No	Yes	No	No	No	No
Valacyclovir	Yes	No	No	No	No	Yes	No

*For treating patients with intolerance of or resistance to other drugs.

cyclovir appear to be more effective than acyclovir. The newer drugs allow for less-frequent administration and provide higher serum drug levels because of their greater oral bioavailability.

Acyclovir is available in an oral suspension for the treatment of children with chickenpox. The drug has a good safety record in this setting.

Acyclovir, famciclovir, and valacyclovir are well tolerated when given orally, and they do not have significant interactions with other drugs. Gastrointestinal disturbances, headache, and rash are the most common side effects. Intravenous administration of acyclovir can produce phlebitis and reversible renal dysfunction.

Penciclovir

Penciclovir, the active metabolite of famciclovir, is now available in a topical cream formulation for the treatment of **herpes labialis**. In a study of patients with a history of frequent herpes labialis episodes, use of penciclovir was found to shorten the time to healing and the duration of pain by about a day. It also was found to decrease the duration of viral shedding.

Ganciclovir and Cidofovir

Ganciclovir and cidofovir are nucleoside analogues used to prevent and treat CMV diseases, including retinitis, esophagitis, and colitis. Both drugs are available for intravenous use, and ganciclovir is also available for oral use. Ganciclovir is usually given initially, whereas cidofovir is generally reserved for diseases that are resistant to ganciclovir or other drugs. Ganciclovir has a relatively low oral bioavailability, so oral administration is used only for long-term suppression of CMV retinitis. Cidofovir can be given intravenously for this purpose.

Ganciclovir is about 100 times more active against CMV than is acyclovir. Ganciclovir, however, produces a much higher incidence of adverse effects than do acyclovir and famciclovir. The most common serious adverse effects of ganciclovir are leukopenia and thrombocytopenia. Severe myelosuppression is more likely if the drug is given concurrently with zidovudine. Other adverse effects of ganciclovir include retinal detachment, liver and renal dysfunction, rash, fever, and gastrointestinal disturbances.

Cidofovir sometimes causes nephrotoxicity, neutropenia, metabolic acidosis, and other serious adverse effects. About 25% of patients have discontinued cidofovir for this reason. The drug is contraindicated in patients who are taking other nephrotoxic drugs, such as aminoglycosides or amphotericin B.

Trifluridine

Trifluridine is administered topically to treat ocular herpesvirus infections. It is the most widely used nucleoside analogue in patients with **herpetic keratoconjunctivitis** and **epithelial keratitis** (inflammation caused by infection of the cornea), and it is usually effective in treating infections that are not responsive to idoxuridine or vidarabine. The drug is generally well tolerated but can cause superficial ocular irritation and hyperemia.

Other Drugs for Herpesvirus Infections

Foscarnet is a pyrophosphate derivative (see Fig. 43–1A). It acts by blocking pyrophosphate-binding sites on viral DNA polymerase and thereby preventing attachment of nucleotide precursors to DNA. Unlike the nucleoside analogues used to treat herpesvirus infections, foscarnet does not require activation by viral or host cell kinases.

Foscarnet is active against CMV, VZV, and HSV. It must be administered intravenously and is used to treat CMV retinitis in patients with AIDS and to treat acyclovir-resistant HSV infections and shingles. Foscarnet can be combined with ganciclovir to treat infections that are resistant to either drug alone.

Adverse reactions to foscarnet include renal impairment and acute renal failure, hematologic deficiencies, cardiac arrhythmias and heart failure, seizures, and pancreatitis. Renal toxicity can be minimized by administering intravenous fluids to induce diuresis before and during foscarnet treatment.

DRUGS FOR HUMAN IMMUNODEFICIENCY VIRUS INFECTION

Remarkable advances have been made in the treatment of HIV infection and AIDS. Many new drugs have been introduced, and the combined use of two or more drugs from different classes has been shown to markedly reduce viral loads and improve survival in many HIV-positive individuals. This type of multidrug treatment for HIV infection has been called **highly active antiretroviral therapy (HAART)**. Initially, HAART regimens were quite complicated and required multiple doses of several drugs throughout the day. In recent years, emphasis has been placed on developing and using drug regimens that only require a few doses a day. This has been accomplished by developing combination drug products and longer-acting drugs.

Sites of Drug Action

Human immunodeficiency virus is an RNA virus that is classified as a **retrovirus**. Its replication and sites of drug action are depicted in Fig. 43–3. HIV replication begins with fusion of the virus to its host cell, the **HIV-specific CD4⁺ T helper lymphocyte** (hereafter CD4⁺ cell). Once HIV enters the CD4⁺ cell, viral RNA serves as a template to produce a complementary doubled-stranded DNA in a reaction catalyzed by viral **reverse transcriptase** (RNA-dependent DNA polymerase). The viral DNA then enters the host cell nucleus and is incorporated into the host genome in a reaction catalyzed by **HIV integrase**. Eventually, the viral DNA is transcribed and translated to produce large, nonfunctional polypeptides called **polyproteins**. These polyproteins are packaged into immature virions at the cell surface. An enzyme called **HIV protease** cleaves the polyproteins into smaller, functional proteins in a process called **viral maturation** as the virions are released into the plasma.

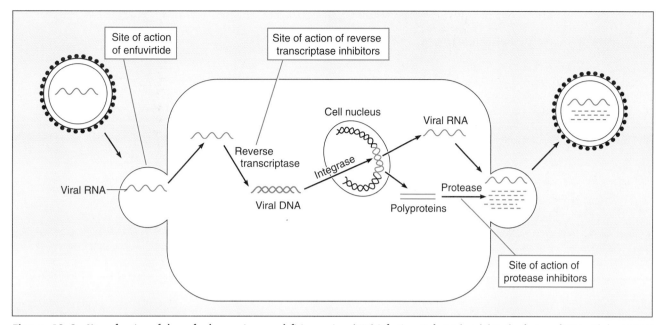

Figure 43-3. Sites of action of drugs for human immunodeficiency virus (HIV) infection. Enfuvirtide inhibits the fusion of HIV with host CD4[+] cell membranes. After the virus penetrates the host cell and becomes uncoated, the viral RNA is transcribed by reverse transcriptase to form viral DNA. Viral DNA is incorporated into the host genome in the cell nucleus by HIV integrase. The viral DNA is then transcribed to RNA. Viral RNA is incorporated into new virions and is translated to synthesize polyproteins. The polyproteins are cleaved into viral proteins by HIV protease as the new virions are released from the cell. Drugs for HIV infection inhibit reverse transcriptase or protease.

The drugs currently available for treatment of HIV infection act by inhibiting viral fusion, reverse transcriptase, or HIV protease. Drugs that act via other mechanisms are being investigated. For example, drugs that inhibit HIV integrase are currently under development.

The two most important types of **reverse transcriptase inhibitors** are the **nucleoside reverse transcriptase inhibitors** (NRTI) and the **nonnucleoside reverse transcriptase inhibitors** (NNRTI). Small amounts of the NRTI are converted to their active triphosphate metabolites by host cell kinases. The triphosphate metabolites (nucleotides) compete with the corresponding endogenous nucleoside triphosphates for incorporation into viral DNA in the reaction catalyzed by reverse transcriptase. Once incorporated into DNA, the NRTI cause DNA chain termination in the same manner as described above for acyclovir (see Fig. 43-2). The NRTI also inhibit host cell DNA polymerase to varying degrees, and this may account for some of their toxic effects (e.g., anemia).

Unlike the NRTI, the nonnucleoside drugs bind directly to reverse transcriptase and disrupt the catalytic site. Hence, the NNRTI do not require phosphorylation for activity. Because they act by different mechanisms, the NRTI and NNRTI exhibit synergistic inhibition of HIV replication when they are given concurrently.

Tenofovir disoproxil fumarate, a diphosphonate diester of a nucleoside drug, is classified as a **nucleotide reverse transcriptase inhibitor** (a nucleotide being a phosphate ester of a nucleoside). As a nucleotide prodrug, tenofovir disoproxil fumarate is hydrolyzed in the body to form tenofovir, and then tenofovir is converted to tenofovir diphosphate by CD4[+] cell kinases. Tenofovir diphosphate competes with deoxyadenosine 5'-triphosphate and is incorporated into

viral DNA by reverse transcriptase, causing DNA chain termination. Hence, tenofovir is similar to the NRTI in its manner of activation and mechanism of action.

Nucleoside Reverse Transcriptase Inhibitors

The NRTI were the first class of drugs developed for the treatment of HIV-positive individuals, and they are included in almost all HIV treatment regimens. Although all NRTI have the same basic mechanism of action, different drugs in the class serve as antimetabolites of different purine and pyrimidine bases of DNA. For this reason, an NRTI is often more effective when it is given in combination with another NRTI than when it is given alone. As shown in Table 43-3, two NRTI are usually combined with either a NNRTI or a protease inhibitor.

Drug Properties

CHEMISTRY. The NRTI are synthetic derivatives of naturally occurring nucleosides (Fig. 43-4). Didanosine is a purine base congener, whereas lamivudine, stavudine, emtricitabine, and zidovudine are pyrimidine base congeners.

PHARMACOKINETICS. All of the NRTI can be given orally, and zidovudine can also be given intravenously. The NRTI cross the blood–brain barrier and are distributed to the cerebrospinal fluid. The drugs are eliminated primarily by renal excretion, and renal impairment will prolong their plasma elimination half-life and may necessitate a reduction in dosage.

SPECTRUM AND INDICATIONS. The NRTI are the foundation of chemotherapy for HIV infection. In addition to inhibiting

Figure 43–4. **Structures of selected nucleoside reverse transcriptase inhibitors.** Each nucleoside reverse transcriptase inhibitor contains a naturally occurring purine or pyrimidine base, which is coupled to a unique carbohydrate moiety (unshaded area). Didanosine is a purine base congener, whereas lamivudine, stavudine, and zidovudine are pyrimidine base congeners.

the replication of human and animal retroviruses, some of the NRTI have demonstrated activity against hepatitis B virus and Epstein-Barr virus.

VIRAL RESISTANCE. Resistance to NRTI can develop during therapy and is more likely to occur in persons receiving

TABLE 43–3.	Drug Regimens for Treating Human Immunodeficiency Virus (HIV) Infection in Adults and Adolescents*

Preferred Regimens for Initial Treatment
Protease Inhibitor-Based
Lopinavir and ritonavir (KALETRA) + (lamivudine or emtricitabine) + zidovudine
Nonnucleoside Reverse Transcriptase Inhibitor-Based
Efavirenz + (lamivudine or emtricitabine) + (zidovudine or tenofovir)

Alternative Regimens

Nonnucleoside Reverse Transcriptase Inhibitor-Based
Efavirenz + (lamivudine or emtricitabine) + (abacavir or didanosine or stavudine)

OR

Nevirapine + (lamivudine or emtricitabine) + (zidovudine or stavudine or didanosine or abacavir or tenofovir)
Protease Inhibitor-Based†
Atazanavir + (lamivudine or emtricitabine) + (zidovudine or stavudine or abacavir or didanosine)

OR

Lopinavir and ritonavir (KALETRA) + (lamivudine or emtricitabine) + (stavudine or abacavir or tenofovir or didanosine)
Nucleoside Reverse Transcriptase Inhibitor-Based‡
Abacavir + lamivudine + zidovudine

*Issued October 29, 2004. For more recent updates see (*http://AIDSinfo. nih.gov*).
†Other protease inhibitor-based regimens can be found at (*http://AIDSinfo. nih.gov*).
‡To be used only when a preferred or alternative protease inhibitor-based or non-nucleoside reverse transcriptase inhibitor-based regimen cannot or should not be used.

single-drug therapy for 6 months or longer. Studies of zidovudine indicate that HIV type I (HIV-1) acquires resistance to the drug in a stepwise manner involving four or five specific mutations in the gene that encodes the reverse transcriptase enzyme. Because the virus undergoes frequent mutations, the only way to prevent resistance is to prevent HIV replication by using combination drug therapy. Resistance to lamivudine is associated with a mutation at codon 184 in HIV reverse transcriptase, which suppresses preexisting resistance to zidovudine in some isolates. Reduced sensitivity of hepatitis B virus (HBV) to lamivudine is related to mutations in the catalytic domain of HBV DNA polymerase.

ADVERSE EFFECTS AND INTERACTIONS. As shown in Table 43–4, the NRTI differ in their major toxicities and in their interactions with other drugs. Zidovudine produces bone marrow suppression and can cause anemia and neutropenia. Didanosine and stavudine can cause pancreatitis, and didanosine can also cause peripheral neuropathy. Abacavir is more likely to cause a hypersensitivity reaction, whereas tenofovir produces renal impairment in some patients.

Specific Drugs

Zidovudine (RETROVIR), also known as **azidothymidine** (AZT), was the first NRTI to be developed, and it is still one of the most widely used drugs in this class. Zidovudine is most often combined today with lamivudine or emtricitabine. It is available in fixed-dose combination products with lamivudine (COMBIVIR) and with lamivudine and abacavir (TRIZIVIR). Zidovudine and stavudine are not used together because they appear to be antagonistic.

Studies indicate that zidovudine treatment significantly reduces the incidence of **in utero transmission of HIV** from infected pregnant women to their offspring. To prevent transmission, zidovudine is administered from the 14th to the 34th week of gestation. Many authorities now recommend combination drug therapy for pregnant women with HIV infection.

Lamivudine (EPIVIR), or **3-thiacytosine** (3TC), appears to cause fewer adverse effects than do other NRTI. Lamivudine is often used in combination with zidovudine or stavudine. Combination therapy with these drugs produces a

TABLE 43-4. Most Important Adverse Effects and Interactions of Drugs for Human Immunodeficiency Virus (HIV) Infection*

Drug	Adverse Effects and Interactions
NRTI	
All NRTI	Lactic acidosis, hepatic steatosis, and lipodystrophy (all higher with stavudine)
Abacavir	Hypersensitivity reactions
Didanosine	**Pancreatitis, peripheral neuropathy,** gastrointestinal intolerance
Stavudine	**Pancreatitis, peripheral neuropathy**
Tenofovir	Headache, gastrointestinal intolerance, renal impairment
Zidovudine	Headache, gastrointestinal intolerance, **bone marrow suppression**
NNRTI	
All NNRTI	Rash, drug interactions
Efavirenz	Neuropsychiatric reactions, teratogenic
Nevirapine	Hepatotoxicity, rash including Stevens-Johnson syndrome, induces metabolism of protease inhibitors and contraceptive steroids
Protease Inhibitors	
All protease inhibitors	Lipodystrophy (fat accumulation), hyperlipidemia, insulin resistance and diabetes, elevated liver function tests, inhibits metabolism of other protease inhibitors
Amprenavir, fosamprenavir	Gastrointestinal intolerance, rash
Atazanavir	Hyperbilirubinemia, PR interval prolongation
Lopinavir and ritonavir	Gastrointestinal intolerance
Ritonavir	Gastrointestinal intolerance, hepatitis, inhibits metabolism of other drugs, including antiarrhythmic drugs, opioids, and tricyclic antidepressants
Fusion inhibitor	
Enfuvirtide	Injection site reactions, hypersensitivity reactions

*NRTI = nucleoside reverse transcriptase inhibitors; NNRTI = nonnucleoside reverse transcriptase inhibitors.

greater reduction in viral load than is obtained with single-drug therapy, and it also decreases the risk for emergence of drug resistance. Lamivudine is also used in the treatment of **hepatitis B.**

Emtricitabine (EMTRIVA), or fluorothiacytidine (FTC), is a newer NRTI that is usually combined with zidovudine or **tenofovir.** A combination product containing emtricitabine and tenofovir intended for once-daily administration is under development.

Other NRTI, including **abacavir, stavudine,** and **didanosine,** usually are used as alternatives to first-line drugs, such as in cases where a first-line drug is not tolerated or when viral resistance occurs. For example, stavudine usually is used as a substitute for zidovudine in persons who cannot tolerate it or fail to respond to it. Didanosine, or **dideoxyinosine** (ddI), is mainly used in combination with lamivudine or emtricitabine plus a protease inhibitor.

Nonnucleoside Reverse Transcriptase Inhibitors

Drug Properties

The NNRTI include efavirenz, nevirapine, and delavirdine. These drugs directly inhibit reverse transcriptase. Unlike NRTI, they do not require metabolic activation, and they are not incorporated into viral DNA. Delavirdine is no longer recommended for most patients with HIV infection because of its modest antiviral activity. Efavirenz is the preferred NNRTI for the initial treatment of patients with HIV infection.

PHARMACOKINETICS. The NNRTI are administered orally and have good oral bioavailability (see Table 43-1). They are highly lipophilic, and the concentrations that they reach in the central nervous system (CNS) are adequate for antiviral activity. The drugs are extensively metabolized before undergoing fecal and renal excretion.

SPECTRUM, INDICATIONS, AND VIRAL RESISTANCE. In vitro studies show that NNRTI act synergistically with NRTI and protease inhibitors against HIV. The NNRTI are never used alone to treat patients with HIV infection, because viral resistance develops rapidly unless they are combined with other drugs.

Preferred and alternative treatment regimens are listed in Table 43-3.

ADVERSE EFFECTS AND INTERACTIONS. NNRTI are moderately well tolerated. **Rash** is the most common side effect. In patients with a mild rash, the drugs can usually be continued or restarted. Patients should be monitored, however, because the rash can progress to Stevens-Johnson syndrome. Efavirenz is teratogenic in primates and should be avoided in pregnant women and women who may become pregnant. Efavirenz can also cause neuropsychiatric reactions. Drug interactions and other common adverse effects of NNRTI are listed in Table 43-4.

Efavirenz

Efavirenz is the most potent NNRTI currently available. Unlike other NNRTI, efavirenz can be taken once a day. For these reasons, it is the preferred NNRTI for initial treatment of most adult patients with HIV infection.

Nevirapine

Nevirapine is most often used in combination with two NRTI (Table 43–3). Nevirapine induces cytochrome P450 and accelerates the metabolism of certain drugs (see Table 43–4). In addition to skin rash, it can also cause hepatotoxicity.

Protease Inhibitors

Human immunodeficiency virus protease cleaves the gag-pol polyprotein precursor to form functional viral proteins essential for the **maturation** of the virus. Protease inhibitors bind to the active site of the enzyme and thereby inhibit proteolytic activity. Inhibition of HIV protease results in the production of immature, noninfectious viral particles.

Saquinavir, the first HIV protease inhibitor (PI), was approved in 1995, ushering in a new era in the treatment of HIV infection and AIDS. Other PI were subsequently developed, including **indinavir, nelfinavir,** and **ritonavir**. More recently, PI that are better tolerated and have better pharmacokinetic properties were introduced, including **atazanavir** and **fosamprenavir**. Because ritonavir inhibits the metabolism of other PI, it is sometimes combined with lopinavir, fosamprenavir, and other PI to increase their plasma levels and duration of action. A fixed dose combination product containing lopinavir and ritonavir (KALETRA) has become the preferred PI for initial treatment of adults with HIV infection (Table 43–3). The administration of ritonavir with another PI is known as **boosted therapy**.

Tables 43–1 and 43–4 compare information on the properties, effects, and interactions of selected protease inhibitors. Fig. 43–3 shows the site of action of these drugs.

Drug Properties

PHARMACOKINETICS. Protease inhibitors are given orally and are extensively metabolized by cytochrome P450 enzymes before undergoing fecal excretion. Two of the drugs, nelfinavir and ritonavir, are available in formulations for administration to pediatric patients.

ACTIVITY, INDICATIONS, AND VIRAL RESISTANCE. Protease inhibitors have synergistic effects with NRTI. The combined use of a PI and two NRTI significantly reduces the viral load, increases $CD4^+$ cell levels, and slows the clinical progression of disease and the emergence of drug resistance. Resistance to PI is associated with the accumulation of mutations resulting in amino acid substitutions at eleven residue positions in the viral protease. Varying degrees of cross-resistance occur between different PI, but cross-resistance between PI and reverse transcriptase inhibitors is rare. The preferred PI and NRTI combinations are listed in Table 43–3.

ADVERSE EFFECTS AND INTERACTIONS. All PI can cause lipid accumulation in tissues (lipodystrophy) and hyperlipidemia, insulin resistance and diabetes, elevated liver function tests, and drug interactions. Ritonavir appears to produce the highest incidence of adverse effects, whereas atazanavir is better tolerated that most other PI and has a lower propensity to cause diarrhea, lipodystrophy, and hyperlipidemia.

Hyperbilirubinemia is a common side effect of atazanavir, but it is largely a laboratory abnormality without physiologic consequences.

Protease inhibitors interact with a number of other drugs (see Table 43–4) via inhibition of cytochrome P450 enzymes. They have the greatest effect on drugs metabolized by the CYP3A4 isozyme, and they can cause a several-fold increase in the plasma concentration of these drugs, including other PI. For this reason, ritonavir has been administered concurrently with saquinavir, indinavir, and lopinavir to increase serum drug levels. The NNRTI also interact with PI. Nevirapine can induce the metabolism and decrease the therapeutic effect of PI.

Lopinavir and Ritonavir

The combination of lopinavir and ritonavir (KALETRA) has become the preferred PI for initial treatment of adults with HIV infection, in combination with zidovudine plus either lamivudine or emtricitabine. The lopinavir and ritonavir combination is highly efficacious and relatively well tolerated.

Atazanavir

Atazanavir is an alternative PI for initial treatment of HIV infection, in combination with two NRTI. Because atazanavir can be dosed once a day, atazanavir-based regimens require fewer pills per day than other PI-based regimens. Moreover, atazanavir is better tolerated than other PI.

Other Protease Inhibitors

Other PI, including **amprenavir, indinavir, saquinavir,** and **nelfinavir**, are less preferred for initial treatment of HIV infection because they require a higher number of pills per day than do atazanavir- and the lopinavir and ritonavir-based regimens, leading to dosing inconvenience, dosing errors, and decreased patient compliance. Because of the complexity of drug regimens for treating HIV infection, the emphasis has shifted in recent years to simplifying therapy by developing regimens that require fewer pills that can be administered once a day. For this reason, many of the original PI are no longer preferred for treatment of HIV infection.

Indinavir has demonstrated excellent clinical effectiveness in combination with lamivudine plus either zidovudine or stavudine. One study found that plasma HIV RNA levels became undetectable after 24 weeks of three-drug therapy and that the levels remained undetectable in almost 80% of patients after 100 weeks of treatment.

Ritonavir is a potent drug with proved clinical efficacy. In recent years, it has often been used in combination with other PI to increase their plasma levels and effectiveness. Ritonavir can be combined with **indinavir, saquinavir,** and **fosamprenavir**, and it is available as a combination drug product with lopinavir (KALETRA). In addition to adverse effects common to all PI (see previous), ritonavir is most likely to cause gastrointestinal distress and hepatitis.

Fusion Inhibitor

Unlike other drugs for HIV infection that work inside the $CD4^+$ T lymphocyte and inhibit HIV replication, **enfuvirtide**

(FUZEON) acts to inhibit the fusion of HIV with host cells before the virus enters the cell and begins its replication process. The HIV virus has two proteins that participate in fusing the virus to the host cell. Glycoprotein-120 attracts the virus to the cell surface and then **glycoprotein-41** (GP41) pulls the virus into the cell. Enfuvirtide is a large synthetic peptide containing 36 amino acids that binds to GP41 and thereby blocks the fusion process. Because it is a large peptide molecule, enfuvirtide must be injected subcutaneously twice daily. This injection often causes injection site reactions, which can be minimized by rotating injection sites. Enfuvirtide is otherwise well tolerated and is approved for use in both adults and children. In clinical trials called TORO-1 and TORO-2, enfuvirtide was given to patients who had developed resistance to other antiretroviral drugs. In these studies, enfuvirtide—in combination with an optimized regimen of antiretroviral agents—caused a significantly greater decrease in viral loads and a significantly greater increase in CD4+ cell counts than did the other antiretroviral agents given alone. Enfuvirtide appears to represent a valuable alternative to other anti-HIV drugs when drug resistance or intolerance occurs.

Treatment Considerations

The decision to initiate therapy for HIV infection is based on several considerations, including the patient's CD4+ count (expressed in terms of the number of T cells per microliter), the patient's viral load (expressed in terms of the number of HIV **RNA copies per milliliter**), and whether the patient has clinical symptoms of disease.

Symptomatic patients should be offered treatment regardless of CD4+ cell count and viral load. **Asymptomatic patients** with less than 200 CD4+ cells/μL should be treated, and those with more than 200 but less than 350 cells/μL should be considered for treatment. For asymptomatic patients with more than 350 cells/μL, some clinicians recommend treatment if the viral load is more than 100,000 copies/mL.

Drug regimens for treating HIV infection in adults are listed in Table 43–3. The preferred regimens for initial drug therapy consist of two NRTI and either a PI or an NNRTI. To determine the response to therapy, viral loads should be measured 2 to 8 weeks after starting therapy and every 3 to 4 months thereafter. The time course of the response is highly variable. Viral suppression can take many months in patients with high viral loads.

The main reasons for changing medication after initiating therapy are treatment failure and drug toxicity. Treatment failure is indicated by increased viral loads and decreased CD4+ cells. If the patient fails to respond to a drug regimen, the new regimen should include at least two new drugs. In some cases, **drug resistance testing** can provide useful information concerning the selection of alternative therapy. Alternative drug combinations are listed in Table 43–3. If dose-limiting or intolerable toxicity occurs, the clinician should choose alternative drugs that cause a lower incidence of the particular adverse effects experienced by the patient.

DRUGS FOR INFLUENZA

Because **influenza** is one of the most common causes of infectious disease-related deaths, efforts have been made to develop methods to prevent and treat illness caused by this RNA virus. Vaccines are available for prevention, and several drugs are available for the prevention and treatment of influenza.

Amantadine and Rimantadine

Drug Properties

CHEMISTRY AND MECHANISMS. Amantadine (SYMMETREL) and rimantadine (FLUMADINE) are synthetic tricyclic amine compounds that have similar structures (see Fig. 43–1B). They prevent the uncoating of influenza A particles following their entry into host cells. These drugs target the **M2 proton-selective ion channel** of influenza A virus, and thereby prevent acidification of the virus and the fusion of endosomes and viral membranes that is required for **uncoating** and transfer of viral nucleic acid into the cytoplasm of the host cell.

PHARMACOKINETICS. Amantadine and rimantadine have good oral bioavailability (see Table 43–1), and both drugs are available in liquid preparations for children. Rimantadine is less lipophilic than amantadine and does not cross the blood–brain barrier. For this reason, rimantadine is associated with fewer CNS side effects. Unlike amantadine, rimantadine is extensively metabolized to inactive compounds before undergoing renal excretion, and doses of rimantadine do not need to be adjusted in persons with renal insufficiency. The half-life of each drug is about 24 hours.

SPECTRUM AND INDICATIONS. Amantadine and rimantadine are active against influenza A but not against influenza B. The drugs are 70% to 90% effective in preventing influenza if they are administered before exposure to the virus. They are also effective in reducing the duration and severity of influenza if they are administered within 48 hours of the onset of clinical illness.

Amantadine and rimantadine are usually administered once or twice a day for 5 to 7 days, but they can be given for longer periods of time during outbreaks of influenza. They are particularly useful in controlling epidemics in institutionalized elderly patients, who have a high risk of influenza-related complications and secondary infections. The drugs are also useful in the management of immunodeficient patients, who may not develop adequate immunity following influenza vaccination.

ADVERSE EFFECTS. Mild CNS side effects caused by amantadine include nervousness, anxiety, insomnia, and difficulty in concentrating. In most cases, these effects diminish with continued drug administration and disappear when the drug is stopped. More serious CNS side effects, including hallucinations and seizures, however, sometimes occur in elderly patients. Rimantadine has a much lower incidence of CNS side effects and may be preferred for the treatment of patients with a higher risk of these adverse effects.

Neuraminidase Inhibitors

Oseltamivir (TAMIFLU) and zanamivir (RELENZA) inhibit the enzyme **neuraminidase (sialidase)** in **influenza A and B** viruses. These drugs were designed to bind to the active site of neuraminidase based on studies of its crystalline structure.

Neuraminidase catalyzes reactions that promote viral spreading and infection. First, neuraminidase catalyzes the **release of virions** from the surface of infected cells following viral replication. Secondly, neuraminidase inactivates respiratory tract mucus that would otherwise prevent **spreading of virions** through the respiratory tract. Neuraminidase accomplishes this by cleaving **sialic acid residues** attached to mucous proteins.

Oseltamivir and zanamivir are active against essentially all influenza A and B viruses. Although drug resistant mutants do occur, such mutants are less virulent than their drug-sensitive predecessors and spread less easily. Oseltamivir can be used for **preexposure prophylaxis** in persons who are at least 13 years of age, and it is indicated for treatment of acute illness in adults as well as in children who are at least 1 year of age. If administered within 48 hours after the onset of symptoms, it decreases **symptom severity** and reduces the **duration of illness.** For treatment of influenza, oseltamivir is administered orally twice a day for 5 days, and it is given once daily for prophylaxis. Zanamivir is administered as a nasal spray twice daily for influenza treatment in adults and children who are at least 7 years of age, but it is not intended for prophylactic use.

The adverse effects of neuraminidase inhibitors are usually mild and transient, consisting of minor respiratory and gastrointestinal reactions.

DRUGS FOR HEPATITIS

Lamivudine inhibits the replication of **hepatitis B virus** and has been approved as the first orally effective drug for patients with HBV. As discussed earlier in this chapter, the drug also inhibits the replication of HIV. Unlike HIV, which is an RNA virus, HBV is a DNA virus. Lamivudine is active against HBV because the replication of this virus depends on reverse transcription of an intermediate RNA. Reverse transcription produces a negative-sense strand of DNA. The negative-sense DNA then serves as a template for synthesis of positive-sense DNA.

As is discussed below, **ribavirin** is active against **hepatitis A and C viruses,** whereas **interferon alfa** is active against **hepatitis B and C viruses.** Hepatitis A and C viruses are both RNA viruses.

DRUGS FOR OTHER VIRAL INFECTIONS

Ribavirin

Drug Properties

CHEMISTRY AND MECHANISMS. Ribavirin is a synthetic guanosine analogue (see Fig. 43–1) that acts by several mechanisms to inhibit the synthesis of viral nucleic acid. Ribavirin is activated by kinases that phosphorylate the drug. The active metabolites disrupt cellular **purine metabolism** by inhibiting inosine monophosphate dehydrogenase and thereby causing a deficiency of guanosine triphosphate. This deficiency, in turn, inhibits the synthesis of viral DNA and RNA. Unlike acyclovir and some reverse transcriptase inhibitors, ribavirin also inhibits the synthesis of host cell nucleic acid, and this may account for some of the toxicity of ribavirin.

PHARMACOKINETICS, SPECTRUM, AND INDICATIONS. Table 43–1 outlines the pharmacokinetic properties of ribavirin.

The drug is a broad-spectrum antiviral drug that is active in vitro against a wide range of RNA and DNA viruses. These include adenovirus, Colorado tick fever virus, Crimean-Congo hemorrhagic fever virus, Hantaan virus, hepatitis A and C viruses, herpesviruses, influenza A and B viruses, Lassa virus, measles virus, Muerto Canyon fever virus, mumps virus, respiratory syncytial virus, Rift Valley fever virus, and yellow fever virus.

Although ribavirin has been successfully used to treat infections caused by several of these viruses, the only US Food and Drug Administration (FDA)-approved indication is for the treatment of **severe respiratory syncytial virus infection.** For the treatment of neonates with this type of infection, ribavirin is administered by aerosol, using a small-particle aerosol generator. Influenza has also been treated by aerosol administration, whereas most other viral infections have been treated by intravenous administration.

ADVERSE EFFECTS AND INTERACTIONS. When ribavirin is given by inhalation, it can cause serious pulmonary and cardiovascular effects, including apnea, pneumothorax, worsening of respiratory status, and cardiac arrest. When the drug is given intravenously, seizures can occur. Ribavirin is teratogenic in animals, and its use is contraindicated in pregnant or lactating women. Ribavirin antagonizes the antiviral effects of zidovudine and zalcitabine, so concurrent therapy with these drugs should be avoided.

Interferons

Interferons are now available through recombinant DNA technology for the treatment of several viral infections, as well as for the treatment of neoplasms and other conditions (see Chapter 45). The interferon preparations available today for treating viral and neoplastic diseases include several alpha interferons (alfa-2a, alfa-2b, and alfa-n3, and pegylated alfa-2b) and a type 1 interferon (alfacon-1). **Pegylated interferon alfa-2b** (peginterferon alfa-2b) consists of a covalent conjugate of recombinant alfa interferon with **polyethylene glycol** (PEG). Pegylation significantly increases the half-life (40 hours) and duration of action of the interferon. Therefore, this preparation is only given once a week for 1 year, rather than several times a week as are other interferon preparations.

Drug Properties

CHEMISTRY AND MECHANISMS. The interferons are a group of naturally occurring proteins produced by host cells in response to a viral infection. The interferons have multiple immunomodulating effects and antiproliferative effects, and their most important mechanisms of action in the treatment of specific disorders are uncertain. The antiviral activity of interferons results in part from induction of proteins that inhibit viral penetration or uncoating, inhibit viral peptide elongation, or degrade viral messenger RNA (mRNA).

PHARMACOKINETICS, SPECTRUM, AND INDICATIONS. The apha interferon preparations are active against **hepatitis viruses** and against some **papillomaviruses.** They are used in the treatment of hepatitis B, hepatitis C, non-A, non-B or non-C hepatitis (chronic, active hepatitis), genital warts (condyloma acuminatum), hairy cell leukemia, chronic myelocytic leukemia, Kaposi's sarcoma, renal carcinoma, malignant melanoma, and multiple myeloma.

Treatment with interferon produces clinical remission in some patients with **hepatitis B** or **hepatitis C** virus. Interferon preparations used in treating patients with hepatitis are interferon alfa-2a, interferon alfa-2b, and pegylated interferon alfa-2b. Except for pegylated interferon, the drugs are administered subcutaneously or intramuscularly three times a week for at least 12 months. In patients with hepatitis C virus, combination therapy with interferon and ribavirin produced a higher response rate than therapy with either drug alone. Some studies showed that pegylated interferon alfa-2b produced better results than conventional alfa-2b.

In clinical studies of chronic hepatitis B, interferon treatment was found to result in loss of hepatitis B antigens, normalization of serum aminotransferase activity, sustained histologic improvement, and a lower risk of progression of liver disease in about one third of the patients. AIDS patients with hepatitis B, however, responded poorly to interferon treatment.

Interferon alfa is also effective in the treatment of **anogenital warts (condylomata acuminata),** which are caused by several types of papillomavirus. For this infection, the interferon is injected directly into the lesions three times a week for 3 weeks, with a repeated course of treatment after 12 to 16 weeks.

ADVERSE EFFECTS. Interferons can cause many serious and unpleasant adverse effects, including hematologic toxicity, cardiac arrhythmias, changes in blood pressure, CNS dysfunction, gastrointestinal distress, chills, fatigue, headache, and myalgia.

SUMMARY OF IMPORTANT POINTS

■ Acyclovir, famciclovir, penciclovir, and valacyclovir are nucleoside analogues used to treat herpes simplex virus (HSV) and varicella-zoster virus (VZV) infections.

■ Trifluridine is a nucleoside analogue used to treat herpetic keratoconjunctivitis.

■ Cidofovir and ganciclovir are nucleoside analogues used for the prevention and treatment of cytomegalovirus (CMV) diseases (e.g., retinitis, esophagitis, and colitis).

■ Valacyclovir is a prodrug that is converted to acyclovir in vivo. It has better oral bioavailability than acyclovir.

■ Acyclovir, ganciclovir, and penciclovir are selectively phosphorylated to their monophosphate metabolites by viral kinases, and then host cell kinases convert them to triphosphates. Other nucleoside analogues, including those for treating human immunodeficiency virus (HIV) infection, are phosphorylated only by host cell kinases.

■ Acyclovir and most nucleoside reverse transcriptase inhibitors (NRTI) cause chain termination when they are incorporated into viral DNA. Ganciclovir and penciclovir inhibit viral DNA polymerase but are not incorporated into viral DNA.

■ Foscarnet is a nonnucleoside drug used to treat CMV retinitis and acyclovir-resistant HSV and VZV infections.

■ Nucleoside and nonnucleoside reverse transcriptase inhibitors (RTI), and protease inhibitors (PI) are three classes of drugs for the treatment of HIV infection. Various combinations of these drugs act synergistically to reduce viral loads and ameliorate symptoms. The most commonly used combinations consist of two nucleoside RTI plus either a PI or a nonnucleoside RTI.

■ Frequently used nucleoside RTI include zidovudine, tenofovir and lamivudine. Zidovudine can cause anemia and neutropenia.

■ Examples of PI include lopinavir and ritonavir. Efavirenz is a frequently used nonnucleoside RTI.

■ Some PI and nonnucleoside RTI interact with a number of drugs via inhibition or induction of cytochrome P450 isozymes.

■ Amantadine and rimantadine are used in the prophylaxis and treatment of influenza A. They act by preventing the uncoating of influenza A virus.

■ Oseltamivir and zanamivir, neuraminidase inhibitors that inhibit the release and spreading of influenza A and B virions, are used in prophylaxis and treatment of influenza.

■ Ribavirin is a broad-spectrum antiviral drug used to treat respiratory syncytial virus infection in neonates, and hepatitis C in combination with interferon alfa.

■ Interferon alfa is used to treat hepatitis B, hepatitis C, and anogenital warts. Lamivudine, an NRTI, is also used to treat hepatitis B.

Review Questions

1. Which of the following drugs inhibits the enzyme that cleaves the gag-pol polyprotein into functional proteins?
   (A) enfuvirtide
   (B) ribavirin
   (C) atazanavir
   (D) efavirenz
   (E) ribavirin

2. Which of the following drug combinations is recommended for the initial treatment of HIV infection in persons with less than 200 CD4+ cells/μL?

(A) abacavir + emtricitabine + efavirenz
(B) stavudine + zidovudine + lopinavir and ritonavir
(C) zidovudine + lamivudine + abacavir
(D) efavirenz + ritonavir + zidovudine
(E) efavirenz + nevirapine + lamivudine

3. Which drug inhibits viral inosine monophosphate dehydrogenase, leading to guanosine triphosphate deficiency?
(A) trifluridine
(B) didanosine
(C) ribavirin
(D) ganciclovir
(E) foscarnet

4. Bone marrow suppression and anemia are most likely to occur in patients receiving which of the following drugs?
(A) lamivudine
(B) zidovudine
(C) efavirenz
(D) rimantadine
(E) acyclovir

5. Which of the following drugs is incorporated into viral DNA and thereby prevents the addition of other nucleotides to the growing DNA chain?
(A) ganciclovir
(B) trifluridine
(C) penciclovir
(D) acyclovir
(E) ribavirin

Answers and Explanations

1. The answer is C: atazanavir. Atazanavir is a protease inhibitor that inhibits HIV maturation by preventing the cleavage of polyproteins (e.g., gag-pol) into functional proteins. Efavirenz is a nonnucleoside reverse transcriptase inhibitor, whereas enfuvirtide inhibits the fusion of HIV and host cells.

2. The answer is A: abacavir + emtricitabine + efavirenz. Abacavir and emtricitabine are nucleoside reverse transcriptase (RT) inhibitors, whereas efavirenz is a nonnucleoside RT inhibitor. Answer (B), stavudine and zidovudine, are antagonistic. The other answers are not recommended for initial treatment of HIV infection, including three nucleoside RT inhibitors (answer C), two protease inhibitors and a nucleoside RT inhibitor (answer D), or a protease inhibitor, a nonnucleoside RT inhibitor and a nucleoside RT inhibitor (answer E).

3. The answer is C: ribavirin. Ribavirin inhibits inosine monophosphate dehydrogenase, thereby leading to a deficiency of guanosine triphosphate and impaired viral nucleic acid synthesis. Ganciclovir, trifluridine, and foscarnet inhibit viral DNA polymerase, whereas didanosine inhibits reverse transcriptase.

4. The answer is B: zidovudine. Zidovudine is the most likely nucleoside reverse transcriptase inhibitor to produce bone marrow suppression and anemia. Concurrent administration of ganciclovir increases the likelihood of this adverse effect.

5. The answer is D: acyclovir. Acyclovir has only a single hydroxyl group on its carbohydrate moiety. For this reasons, it causes DNA chain termination when it is incorporated into a growing strand of viral DNA.

SELECTED READINGS

Anderson, P. L. Pharmacologic perspectives for once-daily antiretroviral therapy. Ann Pharmacother 38:1924–1934, 2004.

Cahn, P. Emtricitabine: a new nucleoside analogue for once-daily anti-retroviral therapy. Expert Opin Investig Drugs 13:55–68, 2004.

De Clercq, E. Antiviral drugs in current clinical use. J Clin Virol 30:115–133, 2004.

Panel on Clinical Practices for Treatment of HIV Infection. Guidelines for the Use of Antiretroviral Agents in HIV-1-Infected Adults and Adolescents. Department of Health and Human Services (USA), October 29, 2004. AIDSinfo Web site (*http://AIDSinfo.nih.gov*).

Patel, I. H., X. Zhang, K. Nieforth, et al. Pharmacokinetics, pharmacodynamics, and drug interaction potential of enfuvirtide. Clin Pharmacokinet 44:175–186, 2005.

CHAPTER 44

Antiparasitic Drugs

CLASSIFICATION OF ANTIPARASITIC DRUGS*

Drugs for Infections Caused by Lumen-and Tissue-dwelling Protozoa
- Metronidazole (FLAGYL)
- Tinidazole (TINDAMAX)
- Paromomycin
- Diloxanide, iodoquinol

Drugs for Infections Caused by Blood-and Tissue-dwelling Protozoa

Drugs for Malaria
- Quinine + doxycycline or mefloquine
- Chloroquine
- Primaquine
- Artesunate
- Atovaquone + proguanil (MALARONE)
- Pyrimethamine + sulfadoxine (FANSIDAR)

Drugs for Toxoplasmosis
- Pyrimethamine + sulfadiazine, spiramycin

Drugs for Other Protozoal Infections
- Melarsoprol, miltefosine, nifurtimox, pentamidine, suramin

Drugs for Helminth Infections

Drugs for Nematode Infections
- Albendazole, mebendazole, thiabendazole
- Pyrantel pamoate
- Diethylcarbamazine, ivermectin

Drugs for Trematode and Cestode Infections
- Praziquantel

Drugs for Ectoparasite Infestations
- Permethrin

*Additional drugs are included in Table 44–1.

OVERVIEW

Endoparasitic infections are extremely common in many parts of the world, particularly in areas where the climate is warm and moist, the sanitation is poor, and insects and other vectors of disease are prevalent. In fact, billions of people in tropical and subtropical regions are infected with **protozoa** (single-cell organisms that dwell in the lumen, tissue, or blood) and **helminths** (worms, including nematodes, trematodes, and cestodes). Factors, such as immigration, an increase in the number of international travelers, and an increase in the number of individuals who have acquired immunodeficiency syndrome (AIDS) and are therefore at greater risk for opportunistic infections, have all increased the probability that physicians will see endoparasitic infections that were rarely found in their usual patient population.

Since 1960, the introduction of new drugs has enabled remarkable advances in the chemotherapy of some endoparasitic infections. Albendazole and mebendazole have significantly improved the treatment of several intestinal nematode infections, whereas praziquantel has revolutionized the treatment of trematode and cestode infections. At the same time, metronidazole and tinidazole have provided more effective and less toxic drugs for the treatment of amebiasis, giardiasis, and trichomoniasis.

Unlike endoparasitic infections, **ectoparasitic infestations** are caused by organisms that live on the skin or hair shafts of patients. The most common examples are the **lice** and **mites** that cause pediculosis and scabies, respectively.

Table 44–1 provides information about the causes and treatment of numerous protozoal infections, helminthic infections, and ectoparasitic infestations. The antiparasitic agents commonly used or represent pharmacologic advances are discussed in this chapter. In some cases, an antibacterial or antifungal agent (e.g., tetracycline or amphotericin B) is listed as either a preferred or alternative drug, and these agents are discussed in earlier chapters. A detailed discussion of other agents listed in the table is beyond the scope of this chapter.

TABLE 44-1. **Causes and Treatment of Parasitic Infections and Infestations**

Condition	Common Pathogens	Primary Drugs	Alternative Drugs
Intestinal protozoal infections			
Amebiasis	Entamoeba histolytica	Metronidazole or tinidazole followed by paromomycin or iodoquinol	Diloxanide
Balantidiasis	Balantidium coli	Tetracycline	Metronidazole
Cryptosporidiosis	Cryptosporidium parvum	Nitozoxanide*	Antidiarrheal medication
Dientamoeba infection	Dientamoeba fragilis	Iodoquinol	Tetracycline, metronidazole, or paromomycin
Giardiasis	Giardia lamblia	Metronidazole or tinidazole	Quinacrine, paromomycin
Microsporidiosis	Encephalitozoon and Enterocytozoon species	Albendazole	Fumagillin
Extraintestinal protozoal infections			
Amebic meningoencephalitis	Naegleria fowleri	Amphotericin B; consider azithromycin†	
Babesiosis	Babesia microti	Atovaquone + azithromycin	Clindamycin + quinine
Leishmaniasis	Leishmania species	Miltefosine	Amphotericin B, antimony drug, fluconazole (cutaneous infections)
Malaria	Plasmodium vivax or P. ovale	Primaquine + chloroquine	Primaquine + quinine and doxycycline
	Chloroquine-sensitive P. falciparum	Chloroquine (if sensitive)	Quinine + doxycycline; mefloquine; halofantrine
	Chloroquine-resistant P. falciparum	Quinine + doxycycline or FANSIDAR‡; atovaquone + proguanil	Artesunate + mefloquine
Toxoplasmosis	Toxoplasma gondii	Pyrimethamine + sulfadiazine; spiramycin	Trimethoprim + sulfamethoxazole
Trichomoniasis	Trichomonas vaginalis	Metronidazole or tinidazole	
Trypanosomiasis (African sleeping sickness)	Trypanosoma brucei	Pentamidine (early disease); melarsoprol (late CNS disease)	Suramin
Trypanosomiasis, American (Chagas' disease)	Trypanosoma cruzi	Nifurtimox	Benznidazole
Intestinal nematode infections			
Ascariasis	Ascaris lumbricoides	Albendazole or mebendazole	Pyrantel pamoate
Capillariasis	Capillaria philippinensis	Mebendazole	Albendazole
Pinworm infection	Enterobius vermicularis	Albendazole or mebendazole	Pyrantel pamoate
Hookworm infection	Ancylostoma duodenale and Necator americanus	Albendazole or mebendazole	Pyrantel pamoate
Strongyloidiasis	Strongyloides stercoralis	Ivermectin	Thiabendazole
Whipworm infection	Trichuris trichiura	Albendazole	Mebendazole
Extraintestinal nematode infections			
Cutaneous larva migrans	Ancylostoma braziliense	Ivermectin	Albendazole
Guinea worm	Dracunculus medinensis	Surgical removal + metronidazole	Mebendazole
Filariasis, lymphatic	Wuchereria bancrofti, Brugia malayi	Ivermectin	Diethylcarbamazine
Filariasis, cutaneous	Loa loa	Diethylcarbamazine	Ivermectin
River blindness	Onchocerca volvulus	Ivermectin + prednisone	
Trichinosis	Trichinella spiralis	Albendazole + prednisone	Mebendazole + prednisone
Trematode infections			
Schistosomiasis	Schistosoma species	Praziquantel	Oxamniquine for S. mansoni
Chinese liver fluke	Clonorchis sinensis	Praziquantel	Albendazole
Sheep liver fluke	Fasciola hepatica	Triclabendazole	Bithionol
Lung fluke	Paragonimus westermani	Praziquantel	Bithionol
Cestode infections			
Beef tapeworm	Taenia saginata	Praziquantel	Niclosamide
Pork tapeworm	Taenia solium	Praziquantel	Niclosamide
Cysticercosis	Larval T. solium	Albendazole for CNS disease + dexamethasone	Praziquantel
Dog tapeworm	Dipylidium caninum	Praziquantel	Niclosamide
Dwarf tapeworm	Hymenolepis nana	Praziquantel	
Fish tapeworm	Diphyllobothrium latum	Praziquantel	Niclosamide
Echinococcosis (hydatid disease)	Echinococcus granulosus	Aspiration + albendazole	

TABLE 44-1. Causes and Treatment of Parasitic Infections and Infestations—cont'd

Condition	Common Pathogens	Primary Drugs	Alternative Drugs
Ectoparasite infestations			
Head lice, crabs	*Pediculus humanus, Phthirus pubis*	Permethrin	Lindane, malathion
Scabies (mites)	*Sarcoptes scabiei*	Permethrin	Lindane, oral ivermectin

*For patients with AIDS, try nitazoxanide, or paromomycin + azithromycin.
†see Goswick and Brenner, 2002.
‡FANSIDAR contains pyrimethamine and sulfadoxine.
CNS = central nervous system.

DRUGS FOR INFECTIONS CAUSED BY LUMEN- AND TISSUE-DWELLING PROTOZOA

Amebiasis, balantidiasis, cryptosporidiosis, giardiasis, and trichomoniasis are examples of infections caused by protozoan parasites that dwell in the lumen and tissues of their human hosts. Among the agents used to treat these infections are metronidazole, tinidazole, iodoquinol, and paromomycin (see Table 44–1).

Metronidazole

Drug Properties

CHEMISTRY AND PHARMACOKINETICS. Metronidazole is a nitroimidazole compound. It is well absorbed from the gut and is widely distributed to tissues and fluids throughout the body, including the liver and central nervous system (CNS). The drug is extensively metabolized before undergoing renal excretion. Metronidazole is usually administered orally, although an intravenous preparation is available for use in patients with severe infections.

SPECTRUM AND MECHANISMS. Metronidazole is active against several anaerobic protozoa that commonly cause infection. These include *Entamoeba histolytica* (the agent of amebiasis); *Giardia lamblia* (giardiasis); *Trichomonas vaginalis* (trichomoniasis); and *Balantidium coli* (balantidiasis). Metronidazole is also active against anaerobic bacteria, including *Bacteroides fragilis*, *Clostridium difficile*, and anaerobic *Peptostreptococcus* and *Streptococcus* species.

Anaerobic protozoa have pyruvate:ferredoxin oxidoreductase, an enzyme that is not found in mammalian cells. In susceptible anaerobic protozoa, this enzyme transfers electrons to the nitro group of metronidazole to form free nitroradicals that attack DNA and proteins and thereby produce a cytotoxic effect.

INDICATIONS. Metronidazole, the drug of choice for **amebiasis, giardiasis,** and **trichomoniasis,** is also used as an alternative drug in the treatment of **balantidiasis.**

Patients with amebiasis can suffer from intestinal infection, with or without dysentery, hepatic abscesses, or other extraintestinal manifestations of disease. Metronidazole acts primarily as a tissue amebicide and is usually given in combination with a luminal amebicide (e.g., iodoquinol) to eradicate intestinal amebas.

Giardiasis causes abdominal discomfort and diarrhea in persons infected with the cyst form of *Giardia*. In the western United States of America (USA), *Giardia* cysts are sometimes present in contaminated streams and ponds and are ingested by campers. The administration of metronidazole for 5 days usually cures the infection.

Trichomoniasis is a sexually transmitted disease that produces vaginitis in women but is usually asymptomatic in men. To prevent reinfection, it is important to treat patients and their sexual partners. Treatment can consist either of a single large dose of metronidazole or of smaller doses taken over a 7-day period.

Metronidazole is also used in the management of several disorders that are not caused by protozoa. For example, it is sometimes used in the treatment of patients with **dracunculiasis (guinea worm infection).** This infection is caused by *Dracunculus medinensis*, a nematode found in India, Pakistan, and parts of Africa. Although metronidazole is not curative, it reduces inflammation and facilitates manual removal of the worm. Metronidazole is considered the drug of choice for **enterocolitis** caused by *C. difficile*, and it is occasionally used to treat infections caused by other anaerobic bacteria. Metronidazole is available in gel or cream form for the topical treatment of **rosacea (acne rosacea),** a skin condition characterized by persistent erythema of the middle third of the face and other areas of the body.

ADVERSE EFFECTS AND INTERACTIONS. Metronidazole is usually well tolerated, but it causes considerable gastrointestinal discomfort in some persons. Other adverse effects include nausea, vomiting, a metallic taste, and transient leukopenia or thrombocytopenia. To reduce the gastrointestinal side effects, patients should take metronidazole with food.

Metronidazole increases the anticoagulant effect of warfarin, so the dosage of warfarin should be adjusted as necessary. Metronidazole also causes a disulfiramlike reaction with ethanol, so patients should avoid drinking alcohol while they are undergoing treatment.

Metronidazole has been shown to be mutagenic in bacteria and mammalian cell cultures. Although retrospective studies of women who took the drug during pregnancy failed to reveal an increased incidence of birth defects or cancer, it appears prudent to avoid using the drug during the first trimester of pregnancy whenever possible.

Tinidazole

Tinidazole (TINDAMAX) is a second-generation nitroimidazole similar to metronidazole but active against metronidazole-resistant strains of *Trichomonas vaginalis.* As with metronidazole it is indicated for the treatment of **trichomoniasis, giardiasis, intestinal amebiasis,** and **amebic liver abscess.** It is also active against *Helicobacter pylori* and anaerobic bacteria, including *Bacteroides fragilis.*

In clinical trials, a single dose of tinidazole cured 93% of patients with giardiasis. In persons with symptomatic intestinal amebiasis, a 3-day course of tinidazole resulted in a cure rate of 86% to 93%, and 2 to 5 days of tinidazole cured 81% to 100% of those with amebic liver abscess. In general, tinidazole produced a higher cure rate in a shorter time period than did metronidazole.

Tinidazole is completely absorbed and widely distributed after oral administration. Its plasma half-life of about 13 hours is considerably longer than that of metronidazole (8 hours). Because it is metabolized by cytochrome P450 3A4, its serum concentrations can be affected by other drugs that inhibit or induce this enzyme. As with metronidazole, tinidazole can cause anorexia, nausea, and vomiting, as well as a bitter taste in the mouth, and it is contraindicated in the first trimester of pregnancy.

Iodoquinol, Paromomycin, and Diloxanide Furoate

Iodoquinol, paromomycin, and diloxanide furoate act as luminal amebicides but not tissue amebicides. A luminal amebicide can be used alone to treat **asymptomatic carriers of E. histolytica,** but it must be used in combination with a tissue amebicide to treat patients with **amebic dysentery or liver abscess.** The preferred combination is usually tinidazole or metronidazole followed by paromomycin or iodoquinol (see Table 44–1).

Paromomycin is sometimes used to treat infections with *Cryptosporidium parvum* in immunocompromised persons. **Cryptosporidiosis** usually presents as chronic diarrhea in immunocompromised persons and has been reported in up to 50% of patients with AIDS. Many treatment methods have been tried, but none is very effective. Paromomycin treatment has produced the greatest clinical response, but high doses of the drug must be used and long-term maintenance therapy is required to prevent relapse. Nitozoxamide (ALINIA) is a new drug for treating cryptosporidiosis in immunocompetent persons, and antidiarrheal medication may be helpful.

Either iodoquinol or paromomycin can be used to treat infections with *Dientamoeba fragilis,* a lumen-dwelling protozoan parasite that causes **diarrhea** and **abdominal pain.**

DRUGS FOR INFECTIONS CAUSED BY BLOOD- AND TISSUE-DWELLING PROTOZOA

Babesiosis, leishmaniasis, malaria, toxoplasmosis, and trypanosomiasis are examples of infections caused by protozoan parasites that dwell in the blood and tissues of their human hosts.

Drugs for Malaria

Malaria, one of the most common infectious diseases in the world today, is believed to be responsible for more deaths than any other infectious disease. Four species of *Plasmodium* cause malaria: *Plasmodium falciparum, Plasmodium malariae, Plasmodium ovale,* and *Plasmodium vivax.* Most cases of malaria are caused by *P. falciparum* or *P. vivax.* The disease is spread via the bites of female *Anopheles* mosquitoes and is primarily found in tropical and subtropical areas. Malaria has largely been eliminated from industrialized countries in temperate regions, so most infections that are diagnosed in people residing in the USA are infections that were acquired during travel in other countries. Nevertheless, periodic outbreaks of mosquito-borne malaria still occur in the USA.

Malaria is transmitted when infected mosquitoes inject *Plasmodium* sporozoites into the blood of the human host (Fig. 44–1). The sporozoites invade the liver, where they undergo schizogony (asexual multiplication) to form tissue schizonts. The multinucleated schizonts divide their cytoplasm to form thousands of merozoites in a process called **exoerythrocytic schizogony.** The merozoites are then released from the liver into the blood, where they infect erythrocytes and undergo **erythrocytic schizogony.** Additional merozoites are subsequently released into the blood by hemolysis.

The synchronous release of merozoites is responsible for the episodic fever observed in patients with malaria. During an infection with *P. falciparum* or *P. vivax,* the fever spikes every other day. The disease produced by *P. falciparum* (malignant tertian malaria) is more severe than that produced by *P. vivax* (benign tertian malaria), partly because *P. falciparum* causes a higher level of parasitemia and produces a persistently higher temperature during the periods between fever spikes. Whereas both *P. vivax* and *P. ovale* have a persistent exoerythrocytic stage, *P. falciparum* and *P. malariae* do not. To eradicate this persistent stage and prevent the relapse of malaria, patients infected with *P. vivax* or *P. ovale* can be treated with primaquine.

Sites and Mechanisms of Action

Fig. 44–1 shows the sites of action of drugs for malaria. As indicated above, primaquine inhibits exoerythrocytic schizogony. In contrast, all of the other antimalarial agents inhibit erythrocytic schizogony.

The mode of action of **primaquine** is uncertain, but the drug appears to act by forming quinoline-quinone intermediates that oxidize schizont membranes. These oxidizing intermediates may also be responsible for the hemolytic effect of the drug.

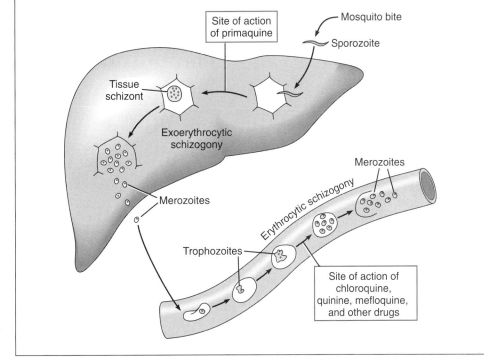

Figure 44–1. Sites of action of drugs for malaria. When a person is bitten by an infected mosquito, *Plasmodium* sporozoites enter the liver, form tissue schizonts, and undergo exoerythrocytic schizogony to produce merozoites. The merozoites that are released from the liver invade erythrocytes and form trophozoites that undergo erythrocytic schizogony. Some trophozoites develop into male and female gametocytes, which must subsequently pass back into a mosquito before they can develop into sporozoites and repeat the infection cycle. Primaquine blocks exoerythrocytic schizogony, whereas other antimalarial drugs inhibit erythrocytic schizogony.

Chloroquine, mefloquine, and **quinine** are believed to inhibit nucleic acid synthesis or function during erythrocytic schizogony, although the exact mechanisms of action are uncertain. Chloroquine may block the synthesis of nucleic acid, and it may also impair the ability of plasmodia to utilize hemoglobin. The selective toxicity of chloroquine can be partly explained by the drug's greater accumulation in infected erythrocytes than in uninfected cells. Quinine appears to form a complex with plasmodial DNA, thereby preventing replication and transcription.

Sulfadoxine is a sulfonamide that acts synergistically with **pyrimethamine** to inhibit the synthesis of folic acid in plasmodia and thereby prevent the synthesis of nucleic acid. The sulfonamides inhibit dihydrofolate formation, whereas pyrimethamine prevents dihydrofolate reduction.

Other drugs used in the treatment of malaria include **artesunate, atovaquone,** and **proguanil.** Proguanil acts by inhibiting folate reductase, and the mechanisms of action of the other drugs are unknown.

Fig. 44–2 shows structures of selected drugs for malaria.

Chloroquine, Quinine, and Quinidine

Quinine, a drug that had been used for centuries to treat malaria, was supplanted by chloroquine after World War II. Until the 1980s, when resistance to chloroquine became widespread, chloroquine remained the drug of choice. Now that drug resistance has severely curtailed the effectiveness of chloroquine, quinine is once again being used to treat malaria in many regions of the world. In addition, other drugs have been introduced.

The only areas where most *P. falciparum* organisms are sensitive to chloroquine are the Caribbean islands, the part of Central America that is west of the Panama Canal, and parts of North and West Africa and the Middle East. In these chloroquine-sensitive areas, chloroquine is still the drug of choice for both the prevention and the treatment of all types of malaria, although it must be used in combination with primaquine (see below) to eradicate vivax or ovale malaria.

The most common adverse effects of chloroquine are gastrointestinal distress, nausea, and vomiting. Toxic doses can cause retinal damage and even blindness. In pregnant women, chloroquine should be used cautiously because fetal damage has been reported.

Patients with **chloroquine-resistant malaria** are usually treated with a combination of quinine sulfate plus either doxycycline or pyrimethamine-sulfadoxine (FANSIDAR). Alternatives include atovaquone-proguanil (MALARONE) and artesunate plus mefloquine.

Mefloquine

Mefloquine (LARIAM) is a newer antimalarial drug that has been used for both the prevention and the treatment of chloroquine-resistant malaria. Because cure rates with this drug have dropped from almost 100% in the 1980s to 40% by 1995, mefloquine is now primarily used to prevent malaria in areas where chloroquine-resistant strains are prevalent. The drug is given orally, undergoes hepatic metabolism, has a half-life of about 14 days, and is eliminated via the bile and feces.

Mefloquine can cause a severe **neuropsychiatric syndrome** characterized by hallucinations, anxiety, confusion, seizures, and coma. It can also cause leukopenia and thrombocytopenia.

For patients who cannot tolerate mefloquine, doxycycline (see Chapter 39) can be used to prevent malaria in areas where chloroquine-resistant organisms are prevalent.

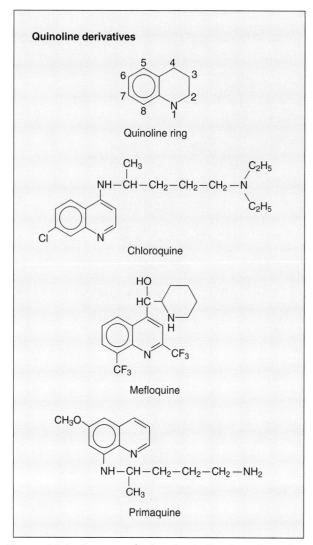

Figure 44–2. Structures of selected quinoline drugs for malaria. Chloroquine is a 4-aminoquinoline derivative, whereas primaquine is an 8-aminoquinoline derivative.

Primaquine

Primaquine is an 8-aminoquinoline derivative that is active against the exoerythrocytic stage of *P. vivax* and *P. ovale.* By eradicating tissue plasmodia, it prevents the reemergence of organisms from the liver and relapse of the infection. Primaquine must be used in combination with other drugs to treat infection with *P. vivax* or *P. ovale,* because primaquine is not active against the erythrocytic stage of these organisms.

Primaquine is converted to oxidizing quinoline-quinone intermediates in the body. These intermediates are believed to be responsible for the antimalarial effects and some of the toxic effects of the drug. In individuals who have **hereditary glucose-6-phosphate dehydrogenase (G6PD) deficiency,** the intermediates may oxidize erythrocyte membranes and thereby cause red cell hemolysis and **hemolytic anemia.** This anemia occurs because G6PD is unable to generate sufficient quantities of reduced nicotinamide adenine dinucleotide phosphate (NADPH) to maintain glutathione in its reduced form and thereby prevent oxidation of erythrocyte mem-

branes. Individuals who experience this type of hemolytic anemia are said to have **primaquine sensitivity.** A number of other drugs with oxidizing properties, including sulfonamides and sulfones, can also cause this reaction.

Pyrimethamine and Sulfadoxine

Pyrimethamine is a folate reductase inhibitor that is generally used in combination with a sulfonamide such as sulfadiazine or sulfadoxine. Pyrimethamine and sulfadiazine are used in the treatment of **toxoplasmosis** (a disease discussed in the next section), whereas pyrimethamine and sulfadoxine (FANSIDAR) are used in the treatment of **malaria.** Some resistance to pyrimethamine-sulfadoxine has been reported in parts of Southeast Asia, the Amazon basin, sub-Saharan Africa, and Bangladesh.

The adverse effects of pyrimethamine-sulfadoxine include anorexia, nausea, vomiting, megaloblastic anemia, leukopenia, thrombocytopenia, hemolytic anemia, and Stevens-Johnson syndrome with epidermal necrolysis.

Proguanil and Atovaquone

Proguanil, or **chloroguanide,** is a biguanide derivative that acts as a **folate reductase inhibitor.** Sometimes combined with atovaquone to treat chloroquine-resistant malaria, it is available as a fixed-dose combination product known as MALARONE.

Atovaquone is a napthoquinone derivative that has a high level of activity against the erythrocytic stage of all *P. falciparum* strains, including the chloroquine-resistant strains. The drug should be used in combination with doxycycline (see Chapter 39) or proguanil for the treatment of malaria, because studies indicate that a high rate of relapse occurs when atovaquone is used alone.

Atovaquone is also used in the treatment of *Pneumocystis jiroveci (carinii)* infections.

Artesunate

The search for new agents to treat multidrug-resistant falciparum malaria led to the identification of **artemisinin** (*qinghaosu*) as the active ingredient of *Artemisia annua,* a plant used in traditional Chinese medicine for over 2 millennia. Two derivatives of artemisinin were subsequently found to have potent activity against the erythrocytic stages of malaria. These sesquiterpene derivatives are called **artemether** and **artesunate.**

Artemether and artesunate have been used effectively in the treatment of millions of cases of falciparum malaria in Southeast Asia, sub-Saharan Africa, and elsewhere. The drugs can be administered orally or parenterally. Artesunate is sometimes combined with mefloquine.

Drugs for Toxoplasmosis

In immunocompetent individuals, *Toxoplasma gondii* infection is common but is rarely symptomatic. Even in cases in which it is symptomatic, treatment is not normally required.

In immunocompromised individuals and congenitally infected neonates, however, *T. gondii* can cause severe damage to many organs. For example, *T. gondii* frequently causes **ocular infections** and **encephalitis** in patients with AIDS and is the most common CNS disease found in these patients. *T. gondii* can cause encephalomyelitis, hydrocephaly, microcephaly, or chorioretinitis in the offspring of women who were infected for the first time during pregnancy. Women who were infected with *T. gondii* before pregnancy are not at risk of transmitting the infection to their offspring.

Although toxoplasmosis is usually treated with **pyrimethamine** plus **sulfadiazine,** this drug combination has some major drawbacks. First, it is not effective against *T. gondii* tissue cysts. Second, the use of pyrimethamine in combination with a sulfonamide drug sometimes induces **folate deficiency** and causes severe hematologic abnormalities and other adverse effects, even when the combination is given in normal doses and for short-term treatment. In patients with AIDS, high doses of pyrimethamine plus sulfadiazine are required to treat toxoplasmosis, and life-long maintenance therapy is often required to prevent reactivation of the disease. In an effort to prevent the adverse hematologic effects of pyrimethamine in these patients, **leucovorin** (folinic acid) can be added to the treatment regimen.

The toxic side effects of pyrimethamine plus sulfadiazine, however, preclude its administration in up to 40% of patients with AIDS. As an alternative, pyrimethamine can be given either with **clindamycin** or with **dapsone.**

Spiramycin is a macrolide antibiotic recommended for fetal infection resulting from acute maternal infection during pregnancy.

Drugs for *Pneumocystis jiroveci* (carinii) Infections

Because **Pneumocystis jiroveci,** *formerly Pneumocystis carinii,* has traditionally been classified as a protozoan parasite, it is discussed in this chapter. Results of several studies, however, support the argument that it is actually a fungus. In addition to causing pneumonia in premature and malnourished infants, the organism causes pneumonia and other diseases in immunocompromised persons, including those with AIDS.

The treatment of choice for *P. jiroveci* infections is **trimethoprim-sulfamethoxazole,** a drug combination discussed in Chapter 40. **Atovaquone** (an antimalarial agent discussed earlier in this chapter), and **pentamidine** are alternatives. Other alternatives include dapsone plus trimethoprim or pyrimethamine. Prednisone, a corticosteroid drug, is also administered to acutely ill patients to reduce pulmonary inflammation.

The antimicrobial agents used to treat *Pneumocystis* infections are also used for prophylaxis and for posttreatment suppression of this infection. Pentamidine is given intravenously for the treatment of *P. jiroveci* infections, but it is administered by inhalation to prevent pneumonia. The adverse effects of pentamidine include hematologic toxicity, ventricular tachycardia, edema, pancreatitis, bronchospasm, and Stevens-Johnson syndrome.

Drugs for Other Protozoal Infections

Pentamidine or suramin, either given alone or in combination with **melarsoprol,** is used to treat **African trypanosomiasis (sleeping sickness),** a disease caused by *Trypanosoma*

brucei. Pentamidine and suramin are used for the early stages of the infection. Melarsoprol is indicated for use in patients with late CNS manifestations of the disease. These drugs must be administered intravenously and can cause serious toxicity.

Nifurtimox is the drug of choice for the treatment of **American trypanosomiasis (Chagas' disease),** a disease caused by *Trypanosoma cruzi.* The effectiveness of nifurtimox is limited. Giving interferon gamma in combination with nifurtimox, however, appears to shorten the acute phase of the illness.

The causes and treatment of **babesiosis** and **leishmaniasis** are outlined in Table 44–1. **Miltefosine** is a new drug for treating **visceral leishmaniasis,** which is also known as **Kala azar.** Miltefosine is a phosphorylcholine ester of hexadecanol, a membrane-active phospholipid. Miltefosine inhibits key enzymes involved in the metabolism of glycolipids found on the surface of *Leishmania* species. It is well absorbed after oral administration and has a half-life of about 8 days. In the past antimonial drug treatments for leishmaniasis had to be given parenterally for prolonged periods and caused considerable toxicity. In contrast, miltefosine given orally for 28 days produced a 94% to 97% cure rate of visceral leishmaniasis in children at the end of treatment and at 6 months follow-up. The most common adverse effects have been vomiting and diarrhea, but they were usually of brief duration and only mild to moderate in severity. A few patients experienced reversible hepatic and renal toxicity. Because of its high efficacy and relatively low toxicity, the availability of miltefosine appears to be a breakthrough in the treatment of visceral and other forms of leishmaniasis.

DRUGS FOR INFECTIONS CAUSED BY HELMINTHS

Helminths can be classified as **nematodes (roundworms), trematodes (flukes),** and **cestodes (tapeworms).** The most common parasites in these groups are listed in Table 44–1 and are responsible for infecting billions of people throughout the world. Effective drugs are available to treat most of the helminthic infections, but the cost of drug treatment is high. Fortunately, the World Health Organization and government agencies have sponsored mass treatment programs that appear to have had a significant impact on some helminthic infections, such as onchocerciasis (river blindness) and schistosomiasis.

Anthelmintic drugs usually act either by inhibiting metabolism in the parasite (as occurs when a benzimidazole drug is used) or by causing muscle paralysis of the parasite (as occurs when ivermectin, praziquantel, or pyrantel is used). The anthelmintic drugs kill the parasites without harming host cells, but the molecular basis for their selective toxicity is not entirely clear. In many cases, a single dose or a few doses of the drug are curative.

Drugs for Nematode Infections
Albendazole, Mebendazole, and Thiabendazole

CHEMISTRY AND PHARMACOKINETICS. Albendazole and related drugs are benzimidazole compounds. Albendazole has poor solubility in water. Only about 5% of an oral dose of the drug is absorbed from an empty stomach. Absorption is markedly improved, however, if the drug is taken with a fatty meal. Albendazole is converted to albendazole sulfoxide by first-pass hepatic metabolism, and this metabolite accounts for the systemic anthelmintic activity of the drug. Sulfoxidation of albendazole also occurs in the intestinal tract. The level of albendazole in cerebrospinal fluid is about 40% of the level in plasma.

About 10% of mebendazole is absorbed from the gut, metabolized in the liver, and excreted in the urine. In contrast to mebendazole and other benzimidazoles, thiabendazole is well absorbed from the gut, and this may partly account for its higher incidence of adverse effects. Thiabendazole is completely metabolized before undergoing renal excretion.

MECHANISMS. The benzimidazoles bind to β-tubulin and thereby inhibit the polymerization of tubulin dimers to form cytoplasmic microtubules in parasites. This action impairs the uptake of glucose by these organisms and leads to depletion of glycogen stores and decreased production of adenosine triphosphate (ATP). Eventually the organisms are immobilized and die.

SPECTRUM AND INDICATIONS. Albendazole and mebendazole are primarily used to treat intestinal nematode infections, including **ascariasis, capillariasis, hookworm infection, pinworm infection,** and **whipworm infection.** For **trichinosis,** the anthelmintic drug is usually given in combination with a corticosteroid (e.g., prednisone) to relieve the inflammation.

As shown in Table 44–1, albendazole is also used to treat two cestode infections: **cysticercosis** and **echinococcosis.** For echinococcosis, surgical aspiration usually is used in conjunction with albendazole therapy. Treatment is not recommended for cysticercosis outside the CNS, which is benign. For cysticercosis in the CNS, albendazole or praziquantel can be effective along with a corticosteroid (e.g., dexamethasone) to control inflammation caused by cyst death.

Albendazole is also used to treat **microsporidiosis,** an infection caused by several species of intestinal protozoans.

PARASITIC RESISTANCE. Resistance to the benzimidazoles is now a worldwide problem in veterinary medicine, but it is not yet a significant problem in human medicine.

ADVERSE EFFECTS AND CONTRAINDICATIONS. The adverse effects of thiabendazole include anorexia, nausea, vomiting, paresthesias, delirium, and hallucinations. Albendazole and mebendazole are well tolerated and produce fewer adverse effects than thiabendazole does. The most common side effects of albendazole and mebendazole are mild gastrointestinal discomfort and constipation or diarrhea. The high doses of albendazole used to treat echinococcosis can cause hepatitis or hematologic toxicity. All of the benzimidazole drugs are contraindicated during pregnancy because of their potential to inhibit mitosis and impair fetal development.

Pyrantel

Pyrantel is a pyrimidine derivative. The drug activates cholinergic nicotinic receptors in the somatic muscles of nematodes and thereby produces a **depolarizing neuromuscular blockade.** In contrast, pyrantel has no marked effect on neuromuscular function in mammalian species. This has led investigators to conclude that the pharmacologic properties of nicotinic receptors of nematode and mammalian species are significantly different.

Pyrantel pamoate (ANTIMINTH) is available as an oral suspension for administration to children and adults who have **ascariasis, hookworm infection,** or **pinworm infection.** The drug is poorly absorbed from the gut and acts primarily within the intestinal tract. It is usually well tolerated, but it can cause abdominal cramps, anorexia, diarrhea, and vomiting.

Ivermectin

CHEMISTRY AND PHARMACOKINETICS. Ivermectin is a semisynthetic derivative of avermectin, an antibiotic obtained from *Streptomyces avermitilis.* Ivermectin has a complex macrocytic lactone structure. The drug is well absorbed from the gut, undergoes hepatic biotransformation, and is excreted in the feces. Its elimination half-life is about 25 hours.

MECHANISMS. Ivermectin increases the chloride permeability of invertebrate muscle cells. This hyperpolarizes the cell membrane and causes paralysis of the pharyngeal muscles in helminths. Ivermectin is believed to activate the **glutamate-gated chloride channel** in invertebrate tissue, but it has no effect on chloride ion permeability in mammalian tissue.

SPECTRUM AND INDICATIONS. Ivermectin is a broad-spectrum anthelmintic drug that is active against a wide range of nematodes. It has been used to treat a number of intestinal helminthic infections in domestic and companion animals. In humans, it is used to treat **strongyloidiasis, onchocerciasis,** and **cutaneous larva migrans.** Ivermectin has revolutionized the management of onchocerciasis. It is active against the microfilariae (skin-dwelling, first-stage larvae) of *Onchocerca volvulus,* even at a very low dosage. When a single dose is administered once a year, it can prevent the ocular form of onchocerciasis, which is called **river blindness.** Repeated treatment is necessary because the drug is not active against the adult parasites and only prevents the maturation of filarial offspring.

Ivermectin is active against all stages of the *Loa loa* parasite and is currently used as an alternative to diethylcarbamazine to treat **loiasis,** a disease that can cause both ocular and skin manifestations. Ivermectin is also active against the microfilariae of *Brugia malayi* and *Wuchereria bancrofti,* parasites that cause **lymphatic filariasis.** Studies show that low doses of the drug kill *W. bancrofti,* whereas higher doses are effective against *B. malayi.* Recently, ivermectin has also been used to treat scabies.

ADVERSE EFFECTS. Ivermectin is usually well tolerated and produces few adverse effects. Uncommonly, it causes constipation, diarrhea, dizziness, vertigo, or sedation.

Diethylcarbamazine

Diethylcarbamazine is a piperazine derivative that is administered orally and is well absorbed from the gut. The drug is partly metabolized and is primarily excreted in the urine. Although it has little activity against the larger nematodes (macrofilariae, such as the pinworm, hookworm, and whipworm), it is active against several microfilariae. Studies suggest that it acts in vivo by inhibiting prostaglandin I_2 (prostacyclin) and prostaglandin E_2, both in host endothelial cells and in filariae. These actions constrict blood vessels and increase aggregation of host granulocytes. Thus, diethylcarbamazine appears to augment the innate immune response to filarial infection.

The administration of diethylcarbamazine produces a rapid filaricidal effect, which sometimes leads to a severe host hypersensitivity response to the dying microfilariae. To prevent such reactions, patients are started on low doses, which are gradually increased as the parasites are eliminated. Otherwise, the drug is well tolerated.

Drugs for Trematode and Cestode Infections

Praziquantel

When praziquantel was introduced in the early 1970s, it revolutionized the treatment of **schistosomiasis,** a disease that can affect a wide range of organs, including the skin, liver, spleen, intestinal and urinary tracts, lungs, brain, and spinal cord. As shown in Table 44–1, it is now the drug of choice for infections caused by several other tissue flukes (trematodes) and by tapeworms (cestodes).

CHEMISTRY AND PHARMACOKINETICS. Praziquantel is an orally effective isoquinoline derivative that is not related to any other antiparasitic drug. In patients taking praziquantel, the drug is widely distributed and enters the CNS. It undergoes some first-pass and systemic metabolism, and the parent drug and metabolites are excreted in the urine.

MECHANISMS. Each schistosome is surrounded by a tegument. Praziquantel acts to increase the calcium permeability of the tegument and thereby cause its depolarization. When the outer bilayer of the tegument is damaged, *Schistosoma* antigens that were previously hidden from host defenses are exposed. This enables host immune cells to move in and attack the schistosomes. Thus, praziquantel acts to facilitate host immunity to these flukes. The drug's mechanism of action in other flukes and in tapeworms is unknown but is thought to be similar to that in schistosomes.

SPECTRUM AND INDICATIONS. Praziquantel is active against most tissue flukes, including the Chinese liver fluke (*Clonorchis sinensis*), the lung fluke (*Paragonimus westermani*), and the various *Schistosoma* species that cause human infections. It is also active against the larval form of the pork tapeworm (the cause of cysticercosis) and against the adult forms of the pork, beef, fish, dog, and dwarf tapeworms.

For patients with **schistosomiasis** or **other fluke infections,** three doses of praziquantel are administered in a single day. For patients with **cysticercosis,** three doses of praziquantel are given each day for a period of 2 weeks. If manifestations of **neurocysticercosis** are present, corticosteroids are given before praziquantel treatment. For patients with **adult tapeworm infections,** a single dose of praziquantel is usually effective.

PARASITIC RESISTANCE. Despite intensive use of praziquantel for over 20 years, few cases of parasitic resistance to the drug have been documented.

ADVERSE EFFECTS. Adverse effects are uncommon but include abdominal discomfort, dizziness, drowsiness, and headache.

Other Drugs

Triclabendazole is the drug of choice for the treatment of **sheep liver fluke infection** (*Fasciola hepatica* infection). Bithionol is an alternative drug for the treatment of sheep liver fluke and **lung fluke infection** (*P. westermani* infection).

Oxamniquine is used as an alternative to praziquantel for *Schistosoma mansoni* infections, but it is not useful in treating infections caused by other *Schistosoma* species.

Niclosamide an alternative to praziquantel for treating cestode infections.

Treatment Considerations

In Africa, Central and South America, and Asia, the use of anthelmintic drugs has evolved from the treatment of individuals to the treatment of populations. This has been possible because of the development of broad-spectrum agents that are effective in a single dose. Albendazole, mebendazole, ivermectin, and praziquantel are examples of drugs that have been successfully used as single-dose therapy to eradicate parasites in a large population.

In most parts of the USA, pinworm infection (enterobiasis) is the most common helminthic infection. It is acquired by ingesting eggs that are initially deposited by the female parasite on the perianal skin and are then transmitted to the mouth via unwashed fingers or fingernails. Contaminated clothing or bedding can also serve as a source of infection. Pinworm infection is often spread to family members, and outbreaks among children are common in day-care settings. For this reason, family members and other close contacts of the patient should be treated at the same time. In cases of pinworm infection, a dose of albendazole, mebendazole, or pyrantel should be followed 2 weeks later by a second dose of the same drug. In cases of whipworm, hookworm, or *Ascaris* infection, a single dose of an appropriate anthelmintic drug (see Table 44–1) is usually effective.

DRUGS FOR INFESTATIONS CAUSED BY ECTOPARASITES

The most common ectoparasites that cause illness in humans are **lice** and **mites.** These parasites cause **pediculosis** and **scabies,** respectively.

Permethrin is the treatment of choice for both types of infestation. The drug is a synthetic pyrethrinlike compound that blocks sodium currents in the neurons of parasites and thereby causes paralysis of the organisms. For pediculosis, a liquid preparation is applied in sufficient volume to saturate the hair and scalp, and then it is rinsed off after 10 minutes. For scabies, a permethrin cream is applied to the skin from head to toe, and it is left on the skin for at least 8 hours before it is washed off. For both types of infestation, a single treatment is usually effective, but it can be repeated in 1 week, if necessary. Alternative drugs are listed in Table 44–1.

SUMMARY OF IMPORTANT POINTS

■ Metronidazole and tinidazole are the drugs of choice for treating symptomatic amebiasis, giardiasis, and trichomoniasis.

■ Primaquine is the only antimalarial drug that blocks exoerythrocytic schizogony. Chloroquine, quinine, and other antimalarial drugs inhibit erythrocytic schizogony.

■ Many strains of *P. falciparum* have become resistant to chloroquine.

■ Chloroquine is used to prevent malaria in geographic regions without chloroquine-resistant plasmodia. Mefloquine or doxycycline is used to prevent malaria in regions with chloroquine-resistant plasmodia.

■ Chloroquine is used to treat all types of malaria caused by chloroquine-sensitive plasmodia. In cases of vivax or ovale malaria, chloroquine is given in combination with primaquine. Primaquine is active against the persistent tissue phase of *P. vivax* and *P. ovale* and prevents relapses of malaria caused by these organisms.

■ Quinine sulfate is usually given in combination with doxycycline or pyrimethamine-sulfadoxine to treat malaria caused by chloroquine-resistant plasmodia.

■ Toxoplasmosis can be treated with pyrimethamine plus sulfadiazine.

■ Pentamidine or suramin with melarsoprol is used to treat African trypanosomiasis, whereas nifurtimox is used to treat American trypanosomiasis (Chagas' disease).

■ Miltefosine is a newer drug for treating visceral leishmaniasis (Kala azar).

■ Most anthelmintic drugs act either by inhibiting mitosis in the parasite (as occurs when a benzimidazole drug is used) or by causing muscle paralysis of the parasite (as occurs when ivermectin, praziquantel, or pyrantel is used). Praziquantel exposes parasite antigens to host cell immune mechanisms.

■ Albendazole, mebendazole, and pyrantel are used to treat intestinal nematode infections.

■ Diethylcarbamazine and ivermectin are used to treat filarial nematode infections, including river blindness (onchocerciasis). Ivermectin is also used to treat strongyloidiasis and cutaneous larva migrans.

■ Praziquantel is the drug of choice for all forms of schistosomiasis and for most tissue fluke infections and tapeworm infections. Triclabendazole is used to treat sheep liver fluke infections.

■ Permethrin is the drug of choice for the treatment of lice and scabies.

Review Questions

1. Which antimalarial drug can cause hallucinations, anxiety, and seizures?
   (A) atovaquone
   (B) artesunate
   (C) mefloquine
   (D) pyrimethamine-sulfadoxine
   (E) primaquine

2. Which anthelmintic activates nicotinic receptors in *Ascaris lumbricoides?*
   (A) pyrantel
   (B) ivermectin
   (C) albendazole
   (D) praziquantel
   (E) diethylcarbamazine

3. Which drug is most likely to cause hemolytic anemia in persons with glucose-6-phosphate dehydrogenase deficiency?
   (A) metronidazole
   (B) primaquine
   (C) praziquantel
   (D) ivermectin
   (E) atovaquone

4. Which drug can be administered to large populations once a year to prevent river blindness (onchocerciasis)?
   (A) diethylcarbamazine
   (B) bithionol
   (C) albendazole
   (D) praziquantel
   (E) ivermectin

5. Diarrhea and abdominal pain caused by *Giardia lamblia* can be effectively treated with a single dose of which drug?
   (A) iodoquinol
   (B) tetracycline
   (C) albendazole
   (D) tinidazole
   (E) diloxanide

Answers and Explanations

1. The answer is C: mefloquine. Mefloquine, particularly when used for chronic prophylaxis of malaria, can cause a neuropsychiatric syndrome that can include hallucinations and seizures.

2. The answer is A: pyrantel. Pyrantel is a nicotinic receptor agonist in intestinal nematodes, leading to depolarizing neuromuscular blockade and worm paralysis.

3. The answer is B: primaquine. Primaquine and other oxidizing drugs can oxidize erythrocyte membrane components leading to hemolysis in persons with glucose-6-phosphate dehydrogenase deficiency. This results from insufficient NADPH to keep glutathione in a reduced state and thereby counteracts primaquine-induced membrane oxidation.

4. The answer is E: ivermectin. Ivermectin kills microfilarial offspring of Onchocerca volvulus, thereby preventing ocular infection caused by these organisms that is responsible for river blindness. Yearly doses must be given because ivermectin does not kill the adult organisms.

5. The answer is D: tinidazole. Tinidazole is a newer nitroimidazole compound that is effective as a single dose to treat diarrhea and pain caused by *Giardia lamblia*. Metronidazole can also be used to treat this infection.

SELECTED READINGS

Centers for Disease Control. Treatment of Malaria (Guidelines for Clinicians), July 28, 2004. (www.cdc.gov/malaria/pdf/clinicalguidance.pdf)

Goswick, S. M., and G. M. Brenner. Activities of therapeutic agents against *Naegleria fowleri* in vitro and in a mouse model of primary amebic meningoencephalitis. J Parasitol 89(4):837–842, 2003.

Manes, G., and A. Balzano. Tinidazole: from protozoa to Helicobacter pylori—the past, present, and future of a nitroimidazole with peculiarities. Expert Rev Antinfect Ther 2:695–705, 2004.

More, B., H. Bhatt, V. Kukreja, et al. Miltefosine: great expectations against visceral leishmaniasis. J Postgrad Med 49:101–103, 2003.

Omura, S., and A. Crump. The life and times of ivermectin—a success story. Nature Rev Microbiol 2:984–989, 2004.

Speare, R., and D. Durrheim. Mass treatment with ivermectin: an underutilized public health strategy. Bull World Health Organ 82(8): 562–562, 2004.

CHAPTER 45

Antineoplastic and Immunomodulating Drugs

CLASSIFICATION OF ANTINEOPLASTIC AND IMMUNOMODULATING DRUGS

DNA Synthesis Inhibitors
Folate Antagonists
- Methotrexate, pemetrexed (ALIMTA)

Purine Antagonists
- Cladribine, fludarabine, mercaptopurine, thioguanine

Pyrimidine Antagonists
- Cytarabine, floxuridine, fluorouracil, gemcitabine (GEMZAR)

Ribonucleotide Reductase Inhibitor
- Hydroxyurea

DNA Alkylating Drugs
Nitrogen Mustards
- Chlorambucil, cyclophosphamide (CYTOXAN), ifosfamide, mechlorethamine, melphalan

Nitrosourea Drugs
- Carmustine, lomustine, streptozocin

Platinum Compounds
- Cisplatin, carboplatin, oxaliplatin

Other DNA Alkylating Drugs
- Busulfan, dacarbazine, mitomycin

DNA Intercalating Drugs
- Bleomycin
- Doxorubicin (ADRIAMYCIN), daunorubicin, idarubicin
- Mitoxantrone, dactinomycin

Mitotic Inhibitors
- Paclitaxel (TAXOL), docetaxel
- Vincristine (ONCOVIN), vinblastine, vinorelbine

Topoisomerase Inhibitors
- Etoposide, teniposide
- Irinotecan, topotecan

Monoclonal Antibodies
- Alemtuzumab, bevacizumab, cetuximab, gemtuzumab ozogamicin, rituximab, trastuzumab

Tyrosine Kinase Inhibitors
- Erlotinib (TARCEVA)
- Imatinib (GLEEVEC)

cytokines and interferons
- Aldesleukin (PROLEUKIN), interferon alpha

Immunosuppressant Drugs
Microbial Products
- Cyclosporine, sirolimus, tacrolimus

Monoclonal Antibodies
- Basiliximab, daclizumab, muromonab-CD3, palivizumab

Other Drugs
- Azathioprine, prednisone
- Thalidomide

OVERVIEW

Cancer occurs after normal cells have been transformed into **neoplastic cells** through alteration of their genetic material leading to the abnormal expression of certain genes. Many neoplastic cells exhibit chromosomal abnormalities and they lose their differentiated properties as they revert to undifferentiated cells that exhibit uncontrolled cell division. In addition, neoplastic cells often invade previously unaffected organs, a process called **metastasis.** This process is dependent on **angiogenesis,** which is the formation of new blood vessels to support the metastatic growth.

The transformation of normal cells into neoplastic cells involves the activation of **oncogenes** and the inhibition of **tumor suppressor genes.** Continued insights into the understanding of these events may eventually lead to the development of drugs that reverse the malignant transformation of cells or that impair the metastatic process by which neoplastic cells invade other organs. Drugs that activate apoptosis, or programmed cell death, may also be developed as anticancer agents. Currently, however, most of the drugs available for cancer treatment act by inhibiting the replication of neoplastic cells. Most antineoplastic drugs inhibit DNA synthesis or alter DNA structure in a manner that prevents DNA replication or transcription. A smaller number of drugs inhibit mitosis and thereby prevent cell division. A growing number of **monoclonal antibodies** are available as anticancer agents. These agents inactivate receptors or proteins involved in tumor cell growth. One of the newer antibodies, bevacizumab, acts to suppress angiogenesis.

Principles of Cancer Chemotherapy

Uses and Goals of Treatment

Antineoplastic drugs are used to treat **hematologic cancers** that cannot be surgically excised, such as **leukemia** and **lymphoma.** They are also used in combination with surgery or radiation therapy to treat **solid tumors.** In patients with solid tumors that can be surgically removed, chemotherapy may eliminate micrometastases and prevent recurrence of the malignant growth. In patients with inoperable tumors, chemotherapy is usually palliative. Palliative therapy is intended to prolong life and reduce incapacitating symptoms but is not curative.

Treatment Regimens and Schedules

Drug regimens for cancer chemotherapy are designed to optimize the synergistic effects of drug combinations while minimizing toxicity. The regimens often use drugs that have different toxicities and different mechanisms of action to maximize cytotoxic effects on tumor cells while sparing host tissue.

In the treatment of some types of cancer, specific drug regimens are used for induction of remission, consolidation therapy, and maintenance therapy. **Induction therapy,** such as that used in acute lymphocytic leukemia, seeks to produce a rapid reduction in the tumor cell burden and thereby produce a symptomatic response in the patient. **Consolidation therapy** seeks to complete or extend the initial remission, and it often uses a different combination of drugs than that used for induction. **Maintenance therapy** aims to sustain the remission as long as possible, and it can use less-frequent courses of chemotherapy and different classes of drugs than were used for induction and consolidation.

Regimens for cancer treatment are among the most complicated forms of drug therapy in use today. These regimens usually employ multiple drugs administered as intermittent courses of therapy rather than as continuous therapy.

Intermittent therapy allows the bone marrow and other normal host cells to recover between treatment courses and reduces the level of toxicity. The dosage rate and frequency of treatment are based on various considerations, including pharmacokinetics, tumor cell cycle kinetics, and circadian variations in host sensitivity to drugs.

Cell Cycle Specificity

Antineoplastic drugs can be classified as cell-cycle-specific and cell-cycle-nonspecific agents. As shown in Fig. 45–1, the **cycle of cell replication** includes the G_1, S, G_2, and M phases. DNA is replicated during the S phase, and mitosis occurs during the M phase. Because early investigators observed no activity occurring between the S and M phases, they referred to the period before S as G_1 (gap 1) and referred to the period before M as G_2 (gap 2). Cytologists now know that cells are extremely active in their preparations for synthesis and mitosis during the G_1 and G_2 phases.

Drugs that act during a specific phase of the cell cycle are called **cell cycle-specific (CCS) drugs,** whereas drugs that are active throughout the cell cycle are called **cell cycle-nonspecific (CCNS) drugs.** CCS drugs include all DNA synthesis inhibitors and mitotic inhibitors. CCNS drugs include all DNA alkylating agents and most DNA intercalating agents.

Limitations of Cancer Chemotherapy

Most of the currently available anticancer drugs have three major limitations: susceptibility to tumor cell resistance, production of host cell toxicity, and an inability to suppress metastasis.

Drug Resistance

Drug resistance is a major cause of cancer treatment failure. As with microbial drug resistance, tumor cell resistance can be innate or acquired. Acquired drug resistance can result from genomic mutations or abnormal gene expression. The mechanisms of tumor cell resistance are similar to those of microbial drug resistance but are more varied. These mechanisms include induction of drug efflux pumps, decreased affinity or overexpression of target enzymes, decreased drug activation or increased drug inactivation, altered expression of proapoptotic and antiapoptotic molecules, and increased tumor cell repair.

Drug resistance can occur through failure of the drug to reach its target because of drug efflux from tumor cells. Two important efflux pumps are the **P-glycoprotein** (Pgp) and the **multidrug resistance protein** (MRP). Both pumps are members of the adenosine triphosphate (ATP)-binding cassette family. Pgp is the product of the multidrug resistance-1 gene and acts to transport many naturally occurring drugs out of neoplastic cells, including anthracyclines, taxanes, and vinca alkaloids (Fig. 45–2). Induction of Pgp by an antineoplastic drug can thereby lead to multidrug resistance. Researchers are searching for drugs that inhibit Pgp and that could be coadministered with antineoplastic agents to prevent efflux-mediated resistance.

Multidrug resistance protein removes drugs from tumor cells after conjugation of drugs with glutathione. The drugs transported by MRP are similar to those transported by Pgp

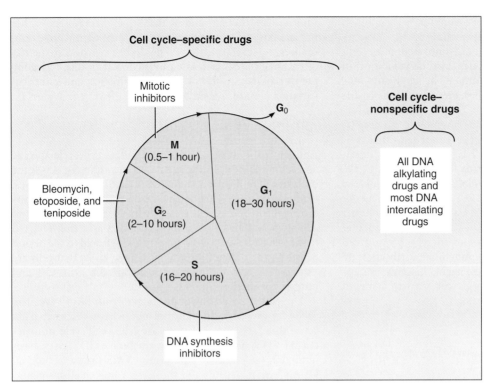

Figure 45–1. Cell cycle activity of antineoplastic drugs. The cycle of cell replication includes the G_1 (gap 1), S (synthesis), G_2 (gap 2), and M (mitosis) phases. Differentiated cells can enter a resting state called G_0. Cell cycle-specific drugs act primarily during the designated phase of the cycle. Cell cycle-nonspecific drugs act throughout the cell cycle.

except that the taxane drugs are poorly transported by MRP. Several drugs that block both Pgp and MRP are undergoing clinical trials as antineoplastic drug enhancers.

Other examples of acquired drug resistance include **topoisomerase mutations** that convey resistance to topoisomerase inhibitors (e.g., etoposide). Resistance to methotrexate can occur through mutations in its target enzyme, dihydrofolate reductase, or through overexpression of the enzyme. Mutations in genes for tubulin or microtubule-associated proteins can cause resistance to the vinca alkaloids and taxane drugs. Finally, expression of **antiapoptotic proteins** (e.g., Bcl-2) can produce resistance to many drugs by interfering with the cell death signal induced by an antineoplastic agent.

Drug Toxicity

The most common toxicities of antineoplastic drugs (Table 45–1) result from inhibition of cell replication in the bone marrow, gastrointestinal epithelium, and hair follicles. Many antineoplastic drugs also stimulate the chemoreceptor trigger zone in the medulla and thereby elicit nausea and vomiting.

The **myelosuppression (bone marrow suppression)** produced by antineoplastic drugs often results in **leukopenia** and **thrombocytopenia,** although **anemia** can also occur. Leukopenia predisposes patients to serious infections, whereas thrombocytopenia can lead to bleeding. The onset of leukopenia is delayed because of the time required to clear circulating cells before the effect that drugs have on precursor cell maturation in the bone marrow becomes evident. With many drugs, including **methotrexate, fluorouracil,** and **cyclophosphamide,** the leukocyte count reaches its nadir in about 7 days and recovery occurs in 2 to 4 weeks. Nitrosourea drugs (e.g., **carmustine**) produce a more delayed and long-lasting suppression of leukocyte production. **Bleomycin, cisplatin,** and **vincristine** produce less myelosuppression than other antineoplastic drugs, so they are often used in combination with myelosuppressive drugs.

Although methods to prevent myelosuppression are not yet available, recombinant forms of hematopoietic growth

Figure 45–2. The P-glycoprotein mechanism of drug efflux. P-glycoprotein utilizes adenosine triphosphate to actively export bleomycin and many other naturally occurring antineoplastic drugs from the cell. Because some agents (e.g., verapamil) inhibit the P-glycoprotein pump and thereby allow antineoplastic drugs to stay in the cell, these agents are being studied as potential adjuncts to cancer chemotherapy. ADP = adenosine diphosphate; ATP = adenosine triphosphate.

TABLE 45–1. **Major Clinical Uses and Adverse Effects of Antineoplastic Drugs**

Drug	Major Clinical Uses	Acute Toxicity	Delayed Toxicity
DNA synthesis inhibitors			
Cladribine	Hairy cell leukemia, non-Hodgkin's lymphoma	Mild nausea and vomiting	Myelosuppression
Cytarabine	AML, non-Hodgkin's lymphoma	Diarrhea, mild nausea and vomiting	Hepatotoxicity, gastrointestinal and oral ulcers, myelosuppression
Floxuridine	Colorectal and hepatic carcinoma	Diarrhea, mild nausea and vomiting	Alopecia, gastrointestinal and oral ulcers, myelosuppression
Fludarabine	CLL, non-Hodgkin's lymphoma	Mild nausea and vomiting	Myelosuppression
Fluorouracil	Breast, colorectal, gastric, and skin cancer	Diarrhea, mild nausea and vomiting	Alopecia, gastrointestinal and oral ulcers, myelosuppression
Gemcitabine	Pancreatic, bladder, and breast cancers	Mild nausea	Myelosuppression and lung cancers
Hydroxyurea	CML, sickle cell anemia	Mild nausea and vomiting	Myelosuppression
Mercaptopurine	AML, ALL, CML	Usually well-tolerated	Hepatotoxicity, myelosuppression
Methotrexate	ALL, breast cancer, non-Hodgkin's lymphoma, osteosarcoma, trophoblastic tumors	Diarrhea, nausea	Gastrointestinal and oral ulcers, hepatotoxicity, myelosuppression, renal toxicity
Pemetrexed	Colorectal cancer, non–small-cell lung cancer	Nausea	Myelosuppression, lung and pancreatic cancers
Thioguanine	AML, ALL, CML	Usually well-tolerated	Myelosuppression
DNA alkylating drugs			
Busulfan	CML	Diarrhea, mild nausea and vomiting	Myelosuppression, pulmonary fibrosis
Carboplatin	Ovarian cancer	Moderate nausea and vomiting	Myelosuppression
Carmustine	Brain tumors, melanoma, myeloma, non-Hodgkin's lymphoma	Severe nausea and vomiting	Myelosuppression, pulmonary fibrosis, renal toxicity
Chlorambucil	CLL	Well tolerated	Myelosuppression, sterility
Cisplatin	Bladder, cervical, ovarian, and testicular cancer; melanoma, myeloma, non-Hodgkin's lymphoma	Acute renal failure, severe nausea and vomiting	Mild myelosuppression, ototoxicity, renal toxicity
Cyclophosphamide	Breast, lung, and ovarian cancer; CLL, ALL, myeloma, neuroblastoma, non-Hodgkin's lymphoma, sarcoma	Nausea and vomiting	Alopecia, hemorrhagic cystitis, myelosuppression, pulmonary fibrosis
Dacarbazine	Hodgkin's disease, melanoma, sarcoma	Severe nausea and vomiting	Alopecia, myelosuppression
Ifosfamide	Sarcoma, testicular cancer	Nausea and vomiting	Alopecia, hemorrhagic cystitis, myelosuppression, pulmonary fibrosis
Lomustine	Brain tumors, non-Hodgkin's lymphoma	Severe nausea and vomiting	Myelosuppression, pulmonary toxicity
Mechlorethamine	Hodgkin's disease, lymphoma	Mild nausea	Alopecia, myelosuppression
Melphalan	Breast and ovarian cancer, myeloma	Severe nausea and vomiting	Myelosuppression
Mitomycin	Bladder, breast, lung, pancreatic, cervical, and stomach cancer	Nausea and vomiting	Alopecia, myelosuppression, pulmonary and renal toxicity, stomatosis
Oxaliplatin	Colon cancer	Nausea and vomiting	Peripheral neuropathy, myelosuppression
Streptozocin	Carcinoid tumor, pancreatic islet cell tumor	Severe nausea and vomiting	Renal toxicity
DNA intercalating drugs			
Bleomycin	Cervical, head, neck, and testicular cancer; Hodgkin's and non-Hodgkin's lymphoma	Fever, mild nausea and vomiting	Alopecia, mild myelosuppression, mucocutaneous toxicity, pneumonitis, pulmonary fibrosis
Dactinomycin	Ewing's sarcoma, trophoblastic tumors, Wilms' tumor	Diarrhea, nausea and vomiting	Alopecia, myelosuppression, oral ulcers
Daunorubicin	ALL, AML	Nausea and vomiting	Alopecia, cardiotoxicity, mucosal ulcers, myelosuppression
Doxorubicin	ALL; bladder, breast, gastric, lung, ovarian, soft tissue, and thyroid cancer; myeloma, neuroblastoma	Nausea and vomiting	Alopecia, cardiotoxicity, mucosal ulcers, myelosuppression

Continued

TABLE 45–1. **Major Clinical Uses and Adverse Effects of Antineoplastic Drugs—cont'd**

Drug	Major Clinical Uses	Acute Toxicity	Delayed Toxicity
Idarubicin	AML	Nausea and vomiting	Alopecia, cardiotoxicity, mucosal ulcers, myelosuppression
Mitoxantrone	AML	Nausea and vomiting	Alopecia, cardiotoxicity, mucosal ulcers, myelosuppression
Mitotic inhibitors			
Docetaxel	Breast and ovarian cancer, non–small-cell lung cancer	Usually well-tolerated	Alopecia, myelosuppression, neurotoxicity
Paclitaxel	Breast and ovarian cancer; non–small-cell lung cancer	Usually well-tolerated	Alopecia, myelosuppression, neurotoxicity
Vinblastine	Bladder, breast, ovarian, and testicular cancer; Hodgkin's and non-Hodgkin's lymphomas	Nausea and vomiting	Alopecia, myelosuppression, stomatitis
Vincristine	ALL; Hodgkin's and non-Hodgkin's lymphoma, lung cancer, myeloma, neuroblastoma, sarcoma	Usually well-tolerated	Alopecia, mild myelosuppression, peripheral neurotoxicity
Vinorelbine	Non–small-cell lung cancer	Nausea and vomiting	Myelosuppression
Topoisomerase inhibitors			
Etoposide	Non-Hodgkin's lymphoma, small-cell lung cancer, testicular cancer, AML	Mild nausea and vomiting	Alopecia, myelosuppression
Irinotecan	Ovarian and colorectal cancer	Diarrhea, mild nausea and vomiting	Alopecia, myelosuppression
Teniposide	ALL, AML	Mild nausea and vomiting	Alopecia, myelosuppression
Topotecan	Lung and ovarian cancer	Mild nausea and vomiting	Alopecia, myelosuppression
Hormones and their antagonists			
Anastrozole, Letrozole	Breast cancer	Nausea and hot flashes	None
Flutamide	Prostate cancer	Nausea and vomiting	Impotence
Leuprolide	Prostate cancer	Nausea and vomiting	Hot flashes, gynecomastia
Prednisone	ALL, breast cancer, CLL, Hodgkin's and non-Hodgkin's lymphoma, myeloma	None	Hyperadrenocortism
Tamoxifen	Breast cancer	Nausea and vomiting	Hot flashes, hypercalcemia
Cytokines, interferons, and monclonal antibodies			
Aldesleukin	Colorectal cancer, melanoma, renal cell carcinoma	Varies with dosage and route of administration	Fluid retention, hematologic deficiencies, hypotension, neuropsychiatric effects, renal dysfunction, skin lesions
Bevacizumab	Colorectal cancer	None	Gastrointestinal bleeding and perforation, pulmonary hemorrhage
Cetuximab	Colon cancer	Nausea	Skin rash, allergic reactions
Interferon alfa	CML, hairy cell leukemia, Kaposi's sarcoma	Flulike illness	Fatigue
Rituximab	Non-Hodgkin's lymphoma	Chills, fever, headache, nausea	Myelosuppression
Trastuzumab	Breast cancer	Chest pain, chills, dyspnea, fever, nausea, vomiting	Unknown

ALL = acute lymphocytic leukemia; AML = acute myeloid leukemia; CLL = chronic lymphocytic leukemia; CML = chronic myeloid leukemia.

factors (e.g., **epoetin alfa, filgrastim,** and **sargramostim**) are used to accelerate recovery from leukopenia or anemia caused by chemotherapy or bone marrow transplantation. These drugs are described more fully in Chapter 17.

The **nausea** and **vomiting** caused by antineoplastic drugs range from mild to severe. Among the antineoplastic drugs, the most emetic are **cisplatin** and **carmustine.** Their adverse effects can be prevented or substantially reduced, however, by pretreatment with a combination of antiemetic drugs, including serotonin antagonists (e.g., **ondansetron**) neuroleptics (e.g., **droperidol**), and corticosteroids (e.g.,

dexamethasone). Another antiemetic, **metoclopramide,** is also useful in preventing chemotherapy-induced nausea and vomiting. The antiemetics are discussed in greater detail in Chapter 28.

Alopecia is a cosmetically distressing but less serious adverse effect of chemotherapy. It is generally reversible after treatment ends, although the hair might differ in texture and appearance from its previous condition.

Several antineoplastic drugs have characteristic organ system toxicities that appear unrelated to inhibition of cell division. For example, use of **doxorubicin** and other anthracyclines can cause **cardiotoxicity;** use of **cyclophosphamide** and **ifosfamide** can cause **hemorrhagic cystitis;** use of **cisplatin** can cause **renal toxicity;** use of **bleomycin** or **busulfan** can cause **pulmonary toxicity;** and use of **vincristine, paclitaxel,** and other vinca alkaloids and taxanes can cause **neurotoxicity.**

Agents have been developed to prevent some of these organ system toxicities. For example, **dexrazoxane** was developed to prevent anthracycline-induced cardiotoxicity. Another cytoprotective drug, **mesna,** was developed to prevent cyclophosphamide-induced hemorrhagic cystitis. Cisplatin-induced renal toxicity can be partly prevented by administering fluids, along with **mannitol** and **sodium thiosulfate.** Mannitol maintains renal blood flow and tubular function, whereas sodium thiosulfate inactivates the drug in the kidneys. No specific agents currently exist to prevent pulmonary toxicity and neurotoxicity; therefore, patients at risk should be closely monitored so that treatment can be discontinued if these toxicities develop.

DNA SYNTHESIS INHIBITORS

Most of the DNA synthesis inhibitors are structural analogues of folic acid or of the purine or pyrimidine bases found in DNA. They act as antimetabolites to inhibit enzymes required for DNA base synthesis. One DNA synthesis inhibitor discussed below, hydroxyurea, is not an antimetabolite; it inhibits the conversion of ribonucleotides to deoxyribonucleotides, a process that is required for DNA synthesis. The uses, adverse effects, and chemical structures of selected DNA synthesis inhibitors are shown in Table 45–1 and Fig. 45–3.

Folate Antagonists

Methotrexate

Nearly 50 years ago, methotrexate (MTX) was used successfully to induce remission in patients with acute childhood leukemia. Today, it is the most widely used antimetabolite in cancer chemotherapy, and it is also used as an immunosuppressive drug in the treatment of rheumatoid arthritis, lupus erythematosus, and other conditions (see Chapter 30).

CHEMISTRY AND MECHANISMS. The structures of MTX and folic acid are similar. MTX, however, has an amino group substituted for a hydroxyl group on the pteridine ring, and it also has an additional methyl group (see Fig. 45–3A).

Methotrexate is actively transported into mammalian cells and inhibits dihydrofolate reductase, the enzyme that normally converts dietary folate to the tetrahydrofolate form required for thymidine and purine synthesis (Fig. 45–4).

PHARMACOKINETICS. MTX can be administered orally or parenterally. The oral bioavailability of the drug is dose-dependent. Low doses are completely absorbed, whereas higher doses undergo significantly less absorption. Because MTX does not penetrate the central nervous system (CNS), it must be administered intrathecally for the prevention or treatment of CNS disease.

Methotrexate is rapidly distributed throughout the total body water, and it is partly degraded in the intestine (by intestinal flora) and in the liver. The drug has a biphasic elimination pattern. It is primarily eliminated as the parent compound and metabolites in the urine. The terminal half-life reflects redistribution from tissues and "third space" fluids, such as ascites and pleural effusions.

INDICATIONS. The use of MTX in the treatment of choriocarcinoma, a trophoblastic tumor, was the first demonstration of curative chemotherapy. Today, MTX has a variety of uses, including the treatment of trophoblastic tumors, breast cancer, non-Hodgkin's lymphomas, and osteosarcoma. It is especially effective for treating acute lymphocytic leukemia and the meningeal metastases of a wide range of tumors.

ADVERSE EFFECTS. The bone marrow and gastrointestinal mucosa are the normal tissues most sensitive to MTX toxicity. Although myelosuppression is the primary dose-limiting toxicity of the drug, severe oral ulceration (stomatitis) can also occur and necessitate dosage reduction. Administration of a fully activated form of folic acid called **leucovorin (folinic acid)** can prevent these adverse reactions, but it cannot reverse them after they have occurred. Leucovorin rescue is normally used with high doses of MTX (doses exceeding 100 mg/m^2 body surface area). Assays for MTX in plasma are readily available, and drug level monitoring provides a useful guide to the duration of leucovorin administration.

Methotrexate can cause hepatotoxicity, especially with long-term low-dose therapy for psoriasis and rheumatoid conditions. At high doses, MTX can crystallize in the urine and cause renal damage. To prevent renal toxicity, dosage reduction is necessary in persons with renal insufficiency.

Pemetrexed

Pemetrexed (ALIMTA) is a novel antifolate drug. It is rapidly metabolized to active polyglutamate forms that inhibit several tetrahydrofolate-dependent enzymes involved in the synthesis of purine and pyrimidine bases, including thymidylate synthase. Although the drug can cause considerable and even life-threatening toxicities when given alone, investigators found that these toxicities can be minimized by giving folic acid and vitamin B_{12} without impairing drug efficacy. Pemetrexed has broad antitumor activity and initial studies found that it prolongs survival in patients with advanced colorectal cancer. Early clinical trials show that it is also active against non–small-cell lung cancer and pancreatic cancer. Neutropenia and other forms of bone marrow suppression are the primary adverse effects of pemetrexed.

Purine Antagonists

Mercaptopurine and Thioguanine

The first purine analogue to be used in cancer chemotherapy was mercaptopurine (6-mercaptopurine, or 6-MP), a drug introduced almost 50 years ago for the treatment of acute lymphocytic leukemia. As with mercaptopurine, thioguanine (6-thioguanine, or 6-TG) is an antineoplastic agent that acts as a purine antagonist.

CHEMISTRY AND MECHANISMS. Mercaptopurine and thioguanine are the thio analogues of the purine bases hypoxanthine and guanine, respectively. The drugs are believed to act

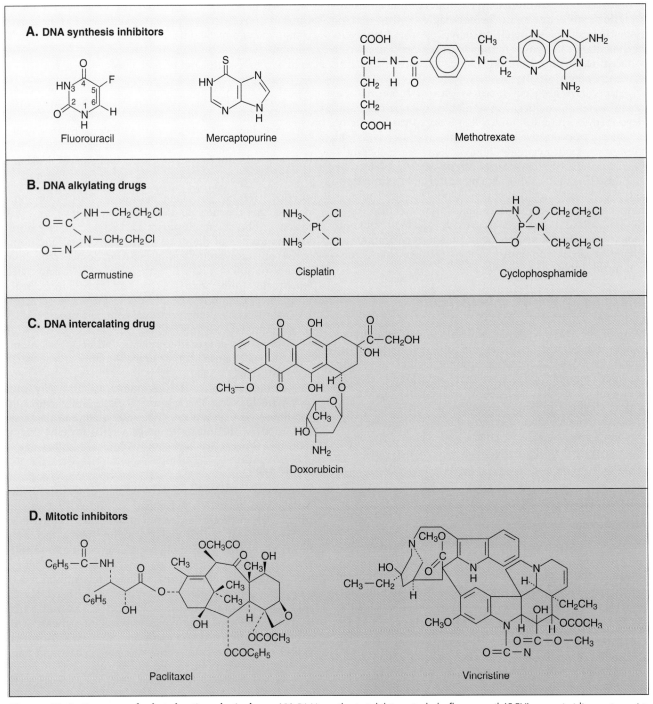

Figure 45–3. Structures of selected antineoplastic drugs. (A) DNA synthesis inhibitors include fluorouracil (5-FU), a pyrimidine antagonist; mercaptopurine, a purine antagonist; and methotrexate, a folate antagonist. **(B)** DNA alkylating drugs include carmustine, a nitrosourea drug; cisplatin, a platinum compound; and cyclophosphamide, a nitrogen mustard. **(C)** Doxorubicin is an anthracycline drug. **(D)** Paclitaxel is a taxane (taxoid), and vincristine is a vinca alkaloid.

similarly to inhibit purine base synthesis, although their exact mechanisms of action are still uncertain. Mercaptopurine and thioguanine inhibit several steps in the biosynthesis of purines and in purine salvage (recycling) pathways that supply purine precursors. Both drugs are activated by conversion to nucleotides through the addition of ribose phosphate. The reactions are catalyzed by hypoxanthine-

guanine phosphoribosyltransferase (HGPRT), and tumor cells that delete this enzyme acquire resistance to the drugs. This probably explains why clinical cross-resistance is usually observed between mercaptopurine and thioguanine.

PHARMACOKINETICS. Mercaptopurine and thioguanine are given orally, and their bioavailability is variable, incomplete,

Figure 45–4. **Inhibition of DNA synthesis by methotrexate and fluorouracil.** Methotrexate inhibits dihydrofolate reductase and the conversion of dihydrofolate to tetrahydrofolate. This reduces the supply of 5,10-methylenetetrahydrofolate, a substance required for the synthesis of deoxythymidine monophosphate (dTMP). The conversion of deoxyuridine monophosphate (dUMP) to dTMP, a critical step in DNA synthesis, is catalyzed by thymidylate synthetase. This enzyme is inhibited by 5-fluorodeoxyuridine monophosphate (5-FdUMP), which is the active form of fluorouracil.

and reduced by food. Both drugs are primarily eliminated by metabolism, although mercaptopurine is partly excreted unchanged in the urine after high doses. Unlike mercaptopurine, thioguanine is not metabolized by xanthine oxidase.

INDICATIONS. Mercaptopurine is used primarily to maintain remission in patients with acute lymphocytic leukemia and is given in combination with MTX for this purpose. It is also used in treating acute and chronic myeloid leukemia. The clinical use of thioguanine includes maintenance of remission in patients with acute lymphocytic and acute myeloid leukemia.

ADVERSE EFFECTS AND INTERACTIONS. Mercaptopurine and thioguanine are usually well tolerated. Myelosuppression is generally mild with mercaptopurine, but can be dose-limiting with thioguanine. Long-term mercaptopurine use can cause hepatotoxicity.

To avoid toxicity, doses of mercaptopurine must be reduced by at least 50% in patients who are taking allopurinol concomitantly. Allopurinol inhibits xanthine oxidase and thereby elevates plasma levels of mercaptopurine. Allopurinol does not interact in this manner with thioguanine, because the latter is not metabolized by xanthine oxidase. Allopurinol is often given to patients undergoing cancer chemotherapy because it inhibits the synthesis of uric acid and thereby prevents hyperuricemia and gout. Cancer chemotherapy places patients at risk for these problems because the rapid destruction of cancer cells leads to excessive purine catabolism and uric acid formation.

Fludarabine and Cladribine

Fludarabine and cladribine are both purine antagonists. Fludarabine is a fluorinated derivative of adenine arabinoside. Adenine arabinoside is an analogue of adenosine in which the ribose moiety has been replaced with arabinose. The active triphosphate form of fludarabine blocks DNA polymerase by causing DNA chain termination. Fludarabine is a highly active agent in the treatment of chronic lymphocytic leukemia and low-grade non-Hodgkin's lymphoma.

Cladribine (2-chlorodeoxyadenosine) acts in a manner similar to fludarabine. It is primarily used for hairy cell leukemia, but it is also active against other leukemias and lymphomas.

Pyrimidine Antagonists

Cytarabine and Fluorouracil

CHEMISTRY AND MECHANISMS. Cytarabine (cytosine arabinoside, or ara-C) and fluorouracil (5-FU) are the most commonly used pyrimidine antimetabolites. Cytarabine is composed of the base cytosine and the sugar arabinose. Arabinose differs from ribose only in the position of one hydroxyl group. Fluorouracil is an analogue of thymine in which the methyl group is replaced by a fluorine atom (see Fig. 45–3A).

Cytarabine and fluorouracil are each converted to active nucleotide metabolites by tumor cell enzymes. The active metabolite of cytarabine is cytarabine triphosphate. It blocks DNA synthesis by several actions, including the inhibition of DNA polymerase and the incorporation into DNA. This incorporation causes DNA chain termination. Fluorouracil has two active metabolites: 5-fluorodeoxyuridine monophosphate (5-FdUMP) and 5-fluorodeoxyuridine triphosphate (5-FdUTP). 5-FdUMP inhibits thymidylate synthetase and prevents the synthesis of thymidine, a major building block of DNA (see Fig. 45–4). 5-FdUTP is incorporated into RNA by RNA polymerase and interferes with RNA function.

PHARMACOKINETICS. Cytarabine can be administered intravenously or subcutaneously, and fluorouracil can be administered intravenously or topically. When the drugs are given parenterally, they are extensively metabolized before undergoing renal excretion. Cytarabine crosses the blood–brain barrier and reaches cerebrospinal fluid levels that are 40% to 50% of plasma levels.

INDICATIONS. Cytarabine is primarily used in combination with daunorubicin or thioguanine to treat **acute myeloid leukemia.** It is less frequently used to treat lymphomas.

Fluorouracil is exclusively used to treat solid tumors, especially breast, colorectal, and gastric tumors and squamous cell tumors of the head and neck. Regional delivery of the drug via the hepatic artery can produce a sustained response in patients whose colorectal cancer has metastasized to the liver. Topical application of fluorouracil is used to treat **actinic keratoses** and noninvasive **skin cancers.**

ADVERSE EFFECTS. Cytarabine and fluorouracil can cause nausea and vomiting, myelosuppression, and oral and gastrointestinal ulceration. Nausea and vomiting are usually mild. With fluorouracil, myelosuppression is more problematic after bolus injections, whereas mucosal damage is dose-limiting with continuous infusions. High doses of cytarabine or fluorouracil can damage the liver, heart, and other organs.

Gemcitabine

Gemcitabine (GEMZAR) is an S-phase specific inhibitor of DNA synthesis. After conversion to gemcitabine diphosphate and triphosphate, these active metabolites inhibit the synthesis of deoxynucleoside triphosphates and the incorporation of deoxynucleoside triphosphates into DNA. In addition, gemcitabine triphosphate itself is incorporated into DNA and terminates DNA synthesis by this mechanism as well. The drug is indicated as a first-line treatment for pancreatic carcinoma and for use with cisplatin as first-line therapy for inoperable, non–small-cell lung cancer. Gemcitabine has also been used for biliary tract, gallbladder, breast, and ovarian cancer. As with other DNA synthesis inhibitors, gemcitabine can cause myelosuppression leading to anemia, leukopenia, and thrombocytopenia. It also causes alopecia and various gastrointestinal disturbances.

Floxuridine

Floxuridine (FUDR) is the deoxyribonucleoside derivative of fluorouracil. It acts as a pyrimidine antagonist and is used in the treatment of colorectal and hepatic carcinoma.

Ribonucleotide Reductase Inhibitors

Hydroxyurea inhibits ribonucleotide reductase, the enzyme that converts ribonucleotides to deoxyribonucleotides. It thereby stops DNA synthesis and causes cells to accumulate in the S phase of the cell cycle.

Hydroxyurea is given orally and is excreted in the urine. It is primarily used to treat chronic myelogenous leukemia, ovarian cancer, and melanoma. Hydroxyurea is also used in the management of **sickle cell anemia.** In this condition, hydroxyurea elevates the concentration of fetal hemoglobin and decreases the frequency of sickle cell crises. The dose-limiting toxicity of hydroxyurea is rapid-onset myelosuppression.

DNA ALKYLATING DRUGS

A DNA alkylating drug is an agent that cross-links DNA strands by forming covalent bonds between alkyl groups of the drug and guanine bases of DNA. The DNA alkylating drugs include nitrogen mustards, nitrosourea drugs, and several other agents. Platinum compounds (e.g., cisplatin) are included in this category because they also cross-link DNA.

Nitrogen Mustards

The nitrogen mustards are nitrogen analogues of the sulfur mustards that were used as chemical warfare agents in World War I. The cytotoxic effects of nitrogen mustards were discovered in the early 1940s, and the drugs were soon introduced into clinical use. They are considered the first effective antineoplastic drugs.

The nitrogen mustards are bifunctional alkylating agents that undergo spontaneous conversion to active metabolites in body fluids or are enzymatically converted to active metabolites in the liver. The strong electrophilic intermediates formed by these reactions attack the N7 nitrogen of guanine and thereby form covalent bonds with this base. Sequential attachment to two guanine residues results in cross-linking of DNA, and this prevents DNA replication and transcription (Fig. 45–5A). The alkylating drugs act throughout the cell replication cycle.

Cyclophosphamide and Ifosfamide

CHEMISTRY AND PHARMACOKINETICS. Cyclophosphamide and ifosfamide are prodrugs that must be converted to active metabolites by hepatic mixed-function oxidase (cytochrome P450) enzymes. The active alkylating metabolite of cyclophosphamide is thought to be phosphoramide mustard. Cyclophosphamide and ifosfamide are each partly converted to acrolein, which is probably responsible for hemorrhagic cystitis, an adverse effect that sometimes occurs with use of these drugs. Either drug can be administered intravenously, and cyclophosphamide can also be given orally. Cyclophosphamide is completely absorbed after oral administration.

INDICATIONS. Cyclophosphamide is the most widely used nitrogen mustard because of its broad spectrum of activity. It is used in the treatment of acute and chronic lymphocytic leukemia; non-Hodgkin's lymphoma; breast, lung, and ovarian cancer; and a variety of other cancers (see Table 45–1). Because cyclophosphamide is a potent immunosuppressant, it is used in the management of rheumatoid disorders and autoimmune nephritis. It is also used in preoperative regimens for bone marrow transplantation.

Ifosfamide is primarily used to treat patients with sarcoma and patients with testicular cancer that is refractory to first-line treatments.

ADVERSE EFFECTS. Adverse effects of cyclophosphamide and ifosfamide include alopecia, nausea, vomiting, myelosuppression, and hemorrhagic cystitis. Nausea and vomiting are usually mild when cyclophosphamide is given orally, but they can be severe when given intravenously. The dose-limiting toxicity of cyclophosphamide is myelosuppression, whereas that of ifosfamide is usually hemorrhagic cystitis. This type of cystitis is characterized by symptoms of urinary frequency and irritation and by blood loss from the bladder. Ingestion of large amounts of fluid and the administration of mesna, a sulfhydryl reagent, can significantly reduce the incidence of cystitis. Mesna binds to acrolein, the toxic metabolite that causes cystitis, and converts it to an inactive substance.

A. Effect of alkylating drugs

Mechlorethamine

B. Effect of intercalating drugs

Doxorubicin → Intercalation between base pairs → Fe and H_2O_2 → Hydroxyl radicals → Strand breaks

Figure 45-5. Mechanisms of action of DNA alkylating drugs and DNA intercalating drugs. **(A)** Mechlorethamine and other bifunctional alkylating drugs form electrophilic intermediates that attack the N7 nitrogen of guanine residues in DNA, thereby cross-linking DNA strands and preventing replication and transcription. **(B)** Doxorubicin and other anthracycline drugs intercalate between DNA base pairs. Anthracyclines are reduced to intermediates that donate electrons to oxygen to form superoxide. Superoxide then reacts with itself to make hydrogen peroxide, which is cleaved in the presence of iron to form the destructive hydroxyl radical that cleaves DNA.

Chlorambucil, Mechlorethamine, and Melphalan

Chlorambucil, mechlorethamine, and melphalan are nitrogen mustards that act via the mechanisms described earlier.

Chlorambucil is orally administered, has selective cytotoxicity for lymphocyte cell lines, and is primarily used to manage **chronic lymphocytic leukemia.** It is well tolerated but can cause dose-limiting myelosuppression and sterility. Long-term therapy is associated with a high incidence of secondary acute leukemia.

Mechlorethamine is a highly reactive and vesicant drug that is rapidly and spontaneously converted to its alkylating intermediate in body fluids after it is given intravenously. Mechlorethamine is used for treating Hodgkin's and non-Hodgkins's lymphomas. Melphalan is a nitrogen mustard that is primarily used to treat multiple **myeloma** (plasma cell myeloma) and breast cancer.

Nitrosourea Drugs

The nitrosourea drugs include **carmustine** (*bis*-chloroethyl nitrosourea, or BCNU), **lomustine** (*cis*-chloroethyl nitrosourea, or CCNU), and a closely related methylnitrosourea called **streptozocin.**

Drug Properties

CHEMISTRY AND MECHANISMS. The structures of nitrosoureas are similar to those of nitrogen mustards (see Fig. 45-3B). The nitrosoureas are bifunctional alkylating drugs, and they spontaneously form active intermediates that cross-link DNA.

PHARMACOKINETICS. Nitrosoureas can be given orally or intravenously. They are highly lipophilic and reach cerebrospinal fluid concentrations that are about 30% of plasma concentrations. The drugs are extensively metabolized before renal excretion.

INDICATIONS. Because of their excellent CNS penetration, carmustine and lomustine have been used to treat brain tumors, such as astrocytomas. Either drug can be used to treat lymphomas, and carmustine is also used to treat melanoma and multiple myeloma. Streptozocin is used only to treat **carcinoid tumor** and **pancreatic islet cell tumor (insulinoma).**

ADVERSE EFFECTS. The nitrosoureas produce delayed and prolonged myelosuppression, with complete recovery taking 6 to 8 weeks. The thrombocytopenia caused by nitrosoureas usually occurs earlier and is more pronounced than the leukopenia produced by these drugs. Although all of the drugs cause nausea and vomiting, these effects are most pronounced with streptozocin treatment. Pulmonary damage occurs when high doses of nitrosoureas are used.

Platinum Compounds

Drug Properties

CHEMISTRY AND MECHANISMS. The drugs **cisplatin, carboplatin,** and **oxaliplatin** are inorganic platinum derivatives. Cisplatin is converted to an active cytotoxic form by reacting with water to form positively charged, hydrated intermediates that react with guanine in DNA. This leads to the formation of intrastrand cross-links between neighboring guanine residues. The intrastrand links cause DNA to bend to distort the normal conformation of DNA and thereby impair its function. Carboplatin and **oxaliplatin** is believed to have a similar mechanism of action.

INDICATIONS. Cisplatin has efficacy against a wide range of neoplasms. It is given intravenously as a first-line drug for testicular, ovarian, cervical, and bladder cancers, and it is also useful in the treatment of melanoma and a number of other solid tumors. Carboplatin has a similar spectrum of activity, but it is approved only for ovarian cancer. Oxaliplatin is used in treating colon cancer.

ADVERSE EFFECTS. Cisplatin produces mild myelosuppression but can cause severe nausea, vomiting, and nephrotoxicity. Pretreatment with an antiemetic (e.g., **ondansetron**) will prevent or significantly reduce the severity of nausea and vomiting. The use of **mannitol** and **sodium thiosulfate** will decrease the severity of nephrotoxicity, an adverse effect associated with loss of potassium and magnesium, reduced glomerular filtration, and renal failure. Mannitol increases urine flow and can reduce binding of cisplatin to renal tubule proteins. Sodium thiosulfate accumulates in renal tubules and neutralizes the cytotoxicity of cisplatin. Renal damage caused by cisplatin is often slowly reversible.

Other DNA Alkylating Drugs

Busulfan

Busulfan is an alkyl sulfonate drug that acts as a bifunctional alkylating agent in the same manner as the nitrogen mustards act. After busulfan is administered orally, it is extensively metabolized. Its metabolites are then excreted in the urine.

Unlike other alkylating drugs, busulfan has greater activity against myeloid cells than against lymphoid cells. For this reason, it has been primarily used in the management of **chronic myeloid leukemia.**

Busulfan causes mild nausea and vomiting and produces dose-limiting myelosuppression. It can also cause pulmonary fibrosis ("busulfan lung"), which occurs in about 4% of patients treated on a long-term basis with the drug. Pulmonary fibrosis usually has its onset about 3 years after treatment begins. It is characterized by a nonproductive cough, dyspnea, and a reticular pattern on chest x-ray film. No treatment has been successful, and the average survival after diagnosis is 5 months.

Dacarbazine

Dacarbazine is an atypical alkylating agent. The drug is converted to active intermediates that can alkylate DNA, although the exact mechanisms are uncertain. Ultimately, the drug inhibits DNA, RNA, and protein synthesis.

Dacarbazine is primarily used to treat Hodgkin's disease. Dacarbazine is administered intravenously and is part of the **ABVD regimen,** which consists of adriamycin (doxorubicin), bleomycin, vinblastine, and dacarbazine.

Mitomycin

Mitomycin (mitomycin C) is an antineoplastic antibiotic that alkylates DNA and thereby causes strand breakage and inhibition of DNA synthesis. After the drug is administered parenterally, it is activated by hepatic reduction reactions to the active alkylating compound. Most of the drug is metabolized, but a small amount of it is excreted unchanged in the urine.

Mitomycin is primarily used in combination with vincristine as salvage therapy for breast cancer. It is also used in the treatment of non–small-cell lung cancer, pancreatic and stomach tumors, and superficial transitional cell carcinomas of the bladder. Although it is administered intravenously for most types of cancer, it is administered intravesically for bladder cancer.

Mitomycin produces delayed and prolonged myelosuppression that preferentially affects platelets and leukocytes. It can also cause severe pulmonary damage and a hemolytic-uremic syndrome characterized by hemolytic anemia, renal dysfunction, and thrombocytopenia. Extravasation can result in severe necrosis.

DNA INTERCALATING DRUGS

The DNA intercalating drugs include the anthracycline drugs, bleomycin, and dactinomycin. These are some of the most widely used antitumor antibiotics. Several of the drugs have a broad spectrum of activity against hematologic cancers and solid tumors, whereas others have a more limited range of clinical uses.

Anthracycline Drugs

Daunorubicin, Doxorubicin, and Idarubicin

CHEMISTRY. Daunorubicin and doxorubicin are antibiotics obtained from *Streptomyces peucetius,* and idarubicin is a semisynthetic derivative. These drugs have a four-membered anthracene ring with attached sugars (see Fig. 45–3C). Two of the four members in the ring are quinone and hydroquinone moieties that enable the compounds to accept and donate electrons and thereby promote the formation of free radicals. The anthracene ring accounts for the intense red color of the drug compounds.

MECHANISMS. Several mechanisms are responsible for the cytotoxicity of the anthracycline drugs: intercalation of DNA, inhibition of topoisomerase, and formation of free radicals. The drugs bind strongly to DNA by inserting themselves between paired bases of double-stranded DNA and thereby causing deformation and uncoiling of the DNA (see Fig. 45–5B). The anthracyclines cause DNA strands to break by interfering with the action of topoisomerase II (an enzyme discussed later in this chapter) and by forming free radicals. The anthracyclines undergo reduction (addition of electrons) to form highly destructive hydroxyl radicals that produce DNA cleavage. The process appears to involve an iron–anthracycline complex that is strongly bound to DNA.

PHARMACOKINETICS. After intravenous administration, the anthracyclines are rapidly distributed to all body tissues except those of the CNS. They avidly bind to tissues and have large volumes of distribution and long half-lives. The drugs are extensively metabolized in the liver, and some metabolites are as pharmacologically active as the parent compounds.

INDICATIONS. Daunorubicin and idarubicin are agents used in induction and consolidation therapy for acute myeloid leukemia. Doxorubicin has a much broader spectrum of activity. It is one of the most active drugs against breast cancer, and it is also useful in the treatment of Hodgkin's disease, bladder cancer, ovarian cancer, gastric carcinoma, and other hematologic cancers and solid tumors (see Table 45–1).

ADVERSE EFFECTS. Among the adverse effects of anthracyclines are myelosuppression and cardiac damage, which are dose-limiting effects; nausea and vomiting, which are dose-related and may be moderate to severe; alopecia, and mucosal ulcerations. Extravasation of the drugs during intravenous infusion can lead to severe localized tissue ulceration and necrosis. These localized reactions can progress over many weeks, and no effective treatment for them currently exists. Hence, exceptional care and specialized training is required for proper administration of anthracycline drugs.

The anthracyclines cause both acute and chronic cardiotoxicity. Manifestations of acute toxicity include sinus tachycardia and ventricular premature beats. These cardiac rhythm disturbances often occur during the first 24 hours and are self-limited. Chronic toxicity leads to congestive cardiomyopathy and limits the cumulative dose of anthracycline that can be given to any patient. The cardiomyopathy appears to result from iron-catalyzed formation of free radicals. Information about this process has led to the development of a cardioprotective drug called **dexrazoxane.** Dexrazoxane is a potent chelator of ferric iron, and it is believed to act by disrupting the iron–anthracycline complex and thereby preventing reactive free radical formation. Dexrazoxane is primarily given to women with breast cancer who might benefit from continued doxorubicin therapy. Another method of preventing cardiotoxicity is to administer doxorubicin as a **liposomal complex** that is not taken up as much by cardiac tissue as is the free drug. This preparation is now approved for the treatment of Kaposi's sarcoma in patients with acquired immunodeficiency syndrome (AIDS), and it is expected to be used in the treatment of other solid tumors.

INTERACTIONS. Drugs that increase the toxicity of doxorubicin include cyclosporine, cyclophosphamide, and mercaptopurine. Verapamil can increase the cytotoxicity of doxorubicin and other anthracycline drugs by inhibition of the Pgp that transports anthracyclines out of cells.

Mitoxantrone

Mitoxantrone is a synthetic anthracene derivative that is primarily used in combination with cytarabine for induction of remission in patients with acute myeloid leukemia. The drug is administered intravenously. As with the anthracycline antibiotics, mitoxantrone intercalates DNA and produces DNA strand breaks, but it has much less potential for free

radical formation. Partly for this reason, mitoxantrone causes less cardiotoxicity, less tissue damage after extravasation, and less nausea, vomiting, mucosal ulceration, and alopecia than do doxorubicin and other anthracycline antibiotics.

Other DNA Intercalating Drugs

Bleomycin

CHEMISTRY AND MECHANISMS. Bleomycin is a mixture of two peptides obtained from *Streptomyces verticillus.* The drug has its greatest effect on neoplastic cells in the G_2 phase of the cell replication cycle. Although bleomycin intercalates DNA, the major cytotoxicity is believed to result from iron-catalyzed free radical formation and DNA strand breakage. The iron-bleomycin complex binds to DNA, which reduces molecular oxygen to oxygen free radicals that cause single strands of DNA to break.

PHARMACOKINETICS. Bleomycin is administered intravenously, is widely distributed, and is primarily eliminated by renal excretion. The drug is inactivated in cells by aminohydrolase, whose low levels in skin and lung may partly account for the toxicity of bleomycin in these tissues.

INDICATIONS. Bleomycin has a broad range of activity and is one of the most widely used antitumor antibiotics. It is useful in Hodgkin's and non-Hodgkin's lymphomas, testicular cancer, and several other solid tumors. It is included in the ABVD regimen for Hodgkin's disease (Table 45–2).

ADVERSE EFFECTS. Bleomycin produces very little myelosuppression. For this reason, it is often combined with myelosuppressive drugs in treatment regimens. The most serious toxicities of bleomycin are pulmonary and mucocutaneous reactions. Patients taking the drug can develop pneumonitis that progresses to interstitial fibrosis, hypoxia, and death. It is important, therefore, to monitor patients carefully for manifestations of pulmonary toxicity, which include cough, dyspnea, rales, and pulmonary infiltrates noted on chest x-ray film. Mucocutaneous toxicity usually presents as mild stomatitis (inflammation of the oral mucosa), skin hyperpigmentation, erythema, and edema.

Dactinomycin

Dactinomycin (actinomycin D) intercalates DNA and thereby prevents DNA transcription and messenger RNA synthesis. The drug is given intravenously, and its clinical use is limited to the treatment of trophoblastic tumors, such as **choriocarcinoma,** and the treatment of pediatric tumors, such as **Wilms' tumor** and **Ewing's sarcoma.**

MITOTIC INHIBITORS

The mitotic spindle that separates the chromosomes during mitosis is made up of hollow tubules called microtubules. The microtubules are formed by the polymerization of the structural protein called tubulin. During mitosis, microtubules are continuously assembled and disassembled by means of tubulin polymerization and depolymerization. As shown in Fig. 45–6, two classes of antineoplastic drugs

TABLE 45–2. **Drugs of Drug Combinations Commonly Used in the Treatment of Selected Neoplastic Diseases**

Disease	Treatment*
Hematologic cancers	
Acute lymphocytic leukemia (ALL)	For induction: vincristine/prednisone. For maintenance: methotrexate/mercaptopurine For central nervous system prophylaxis: methotrexate
Acute nonlymphocytic leukemia (ANLL)	Daunorubicin/cytarabine; cytarabine/thioguanine
Chronic lymphocytic leukemia (CLL)	Chlorambucil: cyclophosphamide; prednisone
Chronic myeloid leukemia (CML)	Busulfan; hydroxyurea; interferon alfa
Hodgkin's disease	ABVD regimen, consisting of Adriamycin (doxorubicin)/bleomycin/vinblastine/dacarbazine
Multiple myeloma	Melphalan; cyclophosphamide/prednisone
Non-Hodgkin's lymphomas	
Histiocytic (high–grade)lymphomas	CHOP regimen, consisting of cyclophosphamide/hydroxydaunomycin (doxorubicin)/Oncovin (vincristine)/prednisone
Nodular (low–grade) lymphomas	CVP regimen, consisting of cyclophosphamide/vincristine/prednisone
Solid tumors	
Bladder cancer	Cisplatin; doxorubicin
Brain tumors	Carmustine; lomustine
Breast cancer	CMF regimen, consisting of cyclophosphamide/methotrexate/fluorouracil; CMF/prednisone; CMF/prednisone/tamoxifen or other hormones
Bronchogenic, small cell lung cancer	Doxorubicin/cyclophosphamide/vincristine
Choriocarcinoma	For gestational use only: methotrexate; dactinomycin
Colorectal cancer	Fluorouracil
Gastric cancer	FAM regimen, consisting of fluorouracil/Adriamycin (doxorubicin)/mitomycin
Malignant melanoma	Dacarbazine; carmustine; cisplatin
Ovarian cancer	Cisplatin/cyclophosphamide; cisplatin/cyclophosphamide/doxorubicin; paclitaxel; docetaxel
Renal cell carcinoma	Aldesleukin
Sarcoma	Doxorubicin/dacarbazine
Testicular cancer	Etoposide/bleomycin/cisplatin; vinblastine/ifosfamide/cisplatin

*Drugs are listed in their general order of use, with the drug or drug combination used most often listed first. Drugs used in combination are separated by the symbol/, such as the combination of vincristine and prednisone, which is listed as vincritine/prednisone. For some diseases, other drugs or drug combinations are also used.

inhibit mitosis and cause metaphase arrest by interfering with microtubule function. The vinca alkaloids bind to tubulin and block tubulin polymerization, whereas the taxanes bind to tubulin and prevent depolymerization. By their action, the taxanes promote the formation of stable but nonfunctional microtubules. The fact that microtubules also have important roles in nerve conduction and neurotransmission may explain why use of mitotic inhibitors can cause neurotoxicity.

Vinca Alkaloids

Vincristine and Vinblastine

CHEMISTRY AND PHARMACOKINETICS. Vincristine (see Fig. 45–3D) and vinblastine are natural alkaloids from the periwinkle plant. Despite their structural similarity and identical mechanisms of action, the two drugs have different antitumor activities and toxicities. The oral absorption of vincristine and vinblastine is unreliable, so the drugs are administered intravenously. Neither drug enters the CNS in significant amounts. Both drugs are extensively metabolized and undergo biliary excretion.

INDICATIONS. Vincristine is often used to treat hematologic cancers, including acute lymphocytic leukemia, Hodgkin's and non-Hodgkin's lymphomas, and multiple myeloma. It

also is used in the treatment of some solid tumors (e.g., small-cell lung cancer, neuroblastoma, and sarcoma). Vinblastine is used for lymphomas and for bladder, breast, ovarian, and testicular cancer. Vinblastine is a component of the ABVD regimen for Hodgkin's disease (see Table 45–2).

ADVERSE EFFECTS. Vincristine produces dose-limiting neurotoxicity. It can cause a form of peripheral neuropathy that is usually distal and symmetric and affects both sensory and motor function. Suppression of deep tendon reflexes, which is often found, may be the earliest sign of neurotoxicity. Paresthesias of the hands and toes are also common. These adverse effects are usually reversible and do not justify discontinuation of vincristine therapy unless they are disabling. Cranial nerve damage can cause hoarseness, facial palsies, or jaw pain, whereas autonomic neuropathies can cause orthostatic hypotension, abdominal pain, and constipation. In contrast to vinblastine, vincristine usually causes little myelosuppression.

The major dose-limiting toxicity of vinblastine is myelosuppression. Vinblastine usually causes little neurotoxicity.

Vinorelbine

Vinorelbine is a new semisynthetic derivative of vinblastine. It has shown good activity against non–small-cell lung cancer and is being used as monotherapy for this disease.

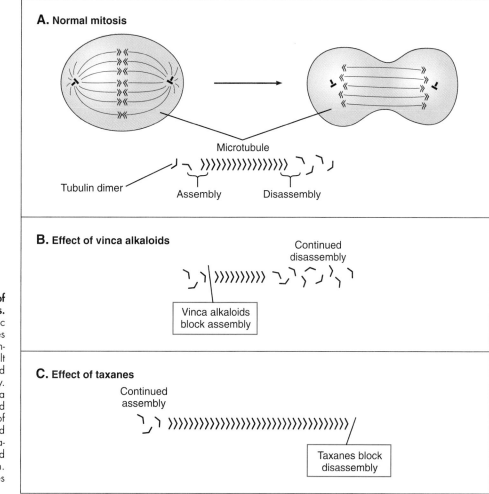

Figure 45–6. Mechanisms of action of mitotic inhibitors. **(A)** In normal mitosis, the mitotic spindle is formed by microtubules that continuously undergo assembly and disassembly as a result of tubulin polymerization and depolymerization, respectively. **(B)** Vincristine and other vinca alkaloids bind to tubulin and prevent the polymerization of tubulin dimers. **(C)** Paclitaxel and other taxanes bind to tubulin, stabilize the tubulin polymer, and thereby prevent depolymerization. As with vinca alkaloids, taxanes cause metaphase arrest.

Taxanes

Drug Properties

CHEMISTRY AND PHARMACOKINETICS. The taxanes (taxoids) are plant alkaloids obtained from yew trees. In 1971, **paclitaxel** (TAXOL) was isolated from the bark of a slow-growing Pacific yew, *Taxus brevifolia*. Because the complex ring structure of paclitaxel cannot be synthesized easily (see Fig. 45–3D) and because harvesting the bark kills the tree, efforts were made to find a more renewable source of this compound. The search resulted in the discovery of **docetaxel** (TAXOTERE), which was isolated from the needles of the European yew, *Taxus baccata*.

Paclitaxel and docetaxel are given intravenously and are eliminated via metabolism and biliary excretion.

INDICATIONS. The taxanes have good activity against several types of cancer (see Table 45–1). Paclitaxel is indicated as first-line therapy for metastatic ovarian cancer in combination with cisplatin, treatment of non–small-cell lung cancer, and treatment of metastatic breast cancer unresponsive to first-line therapy. Docetaxel is approved for locally advanced or metastatic breast cancer, and for metastatic non–

small-cell lung cancer after failure of cisplatin-based chemotherapy.

ADVERSE EFFECTS. The major dose-limiting toxicity of taxanes is myelosuppression, particularly neutropenia. Taxanes can also cause alopecia and neurotoxicity.

TOPOISOMERASE INHIBITORS

The DNA topoisomerases are enzymes that serve to maintain the normal structural topology of DNA. These enzymes relieve the torsional strain that is caused by the unwinding of DNA during the replication or transcription of DNA strands. Topoisomerases work by producing strand breaks that permit the strands to pass through the gap before the breaks are resealed. **Topoisomerase I** breaks and reseals single-stranded DNA, whereas **topoisomerase II** breaks and reseals double-stranded DNA.

Drugs that inhibit topoisomerases cause permanent strand breaks by preventing the resealing of the nicked strands of DNA. The two groups of topoisomerase inhibitors are (1) the podophyllotoxins that inhibit topoisomerase II and (2) the camptothecin analogues that inhibit topoisomerase I.

Podophyllotoxins

Drug Properties

CHEMISTRY AND PHARMACOKINETICS. Podophyllin is a natural substance that is extracted from the mandrake or mayapple plant. Two semisynthetic derivatives of this substance, **etoposide** and **teniposide,** are used as antineoplastic drugs. Both drugs can be given intravenously. Although etoposide can also be given orally, its oral bioavailability varies greatly from patient to patient, so this route of administration can result in significant underdosing or overdosing. Etoposide is primarily eliminated unchanged in the urine, whereas teniposide is extensively metabolized in the liver.

INDICATIONS. Etoposide has a broad spectrum of activity against hematologic cancers and solid tumors. It is especially valuable in the treatment of testicular carcinoma, lung cancer, and non-Hodgkin's lymphoma. It also has value as a preoperative treatment for bone marrow transplantation. Because of its synergy with platinum compounds, etoposide is most frequently administered with cisplatin when it is used in combination therapy. Teniposide has a more limited spectrum of activity than does etoposide, and it is primarily used to treat acute lymphocytic and acute myeloid leukemias.

ADVERSE EFFECTS. Etoposide and teniposide are fairly well tolerated, although they can produce alopecia, mild nausea and vomiting, and dose-limiting myelosuppression. They have also been associated with a low incidence of secondary nonlymphocytic leukemias.

Camptothecin Analogues

Drug Properties

CHEMISTRY AND PHARMACOKINETICS. Camptothecin is an alkaloid obtained from *Camptotheca acuminata.* Although camptothecin is a potent inhibitor of topoisomerase I, it has relatively low clinical efficacy. **Irinotecan** and **topotecan,** synthetic camptothecin analogues that have greater clinical activity and less toxicity than the natural alkaloid, are given intravenously for the treatment of cancer. Irinotecan is rapidly metabolized to an active metabolite called SN-38. This metabolite has from 250 to 1000 times greater antitumor activity than the parent compound. SN-38 is eliminated primarily in the bile, whereas topotecan undergoes renal excretion.

INDICATIONS. Irinotecan is approved for the treatment of colorectal cancer that has recurred or progressed following fluorouracil therapy. It is also active against lymphomas and breast, cervical, gastric, lung, and other tumors. Topotecan is active against glioma, sarcoma, and lung and ovarian tumors.

ADVERSE EFFECTS. The dose-limiting toxicity of both camptothecin analogues is myelosuppression. Irinotecan produces diarrhea in a significant percentage of patients, and both drugs can cause alopecia and mild nausea and vomiting.

HORMONES AND THEIR ANTAGONISTS

Several types of hormone-dependent cancer (especially breast, prostate, and endometrial cancer) respond to treatment with their corresponding hormone antagonists. **Estrogen antagonists** are primarily used to treat breast cancer, whereas **androgen antagonists** are used to treat prostate cancer. **Corticosteroids** are particularly useful in treating lymphocytic leukemias and lymphomas.

The pharmacologic properties of estrogens, androgens, and their antagonists are described in Chapter 34, and those of corticosteroids are described in Chapter 33. The use of these drugs in cancer treatment is summarized below.

Hormones Used in Breast Cancer

Breast cancer is usually estrogen-dependent and can be suppressed by the administration of estrogen antagonists. **Tamoxifen** is the antagonist used most widely. This drug can be given alone to prevent breast cancer in women who have a strong family history of the disease or are otherwise highly predisposed to developing it. Tamoxifen is often used in combination with surgery and other chemotherapeutic drugs for the treatment of breast cancer. In women over 50 years of age, adjuvant use of tamoxifen was found to reduce the annual odds of recurrence by 30%. Long-term survival appears to be greater in women receiving both cytotoxic chemotherapy and tamoxifen.

Aromatase inhibitors that prevent estrogen synthesis, including **anastrozole** and **letrozole,** have moved into first-line therapy for certain forms of breast cancer. The actions and effects of these drugs are described in Chapter 34.

Hormones Used in Prostate Cancer

Prostate tissue is stimulated by androgens and suppressed by estrogens. For this reason, the major drugs for disseminated prostate cancer are androgen antagonists and estrogens. An androgen antagonist (e.g., **flutamide**) will block testosterone stimulation of prostate carcinoma cells. A gonadotropin-releasing hormone agonist (e.g., **leuprolide**) will suppress the release of luteinizing hormone from the pituitary gland and will thereby suppress testosterone production (see Chapter 31).

Corticosteroids

Corticosteroids (e.g., **prednisone**) are primarily used because of their lymphocytotoxic effects in the treatment of lymphocytic leukemias, lymphomas, and multiple myeloma. Corticosteroids are relatively well tolerated and do not produce myelosuppression or other serious organ damage in most patients. For this reason, they are often combined with drugs that inhibit DNA function or mitosis in the treatment of these cancers.

MONOCLONAL ANTIBODIES

Monoclonal antibodies are one of the newest classes of therapeutic agents. Several of these antibodies have been developed for treating malignancies. These particular antibodies bind to receptors or proteins involved in the growth of specific types of neoplastic cells. Other monoclonal antibodies have immunosuppressant effects and these agents are described in the following section of this chapter.

The nomenclature of monoclonal antibodies provides useful information about these agents. The names of monoclonal antibodies end in "mab" or "monab." The letters before mab indicate the source of the antibody: "o" for mouse, "u" for human, and "xi" for chimeric. An internal letter or syllable identifies the therapeutic use of the antibody, for example, "tu" for tumor, "vi" for virus, and "c" or "ci" for circulation. For example, rituximab is a chimeric monoclonal antibody used in treating tumors.

Rituximab (RITUXAN) was the first monoclonal antibody approved for cancer chemotherapy. This chimeric human-murine antibody is used to treat relapsed or refractory B-cell non-Hodgkin's lymphomas. It binds to the CD20 antigen that is found on the surface of over 90% of non-Hodgkin's lymphoma cells, as well as on normal B lymphocytes. CD20 is believed to regulate an early step in cell cycle initiation. The drug is given as an intravenous infusion.

Alemtuzumab (CAMPATH) binds to CD52, a cell surface glycoprotein found on all B- and T-lymphocytes and many other types of leukocytes, leading to cell lysis. It is indicated for the treatment of B-cell chronic lymphocytic leukemia in patients who have been treated with alkylating agents and who have failed fludarabine therapy.

Gemtuzumab ozogamicin (MYLOTARG) is a unique monoclonal antibody conjugated with a **cytotoxic antitumor antibiotic** known as **calicheamicin.** The drug binds to the CD33 antigen expressed by hematopoietic cells, resulting in formation of a complex that is internalized and sequestered in lysosomes, where the calicheamicin is released. Calicheamicin then binds to the cell's DNA, resulting in double strand breaks and cell death. The drug is indicated for treatment of patients with CD33-positive acute myeloid leukemia.

Trastuzumab (HERCEPTIN) is a recombinant human monoclonal antibody to **human epidermal growth factor-2** (HER2). It acts by binding to the extracellular domain of the HER2 receptor on cancer cells and thereby preventing receptor stimulation. Trastuzumab has been approved for the treatment of metastatic breast carcinoma in women whose cancer cells overexpress the HER2 oncogene. Trastuzumab is administered intravenously once a week in combination with doxorubicin and paclitaxel. Its adverse effects include chills, fever, nausea, vomiting, chest pain, and dyspnea.

Cetuximab (ERBITUX) and **Bevacizumab** (AVASTIN) are monoclonal antibodies for the treatment of **colon cancer.** Cetuximab is an antibody that binds to **epidermal growth factor receptor** (EGFR), which is expressed in many normal tissues and is overexpressed in certain human cancers, particularly colon cancer. Overexpression of EGRF in cancer cells is associated with unrestricted cell growth and a poor prognosis. Cetuximab is used in an irinotecan-based regimen for colon cancer. Patients receiving this drug combination had better response rates and increased time to tumor progression than patients not receiving cetuximab. The most common adverse effect of cetuximab is an acne-like skin rash, whereas about 3% of patients experience hypersensitivity reactions during drug infusion. Studies of cetuximab in patients with other types of tumors are ongoing.

Bevacizumab is a recombinant humanized antibody to **vascular endothelial growth factor** (VEGF). The drug prevents binding of VEGF to receptors on endothelial cells and thereby inhibits the formation of new blood vessels. It is the first VEGF **angiogenesis inhibitor** to be approved for cancer chemotherapy, and it is indicated for treating metastatic colon cancer. When bevacizumab is used in a 5-FU regimen, it increases tumor response rates, progression-free survival time, and overall survival time in these patients. The drug can cause gastrointestinal bleeding and perforation, pulmonary hemorrhage, and other thromboembolic events.

TYROSINE KINASE INHIBITORS

A newer group of antineoplastic agents inhibit tyrosine kinase enzymes associated with specific neoplastic cell signal transduction mechanisms. **Imatinib** (GLEEVEC) inhibits the **bcr-Abl tyrosine kinase** expressed by the **Philadelphia chromosome** in **chronic myeloid leukemia** (CML) cells. Bcr-abl is an oncoprotein resulting from a reciprocal chromosomal translocation, t(9;22). Imatinib inhibits leukemic cell proliferation and induces apoptosis. It has produced remarkable rates of hematologic and cytogenetic remission in CML and is a first-line treatment for this disease, especially in patients not suitable for bone marrow transplantation. Imatinib also inhibits c-kit activity and is used to treat gastrointestinal stromal tumors with c-kit mutations.

Erlotinib (TARCEVA) is a reversible and highly specific inhibitor of EGFR tyrosine kinase. It has been approved as a second-line therapy for non–small-cell lung cancer in patients who have failed at least one chemotherapy regimen. Clinical trials have shown that it produces modest increases in median survival time and 1-year survival compared with placebo. It is metabolized by cytochrome P450 3A4, and drugs that inhibit or induce this enzyme can alter plasma levels of erlotinib.

CYTOKINES AND INTERFERONS

Interferons are endogenous proteins that increase the activity of various cytotoxic cells in the immune system and directly inhibit the proliferation of neoplastic cells. **Interferon alpha** is an immunomodulating drug that can be administered intramuscularly, intravenously, or subcutaneously. It is used to treat Kaposi's sarcoma in patients with AIDS. In addition, it is used to treat hairy cell leukemia and chronic myelogenous leukemia and produces a clinical response in about 70% of patients with either of these diseases. In about 30% of patients with chronic myeloid leukemia, interferon therapy causes a cytogenetic response that is characterized by loss of a chromosome called the Philadelphia chromosome.

Aldesleukin (interleukin-2, or IL-2) is a lymphokine formerly known as T-cell growth factor. Aldesleukin activates IL-2 receptors and promotes B- and T-cell proliferation and differentiation. The antitumor effect of the drug is primarily caused by increased numbers of cytotoxic T cells that can recognize and destroy tumor cells without damaging normal cells. These cytotoxic cells include natural killer cells, lymphokine-activated killer cells, and tumor-infiltrating cells.

Aldesleukin can be administered intramuscularly, intravenously, or subcutaneously. It is primarily used to treat metastatic **renal cell carcinoma,** but it also has activity against malignant melanoma and colorectal cancer. In about 20% of patients with renal cell carcinoma, it produces a good response, which in some cases persists for several years without further therapy.

In low doses, aldesleukin is often well tolerated and can be given as outpatient therapy. In higher doses, the drug can be very toxic. The most common dose-limiting toxicities are hypotension, fluid retention, and renal dysfunction. Other toxicities include a broad range of hematologic deficiencies, skin lesions, and neuropsychiatric changes. The toxicities are usually reversible and can be prevented or managed by giving corticosteroids before aldesleukin therapy and providing vigorous supportive care. Prolonged infusions of aldesleukin appear to be less toxic than high-dose bolus injections.

Alpha-interferons have anti-proliferative effects in various neoplastic cells where they act to alter nucleic acid and protein synthesis expressed by oncogenes. They also have immunomodulatory actions that can contribute to their antineoplastic effects. In addition their use in treating viral infections, several interferon-alpha preparations are available for treating hairy cell leukemia, Kaposi's sarcoma, bladder or renal carcinoma, chronic myeloid leukemia, malignant melanoma, and multiple myeloma. Interferon preparations are administered intramuscularly. The most common adverse effects of interferons include leukopenia, thrombocytopenia, a flulike syndrome, nausea or vomiting, tiredness, altered taste, and diarrhea.

IMMUNOMODULATING DRUGS

Drugs that affect the immune system are called **immunomodulators** or **biologic response modifiers.** These drugs can be classified as **immunostimulants** or **immunodepressants.** Most of these drugs suppress immune mechanisms and are used to treat autoimmune diseases or to prevent **allograft rejection** following organ or bone marrow transplantation. In the latter case, these drugs act by inhibiting the immune response to the foreign antigens contained in an allograft, which is a graft of tissue between individuals of the same species but of disparate genotypes. A few drugs, including thalidomide and palivizumab, act to enhance host immunity.

Monoclonal Antibodies

Daclizumab (ZENAPAX) and **basiliximab** (SIMULECT) are monoclonal antibodies to the high-affinity **interleukin-2 receptor** that is expressed on activated T cells. These antibodies bind to the α-subunit of the receptor and prevent IL-

2 binding. By this action, IL-2–mediated activation of lymphocytes is prevented and the response of the immune system to antigens (e.g., those present in transplanted allografts) is impaired. Daclizumab and basiliximab are used in combination with cyclosporine and prednisone to prevent rejection of **renal transplants.**

Muromonab-CD3 (ORTHOCLONE OKT3) is a monoclonal antibody to the CD3 glycoprotein that is part of the **T-cell antigen recognition receptor.** The antibody prevents antigen access to the receptor and thereby prevents T-cell activation. Muromonab-CD3 is used to treat **acute allograft rejection** in renal transplant patients. In addition, it is used to reverse bone marrow, cardiac, hepatic, kidney, and pancreatic transplant rejection episodes that are resistant to conventional drugs (e.g., cyclosporine).

Palivizumab (SYNAGIS) is a human monoclonal antibody to the fusion protein of **respiratory syncytial virus** (RSV). It is approved for prevention of RSV infection in infants with bronchopulmonary dysplasia and in **premature infants** whose gestational age is under 35 weeks. It is given as five monthly intramuscular doses.

Microbial Products

Cyclosporine (SANDIMMUNE), **tacrolimus** (PROGRAF, PROTOPIC), and **sirolimus** (RAPAMUNE) are examples of immunosuppressants that are derived from microbes. Cyclosporine is a complex fungal polypeptide, whereas tacrolimus and sirolimus are macrolide antibiotics produced by *Streptomyces* species. Cyclosporine and tacrolimus inhibit the production and release of IL-2 that is required for activation of cytotoxic T-lymphocytes in response to alloantigenic challenge. Specifically, cyclosporine and tacrolimus bind to intracellular proteins called immunophilins (cyclophilin and FK506-binding protein, respectively). The drug–immunophilin complex then binds the phosphatase enzyme called **calcineurin** and inhibits calcineurin-mediated transcription of the IL-2 gene.

Sirolimus, also called **rapamycin,** forms a complex with FK binding protein-12, which then inhibits a key regulatory kinase (**mammalian Target of Rapamycin,** mTOR) involved in cytokine-driven T-cell proliferation (cell-cycle progression).

Cyclosporine, tacrolimus and sirolimus can be used to prevent rejection of organ transplants and are usually given in combination with corticosteroids or other drugs. For example, sirolimus is given in combination with cyclosporine and a corticosteroid (e.g., prednisone). Cyclosporine can also be used to treat **psoriasis** and severe autoimmune diseases that are resistant to other therapeutic agents, such as **rheumatoid arthritis** that does not respond to MTX. In addition to these indications, sirolimus and tacrolimus have been incorporated into vascular stents that slowly release the drugs to inhibit the proliferation of vascular smooth muscle cells and other vascular cells that otherwise cause restenosis of coronary arteries following stent placement. The use of drug-releasing stents has dramatically reduced the incidence of coronary restenosis in this setting.

Cyclosporine frequently causes nephrotoxicity, hypertension, hirsutism, gingival hyperplasia, and muscle tremor. Cyclosporine is metabolized by CYP3A, a cytochrome P450 enzyme, and interacts with other drugs that inhibit or induce this enzyme. CYP3A inhibitors can increase the plasma levels and toxicity of cyclosporine, and these include erythromycin and other macrolide antibiotics, azole antifungal drugs, calcium channel blockers, and grapefruit juice. CYP3A inducers can decrease the plasma levels of cyclosporine, and these include carbamazepine, phenytoin, and rifampin.

Corticosteroids

Prednisone and other corticosteroids inhibit T-cell proliferation and the expression of genes encoding various cytokines. They are used with other immunosuppressive drugs to prevent organ transplant rejection and to prevent graft-versus-host disease in patients who have undergone bone marrow transplantation. Corticosteroids are frequently used to treat various autoimmune disorders, including lupus erythematosus and rheumatoid arthritis. Their anti-inflammatory actions are also very beneficial in these disorders (see Chapter 30).

Other Drugs

Azathioprine, Cyclophosphamide, and Methotrexate

In the body, azathioprine is converted to 6-mercaptopurine. As with methotrexate, 6-mercaptopurine acts by inhibiting DNA synthesis. Cyclophosphamide acts by alkylating DNA. Because these agents prevent the proliferation of B- and T-lymphocytes, they are used to prevent organ graft rejection and treat autoimmune disorders and collagen diseases. Cyclophosphamide and MTX are also used in the treatment of cancer (see previous).

Azathioprine is often given in combination with corticosteroids and cyclosporine or tacrolimus to patients with tissue transplants, and it is also useful in the treatment of patients with inflammatory bowel disease, rheumatoid arthritis, or lupus erythematosus. Cyclophosphamide is used primarily to treat lupus erythematosus and other autoimmune diseases and is usually given in combination with corticosteroids. MTX has anti-inflammatory effects that make it especially useful in the management of rheumatoid arthritis (see Chapter 30). It is also useful in the treatment of psoriasis and severe asthma.

Thalidomide

Thalidomide was once banned because of its potential to cause phocomelia and other congenital malformations. It was subsequently discovered to have immunomodulating effects, and it is now being used to treat cancer, recurrent aphthous ulcers (canker sores), tuberculosis, leprosy, erythema nodosum leprosum, and the AIDS-associated wasting syndrome (cachexia).

Thalidomide acts, in part, by inhibiting **angiogenesis,** the formation of new blood vessels. This action appears to account for its teratogenic effects, because the drug prevents vascular growth during fetal limb development. The antiangiogenesis actions of the drug and its analogues are now being evaluated in the treatment of cancer, and early trials are encouraging.

Thalidomide has both immunosuppressant and immunostimulant effects. It inhibits the production of IL-2, tumor necrosis factor alpha (TNF-α), and other cytokines. Although thalidomide inhibits lymphocyte proliferation stimulated by alloantigens, some studies show that it stimulates CD8$^+$ cells in vitro. The mechanism of action of thalidomide in specific diseases continues to be investigated.

SUMMARY OF IMPORTANT POINTS

■ Most antineoplastic drugs inhibit DNA synthesis or disrupt DNA structure and function.

■ DNA synthesis inhibitors include folate antagonists (methotrexate and trimetrexate), purine antagonists (mercaptopurine, thioguanine, and others), pyrimidine antagonists (cytarabine, floxuridine, and fluorouracil), and a ribonucleotide reductase inhibitor (hydroxyurea).

■ DNA alkylating drugs that cross-link DNA include nitrogen mustards (cyclophosphamide and others), nitrosoureas (carmustine and others), and miscellaneous drugs (busulfan, dacarbazine, and mitomycin). Platinum compounds (cisplatin and others) also cross-link DNA strands.

■ DNA intercalating drugs include the anthracycline drugs (doxorubicin and others), bleomycin, and dactinomycin.

■ Inhibitors of mitosis include vinca alkaloids (vincristine and others) and taxane drugs (docetaxel and paclitaxel).

■ Topoisomerase inhibitors include podophyllotoxin drugs (etoposide and teniposide) and camptothecin analogues (irinotecan and topotecan).

■ Biologic response modifiers used in the treatment of cancer include interferon alfa, aldesleukin, and monoclonal antibodies (bevacizumab, cetuximab, rituximab, and trastuzumab).

■ Myelosuppression is the dose-limiting toxicity of most antineoplastic drugs.

■ Doxorubicin and other anthracycline drugs produce cardiotoxicity; cyclophosphamide and ifosfamide cause hemorrhagic cystitis; bleomycin and busulfan produce pulmonary fibrosis; vincristine, docetaxel, and related drugs cause neurotoxicity; and cisplatin produces renal toxicity.

■ Hormonal agents are used to treat some cancers, especially estrogen antagonists to treat breast cancer, androgen antagonists to treat prostate cancer, and corticosteroids (e.g., prednisone) to treat lymphocytic leukemias and lymphomas.

■ Immunosuppressant drugs used to prevent organ transplant rejection or to treat autoimmune diseases include monoclonal antibodies (basiliximab, daclizumab, and muromonab-CD3), microbial products (cyclosporine, sirolimus, and tacrolimus), corticosteroids (e.g., prednisone), and cytotoxic drugs (e.g., azathioprine).

Review Questions

1. After receiving several courses of chemotherapy for breast cancer, a woman complains of fatigue, shortness of breath, and exercise intolerance. Her examination reveals cardiomegaly. Which one of the following drugs most likely caused of this adverse drug reaction?
   (A) cyclophosphamide
   (B) methotrexate
   (C) vincristine
   (D) doxorubicin
   (E) cisplatin

2. Deletion of hypoxanthine:guanine phosphoribosyl transferase from tumor cells can confer resistance to which drug?
   (A) fluorouracil
   (B) cytarabine
   (C) mercaptopurine
   (D) pemetrexed
   (E) gemcitabine

3. Which drug acts to prevent the depolymerization (disassembly) of tubulin in tumor cells?
   (A) docetaxel
   (B) etoposide
   (C) bleomycin
   (D) vinblastine
   (E) carmustine

4. Which monoclonal antibody binds to the human epidermal growth factor-2 in certain tumor cells?
   (A) trastuzumab
   (B) rituximab
   (C) bevacizumab
   (D) cetuximab
   (E) daclizumab

5. Mutations in tumor cell topoisomerase II can confer resistance to which drug?
   (A) vinorelbine
   (B) teniposide
   (C) paclitaxel
   (D) vincristine
   (E) bleomycin

Answers and Explanations

1. The answer is D: doxorubicin. Cardiac toxicity leading to heart failure is the dose-limiting toxicity of doxorubicin. This toxicity is partly caused by iron-catalyzed free radical formation and can be mitigated by administration of the iron chelator called dexrazoxane.

2. The answer is C: mercaptopurine. Mercaptopurine and thioguanine are activated to the nucleotide form by addition of ribose and phosphate groups catalyzed by hypoxanthine:guanine phosphoribosyl transferase. Deletion of this enzyme from tumor cells confers resistance to these drugs.

3. The answer is A: docetaxel. The taxanes (e.g., docetaxel and paclitaxel) act by preventing the depolymerization of tubulin dimers of microtubules of the mitotic spindle that is required for separation of the chromosomes during mitosis.

4. The answer is A: trastuzumab. Trastuzumab binds to human epidermal growth factor-2 (HER-2) that is overexpressed in some breast cancer cells. The drug acts to inhibit proliferation of the cells and is used to treat metastatic breast cancer.

5. The answer is B: teniposide. Teniposide and etoposide inhibit mammalian topoisomerase II and thereby cause DNA strand breaks and tumor cell death. Mutations in this enzyme can confer resistance to these drugs.

SELECTED READINGS

Brennen, W. N., C. R. Cooper, S. Capitosti, et al. Thalidomide and analogues: current proposed mechanisms and therapeutic range. Clin Prostate Cancer 3:54–61, 2004.

Calvert, A. H. Biochemical pharmacology of pemetrexed. Oncology (Huntington) 18(13 Suppl 8):13–17, 2004.

Sawicka, M., M. Kalinowska, S. Skierski, et al. A review of selected antitumour therapeutic agents and reasons for multidrug resistance occurrence. J Pharm Pharmacol 56:1067–1081, 2004.

Sawyer, T. K. Cancer metastasis therapeutic agents and drug discovery: emerging small-molecule protein kinase inhibitors. Expert Opin Investig Drugs 13:1–19, 2004.

Tsuruo, T., M. Naito, A. Tomida, et al. Molecular targeting therapy of cancer: drug resistance, apoptosis and survival signal. Cancer Sci 94:15–21, 2003.

INDEX

Note: Page numbers followed by b indicate material in boxes; page numbers followed by f indicate figures; and page numbers followed by t indicate tables.

A

Abarelix, 350
Abbreviated new drug application (ANDA), 37
Abciximab, 169t, 174
Abnormal impulse conduction, 141b–142b, 142–143
Abnormal impulse formation, in arrhythmias, 140–142, 141b–142b
Absence seizures, 209, 211, 211t
  generalized, EEG patterns during, 210f
Absorption, drug, 9–12, 10f, 11b–12b. *See also* Drug(s), absorption of
Abuse
  drug. *See also* Drug abuse
  drugs of, classification of 274, 274–285, 275. *See also* Drugs of abuse
Acamprosate calcium, 284
Acarbose, 394
ACCOLATE. *See* Zafirlukast
ACE inhibitors. *See* Angiotensin-converting enzyme inhibitors
Acebutolol, 83t, 87t, 88
Acetaminophen, 337–338, 337f
  for viral rhinitis, 308
Acetaminophen with codeine, for migraine, 328
Acetazolamide, 132t, 134t, 137
  structure of, 132f
Acetylation, in drug biotransformation, 15
  variations in, 15–16
Acetylcholine (Ach), 47, 47f, 186, 187t, 188f
  chemistry and pharmacokinetics of, 57
  clinical uses of, 56t
  indications for, 57
  properties of, 56t
  receptors for, 49
  side effects of, 57
    drugs augmenting, 62
Acetylcholine (Ach) receptor antagonists, for Parkinson's disease, 268t, 269
N-Acetylglucosamine (GlcNAc), 421, 422f
N-Acetylmuramic acid (MurNAc), 421, 422f
Ach. *See* Acetylcholine (Ach)
Acid(s)
  amino, 186–188, 187t
  ethacrynic, 132t, 134t, 136
  fatty, omega-6, 293
  folic, 178–179, 179f
    structure of, 179f
  nicotinic, for hypercholesterolemia, 159t, 160t, 164
  salicylic, 11, 12, 334–336, 342
  weak, absorption of, pH effects on, 9, 11b, 12
  zoledronic, 400, 401
Acidity, gastric, drugs that reduce, 312–315, 312f, 313f, 313t

Acne vulgaris, 438
Acromegaly, 349
ACTHRELIA. *See* Corticorelin ovine triflutate
ACTIVASE. *See* Alteplase
Activated partial thromboplastin time (aPTT), 171
Active transport, 9
Active tubular secretion, in drug excretion, 17, 19b
ACTONEL. *See* Risedronate
ACTOS. *See* Pioglitazone
ACULAR. *See* Ketorolac
Acute angle-closure glaucoma, 57
Acute gastroparesis, 311
Acute tubular necrosis, 436
Acyclovir
  for herpesvirus infections, 469–472, 469f, 470f, 471t
  structure of, 469f
Adalimumab, 341
Adaptive response, 196
Addiction, drug, 275
Additive effect, 39
Adehyde dehydrogenase, 109, 110
Adenohypophysis, 346, 347f
Adenosine, 49, 144t, 146t, 150, 191
Adenosine triphosphate (ATP), 49, 191
Adjustment disorder, 197
Adrenal androgens, 367
Adrenal insufficiency, glucocorticoids for, 365
Adrenal steroids, 360–369
  binding to receptors, 362
  biosynthetic pathways for, 361f
  classification of, 360
  inhibitors of, 367
  pharmacologic properties of, 363t
  preparations of, 362–367, 363f, 363t, 364f
  secretion of, 360, 362f
  structures of, 363f
  synthesis of, 360, 361f
  uses of, 362
Adrenergic neurotransmission, drug action effects of, 49t, 50f, 51
Adrenergic receptor(s), 49, 71–73, 72f, 72t
  signal transduction in, 73
α-Adrenergic receptor(s), 71–72, 72f, 72t
β-Adrenergic receptor(s), 72–73, 72f, 72t
Adrenergic receptor agonists, 71–80
  catecholamines, 74–79, 74t, 75f
  classification of, 71, 73–74, 73f
  clinical uses of, 74t
  direct-acting, 51, 74–79, 74t, 75f, 76f
  indirect-acting, 51, 79
  mixed-acting, 79
  noncatecholamines, 77–79
  pharmacologic effects of, 74t
  structures of, 75f

β-Adrenergic receptor agonists
  in heart failure management, 122, 122t, 123t
  for respiratory tract disorders, 303–304, 304f, 305f, 305t
Adrenergic receptor antagonists, 51, 81–89
  classification of, 81
  clinical uses of, 83t
  for hypertension, 97, 98t, 99
  mechanism of action of, 83t
  pharmacologic effects of, 83t
  structures of, 86f
α-Adrenergic receptor antagonists, 81–84, 82f–86f, 83t
  nonselective, 81–82, 82f
    for hypertension, 97, 98t
β-Adrenergic receptor antagonists, 84, 85f, 86–88, 87t, 357. *See also* β-Blockers
  for angina pectoris, 112
  in heart failure management, 124–125
  for hypertension, 97–99, 98t
  for migraine, 324t, 326
α_1-Adrenergic receptor antagonists, urinary bladder effects of, 86f
ADVAIR. *See* Fluticasone
Aerosols, 6
Affective disorders, 233, 241–243
  causes of, 241–243
  clinical findings in, 241
  pathogenesis of, 241–243
Affinity, in drug–receptor interactions, 28–29, 29f
African trypanosomiasis, pentamidine for, 482t, 487
African-American Heart Failure Trial, 124
Afterdepolarization, 119, 121f, 141b, 142
Age, as factor in drug safety, 42, 42t
AGGRASTAT. *See* Tirofiban
Agonist(s), 29–30
  full, 30, 32
  inverse, 30
  partial, 30, 32
Agoraphobia, 197
Airway obstruction, causes of, 300
Akathisia, 238
Albuterol, 78, 303, 305t
  effects on heart rate and pulmonary function in asthmatic patients, 305f
  structure of, 75f, 304f
Alcohol(s), 275–278, 276t, 277f, 277t
  isopropyl, 278
  methyl, 278
  withdrawal from, signs and symptoms of, 277t
  wood, 278
Aldosterone, structure of, 132f
Aldosterone antagonists
  in heart failure management, 125
  structures of, 132f